Health
&
Wellness

The Jones and Bartlett Series in Health Sciences

Health & Wellness

A Holistic Approach

Gordon Edlin
UNIVERSITY OF CALIFORNIA, DAVIS

and

Eric Golanty
UNIVERSITY OF CALIFORNIA, DAVIS

Jones and Bartlett Publishers
Boston • Portola Valley

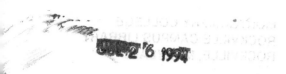
Editorial, Sales and Customer Service Offices
Jones and Bartlett Publishers
20 Park Plaza
Boston, MA 02116

Printed in the United States of America
10 9 8 7 6 5 4 3 2

Library of Congress Cataloging-in-Publication Data

Edlin, Gordon, 1932–
 Health & wellness.

 1. Health.   2. Holistic medicine.   I. Golanty, Eric.   II. Title.
III. Title: Health and wellness.
RA776.E24   1988   613   87-31205
ISBN 0-86720-091-X

ISBN 0-86720-091-X

Production and typesetting: PC&F, Inc.

Designer: Rosedesign Associates

Copyeditor: PC&F, Inc.

Cover design: PC&F, Inc.

Cover photograph: H. Armstrong Roberts, Inc.

ACKNOWLEDGMENTS

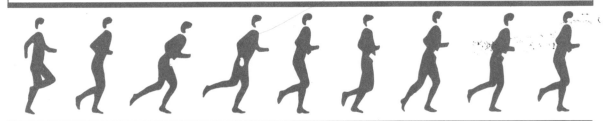

The authors would like to extend a special thanks to all the people who participated in the assembling of the art program for *Health & Wellness*.

Louis Neiheisel, Eldon P. Slick, art direction
Karl Nicholason, Everett Peck, Denise Hilton Putnam, illustrations and cartoons
John Odam, silhouettes
William Call, photography
Alice Harmon, charts and graphs
Lindsay Kefauver, photo research
Maureen Cunningham-Neumann, Director of Production

PHOTO CREDITS   94: H. Armstrong Roberts; 108: Larry Ford; 134: The Image Works; 200: Robert Eckert/EKM-Nepenthe; 308: Courtesy of Fay Foto/Boston; 330: H. Armstrong Roberts; 394: Andrea Beseman; 476: George Tooker, "Mirror II," Addison Gallery of American Art, Phillips Academy, Andover, Massachusetts; 522: H. Armstrong Roberts; 524: Environmental Protection Agency; 532: Courtesy Environmental Protection Agency.

TEXT CREDITS   8–9: Excerpted from the book *Mind as Healer, Mind as Slayer: A Holistic Approach to Preventing Stress Disorders*. Copyright © 1977 by Kenneth R. Pelletier. Reprinted by permission of Delacorte Press/Seymour Lawrence.

CONTENTS

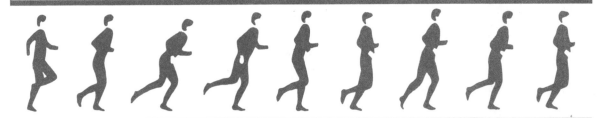

PREFACE

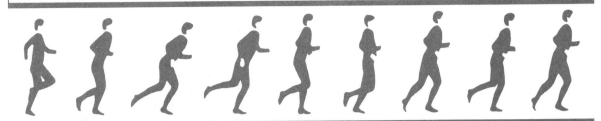

When we were writing the first edition of *Health and Wellness* between 1979 and 1981, we had no idea that our book would be received so warmly and enthusiastically by hundreds of instructors and thousands of students. We were particularly gratified by the many students who conveyed to us that *Health and Wellness* made a profound impact on their well-being. Many students have told us that the broad coverage and scientifically documented presentation made them want to keep the book as part of their permanent library. To all of the students and instructors who chose our text, we say thank you very much.

In the second edition we added two completely new chapters, one on weight control and eating disorders and another on psychoactive drug use. Both topics are of considerable interest to college students and pose significant health concerns.

In this third edition we have updated all of the relevant health statistics and recent scientific findings. We have also added a new chapter on AIDS that includes up-to-date information on this tragic epidemic that will become increasingly serious in the years ahead.

In this edition we also introduce a major new theme and discuss its relevancy to health throughout the book. Advertising of health care products and services as well as products detrimental to health has become so pervasive and persuasive in our society that countermeasures are needed. We alert readers to the many useless products, dangerous substances that are heavily advertised, and unnecessary surgeries and services. As one physician recently wrote, "Advertising in medicine has become a reality. . . . Protection may be even more necessary now that consumers are selecting health care on the basis of information supplied by the advertising industry."

More money is spent on advertising cigarettes and alcohol than on any other products. So-called "light" foods and beverages as well as nutritionally useless products are aggressively advertised. Newspapers and magazines now carry ads for do-it-yourself medical kits, surgery to cure impotence, liposuction for fat removal, radial keratotomy to correct nearsightedness, as well as the usual ads for fad diets and miracle cures. To alert readers to potential dangers of procedures and products that are advertised, we present cautionary examples throughout. In this age of deregulated health care even hospitals and physicians may push services and operations solely to boost profits.

We continue to emphasize self-responsibility and a holistic approach to wellness and illness. The cost of conventional medical care continues to increase uncontrollably, and there are even more people dissatisfied with their health care now than when we wrote the first edition. Thus, we feel it is worth reiterating the health philosophy of this text.

Many people think of "health" as having to do with doctors, the absence of illness or pain, medications of one sort or another, the prolongation of life, and sometimes even escape from death. In other words, health is what people have when they're not sick or dying. We believe that health is a feeling of whole and complete well-being, not just the absence of illness or pain. Health is a feeling of physical, mental, emotional, and spiritual harmony that each of us can experience—and that many of us do experience—even if for only short periods of time. Health is feeling that you have enough energy to do whatever you want to do and that you have confidence to approach life enthusiastically. These elements are part of the *holistic* view of health.

It is our view that most people are programmed from early childhood to believe that symptoms, disabilities, pain, and sickness are their lot and that the best they can do is recognize the symptoms and seek treatment from a member of the medical establishment. Although it is true that people get sick and may need professional help to recover, we believe that people have the personal power to influence their state of health in positive ways.

We believe that you can determine your state of health to a large degree. There are many things in life over which you have little influence and that you cannot easily change. But instead of lamenting and complaining, you can spend your time and energy more productively by getting in touch with how you can improve your health and well-being.

The way to achieve a healthy life is simply to live healthfully: to apply some of the principles of health science coupled with some understanding of how your mind, body, and emotions interrelate; to set some health goals for yourself, and then to follow through in achieving your goals.

Take responsibility for your health. Take responsibility for your feelings, your relationships, your diet, your level of physical activity, your drug-taking behavior (including smoking cigarettes and drinking alcohol), and your social environment (where you live, work, or go to school and the stresses that may result). All these factors are within your power to control, change, or accept, depending on what you want out of life.

Supplementary Materials

A variety of instructor aids and other material is available as described below.

1. An Instructor's Manual containing detailed chapter outlines, multiple-choice and true-false questions, essay topics, classroom activities, and film suggestions.

2. A 178-page workbook containing more than thirty exercises and study suggestions that students can use along with reading from the text.

3. A computerized set of test questions is available. Information on use of these questions can be obtained from the publisher.

4. A series of transparencies of many of the figures, tables, and graphs in the text is available from the publisher. These are suitable for use with overhead projectors.

5. In addition, the publisher will help defray the costs of renting films. For each one hundred copies of the text that are adopted, the publisher will grant an allowance of $25 per film up to maximum of three films.

Of the many people who reviewed all or part of the first, second, or third editions of our book, we particularly want to thank the following:

David Anspaugh, Memphis State University
Nancy J. Binkin, M.D., Centers for Disease Control, Atlanta
Barbara Coombs, San Francisco City College
Linda Chaput, W. H. Freeman, New York
Sherry Hineman, University of California, San Diego
Stanley Inkelis, M.D., Harbor General Hospital, Los Angeles
Will Lotter, University of California, Davis
Roland Marchand
Mary C. Martin, M.D., University of California, San Francisco
Marion Nestle, University of California, San Francisco
David Phelps, Oregon State University
Richard Plant, South Middlesex Community College, New Jersey
Carol Rinklieb, Berkeley, California
Sam Singer, M.D., University of California, Santa Cruz

Seymour Eiseman, California State University, Northridge
Leo E. Hollister, M.D., Stanford Medical Center
Dorothy Coltrin, De Anza College
John Struthers, Planned Parenthood of Sacramento County
Dwayne Reed, M.D., Director, Honolulu Heart Program
N. K. Bhagavan, University of Hawaii Medical School

We would especially like to thank Arthur Bartlett and Don Jones, our publishers, for their enthusiasm and support. We are also appreciative of the many talents and services provided by Anne Gingras. Finally, we would like to thank Nancy Sjoberg, Jackie Estrada, and all the Del Mar Associates for their enthusiasm and devotion to this project, and to Maureen Cunningham-Neumann for producing this third edition.

GORDON EDLIN
ERIC GOLANTY
Davis, California

UNIT ONE

Wellness

CHAPTER ONE

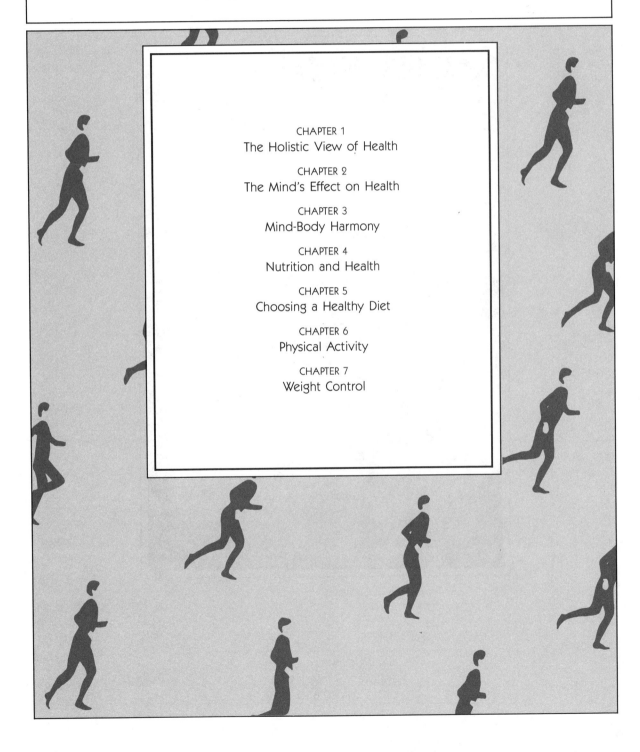

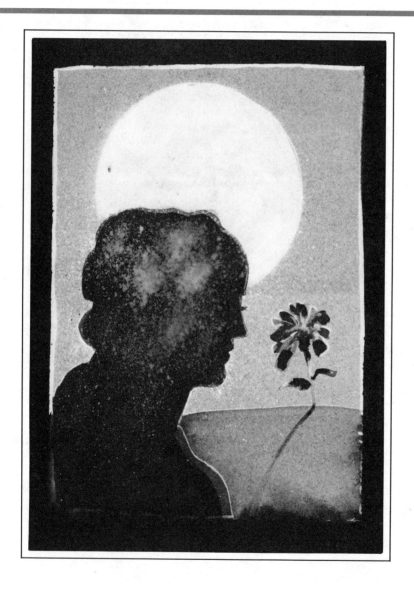

Health comes from the
harmonious integration of
body, mind, and spirit.

The Holistic View of Health

You the individual can do more for your own health and well-being than any doctor, any hospital, any drug, any exotic medical device.

Joseph A. Califano
Former U.S. Secretary of Health, Education, and Welfare

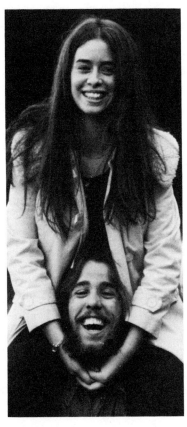

Figure 1-1
Health—that condition of the individual that makes possible the highest enjoyment of life. (Courtesy of the Environmental Protection Agency.)

Many people think of health in terms of disease. For them, a discussion of health is primarily about the presence or absence of symptoms and illness. They view health as what people have when they're not sick or dying.

It's true that not being sick is one aspect of a healthy existence. Just as important, however—and perhaps even more important—is the idea that health is a sense of optimum well-being that all people can attain by reducing their exposure to health risks and by living in harmony with themselves and their environment as much as possible.

In this book we present the view that health has much more to do with the quality of life and the attainment of well-being than with the medical repair of various body parts. We use the word "holistic" to emphasize that health is affected by every aspect of life: Health encompasses not only your body but also your emotions, thoughts, attitudes, and feelings. Health also depends on the quality of your physical surroundings, including the state of health of your family, friends, and acquaintances, the satisfaction and enjoyment you get from your daily activities, and the success of your relationships with others.

Health care is not simply another business. We must find ways to maintain and increase both the quality of care and the viability of the health care organizations.

Jean Mayer
President, Tufts University

Traditional Definitions of Health

Health, like love or happiness, is a quality of life that is difficult to define and virtually impossible to measure. For the purposes of health planning and medical record keeping, health is usually defined in terms of one or more measures of sickness. The United States Public Health Service (USPHS) and the World Health Organization (WHO) collect extensive data on the number of illnesses reported by doctors and hospitals and the number of deaths attributable to particular causes in the United States and other countries. From these data, known as **vital statistics,** such information as infant mortality rates, maternal mortality rates in childbirth, the incidence of influenza, or the number of deaths from heart disease and other illnesses can be ascertained and used as a measure of health in a population.

Another sickness-related way health is measured involves researchers directly asking a random sample of the population how frequently and for what reasons they become ill. These measures differ from those based on vital statistics because people who are sick do not always see doctors whenever they feel ill.

All these are ways of measuring health in a negative sense. They measure the "5 d's"—death, disease, discomfort, disability, and dissatisfaction. The assumption underlying this approach is that a person who is not sick is in the best state of health he or she can attain. To consider health merely as the absence of illness, however, severely limits our con-

ception of what true health is. Jesse Williams (1934), one of the founders of modern health education, wrote that health is "that condition of the individual that makes possible the highest enjoyment of life, the greatest constructive work, and that shows itself in the best service to the world. . . . Health as freedom from disease is a standard of mediocrity; health as a quality of life is a standard of inspiration and increasing achievements."

Health as Positive Wellness: The Holistic View

If freedom from sickness isn't all there is to health, then what else is involved? The World Health Organization has defined health as "a state of complete physical, mental, and social well-being, and not merely the absence of disease or infirmity." This definition is so broad and covers so much that it is said by some to be meaningless. But its universality is exactly right. People's lives, and therefore their health, are affected by everything they interact with—environmental influences such as climate; the availability of nutritious food, comfortable shelter, clean air to breathe, and pure water to drink; and other people, including family, lovers, employers, co-workers, friends, and associates of various kinds.

The WHO definition of health takes into account not only the condition of your body but also the state of your mind. Your mental processes are perhaps the most important influences on your

> To a greater extent than most of us are willing to accept, today's disorders of overweight, heart disease, cancer, blood pressure, and diabetes are by and large preventable. In this light, true health insurance is not what one carries on a plastic card, but what one does for oneself.
>
> **Lawrence Power, M.D.**
> **Health columnist**

health, for they determine how you deal with your physical and social surroundings, what your attitudes about life are, and how you interact with others.

Seeing health as the totality of a person's existence is the **holistic view** of health. Such a view recognizes the interrelatedness of the physical, psychological, emotional, social, spiritual, and environmental factors that contribute to the overall quality of a person's life. No part of the mind, body, or environment is truly separate and independent.

The philosophy of holistic health is not incompatible with the practice of conventional medicine. Rather, it emphasizes a view that has gained wide acceptance among members of the medical community: that each person has the capacity and the responsibility for optimizing his or her sense of well-being, for self-healing, and for the creation of conditions and feelings that can help prevent disease. Holistic health is hardly a revolutionary idea—even the Old English root of our word "health" (*hal,* meaning sound or whole) implies that there is more to health than freedom from sickness.

The holistic view of health embraces the concept of **positive wellness,** which, according to Lester Breslow (1972), professor of public health at the University of California, Los Angeles,

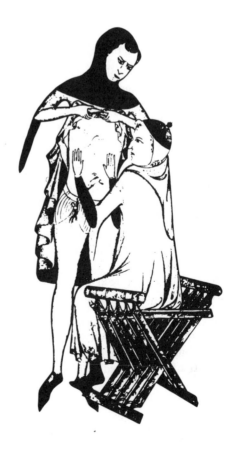

focuses attention on the living state rather than on categories of disease that may cause morbidity (disease) or mortality (death). It recognizes that life, at least in some parts of the world, has extended to the point where its finer differentiation deserves attention—

> We must always follow somebody looking
> for truth, and we must always run away
> from anyone who finds it.
>
> **Andre Gide**

not merely its existence and freedom from gross specific diseases. Sometimes called "positive" to distinguish it from the "negative" or pathologic concept, the emerging view is a generic one expressed in the WHO (World Health Organization) definition.

Positive wellness involves (1) being free from symptoms of disease and pain as much as possible, (2) being able to be active—able to do what you want and what you must at the appropriate time, and (3) being in good spirits most of the time. These characteristics indicate that health is not something that is suddenly achieved at a specific time, like getting a college degree. Rather, health is an ongoing *process*—indeed, a way of life—through which you develop and encourage every aspect of your body, mind, and feelings to interrelate harmoniously as much of the time as possible. M. Barry Flint (1986), executive director of the Institute for the Advancement of Health, gives a realistic view of the goals of holistic medicine:

> There is no quick holistic fix. We're so used to the quick foods, quick weight loss diets, quick beauty, and quick self-help advice that are part of our hurried, achievement-oriented lives that we expect a quick cure when we're sick. We see illness as something to get rid of so we can get back to work as soon as possible, rather than viewing it as a warning signal. Holistic medicine . . . focuses on creating health, not on simply curing illness.

The Holistic Health Philosophy in Practice

The philosophy of holistic health emphasizes the unity of the mind, spirit, and body. Therefore, symptoms of illness and disease may be viewed as an imbalance in a person's total state of being and not simply as the malfunction of a particular part of the body. Consider, for example, a common minor illness: the headache. About 80 to 90 percent of American adults experience at least one headache each year. Although a headache can be the result of brain injury or the symptom of another illness, more often it is caused by emotional stress that produces a tightening of the muscles in the head and neck (see Box 1-1). These contracting muscles increase the blood pressure in the head, thereby causing the pain of headache. Most people try to relieve a headache by taking aspirin or some other analgesic drug that can alter the physiological mechanisms that produce the pain. In contrast, someone using the holistic approach would first try to determine the *source* of the tensions—such as worry, anger, or frustration—and then work to reduce or eliminate the tensions. Similarly, an upset stomach cannot be regarded as simply the result of excessive stomach-acid secretion, requiring only some antacid preparation to bring relief. In many cases, the upset results from unexpressed hostility or fear. You are probably aware that such common events as taking an examination or having a dispute with someone can cause uncomfortable feelings in the stomach.

BOX 1-1

OH MY ACHING HEAD!

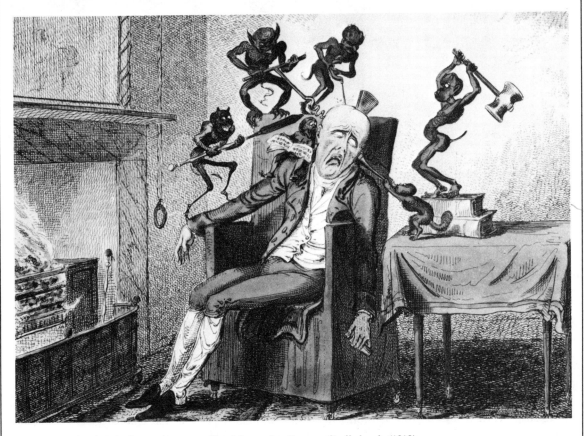

The agony of a headache, as conceptualized by artist George Cruikshank (1819). (Reproduced by permission of the Philadelphia Museum of Art.)

Headaches are one of the most common causes of human discomfort. Although headaches can be a symptom of a brain disease or injury, the vast majority of headaches are caused by anxiety, tension, and emotional distress.

Tension headache is the most common type of headache. It is caused by persistent contractions of the muscles in the neck and scalp, brought on by anxiety, stress, or allergic reactions to drugs and foods. Tension headaches may last for hours, may occur frequently, and may be a problem over the course of several years. The pain of a tension headache often can be relieved by experiencing a few minutes of deep mental relaxation or by massaging the tense muscles in the neck and scalp.

Migraine headache, or vascular headache, is characterized by throbbing pain that can last for hours and even days. Migraine headaches are accompanied by altered blood flow to the brain's blood vessels. Massaging the neck and scalp can help relieve the pain, as can mental relaxation and visualizing normal blood flow to the head. Autosuggestion and visualizing the hands becoming warmer may also help relieve pain because some blood flow is diverted from the brain to the hands, thereby reducing blood pressure in the brain.

Identifying and eliminating the sources of tension and anxiety in your life is the surest way to prevent headaches. Some people have learned to use "having a headache" as a means of avoiding unpleasant situations, such as school or work obligations. As children they may have observed their parents coping with tension and stress by "getting a headache," and so they too learned that "having a headache" can be used to avoid anxiety-provoking experiences. Have you developed such an avoidance mechanism?

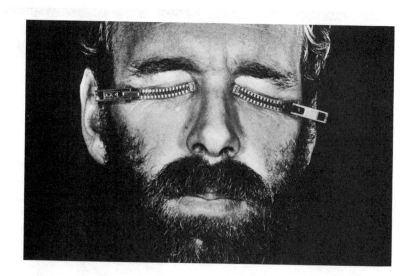

The subjective experience of a headache—some people feel it right behind the eyes.

Sometimes a holistic approach to such symptoms must consider the life situation of the distressed person as a first step in reducing or eliminating the problem that is creating the stress or fear. Consider the case of Eileen M., a 29-year-old married social worker. While on a two-week stay with her husband's parents in another city, she had to be rushed to a hospital for emergency treatment of sudden and unexpected bleeding from her gastrointestinal tract. Fortunately, the surgeon on duty was able to stop the bleeding and to give proper medical treatment so that Eileen was able to leave the hospital within a few days. Upon her return home, Eileen visited a specialist in gastrointestinal illness who diagnosed her problem as ulcerative colitis. The specialist prescribed certain foods as well as medications, and he carefully monitored her recovery. He found no underlying physical problem associated with Eileen's colitis, and within a few weeks she seemed fully recovered.

The specialist advised Eileen to visit her family physician periodically to be sure her recovery was permanent. On one of these visits, the physician asked her, "Do you want this bleeding business to happen again?" Of course, Eileen said she didn't. The two women began to talk about what might have caused or contributed to Eileen's illness, and the doctor quickly learned that Eileen had been nervous and worried about visiting her in-laws for several months before the trip. She had always felt that her mother-in-law was severely critical of her, and she had once overheard the woman say that

Eileen wasn't good enough for her son. Eileen had dreaded spending the two weeks with a person she had grown to dislike intensely but had said nothing for fear of hurting her husband's feelings.

After talking about this situation for a while, Eileen and her physician agreed that the suppression of her hostile feelings for her mother-in-law had probably caused her gastrointestinal problems. Eileen's physician pointed out that unless she learned to deal with her hostile feelings for her mother-in-law, the next time she paid a visit the sudden bleeding might recur—possibly with fatal results. Eileen agreed. She acknowledged that these feelings made her unhappy and that she would like to overcome them. Eileen's physician recommended that she see a psychological counselor who could help her find ways of dealing with the problem.

Fortunately for Eileen, her doctor was not content merely with her recovery from her physical symptoms but instead insisted on determining their underlying cause. In so doing, the physician was practicing **holistic medicine.** This approach to healing is described by Kenneth Pelletier (1977b), a professor of psychiatry at the University of California, San Francisco, School of Medicine:

> The going model of disease is that of infection or trauma, in which there is a single cause for a given disorder. However, when we get sick, it is the outcome of the complex interaction of social factors, physical and psychological stress, and our inability to

> Far from being simply the absence of disease,
> health is a dynamic and harmonious equilibrium
> of all the elements and forces making up and
> surrounding a human being.
>
> **Andrew Weil, M.D.**

adapt to these pressures. All illness signals excessive strain of some sort. While medical remedies may clear up a person's symptoms, they leave untouched the strains that have made him susceptible to these symptoms. A more total cure requires that we consider more than a single obvious cause.

The holistic approach does just this; it emphasizes healing, the maintenance of health, and the prevention of illness rather than the treatment of single disorders. This approach is by no means antagonistic to modern medicine. The strengths of medical technology are unquestionable. *Holistic medicine* simply integrates this technology into a broader approach to disease that looks not only at a person's symptoms, but also at the sources of stress in his life that have thrown him out of harmony.

From the holistic point of view, illness is the result of some imbalance in the desirable harmonious interaction of the body, mind, and environment. Thus, to the extent that we can follow a program of positive wellness and create a healthy environment, we can be free of disease.

Some of the great advances in medicine have resulted from considering illness solely in terms of the affected bodily organ. Indeed, devoting medical attention to one specific ailing part of the body is sometimes the most efficient way to treat a medical problem, which is why we have specialists who

are experts in treating diseases of different body parts—heart specialists, gastrointestinal specialists, and so on. But as we saw in Eileen M.'s case, consideration of a person's thoughts, feelings, and life situation is sometimes a better route to a cure. This realization is not new to medical practice. But in an age when highly specialized technology governs many medical decisions, it is sometimes disregarded.

Some health professionals have been critical of those who advocate holistic health practices and holistic medicine, arguing that the concepts and methods are anti-scientific and hence harmful (Glymour and Stalker, 1983). Holistic health is not anti-scientific. By encouraging individuals to take personal command of their health, including how they utilize medical services, holistic health practices are likely to be less harmful than some traditional medical practices, including unnecessary surgery. Criticism is useful but some people resist change because the changes are perceived as threats to their personal convictions or financial security.

The Health Care Industry

The philosophy and practice of holistic health—emphasizing as it does prevention of illness and disease, self-responsibility for health, and reduced use of drugs and medical care for conditions that are better served by exercise, stress reduction, and improved nutrition—threatens well-established and powerful economic interests represented by hospitals, pharmaceutical companies, and other providers

> Health has become one of America's biggest businesses. It is the nation's second-largest employer, after education, and third-largest industry in consumer spending, behind only food and housing.
>
> **Joseph A. Califano**
> **Former U.S. Secretary of Health, Education, and Welfare**

of medical equipment, supplies, and services, all of which make up what is referred to as the medical-industrial complex. Whereas these businesses are presumably dedicated to caring for the sick, their actual purpose is to make money. The companies that do well at making money are rewarded by having shares of their stock trade at high prices and their executives compensated extremely well. For example, in 1984, the second-highest-paid corporate executive in America ($17 million) was David A.

Figure 1-2
The annual cost of medical care rose dramatically between 1950 and 1985 — and it is still rising. (Data from U.S. Department of Health and Human Services.)

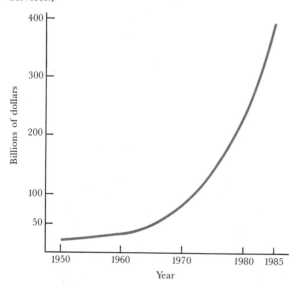

Jones of Humana Incorporated, which owns a large chain of hospitals and which sponsors most of the research on artificial hearts.

The modern health care system, which is actually a sickness care system since very little attention is given to illness prevention and health promotion, is a major growth industry in the U.S. Throughout the 1970s and continuing to the present, the costs of medical goods and services have increased at a rate exceeding the rate of growth of the U.S. economy. Since the mid-1960s health care costs in the U.S. have risen from 5 to 11 percent of the gross national product to an annual total of more than $400 billion (see Figure 1-2). Doctors, hospitals, health maintenance organizations, pharmaceutical companies, and other medical-related businesses compete vigorously for these billions of dollars. Giant corporate hospital chains, such as Hospital Corporation of America, National Medical Enterprises, American Medical International, and Humana Incorporated own over 1000 hospitals and already garner about 5 percent of the $400 billion total. They hope to increase that share to at least 20 percent over the next several years.

The persistent and alarming increase in medical care costs has forced those who pay for medical services — government, insurance companies, company health plans, and individuals — to devise ways to reduce health care costs. For example, the federal government now limits the amount of money Medicare programs will pay for specific treatments. Health insurance companies are devising ways to reduce payments to suppliers of medical products

> In search of a healthy state, the nation squanders $400 billion, allocating no more than 2 percent to prevention. The mad symbol of our plight is the ordeal of attaching an artificial heart to a man at the end of his life. . . .
>
> **Quentin D. Young, M.D.**
> **Editor, *Health and Medicine***

and services. Also, some corporations and government agencies have initiated health promotion programs for their employees. Such programs provide health education and opportunities to maintain physical fitness, improve nutrition, reduce stress, stop smoking, and manage alcohol and drug abuse.

Basing the delivery of medical services on profit motives has both advantages and disadvantages. Proponents point out that a for-profit system stimulates competition and efficiency, which meets consumer demands quickly and at lower cost than governmental programs. Critics argue that a for-profit system provides access to medical services based on the ability to pay rather than need, and hence a large number of people, particularly the elderly, the poor, the unemployed, and employed persons without health insurance (about 11 percent of the U.S. population) have limited access to the system. Furthermore, they point out that profit rather than humanitarian motives does not necessarily lead to lower costs, as providers find ways to order unnecessary diagnostic tests or perform unnecessary surgery (Margo, 1986). Critics also point out that the for-profit system can compromise the delivery of good medical care by forcing practitioners to make decisions based on financial gain or loss rather than on patients' welfare.

Surveys indicate that people want a more holistic and humanistic approach to health care, and that they want more information from their personal physicians. Although the Latin root of the word doctor, *docere,* means "to teach," very few physicians have the time, training, or skills to discuss health promotion or medical alternatives with their patients. Most physicians have been trained to practice "high-tech" medicine such as CAT and ultrasound scans or sophisticated surgery. Along with other health experts, Joseph A. Califano (1986), former U.S. Secretary of Health, Education, and Welfare, believes that medical education must change to meet current needs:

> Medical schools should train students and prod practitioners to count to ten before employing spectacular—and extraordinarily expensive—technology, whatever the marginal benefit, beyond the point at which it fosters the mental, spiritual, and physical capacity or human dignity of the patient, and teach them to be more skeptical in resorting to surgery and less promiscuous in dispensing pills.

Patients also must change their excessive demands for hospital, drug, and medical care. People must realize that their expectations of doctors and drugs to prevent and cure disease far exceed the abilities of physicians or the power of pills. The medical industry, academic research institutions, and even charities such as the Muscular Dystrophy Association, the American Heart Association, and the American Cancer Society promise breakthroughs and miracle cures that are difficult or impossible to achieve. We all have become skeptical of advertising claims for various consumer products and the promises of political candidates, but we still tend

> All worldly pursuits have but one unavoidable
> and inevitable end, which is sorrow: acquisitions
> end in dispersion; buildings in destruction;
> meetings in separation; births in death.
>
> **Milarepa**
> **Buddhist priest**

to take seriously the promises made by the medical-drug industry. And when doctors and drugs fail, people have been encouraged to take legal action, which creates additional problems for the health care system.

We are going to have to accept that the best medical care does not use every experimental drug, heroic interventions, and artificial hearts. We are going to have to accept the fact that physicians are fallible and that mistakes will be made despite the best efforts and precautions. The best health care emphasizes prevention and self-responsibility, which is something we are all capable of.

Diseases—Past and Present

Not so many years ago, people were subject to a variety of diseases over which they had little control. In the early part of the twentieth century, diseases caused by viruses, bacteria, and parasites were the leading causes of death in the U.S. because modern sanitation, public health methods, and antibiotic drugs had not been developed. Because people did not have the considerable health knowledge we now possess, it was not possible for them to prevent many illnesses, and for those who became ill, there was usually little that could be done to help. In 1918, millions of people died from a worldwide influenza epidemic that ran its course virtually unabated. In the 1980s, a viral disease called AIDS is killing thou-sands of people with no cure in sight, so infectious diseases still have not been conquered (see Chapter 18).

Today, however, many of the most serious illnesses are a product of our patterns of day-to-day living. In other words, in many instances we make ourselves sick by the way we live. Ours is a technologically complex, highly competitive culture that for many is highly stressful. Tensions and worries about work and career can make people anxious and depressed. So can frustrations and angers stemming from relationships with others. Tension and worry can also predispose people to any of several stress-related illnesses, including ulcers and hypertension (high blood pressure).

Tensions, worries, and frustrations are also largely responsible for the excessive demands placed on the medical care system. Several studies have shown that people tend to visit physicians when they are psychologically unwell, whether or not they are suffering from something that a physician can diagnose as a particular disease (Tessler and Mechanic, 1978). Many studies show that 50 percent or more of the people doctors see as outpatients have no discernible illness. Rather, such patients are experiencing some life situation that is making them feel bad and that may even be producing symptoms such as an upset stomach, diarrhea, insomnia, low energy, headaches, or loss of appetite. Yet a physical examination reveals no underlying physical problem. The bad feelings and the symptoms are the result of an emotionally upsetting life situation, not a disease. In their attempt to get help, these people visit the

> I want to find out how to be happy in spite
> of everything I know about us.
>
> **Alan Alda**

doctor. But few physicians are trained to deal with emotional problems, and often the only therapy offered is a tranquilizer, which does not provide a solution to the life situation causing the problem.

Certain habits of living are also associated with the most common causes of death. Most of the major causes of death in the U.S., Canada, and other industrialized nations are chronic (long-continued) degenerative diseases (see Figure 1-3), and many of these diseases are caused by particular behaviors or living practices. For example, a sedentary lifestyle, emotional stress, high blood pressure, cigarette smoking, and obesity all increase the risk of developing heart disease and diseases of the blood vessels. There is no "heart disease bacterium" responsible for the almost one million American deaths each year from these disorders.

Living habits also contribute to the development of other diseases that are major causes of death, including suicide and homicide; some types of cancer (cigarette smoking, environmental pollution, poor nutrition); injuries from automobile collisions and other accidents (alcohol abuse, excessive stress); lung disease (cigarette smoking, breathing polluted air, damage to lungs in certain occupations); and cirrhosis of the liver (alcohol abuse) (see Figure 1-4).

Traditionally, we have depended on doctors and other trained health practitioners to help us get well when we are sick. But medically very little can be done to help someone afflicted with one of the chronic degenerative diseases. By the time someone has developed clear-cut symptoms of heart disease, cancer, diabetes, arthritis, or emphysema, it is usually too late for medical care to reverse the dis-

Figure 1-3
Death rates for the leading causes of death in the U.S., 1983. Heart disease, cancer, stroke, diabetes, cirrhosis, and arteriosclerosis are chronic degenerative diseases. (Data from National Center for Health Statistics.)

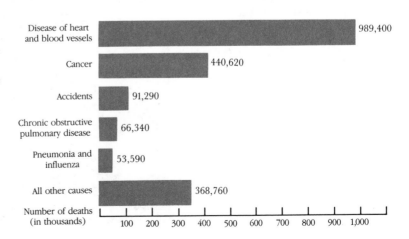

> We are killing ourselves by our own careless habits. We are killing ourselves by carelessly polluting our environment. We are killing ourselves by permitting harmful social conditions to persist—conditions like poverty, hunger, and ignorance— which destroy health.
>
> **Joseph A. Califano**
> **Former U.S. Secretary of Health, Education,**
> **and Welfare**

ease process and restore normal functioning. That is why these illnesses are called chronic and degenerative: once they get started, they tend to persist for life, often becoming progressively worse. The only effective way to deal with these diseases is to prevent them, which in many instances involves improving living habits, especially early in life.

In our consumer-oriented society we have come to think of health as something we can buy from the medical establishment—doctors, the pharmaceutical industry, hospitals and clinics, insurance companies. Many people also depend on the government to make health decisions for them and to help them care for their illnesses. But health cannot be purchased from anyone inside or outside the medical profession. Personal responsibility for health involves establishing attitudes and behaviors that promote positive wellness and spiritual harmony, by eating sensibly and exercising regularly, by not smoking, by not drinking alcohol excessively, and by becoming a knowledgeable consumer of medical care services. If individuals accept this responsibility, they will be free from illness much more of the time. They will be less dependent on doctors and will have fewer medical expenses. They will also feel a lot better.

Figure 1-4
Certain living habits, such as cigarette smoking, excessive alcohol consumption, sedentary living habits, and poor nutrition can contribute to ill health. (Courtesy Kaiser Permanente, Oakland, California.)

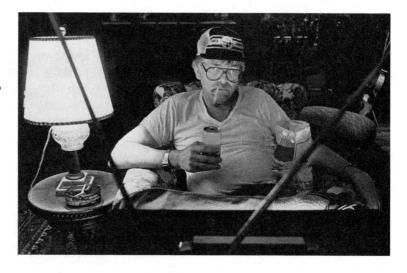

> Your religion is how you really get along with folks—not what you may claim your religion is.
>
> **Stephen Gaskin**
> *This Season's People*

Spirituality and Health

The holistic approach to health recognizes that for many people spiritual feelings and experiences—those which are not necessarily achieved by the application of logic and critical thought but which are more intuitive and subjective—can affect a person's state of wellness. This idea is contrary to much of our culture's traditional thinking about health, which tends to view states of wellness and illness as being affected only by physical processes that are amenable to objective, scientific study. The holistic view acknowledges that an objective, scientific explanation of the workings of the physical body contributes to a greater understanding of the mechanisms of disease and hence illness prevention and the attainment of health. But it also recognizes that many people have inner experiences that are subjective, mystical, and for some religious, and that these experiences may affect health as well.

By recognizing that the spiritual aspects of being can be important to health, the holistic health philosophy is in accord with such centuries-old traditional philosophies as the Hinduism of India, Taoism of China, and Buddhism of Tibet, Japan, and other Asian countries.

The holistic health outlook shares with Eastern philosophies the belief that spiritual experiences can engender feelings of compassion, peace of mind, and harmony with the environment. These feelings are believed to be the cornerstone of health, for they represent a balance between the inner and outer aspects of human experience. Yeshe Dhonden, a Tibetan Buddhist priest and physician, describes the essence of the Buddhist view of health:

> Health is the proper relationship between the microcosm which is man and the macrocosm which is the Universe. Disease is the disruption of this relationship. Tibetan medicine does not limit man to sensory perception. Within and beyond the visible man there is the vast area of invisible forces, currents, and vibratory structures, inaccessible to the senses, but nevertheless entirely real, concrete, and essential for the proper functioning of the body and mind. (Dhonden and Tschering, 1976)

The significance of the similarity of the holistic view and that of Eastern philosophies, as represented in Yeshe Dhonden's statement, is not that health requires belief in suprasensory forces but that to the extent that you feel in harmony with your inner and outer experiences you will be healthy.

In the practice of holistic health, as in the practice of Eastern philosophies, introspection and intuition are paths to spiritual experiences. Because so much of our cultural tradition and nearly all of our educational methods are based on cognitive, rational appraisals of experience, many of us neither understand nor appreciate subjective, intuitive, or spiritual modes of experience. Therefore, in the fol-

> Heavy thoughts bring on physical maladies;
> when the soul is oppressed so is the body.
> **Martin Luther**

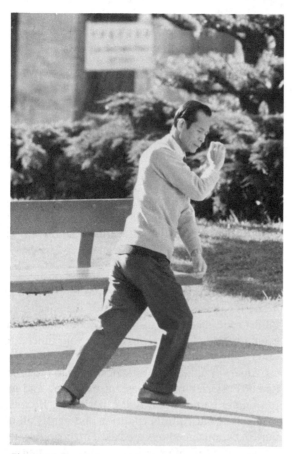

Figure 1-5
The practice of t'ai chi ch'uan fosters inner harmony and calm.

lowing chapters, as we discuss wellness and illness in the modern scientific terms of chemistry, genetics, physiology, and psychology, we will also consider the role of spiritual awareness in promoting health.

Many religious and psychological methods can help people experience spiritual realms of existence. Insofar as these methods foster feelings of inner peace and harmony, which we consider essential to health, they, too, will be discussed in this book. These methods include the many forms of meditation, yoga, and the ancient Chinese dancelike exercise, **t'ai chi ch'uan**. Of course, these methods of the Eastern philosophies are not the only routes to feelings of inner peace and harmony. Western religious traditions of prayer and meditation, as well as many artistic, musical, and even athletic activities, foster transcendent or spiritual experiences.

Becoming more spiritually aware, regardless of the chosen method, can lead to a healthier life. Being in touch with your spiritual feelings helps you handle life's ups and downs with understanding and compassion for yourself and others. You become open to love in the higher sense of its meaning, which is acceptance and tolerance. You begin to love yourself despite your problems and hangups. You love your family and friends even when relations are strained. You see beauty and harmony in more and more aspects of living. And occasionally—however fleetingly—you may experience the truly wondrous feeling of being completely and joyfully alive.

Supplemental Readings

Califano, J. A., Jr. *America's Health Care Revolution.* New York: Random House, 1986. A factual and scathing account of the U.S. health care industry.

Grossman, Richard. *The Other Medicines.* New York: Doubleday, 1985. A good introduction to alternative therapies.

Hastings, A. C., Fadiman, J., and **Gordon, J. S., eds.** *Health for the Whole Person — The Complete Guide to Holistic Medicine.* Boulder: Westview Press, 1980. A comprehensive guide to holistic health ideas and alternative therapies by experts in the fields.

Nolen, William A. *Healing: A Doctor in Search of a Miracle.* New York: Random House, 1985. A famous physician describes how he became more open-minded to medical alternatives.

Siegel, B. S. *Love, Medicine, and Miracles.* New York: Harper & Row, 1986. A cancer physician describes how he learned to practice healing as well as medicine.

Weil, A. *Health and Healing.* Boston: Houghton Mifflin, 1983. A personal view of holistic health and alternative medical therapies by an outspoken physician.

Summary

The holistic view of health emphasizes that health is a state of optimal well-being and not simply the absence of disease. From the holistic viewpoint, health is a way of life in which people seek positive wellness — a maximization of individual potentialities to make life as meaningful and harmonious as possible.

Analysis of the health status of our population shows that many people do not feel as healthy as they could feel and that much of this ill-feeling is the result of styles of living that create sickness. Excess smoking, obesity, emotional stress, and environmental pollution are among the lifestyle factors that produce many of today's sicknesses, including heart disease, stroke, cancer, and the emotional upsets that make tranquilizers and ulcer medications among the most frequently prescribed by physicians.

In our consumer-oriented society we've come to think of health as something to buy from the medical establishment — physicians, the pharmaceutical industry, hospitals and clinics, and insurance companies. Many people also depend on the government to make health decisions for them. In contrast, the holistic health approach provides a framework for relying on yourself to create a life in which the inner self is more in harmony with everything in the environment.

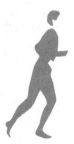

FOR YOUR HEALTH

Complete the following Health and Wellness Inventory to gauge your present degree of wellness. Then make a contract with yourself to begin to make appropriate changes in those categories in which you would like to improve. List the changes you wish to make, set a time to begin making them, and decide when you want the change to be fully integrated into your life. For example:

Change Desired
quit smoking
take up meditation
record dreams

Begin Change
in one week
immediately
after quitting smoking

Time Allotted
one month
two weeks
one week

Do not try to make all the changes on your list at the same time. Select either the one or two most important, or the one or two you know you can accomplish as places to begin. Then make one or two changes at a time after that.

Health and Wellness Inventory
For each of the questions, circle the number
5 if the statement is ALWAYS true
4 if the statement is FREQUENTLY true
3 if the statement is OCCASIONALLY true
2 if the statement is SELDOM true
1 if the statement is NEVER true

1. I am able to identify the situations and factors that overstress me. 5 4 3 2 1
2. I eat only when I am hungry. 5 4 3 2 1
3. I don't take tranquilizers or other drugs to relax. 5 4 3 2 1
4. I support efforts in my community to reduce environmental pollution. 5 4 3 2 1

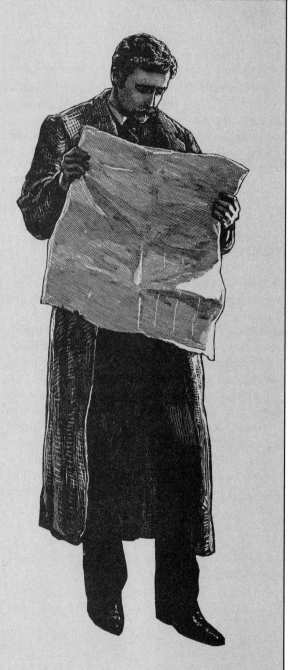

(Continued on next page.)

FOR YOUR HEALTH

5.	I avoid buying foods with artificial colorings.	5	4	3	2	1
6.	I rarely have problems concentrating on what I'm doing because of worrying about other things.	5	4	3	2	1
7.	My employer (school) takes measures to ensure that my work (study) place is safe.	5	4	3	2	1
8.	I try not to use medications when I feel unwell.	5	4	3	2	1
9.	I am able to identify certain bodily responses and illnesses as my reactions to stress.	5	4	3	2	1
10.	I question the use of diagnostic x-rays.	5	4	3	2	1
11.	I try to alter personal living habits that are risk factors for heart disease, cancer, and other lifestyle diseases.	5	4	3	2	1
12.	I avoid taking sleeping pills to help me sleep.	5	4	3	2	1
13.	I try not to eat foods with refined sugar or corn sugar ingredients.	5	4	3	2	1
14.	I accomplish goals I set for myself.	5	4	3	2	1
15.	I stretch or bend for several minutes each day to keep my body flexible.	5	4	3	2	1
16.	I support immunization of all children for common childhood diseases.	5	4	3	2	1
17.	I try to prevent friends from driving after they drink alcohol.	5	4	3	2	1
18.	I minimize extra salt intake.	5	4	3	2	1
19.	I don't mind when other people and situations make me wait or lose time.	5	4	3	2	1
20.	I walk four or fewer flights of stairs rather than take the elevator.	5	4	3	2	1
21.	I eat fresh fruits and vegetables.	5	4	3	2	1
22.	I use dental floss at least once a day.	5	4	3	2	1
23.	I read product labels on foods to determine their ingredients.	5	4	3	2	1
24.	I try to maintain a normal body weight.	5	4	3	2	1
25.	I record my feelings and thoughts in a journal or diary.	5	4	3	2	1
26.	I have no difficulty falling asleep.	5	4	3	2	1
27.	I engage in some form of vigorous physical activity at least three times a week.	5	4	3	2	1
28.	I take time each day to quiet my mind and relax.	5	4	3	2	1
29.	I am willing to make and sustain close friendships and intimate relationships.	5	4	3	2	1
30.	I obtain an adequate daily supply of vitamins from my food or vitamin supplements.	5	4	3	2	1
31.	I rarely have tension or migraine headaches, or pain in the neck or shoulders.	5	4	3	2	1
32.	I wear a safety belt when driving.	5	4	3	2	1
33.	I am aware of the emotional and situational factors that lead me to overeat.	5	4	3	2	1
34.	I avoid driving my car after drinking any alcohol.	5	4	3	2	1

(Continued on next page.)

FOR YOUR HEALTH

35. I am aware of the side effects of the medicines I take. 5 4 3 2 1
36. I am able to accept feelings of sadness, depression, and anxiety, knowing that they are almost always transient. 5 4 3 2 1
37. I would seek several additional professional opinions if my doctor recommended surgery for me. 5 4 3 2 1
38. I agree that nonsmokers should not have to breathe the smoke from cigarettes in public places. 5 4 3 2 1
39. I agree that pregnant women who smoke harm their babies.
40. I feel I get enough sleep. 5 4 3 2 1
41. I ask my doctor why a certain medication is being prescribed and inquire about alternatives. 5 4 3 2 1
42. I am aware of the calories expended in my activities. 5 4 3 2 1
43. I am willing to give priority to my own needs for time and psychological space by saying "no" to others' requests of me. 5 4 3 2 1
44. I walk instead of drive whenever feasible. 5 4 3 2 1
45. I eat a breakfast that contains about one-third of my daily need for calories, proteins, and vitamins. 5 4 3 2 1
46. I prohibit smoking in my home. 5 4 3 2 1
47. I remember and think about my dreams. 5 4 3 2 1
48. I seek medical attention only when I have symptoms or feel that some (potential) condition needs checking, rather than have routine yearly checkups. 5 4 3 2 1
49. I endeavor to make my home accident free. 5 4 3 2 1
50. I ask my doctor to explain the diagnosis of my problem until I understand all that I care to. 5 4 3 2 1
51. I try to include fiber or roughage (whole grains, fresh fruits and vegetables, or bran) in my daily diet. 5 4 3 2 1
52. I can deal with my emotional problems without alcohol or other mood-altering drugs. 5 4 3 2 1
53. I am satisfied with my school/work. 5 4 3 2 1
54. I require children riding in my car to be in infant seats or in shoulder harnesses. 5 4 3 2 1
55. I try to associate with people who have a positive attitude about life. 5 4 3 2 1

(Continued on next page.)

FOR YOUR HEALTH

56. I try not to eat snacks of candy, pastries, and other "junk" foods.	5 4 3 2 1
57. I avoid people who are "down" all the time and bring down those around them.	5 4 3 2 1
58. I am aware of the calorie content of the foods I eat.	5 4 3 2 1
59. I brush my teeth after meals.	5 4 3 2 1
60. (for women only) I routinely examine my breasts.	5 4 3 2 1
(for men only) I am aware of the signs of testicular cancer.	5 4 3 2 1

How to Score

Enter the numbers you've circled next to the question number and total your score for each category. Then determine your degree of wellness for each category using the wellness status key.

Emotional health	Fitness and body care	Environmental health	Stress	Nutrition	Medical self-responsibility
6____	15____	4____	1____	2____	8____
12____	20____	7____	3____	5____	10____
25____	22____	17____	9____	13____	11____
26____	24____	32____	14____	18____	16____
36____	27____	34____	19____	21____	35____
40____	33____	38____	28____	23____	37____
47____	42____	39____	29____	30____	41____
52____	44____	46____	31____	45____	48____
55____	58____	49____	43____	51____	50____
57____	59____	54____	53____	56____	60____
Total____	Total____	Total____	Total____	Total____	Total____

Wellness Status

To assess your status in each of the six categories, compare your total score in each to the following key: **0–34** Need improvement; **35–44** Good; **45–50** Excellent.

CHAPTER TWO

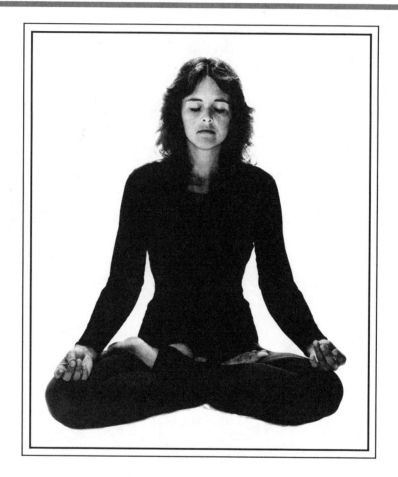

How the mind can be used to help
maintain health.

The Mind's Effect on Health

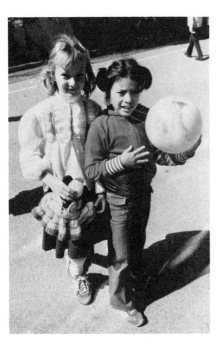

(Courtesy Environmental Protection Agency.)

The holistic view of health recognizes that the human mind and body make up a single, unified organism. No body exists without a mind; no mind exists without a body. That people are integral mind-body entities has considerable importance to health and well-being, for what goes on in the mind can produce changes in the body's tissues and organs that may either increase or decrease one's overall state of health and wellness. As we describe in detail in Chapter 3, thoughts and feelings can alter body physiology and chemistry because thought and feeling centers in the brain influence the activity of the nervous system, endocrine (hormone) system, and immune system, each of which in turn influence body physiology. Therefore, people can affect their health by what they think and feel.

The mind is a healer. Indeed, there is no medicine or treatment more effective or more capable of healing than the human mind. Therefore, you can use your mind to heal your body and to improve your health. In order to do so most effectively, you must know something about how the mind functions and how physiology—the workings of the body—can be affected by your mental state.

In our culture we are accustomed to thinking of health and the healing of disease in terms of medicines, surgery, and other physical interventions, but in many other cultures, past and present, healing has been accomplished by magic, ritual, faith, and other nonmedical methods. Even in our own culture we recognize the role of the mind in healing when we talk about a patient's "will to live." All physicians are aware that a sick person's attitude greatly affects his or her chances for recovery. We wish to emphasize in this chapter (and throughout this book) that there is no magic in the success of nonmedical healing practices; they can be effective because they *do* affect body physiology and chemistry.

Jerome Frank, emeritus professor of psychiatry of the Johns Hopkins University School of Medicine, discussed the effectiveness of nonmedical healing in his book *Persuasion and Healing* (1973). He observed:

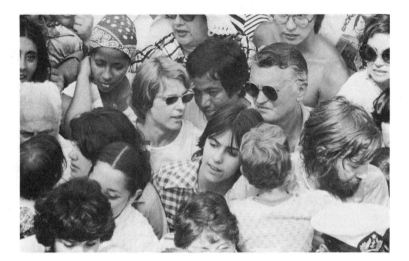

Figure 2-1
Whatever our age, sex, race, or ethnic background, we are thinking, feeling human beings who can use our minds to influence healthful physiological functioning. (Photos by Owen Franken/Stock, Boston.)

Nonmedical healing of bodily illness highlights the profound influence of emotions on health and suggests that anxiety and despair can be lethal; confidence and hope, life-giving. The current assumptive world of Western society, which includes mind-body dualism, incorporates this obvious fact with difficulty and, therefore, tends to underestimate its importance.

However, these views are still regarded with skepticism by other physicians. Based on a study of the survival of cancer patients and their attitudes, Barrie Cassileth (1985) concluded, "It is time to acknowledge that our belief in disease as a direct reflection of mental state is largely folklore." Despite this pessimistic view, an increasingly large body of research supports the idea that the human mind can be extremely effective in altering physiology. All of

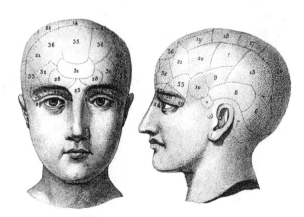

us can use our thoughts, feelings, and beliefs to prevent illness, to help cure ourselves of disease, and to promote positive well-being and optimum health.

Psychosomatic Illness

The powerful effect of the mind on the body is dramatically demonstrated by maladies called **psychosomatic illnesses**. These illnesses are caused by negative mental states and attitudes that harmfully change physiology—hence the description *psycho-* ("mind") *somatic* ("body"). Many people have the idea that a psychosomatic illness is imaginary—that the person feels sick but doesn't actually have a disease. But psychosomatic illnesses are real—as real as appendicitis or an infected lung. Tissues and organs can be damaged by infectious organisms or toxic chemicals. The distinctive feature of psychosomatic diseases is that psychological, social, and environmental factors seem to contribute in a large part to their onset. The case of Eileen M., cited in Chapter 1, is a clear instance of psychosomatic illness.

Table 2-1 lists six common psychosomatic diseases and several other less serious disorders that are principally of psychosomatic origin. All of them can be cured or relieved by changes in a person's mental state, by a change of environment, or by a combination of both.

The capacity of the human mind to cause disease and also to heal is often neglected or deemphasized in present-day medical care. But as we pointed

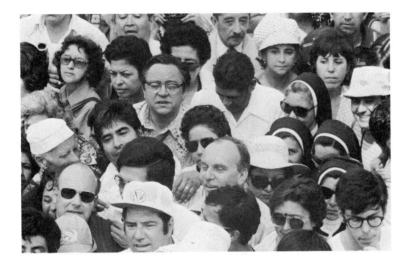

out in Chapter 1, there is no fundamental disagreement between modern medical ideas about the origin of disease and views about illness embodied in Eastern religions and philosophies. Chogyam Trungpa (1977), a well-known Tibetan priest who now resides in the United States, interprets the Buddhist view of disease:

> A person cannot get sick without some kind of loss of interest. Whether you are run down by a car or you catch a cold, there is some gap in which you do not take care of yourself, an empty moment in which you cease to relate properly to things. There is no ongoing sense of awareness of your psychological state. So to the extent that you have to invite it, *all* sickness is psychological, not just the diseases traditionally considered to be psychosomatic. All diseases are instigated by your state of mind.

This view does not mean that all sickness is caused *just* by a person's state of mind but that the mind is a factor—sometimes the most important one—in the onset of disease.

Many people intuitively understand that their thoughts and feelings play an important role in their health, but they usually do not know *what* to do to improve their mental and emotional states. Nor do they know *how* to do it. So they look to outside sources for solutions to their health problems. Some turn to physicians or psychologists for help; others seek counsel from faith healers, gurus, or herbalists. We would like to advance the idea—strongly supported by a wealth of evidence—that the solution

Table 2-1
Psychosomatic Diseases and Disorders

Six common psychosomatic diseases

Peptic ulcer
Essential hypertension
Bronchial asthma
Hyperactive thyroid
Rheumatoid arthritis
Ulcerative colitis

Other disorders that are partially or wholly psychosomatic

Hay fever
Asthma
Acne
Diarrhea
Impotency
Menstrual problems
Warts
Eczema
Tinnitus (ringing in one or both ears)
Bruxism (grinding of teeth)
Nail biting
Tension headaches
Back pain
Urinary problems
Insomnia

to many illnesses resides within ourselves. However, if an individual *believes* that the illness, whatever the cause, can be cured by someone or something outside of himself, then that belief (which itself initiates an internal healing process) can also produce the cure.

> Faith.
> You can do very little with it
> and nothing without it.
> **Samuel Butler**

Placebo Effects

The healing that results from a person's belief in substances or treatments that have no medicinal value in themselves is called a **placebo effect**. Even though the term "placebo," which comes from the Latin meaning "to please," usually refers to an inert substance administered to someone, "placebo effect" also has a broader meaning. Anything that a person strongly believes is able to cure can produce the placebo effect. Superstition, sugar pills, mineral water, health spas—even laughter—can initiate an internal healing process.

Placebo effects have been studied scientifically since 1952 when a survey of medical prescriptions in England showed that at least 30 percent of the drugs used by people were placebos, since the drugs were known to have no pharmacological effect on the condition for which they were prescribed. Almost any physiological or psychological illness responds to placebos—pain, cough, blood cell counts, blood pressure, hormone levels, insomnia, contraception, asthma, depression, headache, dermatitis, serum lipoprotein levels, and pupil dilation. In many instances as much as 50 percent of a drug's effectiveness is due to a placebo effect (see Table 2-2). The biological and psychological mechanisms responsible for placebo effects are still unknown. Hypnosis, the power of suggestion, shared expectations, and conditioned responses have all been invoked to explain how placebos act to relieve pain and other symptoms of disease. Whatever the correct explanation, placebos are invaluable. As pointed out by Frederick J. Evans (1984), "Far from being a nuisance, the placebo should be considered a potent therapeutic intervention in its own right. . . . "

Placebo effects are also produced by the words and touches of charismatic healers. Again, the power of healing does not reside so much in the healer as in the belief of the patient or supplicant. The cures that result from placebo effects sometimes seem miraculous but actually are caused by physiological changes brought about by people's beliefs and mental states. The mind is healer.

The most frequent use of placebos today is in testing the efficacy of new drugs and treatments. To determine how effective a drug is in relieving a particular symptom or in curing a disease, a group of people—called the subjects of the experiment—is given either a new drug or a placebo. Neither the

Table 2-2

A Comparison of Placebos with Pain-Relieving Drugs in Double-Blind Studies

Placebo compared with	Percent effectiveness
Aspirin	54
Codeine	56
Darvon	54
Morphine	56
Zomax	55

Data from F. J. Evans, "Unravelling Placebo Effects." *Advances,* 1 (1984).

> The fact that the placebo effect has been identified in thousands of drug studies is stark and incontrovertible testimony to the role of the imagination in health.
>
> **Jeanne Achterberg**
> *Imagery in Healing*

subjects nor the doctor knows which persons receive the drug or the placebo; hence, these clinical drug tests are called "double-blind" studies.

Amazingly, many such drug-effectiveness studies show that a large percentage of all those who receive a placebo experience relief of symptoms or improvements to the same degree as patients receiving the actual drug (see Figure 2-2). At one time or another placebos have been used successfully for treating virtually every disease, as well as for a wide variety of symptoms including pain, depression, headaches, and allergies. Placebos have even been used to treat heart disease and cancer—although such use would be regarded as unethical by most people today.

Norman Cousins, who for years was the editor of *Saturday Review* magazine, became interested in the effects of placebos after using a variety of them (including laughter induced by watching old-time comedy films) to cure himself of ankylosing spondylitis, a form of arthritis of the spine that physicians had told him was progressive and incurable. In an article titled "The Mysterious Placebo" (1977), he described how placebos work:

> The placebo, then, is not so much a pill as a process. The process begins with the patient's confidence in the doctor and extends through to the full functioning of his own immunological and healing system. The process works not because of any magic in the tablet but because the human body is its own best apothecary and because the most successful prescriptions are those filled by the body itself.

After being cured of what was thought to be an incurable disease, Cousins compiled a long list of diseases that had been successfully treated by the use of placebos (see Box 2-1 for excerpts from the list). Because of the sick person's *belief*—whether in the placebo, the physician, or the healing process—his or her body and brain chemistry are changed. Symptoms disappear. Illness vanishes. Well-being is restored. Scientists are just beginning to unravel the complex changes in body chemistry that can be initiated in the mind. The placebo effect demonstrates quite convincingly that for many people a belief that they have been administered an effective drug is sufficient to provide relief or even to cure their disease. So, all people carry within them a powerful source of healing—the beliefs in their minds.

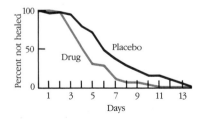

Figure 2-2
Placebo effects. When patients with genital herpes were treated with a drug or with a placebo, the drug-treated group healed only slightly faster than the placebo group.

BOX 2-1

PLACEBOS CURE ALMOST ANYTHING!

The late Dr. Henry K. Beecher, noted anesthesiologist at Harvard, considered the results of 15 studies involving 1082 patients. He discovered that across the broad spectrum of these tests, 35 percent of the patients consistently experienced "satisfactory relief" when placebos were used instead

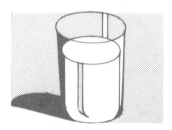

of regular medication for a wide range of medical problems, including severe postoperative wound pains, seasickness, headaches, coughs, and anxiety. Other biological processes and disorders affected by placebos, as reported by medical researchers, include rheumatoid and degenerative arthritis, blood-cell count, respiratory rates, vasomotor function, peptic ulcers, hay fever, hypertension, and spontaneous remission of warts.

Dr. Stewart Wolf wrote that placebo effects are "neither imaginary nor necessarily suggestive in the usual sense of the word." His comments were connected to the results of a test in which a placebo induced eosinophilia—a blood condition in which specialized blood cells called eosinophils accumulate beyond their normal numbers and circulate throughout the system. Wolf also reported a test by a colleague in which a placebo reduced the amount of fat and protein in the blood.

When a patient suffering from Parkinson's disease was given a placebo but was told he was receiving a drug, his tremors decreased markedly. After the effects of the placebo wore off, the same substance was put into his milk without his knowledge. The tremors reappeared.

During a large study of mild mental depression, patients who had been treated with sophisticated stimulants were taken off the drugs and put on placebos. The patients showed exactly the same improvement as they had gained from the drugs. In a related study, doctors gave placebos to 133 depressed patients who had not yet received a drug. One-quarter of them responded so well to placebos that they were excluded from further testing of actual drugs.

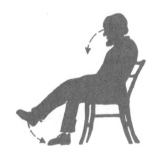

When a group of patients were given a placebo in place of an antihistamine, 77.4 percent reported drowsiness, which is characteristic of antihistamine drugs.

In a study of postoperative wound pain by Beecher and Lasagna, a group of patients who had just undergone surgery were alternately given morphine and placebos. Those who took morphine immediately after surgery registered a 52 percent relief factor; those who took the placebo first, 40 percent. The placebo was 77 percent as effective as morphine. Beecher and Lasagna also discovered that the more severe the pain, the more effective the placebo.

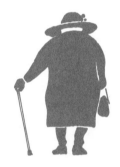

Eighty-eight arthritic patients were given placebos instead of aspirin or cortisone. The number of patients who benefited from the placebos was approximately the same as the number benefiting from the conventional antiarthritic drugs. Some of the patients who had experienced no relief from the placebo tablets were given placebo injections. Sixty-four percent of those given injections reported relief and improvement. For the entire group, the benefits included not just pain relief but general improvement in eating, sleeping, elimination, and even reduction in swelling.

From "The Mysterious Placebo" by Norman Cousins, *Saturday Review,* October 1, 1977. Reprinted by permission of the *Saturday Review.*

> The apparent success of healing methods based on various ideologies and methods compels the conclusion that the healing power of faith resides in the patient's state of mind, not in the validity of its object.
>
> **Jerome Frank, M.D.**
> *Persuasion and Healing*

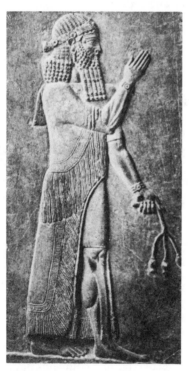

Figure 2-3
An Assyrian priest-physician. In the antique world, one man played both roles. (Courtesy World Health Organization.)

Healing by Faith: A Placebo Effect

Thousands of years ago the priest-healers of ancient civilizations and the shamans of primitive tribes used the beliefs of their people to heal by incantation, to exorcise evil spirits, to vanquish devils and demons. The existence of shamans, faith healers, and medicine men in cultures throughout history suggests that their healing methods must have been successful to some degree. Recently discovered papyri show that although Egyptian priest-physicians prescribed herbs and performed surgery, their treatments relied primarily on the beliefs of the Egyptian people in the healing power of the gods and priests. The priest-physicians used suggestions, dreams, and magic, along with herbs and other treatments. It is impossible for us to measure accurately how successful these treatments were, but many people must have felt better; many were probably even cured.

The Greeks and Romans also had gods, oracles, and temples of healing. Their priest-physicians would induce trance and sleeplike mental states in which the mind was particularly receptive to healing suggestions. Sometimes "miraculous cures" resulted from healing suggestions. Greek and Roman emperors, kings, and priests effected cures by "laying on of hands" or by other forms of touch—King Pyrrhus of Epirus is reputed to have cured persons suffering from colic solely by the touch of his big toe.

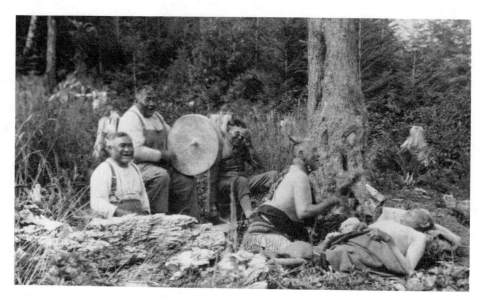

Figure 2-4
Shamanistic healing ritual. (Courtesy National Museums of Canada.)

These stories may sound outlandish, but all religions embody concepts of spiritual healing. The New Testament recounts in many places the healing power of Jesus. For example:

That evening they brought to him many who were possessed with demons, and he cast out the spirits with a word, and healed all who were sick. (Matthew 8:14)

And great crowds came to him, bringing with them the lame, the maimed, the blind, the dumb, and many others, and they put them at his feet, and he healed them, so that the throng wondered, when they saw the dumb speaking, the maimed whole, the lame walking, and the blind seeing; and they glorified the God of Israel. (Matthew 15:29)

And he said to her, "Daughter, your faith has made you well; go in peace and be healed of your diseases." (Mark 5:34)

Mary Baker Eddy (1890), the founder of Christian Science, which emphasizes healing by spiritual means, told her followers:

To prevent disease or to cure it, the power of Truth, of divine Spirit, must break the dream of the material senses. To heal by argument, find the type of ailment, get its name, and array your mental plea against the physical. Argue at first mentally, not audibly, that the patient has no diseases, and confirm the argument so as to destroy the evidence of disease. Mentally insist that harmony is the fact, and that sickness is a temporal dream. Realize the presence of health and the fact of harmonious being, until the body corresponds with the normal conditions of health and harmony.

Many present-day religious and spiritual leaders— including Billy Graham, Oral Roberts, and other evangelists—employ the power of belief and suggestion in the healing process.

The physician today who tells a patient, "I'm sure you'll feel better in a couple of days" or "Take these pills and you'll feel as good as new in no time at all" is practicing healing by the power of suggestion. Today's patient has faith in the knowledge and medicines of the physician, just as the people in ancient civilizations had faith in their priests and herbs. The improvement in the patient's condition is often as much a result of the *faith* in his or her mind as it is the effects of the medicine. Placebo effects play an important role in the practice of modern medicine; in fact, they may be just as important as the prescription of modern drugs.

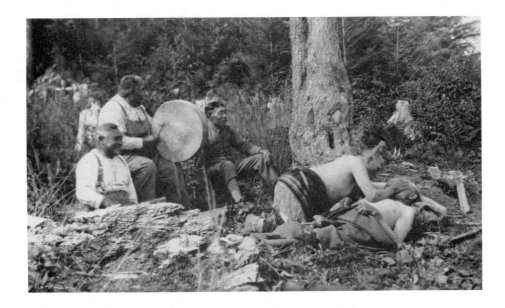

Healing Through Suggestion and Relaxation

In the late nineteenth century, two French physicians showed that healing could be accomplished solely by means of suggestion and of the sick person's expectation of being cured. Ambroise-Auguste Liébeault and Hippolyte-Marie Bernheim successfully treated over 12,000 patients with hypnosis, or **hypnotherapy,** as it is now referred to medically. Bernheim believed that the cures were actually accomplished by suggestion, to which the hypnotized patient was especially receptive.

At the beginning of this century the idea that the mind could heal and cure disease by the power of suggestion was used with great success by many health practitioners. Emile Coué, a French pharmacist, opened a clinic in 1910 and expanded on Bernheim's philosophy of "healing through suggestion." Coué employed **autosuggestion** (a form of self-hypnosis). According to his method, which he called "conscious autosuggestion," the responsibility for the healing process rests with the patient and can only be encouraged by the healer. Coué became world-famous for the autosuggestion that he recommended people recite to themselves daily: "Day by day in every way I am getting better and better."

Today hypnotherapy and healing by suggestion are used by many physicians to help treat a variety of illnesses. Descriptions of the successful treatment of arthritis, obesity, and warts by the use of present-day hypnotherapy are provided in Box 2-2. This is not to suggest that *all* cases of such problems can be cured by suggestion or hypnosis. But the fact that many diseases and disorders can be cured solely by a change in the individual's mental state should encourage people to rely more on their own mental powers to reduce illness and to increase health and wellness.

Effective use of suggestion in healing seems to depend on the degree of mental relaxation involved. For most people, the day is filled with a whirl of thoughts, ideas, plans, and concentration on certain tasks. For reasons that are not entirely clear, a mind engaged in conscious thought is not as open to suggestion as one relaxed or focused inward.

Many people have difficulty relaxing their minds because they mistakenly think that relaxation is something that requires effort. People *try* to relax in much the same way that they might try to solve a tough math problem, but the harder they try, the less relaxed they become. Mental (and physical) relaxation is best accomplished by "letting go" and by not trying to accomplish anything.

Nearly everyone has experienced daydreaming. Now and again—even while engaged in some complicated physical or mental task—the mind chooses to "take a trip"; its attention is elsewhere. Although there are occasions when daydreaming might be

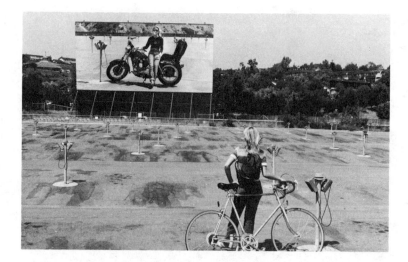

dangerous—while driving on a winding mountain road or when using a chain saw, for example—there are many opportunities for daydreaming. Students who become bored with a lecture often let their minds wander. Allowing the mind to go where it chooses is one example of letting go.

Both Bernheim and Coué taught their patients in Europe to relax through the use of hypnosis and suggestion (see Figure 2-5). In 1929 a Chicago physician named Edmund Jacobson introduced a method he called **progressive relaxation.** Jacobson taught people to relax specific parts of their bodies by first tightening the muscles, such as clenching a fist or tensing the muscles in the face, and then relaxing them. After being tightened, a muscle's normal response is to relax, and Jacobson used this principle to create whole body relaxation (see Box 2-3).

Autogenic Training

Around 1930 one of the most comprehensive methods for producing deep relaxation by autosuggestion was developed in Germany by Johannes H. Schultz. This method, which Schultz called **autogenic training,** has been used by thousands of people during the past fifty years with great success. The basic autogenic exercises, which are really autosuggestions, are designed to establish a balance between the mind and the body through changes in the autonomic nervous system (see Chapter 3 for a more detailed description of how the autonomic nervous system controls body functions).

Autogenic relaxation is achieved as the patient learns to concentrate on one of six basic autosuggestive phrases for a few minutes each day for a week or more. After weeks or months of practice, the person is able to attain deep states of relaxation, often within seconds, which can result in healthful changes in physiology.

The six basic autogenic suggestions designed by Johannes Schultz and Wolfgang Luthe (1959) are:

My arms and legs are heavy.

My arms and legs are warm.

My heartbeat is calm and regular.

My lungs breathe me.

My abdomen is warm.

My forehead is cool.

Each of these suggestions repeated over and over in the mind can have profound effects on body physiology. The exact phrasing of any suggestion is not critical, and there is no magic in the words themselves. Any suggestion can be rephrased so that it becomes comfortable, believable, and acceptable to the individual's mind.

Figure 2-5 ▶
All hypnosis is self-hypnosis. (Courtesy King Features Syndicate.)

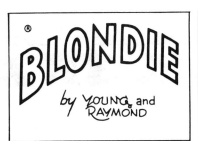

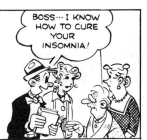

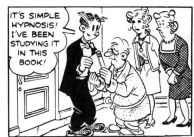

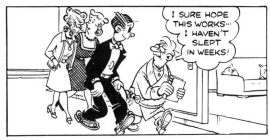

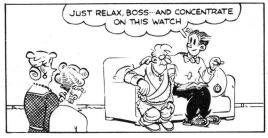

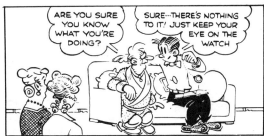

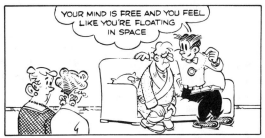

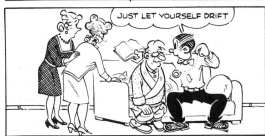

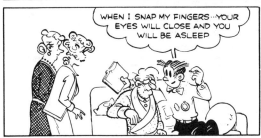

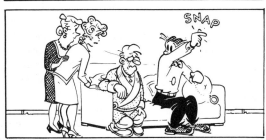

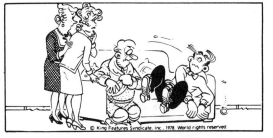

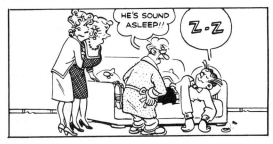

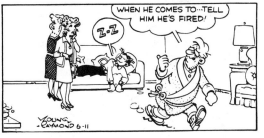

<table>
<tr><td colspan="3" align="center">BOX 2-2</td></tr>
</table>

HYPNOTHERAPY: THREE SUCCESSFUL APPLICATIONS

Juvenile Rheumatoid Arthritis

A 10-year-old girl in whom a diagnosis of juvenile rheumatoid arthritis was made by a rheumatologist responded minimally to large doses of salicylates and physical therapy over seven weeks. Three sessions of hypnotherapy were given. Despite resistance to the first session, questionable improvement ensued. At the time of the second session, one month after the first, the patient still had to be carried frequently by her mother. Four hours after the second session, she rode her bicycle, and was without pain, for the first time in 12 weeks. Two reinforcing hypnotherapy sessions were added. School work and social adjustment improved markedly. The child has remained well for the ensuing 31 months. Hypnotherapy appears to have initiated an attitudinal change, at a level sufficiently deep to accelerate remission.

From F. J. Cioppa and A. D. Thal, "Hypnotherapy in a Case of Juvenile Rheumatoid Arthritis," *American Journal of Clinical Hypnosis,* 18 (October 1975).

Obesity

A physician's wife in her late forties entered the office and explained that she wished a single interview during which hypnosis was to be employed to correct her obesity. She added that her normal weight was 120 pounds, but that her present weight was 240, and that for many years she had weighed over 200 pounds despite repeated futile attempts to reduce under medical supervision. She stated that in recent years she had been slowly gaining to her present weight, and that she was distressed about her future because, "I enjoy eating—I could spend all the time in the world just eating." . . .

She was found to be an unusually responsive subject, developing a profound trance almost immediately. In this trance state an understanding of time distortion as a subjective experience, particularly time expansion, was systematically taught to her. She was then instructed to have her physician husband prescribe the proper diet for her and to supervise her weight loss. She was henceforth to eat each meal in a state of time distortion, with time so expanded and lengthened that, as she finished each portion of food her sense of taste and feeling of hunger for that item would be completely satiated as if she had been eating for "hours on end with complete satisfaction." All of this instruction was given repetitiously until it seemed certain she understood fully, whereupon she was aroused and dismissed.

The patient, together with her husband, was seen nine months later. Her weight had been 120 lbs. for the past month, and her husband declared that her weight loss had occurred easily and without any medical complication. Both she and her husband spoke at length about their improved personal, social, and recreational activities, and she commented that, even though she ate much less, her eating pleasures had been intensified, that her sense of taste and smell were more discerning, and that a simple sandwich could be experienced with as much subjective pleasure as a two-hour dinner.

From M. H. Erickson, "The Utilization of Patient Behavior in the Hypnotherapy of Obesity," *American Journal of Clinical Hypnosis,* 3 (October 1960).

Warts

A 12-year-old girl had been treated with Prednisone since age six (1968), when a diagnosis of juvenile rheumatoid arthritis was made. . . . During the second year of her treatment she began to develop warts on her hands, legs and face. Since 1972 she was treated unsuccessfully with topical liquid nitrogen, trichloroacetic acid and electrocauterization.

She was first seen for hypnosis on February 7, 1974. She was a "moon faced" child who was very distressed because of the many warts on her face. One of these irritated her eyelid whenever she blinked. This wart was surgically removed under hypnosis during the first visit. The standard suggestion was made during this hypnosis experience for the warts to disappear. She experienced no pain during the surgical procedure and was totally amnesic postoperatively. Regression in all her lesions was noted during a second visit one month later. Three months after the first hypnotic session she was wart free for the first time in four years. There was no recurrence of warts at the eight month follow-up examination.

From M. F. Tasini and T. P. Hackett, "Hypnosis in the Treatment of Warts in Immunodeficient Children," *American Journal of Clinical Hypnosis,* 19 (January 1977).

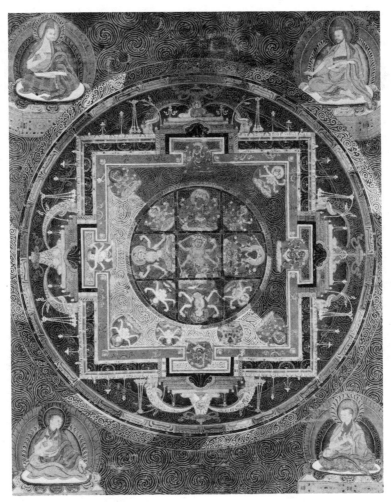

Figure 2-6
An eighteenth-century Tibetan mandala, used in meditation.
(Courtesy the Asian Art Museum of San Francisco, the Avery
Brundage Collection.)

Meditation

Meditation is another technique that people can use
to relax their mind and body, and also to seek
spiritual enlightenment. In a popular form of meditation, called **transcendental meditation** (TM), the
participant pays attention to an internally repeated
sound called a **mantra**. Keeping your mind focused
on the particular sound — especially if you have paid
money to learn it and have been told that it has
secret, magical properties — can induce relaxation
and stress-reducing physiological changes. Among
Western religions, use of rosary beads and chanting serve a similar purpose in focusing attention and
calming the mind. Other meditation techniques

focus the mind's attention on breathing (as in Zen
and yoga) or on religious symbols (such as the **man-
dalas** used in Buddhist meditation — see Figure 2-6).
The daily use of a meditation or relaxation technique can be of great benefit (see Box 2-4).

Focusing the Mind's Attention

All techniques that produce states of deep relaxation, such as hypnosis, autosuggestion, autogenic
training, and meditation, rely on narrowing or
focusing the mind's attention. Once the mind becomes focused, the process of relaxation follows automatically.

BOX 2-3

PROGRESSIVE RELAXATION

The voluntary tightening of a muscle or group of muscles produces a corresponding relaxation when the tension is released. Edmund Jacobson used this principle in developing a method of relaxing outlined in his book *Progressive Relaxation* (1938). Jacobson's technique requires you to lie on your back in quiet, comfortable surroundings, with feet slightly apart and palms facing upward. Before beginning the relaxation exercises, close your eyes, breathe naturally, and allow the thoughts of the day to leave your consciousness. Then you are ready to begin.

1. Close your eyes and then squeeze your lids shut as tightly as you can. Hold them shut for a count of five and then slowly release the tension. Notice how relaxed your eyes feel. Keep the eyelids lightly closed and continue to breathe normally.

2. Turn your palms down. Bend your left hand back at the wrist, keeping your forearm on the floor. Bend your hand as far as it will go until you feel tension in your forearm muscles. Hold for five seconds and then release the tension. Notice the warm, relaxed sensations in your wrist. Do the same with the other hand.

3. With palms up, bend your left hand at the wrist toward you, tightening the muscles in your forearm. Release the tension by letting your hand drop to its normal position. Repeat with the right hand.

4. Focus your attention on your left leg and slowly bring the top of your foot as far forward as you can while still keeping your heel on the floor. Notice the tension in the muscles of your lower leg. Hold for five seconds and release the tension. Repeat with the other leg.

5. Point the toes in your left foot away from you as far as you can. Notice the tension in your calf muscles. Release the tension after five seconds. Repeat with the other foot.

   Similar tensing and relaxing exercises can be performed with other parts of the body and with other muscles.

Your attention can be focused by virtually anything you agree to focus on, whether a conversation, a body massage, music, or dancing. The mind's activity can be focused by concentrating on a repetitious thought or internal sound, a particular feeling, a part of the body, or an external object or sound. For example, movies and television can capture and focus your attention with sounds and images. When your attention is focused on a movie or a television program, you become temporarily unaware of your problems or worries, and are distracted from unpleasant thoughts. For most people, such distraction is comforting and relaxing. That is the reason why many people seek escape from "reality" by watching a TV show or by going out to a movie.

However, when you have allowed your mind to be focused by a device such as the TV set, it becomes quite uncritical and open to other people's suggestions and ideas. Advertisers know how to take advantage of a viewer's suggestible, hypnotic-like state of mind. Most people believe they are not affected by TV and newspaper advertising, but marketing studies indicate otherwise. Some advertisements may even influence people to own, taste, or experience things that may not be in their best interest. The cosmetics industry, for example, often plays on anxieties about how people look and smell, and manipulates these fears to create needs for new beauty-aid products. As the authors of *Consumer Guide to Cosmetics* point out:

> After exploiting our fears about body odor in order to market underarm deodorant, advertisers began pushing vaginal sprays. The strategy worked. By creating a new anxiety—along with a product to allay it—vaginal spray makers increased sales in 1969 by 258 percent over what they'd been the year before. . . . Advertisers delight in an au-

dience that believes ads to be harmless nonsense, for such an audience is rendered defenseless by its belief that there is no attack taking place. (Conry et al., 1980)

Promoting products through scare tactics is nothing new for cosmetic or other companies (see Figure 2-7). Because advertisements focus the mind's attention, even if only briefly, the suggestions in the ad are often accepted by the mind.

If you think about the number of ways that the mind's attention can be focused, you can begin to understand how your behaviors and even your health are influenced by suggestion. But it is worth remembering that nothing—neither another person's ideas nor a TV program nor a commercial—can affect your mind unless you *agree* to let it be changed or influenced. You must first allow your mind to be focused before it can be influenced by the suggestions of others. Some people mistakenly believe that if they are hypnotized they can be made to do something contrary to their principles or against their will. This notion is incorrect. Most investigators of hypnosis agree that all hypnosis is self-hypnosis, or autohypnosis. Your mind has the final responsibility for its beliefs and mental states.

As long as you remember that your mind is responsible for all of its mental states, including desires and needs, you can determine what is best for your own mental, emotional, and physical health and can act accordingly.

The Relaxation Response

In recent years Herbert Benson (1975) of the Harvard Medical School and his colleagues have studied the effects of various relaxation techniques on human physiology. A summary of their findings (see Table 2-3) shows that most relaxation methods affect the body in the same way. Therefore, it appears that regardless of the specific technique employed to induce relaxation, the body responds in the same way. Benson calls this the **relaxation response.** The relaxation response has four essential elements: (1) a quiet environment; (2) mental repetition of a specific word or phrase that serves to focus the

Figure 2-7
Advertisements that carry scare messages. These ads appeared in the 1930s.

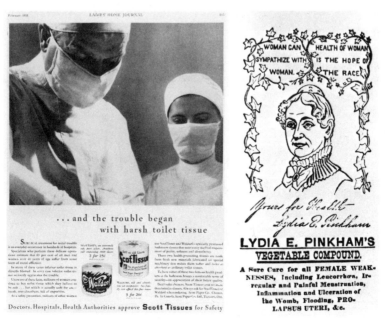

> Mental practice is more
> effective if the visualizer "feels"
> as well as "sees"
> the activity he is symbolically practicing.
> **Allan Richardson**

mind's attention; (3) a passive, accepting mood; and (4) a comfortable physical position.

It is not necessary to pay a lot of money for a course in meditation or to become a disciple of a guru in order to learn to relax. You can learn a relaxation technique that you are comfortable with on your own, perhaps using books or cassette tapes for guidance.

Image Visualization

One of the most effective ways to use the mind to generate health, to improve physiological functions, and even to change behaviors and habits is through the use of **image visualization.** Many therapeutic and healing techniques encourage and teach people to visualize past experiences. For example, fearful childhood experiences recorded by the subconscious mind may be the cause of disease and illness in later life. By reexperiencing frightening memories in a relaxed, calm state of mind, one can often make symptoms disappear. Mental images can also reduce or control pain, change the functioning of body physiology, improve study habits or sports performance— even assist in destroying cancer cells in the body (discussed in Chapter 17).

At one time or another each of us runs an "internal movie." We mentally project fantasies and fears, hopes and desires, scenes and memories onto

Table 2-3
Effects of Relaxation Techniques

Relaxation technique	Oxygen consumption	Respiratory rate	Heart rate	Blood pressure	Muscle tension
Progressive relaxation	— — —*	— — —*	— — —*	— — —*	Decreases
Autogenic training	— — —*	Decreases	Decreases	— — —*	Decreases
Hypnosis with suggested deep relaxation	Decreases	Decreases	Decreases	— — —*	— — —*
Zen and yoga	Decreases	Decreases	Decreases	Decreases	— — —*
Transcendental meditation	Decreases	Decreases	Decreases	Decreases	— — —*

*A blank indicates that the particular response has not been measured or that the results are inconclusive.
Data from H. Benson, *The Relaxation Response* (New York: Wm. Morrow, 1975).

BOX 2-4

A MOTHER'S MORNING MEDITATION

I have learned to relax through meditation and I have learned the basic elements I need to help myself relax. The first element is a quiet environment. I can "turn off" not only internal stimuli but also external distractions. I have found a quiet room in my home and a place outdoors where I can go to be alone with myself. The second element is a scene to dwell on with my mind. I have a special memory of a peaceful sensation I experience when I am in the mountains, lying in a floating chair in a cool pool of water with the warm rays of the sun on me and the sight of green trees in the distance as still as in a photograph. This is a very strong image for me, since I have actu-

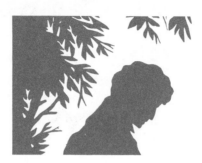

ally been there and will return again and again. The third element is a passive attitude. I can empty my mind of all thoughts and distractions. Thoughts drift in and out of my mind freely, until I have reached a total state of relaxation, actually a kind of not-feeling. The fourth element is a comfortable position. I find that

lying down on my back is most comfortable for me—I feel freer to just let go.

I meditate soon after I awaken. In the past I found it difficult to face the prospect of preparing the children for their day and mapping out my day's activities while trying to get breakfast. I now begin the day feeling energetic and really tuned into what everyone in the family is saying, and more important, what they are feeling. My meditations help me deal with the distressing aspects of my life, and they seem to have a positive effect on the rest of the family, too.

This account was excerpted from a paper written for a college health course.

---

a mental screen. We visualize when we daydream, night-dream, or simply let our thoughts wander without direction or effort. The process of visualization can affect many physiological processes, including body temperature, blood flow, heart rate, breathing, and hormone production (discussed in Chapter 3).

Many modern techniques for improving sports performance rely on visualization—the so-called "inner game" of tennis, golf, or skiing. The principle underlying these techniques is that what your mind visualizes, the muscles of your body will be able to accomplish. According to this principle, once you have acquired a satisfactory basic tennis stroke, for example, you can spend 15 minutes a day in a quiet place visualizing yourself hitting the ball and mentally seeing it land at the baseline on the opponent's side of the net. Visualization can also be used to improve sexual enjoyment and sexual response. The sex organs are particularly responsive to images

and thoughts—sexual arousal occurs first in the mind.

In her book *Imagery in Healing* Jeanne Achterberg (1985) describes imagery as being the oldest of all healing resources:

Imagery, or the stuff of the imagination, affects the body intimately on both seemingly mundane and profound levels. Memories of a lover's scent call forth the biochemistry of emotion. The mental rehearsal of a sales presentation or a marathon race evokes muscular change and more: blood pressure goes up, brain waves change, and sweat glands become active.

A sample visualization exercise is presented in Box 2-5. Spending a brief time each day visualizing yourself the way you really want to be can help you realize your goals and enhance your health.

> The mind freeing
> itself from the known is
> meditation. Meditation is the
> total denial of everything that the
> mind has accumulated.
> Meditation is the
> action of
> silence.
> **Krishnamurti**

Learning to Use the Mind

Because many of the ideas of mental healing and relaxation presented in this chapter may be new to you, we now summarize the steps that we think are essential for producing healthful changes. The following suggestions are merely guidelines to assist you in learning how to use your own mind to improve your health; they are not absolute rules.

1. Become aware that your mind has the power to promote your personal wellness and to accelerate healing processes. Remember that faith and belief have been instrumental in healing rituals for thousands of years and that a person's *belief* in a particular treatment or cure helps healing over and above the treatment itself.

2. Become aware of the power of your mental images and thoughts on how you feel. By dwelling on negative thoughts and images, such as "I feel lousy," "I'm too tired," or "I can't do that," you program yourself into feeling just that way. On the other hand, thinking positive thoughts such as "I feel fine" or "today is a good day" can create positive feelings and beneficial outcomes.

Sometimes just repeating a positive word, such as "calm," "love," or "smile," can improve feelings. You can reverse the trend of a "bad" day by suggesting to yourself that the negative aspects of the day are now going to stop and that as the day progresses you are going to feel better and better.

3. Accept the idea that you can put healing suggestions into your mind and that they can be effective. For example, you can suggest to yourself that a headache will disappear in an hour or so, a cold will be mild and its symptoms will cause little discomfort, or a cut or burn will heal rapidly and completely in just a few days.

4. Allow your mind to dwell in a quiet, relaxed state for a brief period each day. This is especially necessary if you are worried or are living and working in a stressful situation. The moments just before falling asleep and also just on awakening are excellent times to focus your mind on positive, constructive suggestions. For example, as you awake, think how much energy and vitality you will have all day; think how much you'll be able to accomplish; think of pleasant experiences you expect to have.

The extraordinary functioning
exhibited by hypnosis subjects and
yogis supports the belief that the body
can be altered in almost any way whatsoever
if only the brain can be made to accept the
suggestions or instructions given it.

Robert Masters and Jean Houston
Listening to the Body

BOX 2-5

A VISUALIZATION EXERCISE

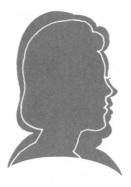

Find a quiet, pleasant spot where you can sit or lie down comfortably. Remove any uncomfortable clothing, eyeglasses, or contact lenses. Give yourself permission to relax and decide what you are going to visualize. It's probably best to begin with something specific. You can visualize yourself being thinner, giving up cigarettes, being successful in an upcoming job interview, or taking an exam while feeling confident and sure of the answers. You can visualize yourself becoming physically stronger or an area of your body becoming well.

Allow your eyes to close, and relax the muscles in the eyelids all the way—to the point where they are so relaxed and comfortable that you feel you are unable to pull your eyelids open. Then let your mind transfer that same comfortable, relaxed feeling to all the other parts of the body, one by one, from top to bottom—head, chest, arms, hands, back, stomach, legs, feet.

Imagine that you are floating on a white cloud bathed in warm sunlight. Everything is quiet and peaceful. You are warm and comfortable and serene. Allow your mind to visualize whatever scene or image it chooses that is related to what you want to improve or heal. Accept your mind's images. They are helping you to change, to feel better. Allow yourself to remain in this relaxed state while your mind continues to create pleasant, positive, beneficial images. Begin to notice how relaxed your body is and how good it feels.

Whenever your mind decides it wants to return to a fully awake state, you will automatically open your eyes and be fully aware of your surroundings. Notice how refreshed and relaxed you feel!

Supplemental Readings

Achterberg, Jeanne. *Imagery in Healing.* Boston: New Science Library, 1985. An excellent introduction to the power of imagery in shamanistic healing as well as in modern medicine.

Benson, Herbert. *The Relaxation Response.* New York: Wm. Morrow, 1975. A good introduction to the health benefits of relaxation and to ways of achieving relaxation.

Frank, Jerome. *Persuasion and Healing.* Baltimore: Johns Hopkins University Press, 1973. A scholarly discussion of how the mind affects healing.

Hales, D. "Mind Over Body: Old Theories, New Proof." *Medical World News,* October 10, 1983. An article that discusses the evidence for the mind's effect on the immune system, hormones, and health.

Harner, Michael. *The Way of the Shaman.* New York: Bantam Books, 1982. Describes the basis of shamanistic healing and how to become a modern shaman.

LeShan, L. *How to Meditate.* New York: Bantam, 1975. A discussion of the psychology and physiology of various meditative practices.

Summary

The human mind can cure illness and improve health as well as cause disease. Health and well-being begin with your state of mind. If you are angry, frightened, tense, or depressed, you can initiate physiological changes in the body that may result in disease. If your mind is relaxed—at peace with itself and with your environment—the functioning of your body will be more harmonious and enhance wellness. Many techniques can be used to achieve relaxed mental states and to increase mind-body harmony. Self-hypnosis, relaxation, autogenic training, meditation, and positive mental imagery can all stimulate beneficial changes in physiology, improve behavior, and change unhealthy habits.

Psychosomatic diseases are caused by fear, anxiety, and stress. They can often be cured or greatly alleviated by dealing with the causes of the stress and practicing mental and physical relaxation. Placebo effects can produce healthy changes because of a person's belief in the particular placebo employed. Belief, faith, and suggestion all have the capacity to heal and to prevent illness.

Because your state of mind is an important factor influencing your health, you should be aware of how open to suggestion your mind is and should consider carefully the programs you watch on TV, the movies you see, and the ideas you accept without scrutiny.

Learn and practice a relaxation technique—it will help keep you healthy throughout life.

FOR YOUR HEALTH

A Relaxation Guide

To free your mind's considerable power to promote wellness and help cure disease, you must be relaxed and open to positive thoughts and healing suggestions. Take the opportunity now to incorporate mental and physical relaxation into your daily life to promote wellness. Beginning a relaxation program involves three steps: (1) discovering a suitable time and place for relaxation, (2) choosing a relaxation technique you are comfortable with, and (3) daily practice.

(Continued on next page.)

FOR YOUR HEALTH

1. *Discovering a place and time.* Spend a few days experimenting with various settings, either indoors or outdoors, and times of the day or night to discover those in which you feel the most comfortable, quiet, relaxed, and free of interruption. Your feelings of comfort and inner peace will tell you which places and times are best for your relaxation exercises.

   When trying out various places and times for relaxation, practice this simple relaxation exercise (or some other of your choosing) in each one. Sit or lie quietly, close your eyes, and repeat to yourself "I am relaxed" over and over again. Say or imagine the words, "I am" as you inhale and "relaxed" as you exhale. Do this exercise for about five minutes. Another test is to imagine a peaceful scene instead of saying "I am relaxed." Imagine yourself under a calm blue sky along the shore of a calm ocean, lake, or stream. Imagine the soothing feelings created by a gentle wind and warm sunlight.

2. *Choosing a relaxation technique.* After finding a suitable place and time for relaxation exercies, practice one of the techniques discussed in this chapter (progressive relaxation, autogenic training, meditation, image visualization) for about 30 minutes a day for about two weeks. You may want to consult a self-help book for details on a particular relaxation method. And you may want to experiment with more than one technique to see which is most suitable for you. As you use the relaxation techniques, try to become aware of the changes that occur in your mind and body.

3. *Daily practice.* Practice once or twice a day for 15 to 30 minutes is the surest way to receive the full benefit from relaxation exercise.

TV Ads and Your Health

Each year television advertisers spend billions of dollars trying to influence some of your health decisions. Some advertisements, such as those for toothpaste, are probably beneficial insofar as they may encourage dental care. Many advertisements, however, suggest strategies for dealing with illness and in so doing program people into following one particular course of action—usually taking a drug—when better alternatives may be available. For example, TV ads can influence people to take aspirin or some other product to relieve a headache when a better solution might be to relax for five minutes or to eliminate the source of the tension that caused the headache in the first place.

How much does television advertising influence your health behavior? As you watch TV, keep a list (example below) of health-related advertisements and the claims that are made. List alternative methods for handling the same problem. Then note whether your health decision making has been influenced by some ads.

Product advertised	Claimed remedy for	Possible alternatives	Am I influenced?		
			often	sometimes	never
aspirin	headache	relaxation	☐	☐	☐
laxative	constipation	change in diet	☐	☐	☐
antacids	upset stomach	image visualization	☐	☐	☐

CHAPTER THREE

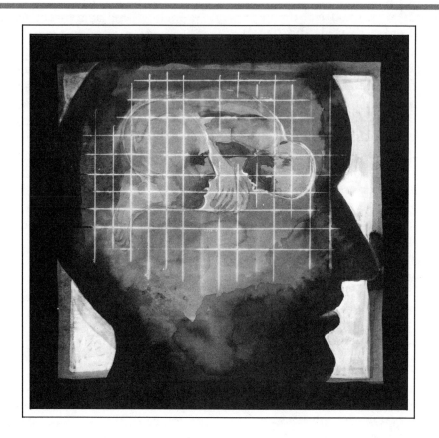

How the mind and body
communicate and interact to maintain
wellness and promote healing

Mind-Body Harmony

Science does not rest upon solid bedrock. The bold structure of its theories rises, as it were, above swamp. It is like a building erected on piles. The piles are driven down from above into the swamp, but not down to any natural or "given" base; and if we stop driving the piles deeper, it is not because we have reached firm ground. We simply stop when we are satisfied that the piles are firm enough to carry the structure, at least for the time being.

Karl Popper

For centuries visitors have returned from India, Tibet, China, and other Eastern countries with stories about individuals (yogis, gurus, swamis, fakirs) who could perform incomprehensible feats of mind and body control. Many of these feats seemed to violate the known laws of nature. Some involved profound changes in body physiology: reducing metabolism almost to the point of death; increasing or decreasing the heart rate on command; maintaining a particular posture for days without apparent effort or discomfort.

Because descriptions of such feats—and equally amazing stories of miraculous healing—were often intermixed with tales of objects floating in the air or being materialized out of nothing, sensible people were inclined to discount all reports of remarkable physiological control and seemingly miraculous healings.

Today we know that many such reports were quite true. In recent years psychologists and medical researchers have been able to verify that some individuals do in fact have extraordinary control over their mental and physiological processes.

But what is the significance of these findings for individual health? Simply this: they indicate that everyone can learn to consciously control supposedly "unconscious" mental and physiological processes, at least to some degree. Although some people are able to learn such control without understanding the biological mechanisms that serve to connect the mind and body, for most people increased knowledge of the body's functions (of physiology) will assist in improving health. Understanding how the body's physiology responds to thoughts and feelings can help you make desirable changes. The brain, along with the rest of the nervous system and the endocrine system, ultimately controls nearly all of the body's physiological responses. And in so doing it strongly influences states of wellness and illness.

In this chapter we will discuss some of the brain-body mechanisms that maintain correct functioning of physiological processes. Disruption of the harmonious interactions of these mechanisms, whether through improper nutrition, emotional upset, stress, or other imbalancing influences, can produce poor health and disease. On the other hand, harmonious functioning of mind-body regulatory mechanisms is likely to produce health and well-being.

As you read this chapter, remember that its overall purpose is not to make you an expert neurophysiologist but rather to demonstrate that your physiology and your health *are* under your control—that positive mental states can increase health and wellness and also promote any healing process.

Homeostasis: Balancing Life Energy

Many of the vital functions your body carries out, such as breathing, heartbeat, blood circulation, and digestion, require no conscious effort on your part. Rarely do you think about when to breathe or whether your heart needs to beat faster or slower. Your body has ways of controlling and integrating its many functions automatically—without conscious control—so that it retains a relatively constant internal environment and regulates physiological processes within certain limits for optimum functioning.

The tendency for body systems to interact and to be regulated in such a way as to produce a relatively constant physiological state is called **homeostasis.** Homeostatic mechanisms maintain the normal blood pressure of most people within the limits of 70 and 130 mm Hg, internal body temperature near 37°C, heart rate between 60 and 90 beats per minute, and blood glucose (sugar) level around 80 mg per 100 ml of blood.

Homeostatic processes also affect behavior. Centers in the brain monitor the amounts of nutrients in the blood and the amount of water in the body. When nutrients are low or the body is in need of water, these centers become activated, and you experience feelings of hunger and thirst that motivate you to eat and drink.

When you are healthy, your body systems function harmoniously, much as the various members of an athletic team function in a coordinated way to accomplish the tasks involved in playing a game. But if one of your organ systems is not functioning properly, the others may not be able to function properly either, and you may become ill. Thus, illness may be viewed as the disruption of homeostasis, or internal disharmony.

The idea of homeostasis was first conceived in the second half of the nineteenth century by the French physiologist Claude Bernard (although he did not use that word). Bernard discovered that the liver releases glucose into the blood when the blood's glucose level is low. He reasoned that the liver must have responsibility for monitoring the blood's glucose level and keeping it constant. And he went beyond this reasoning to formulate the general idea of an internal environment that remains constant—or, more precisely, that always returns to a constant state after any departure.

In the 1930s Walter B. Cannon, a professor of physiology at Harvard, further developed Bernard's concept of a stable physiological environment. He stressed the crucially important point that such sta-

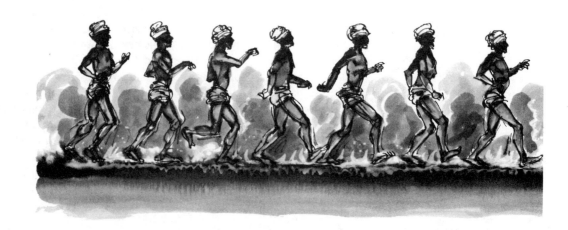

A sound mind
in a sound body
is a short but full description of
a happy state in the world.

John Locke

bility could be achieved only by carefully coordinated physiological processes, and he named this coordination "homeostasis." Cannon (1932) summarized homeostasis in this way:

> We find the organism liberated for its more complicated and socially important tasks because it lives in a fluid matrix, which is automatically kept in a constant condition. If changes threaten, indicators at once signal the danger, and corrective agencies promptly prevent the disturbance or restore the normal when it has been disturbed. The correc-

tive agencies act, in the main, through a special portion of the nervous system which functions as a regulatory mechanism. For this regulation it employs, first, storage of materials as a means of adjustment between supply and demand, and, second, altered rates of continuous processes in the body. These devices for maintaining constancy in the organism are the result of myriads of generations of experience, and they succeed for long periods in preserving a remarkable degree of stability in the highly unstable substance of which we are composed.

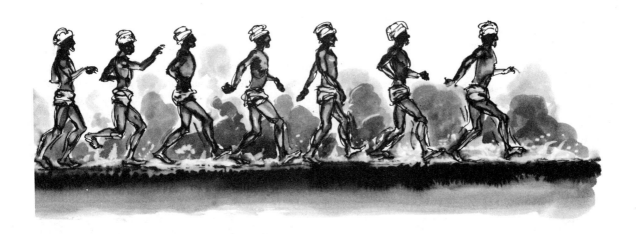

The constancy of the "milieu interieur" is the condition of a free and independent existence.

Claude Bernard

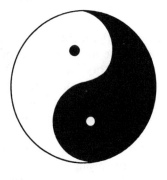

Figure 3-1
The Yin/Yang symbol. This symbol represents the harmonious balance of forces in nature and in people. According to ancient Chinese philosophy, every living organism is composed of complementary but opposite forces called Yin (the dark portion of the symbol) and Yang (the light portion). The relation between the forces is always dynamic—each blends into the other, and the balance is always changing. When the two forces are in balance, an individual is healthy and in harmony with nature. The white and dark dots show that there is always some Yin in a person's Yang component and vice versa. The goal in life and nature, according to the Chinese view, is to maintain a harmonious balance between Yin and Yang forces.

Taoist philosophy and traditional Chinese medicine embody ideas of energy (*ch'i*), balance, and harmony that are, in some respects, analogous to the Western concept of homeostasis. Yin and Yang, which are expressed by the symbol in Figure 3-1, represent the opposing and complementary aspects of the universal ch'i that is in everything. Yang forces are characterized as light, positive, creative, full of movement, and with the nature of heaven. Yin forces are characterized as dark, negative, quiet, receptive, and with the nature of earth. Chinese medicine classifies the organs of the body as being Yin or Yang: hollow organs such as the stomach, intestines, and bladder are Yang; solid organs such as the heart, spleen, liver, and lungs are Yin. Food and herbs are also classified as having predominantly Yin or Yang properties. When Yin and Yang forces are in balance in an individual, a state of harmony exists and the person experiences health and well-being. If, however, either Yin or Yang forces predominate in a person, a state of disharmony, or disease, may result.

Asian philosophies embodying the idea of Yin and Yang do not differentiate between physical harmony and mental harmony. Body and mind are regarded as inseparable. Thus, illness and its treatment involve the whole person and not simply a part of the body. The healing techniques of Asian medicine are designed to foster total harmony and well-being—that is, to restore the harmonious balance of the Yin/Yang forces. A Western physician might describe such techniques as ways that help restore homeostasis.

Glands and hormones	Function
Pituitary gland	
Growth hormone	Stimulates growth of bones and other structures
Adrenocorticotropic hormone (ACTH)	Stimulates release of hormones from the adrenal glands
Thyroid-stimulating hormone	Stimulates growth of the thyroid gland and release of thyroxin
Luteinizing hormone	Stimulates ovaries and the release of ovarian hormones in women; stimulates testes to produce hormones in men
Follicle-stimulating hormone	Stimulates ovum production in women; stimulates sperm production in men
Prolactin	Stimulates milk production in breasts
Testes	
Testosterone	Controls maleness
Ovaries	
Estrogen	Controls aspects of female sexuality and reproduction

Glands and hormones	Function
Progesterone	Controls aspects of female sexuality and reproduction
Pancreas	
Insulin	Regulates blood sugar
Thyroid gland	
Thyroxin	Regulates metabolism
Parathyroid glands	
Calcitonin	Regulates calcium and phosphorus
Adrenal glands	
Aldosterone	Regulates water balance in the body
Cortisol	Increases blood glucose
Stomach	
Gastrin	Increases secretion of digestive juices in the stomach
Small intestine	
Secretin	Increases digestive functions of pancreas

Nerves, Hormones, and Homeostasis

Homeostasis and well-being are achieved when the nervous system and the endocrine (hormone-producing) system coordinate and integrate the functions of the body's various organs so that all is in balance. The nervous system is made up of the brain and the many nerves that connect it to nearly all the parts of the body. The endocrine system is made up of several hormone-producing glands located at various body sites (see Figure 3-2). Both the nervous and endocrine systems help maintain homeostasis by initiating physiological changes in response to the external and internal environments. For example, when your body temperature increases (say, during vigorous exercise), your nervous system causes the blood vessels in your skin to dilate, which in turn causes you to sweat in order to cool off; when your body temperature drops, the nervous system causes body muscles to contract, which generates heat through shivering. When you eat a candy bar, the pancreas releases the hormone insulin into the blood to keep the blood sugar level within normal limits.

The nervous system governs brain-body communication by means of electrical and chemical signals. For an electrical signal to travel from your brain to your toes in a fraction of a second, for example, thousands of individual nerve cells (**neurons**) generate electrical impulses that are transmitted from neuron to neuron. An electrically stimulated neuron releases chemical substances called **neurotrans-**

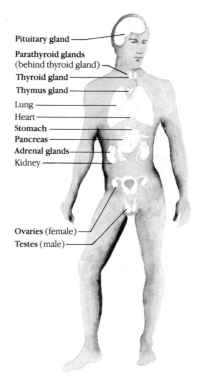

Figure 3-2
The principal endocrine glands in the body and their functions.

Pituitary gland
Parathyroid glands (behind thyroid gland)
Thyroid gland
Thymus gland
Lung
Heart
Stomach
Pancreas
Adrenal glands
Kidney
Ovaries (female)
Testes (male)

Figure 3-3

The transmission of a nerve impulse from neuron to neuron. When an electrical impulse reaches the end of an axon (the "sending" part of the neuron), neurotransmitter molecules are released. They flow across the **synapse,** the tiny space between nerve cells, and bind to receptor sites on the receiving neuron. This chemical message acts to either excite or inhibit the second neuron. Without neurotransmitters and receptor sites on neurons, the nervous system could not function.

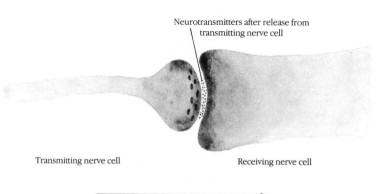

Neurotransmitters after release from transmitting nerve cell

Transmitting nerve cell

Receiving nerve cell

Direction of impulse transmission

mitters that can trigger an electrical impulse in an adjoining neuron (see Figure 3-3). This sequential process (electrical impulse → chemical release → electrical impulse) is repeated along every nerve fiber. Electrical impulses in neurons can be initiated or inhibited by many different neurotransmitters. Through electrical impulses and neurotransmitters the brain and nervous system communicate with all the parts of the body.

Neurotransmitters are synthesized in the body's nerve cells from amino acids and other nutrients in food (discussed in Chapter 4). That is why your thoughts, feelings, and mental states can be affected by your nutritional state. Optimal functioning of the brain and nervous system depends on more than a dozen different neurotransmitters and certain brain hormones whose synthesis can be affected by diet and other factors.

Two amino acids present in dietary protein are used by the body to synthesize neurotransmitter chemicals that are essential to normal functioning of the brain and nervous system. The amino acid

tyrosine (about 5 percent of protein) is converted to three different neurotransmitters—dopamine, norepinephrine, and epinephrine—by enzymes in various cells of the body (see Figure 3-4). Each different neurotransmitter binds to specific receptor sites for that neurotransmitter on nerve cells, thereby regulating signals of the nervous system. Another amino acid, tryptophan (about 1 percent of protein), is used for the synthesis of the neurotransmitter serotonin. Both tryptophan and serotonin have chemical structures that are similar to the chemical structures of particular hallucinogenic drugs, such as mescaline and psilocybin. Because of the chemical relatedness of neurotransmitters and hallucinogenic drugs, the drugs can bind to nerve cells in the brain and can change thoughts and feelings (see Chapter 13).

Amino acids and other chemicals in the food we eat alter the way we think and feel. Richard Wurtman, a neuroendocrinology researcher at the Massachusetts Institute of Technology, has been investigating the effects of nutrition on neurotransmitter synthesis and function for many years. He

Figure 3-4

The neurotransmitters dopamine, norepinephrine, and epinephrine are synthesized in the body from the amino acid tyrosine, which is present in dietary protein.

Tyrosine

Norepinephrine

Dopamine

Epinephrine

Figure 3-5
The principal control centers of the brain. Although all areas of the brain are interconnected, certain functions are localized to some degree in particular brain regions.

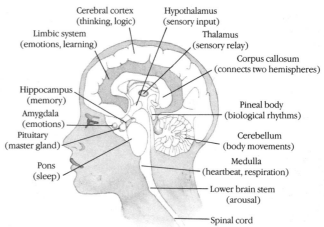

Cerebral cortex (thinking, logic)
Hypothalamus (sensory input)
Limbic system (emotions, learning)
Thalamus (sensory relay)
Corpus callosum (connects two hemispheres)
Hippocampus (memory)
Pineal body (biological rhythms)
Amygdala (emotions)
Pituitary (master gland)
Cerebellum (body movements)
Pons (sleep)
Medulla (heartbeat, respiration)
Lower brain stem (arousal)
Spinal cord

has found that tryptophan and serotonin levels may affect appetite, sleep, and sensitivity to pain. Tyrosine and the neurotransmitters synthesized from it may be involved in people's response to stress and may play a role in certain mental disorders (Weisburd, 1984).

Hormones are chemical substances produced by the endocrine glands. Hormones affect a wide variety of physiological processes, including body growth, the development of male and female sex characteristics, the menstrual cycle, the workings of the stomach and intestine, and the level of sugar in the blood, to mention but a few. Hormones are synthesized and released in response to a variety of environmental stimuli. Release is often initiated by signals from the brain and nervous system in response to what a person experiences.

Whatever you are experiencing, whether it is something in the environment that is detected by your senses (sight, hearing, touch, taste, smell) or whether it is an internal mental experience such as a fantasy or meditation, your brain is processing the information from the experience and transmitting nerve signals to brain centers that control physiology. In turn, neurotransmitters and hormones are released and they direct responsive changes in other parts of the body. For example, when the brain interprets a situation as threatening, regardless of whether there is a real danger or merely an imagined one, neurotransmitter and hormone signals are sent throughout the body, producing the familiar physiological responses to fear: increased heart rate, increased blood pressure, sweaty palms, butterflies in the stomach, and so forth. **Epinephrine** (also called adrenalin), which acts as both a neurotransmitter and a hormone, initiates the physiological changes that you feel in response to a frightening experience.

The Brain Controls Physiology

Whatever interpretation your mind puts on your experience—pleasant or unpleasant, dangerous or delightful—is passed to various parts of the brain, which then determine what, if any, physiological changes are required. Figure 3-5 shows the location of several physiological and behavioral control centers of the brain. Although it may appear from this diagram that the brain has separate parts with separate functions, remember that all the brain's functions are coordinated; all of its components interact with each other to produce the appropriate responses.

It is important to realize that your thoughts and emotions directly influence your physiology through these regulatory centers in the brain. Perhaps you can now see why many of the relaxation and autosuggestion techniques discussed in Chapter 2 do promote healing and well-being—putting the mind in a relaxed, peaceful, harmonious state leads to a similar state in the brain centers that control physiological responses. Conversely, you should be able to see why stress and emotional turmoil can lead to illness. C. Norman Shealy emphasizes this point in his book *90 Days to Self-Health* (1978):

> Anger, frustration, depression, hatred, anxiety, fear, and guilt are real stresses. They create physical disease. They weaken the system of immunity. They stimulate the body to produce excess adrenalin and cortisone, and, in general, they upset the homeostasis—the balance—of the various functions of the body.

> Persons who lack curiosity about life, who find minimal joy in existence, are all too willing, subconsciously, to cooperate with—and attract—disease, accident, and violence.
>
> **Tom Robbins**
> *Jitterbug Perfume*

Realizing that you have tremendous powers to affect your health by emotional and mental processes is one of the most important concepts in holistic health.

The Autonomic Nervous System

The power of the mind to influence health and healing is mediated largely through a special group of nerves that connect the physiological control centers of the brain with virtually all of the body's tissues and organs. This group of nerves, called the **autonomic nervous system** (ANS), is responsible for the physiological responses shown in Figure 3-6.

The ANS has two divisions, the **sympathetic division** and the **parasympathetic division**. In the broadest terms, these two divisions tend to work in opposition to each other on various body functions. For example, sympathetic division activity tends to increase heart rate; parasympathetic activity tends to reduce it. Sympathetic activity tends to decrease digestive activity; parasympathetic activity tends to increase it.

The autonomic nervous system derives its name from the fact that the activities of both the sympathetic and parasympathetic divisions normally operate without conscious control. In other words, you don't have to think about how fast you want your heart to beat or to consciously direct the minute-to-minute operation of your digestive tract after you've eaten dinner. Control over the internal organs is relatively automatic; the built-in mechanisms in the brain maintain homeostasis.

Figure 3-6
The autonomic nervous system consists of nerve cells and fibers organized into two divisions: the sympathetic and the parasympathetic. These two divisions act together to regulate the various organs and tissues. Some of their opposing and balancing functions are illustrated here.

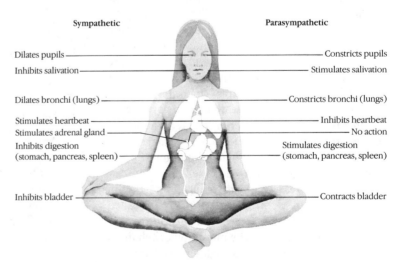

Sympathetic | Parasympathetic

Dilates pupils — Constricts pupils
Inhibits salivation — Stimulates salivation
Dilates bronchi (lungs) — Constricts bronchi (lungs)
Stimulates heartbeat — Inhibits heartbeat
Stimulates adrenal gland — No action
Inhibits digestion (stomach, pancreas, spleen) — Stimulates digestion (stomach, pancreas, spleen)
Inhibits bladder — Contracts bladder

> There are mysteries,
> above all the mystery
> of the relationship of mind and body,
> that will never be explained,
> not by the most brilliant doctors,
> the wisest of scientists
> or philosophers.
>
> **Stewart Alsop**

That the ANS can function without conscious control does not mean that its activity cannot be affected by thoughts and feelings. A clear-cut demonstration of how mental processes influence the ANS and physiology can be found in the way **galvanic skin response** (GSR) is affected. The GSR is one measure of so-called lie detector tests. Also monitored are blood pressure, pulse rate, and respiration, since these physiological processes are affected by emotional states mediated through the ANS. To monitor GSR, two wires are attached to a person's skin — usually a finger — and a tiny electric current is directed down one wire, is passed through the skin separating the two wires, and returns through the other wire to a recording device. Although the amount of electricity is too small to be felt, it is enough for measuring the electrical resistance in the patch of skin.

After a person's normal GSR is established, it is a simple matter to observe how the GSR changes in response to questions, suggestions, or other stimuli. When a person becomes aroused — excited, emotionally upset, frightened, or just more alert — he or she perspires more, and the resulting moisture lowers the skin's electrical resistance. Such reactions may occur when a person is consciously lying. However, many people who are asked to take a lie detector test are likely to be upset or frightened by the test itself, even if they have nothing to hide. And since the test really measures GSR, not truth-telling, the lie detector or the person interpreting the result may be the "liar" if the person fails the test. In fact, recent studies of "lie detector" tests show that the test are wrong at least one-third of the time, that

they are biased against innocent persons, and that they can be "beaten" by liars who are trained to deceive the instruments (Lykken, 1984). For these reasons, the results of lie detector tests are not accepted as evidence in many courts of law.

As indicated in Figure 3-6, the ANS, responding to thoughts and emotions, can cause constriction of blood vessels, can affect heart contractions, and can alter the secretion of various hormones. If such changes are drastic enough, or if abnormal physiological responses persist over a period of time, minor complaints such as headache or upset stomach may result. Even more serious diseases can result from ANS-mediated reactions to stress (see Chapter 10).

Voluntary Control of the ANS

To realize the extent to which thoughts and feelings can produce physiological changes, it is useful to consider some cases reported by Elmer Green, director of the biofeedback laboratory at the Menninger Clinic in Topeka, Kansas. He has conducted extensive studies on the ability of exceptional individuals such as Swami Rama (an Indian yogi) and Jack Schwarz (a Dutch hypnotist and healer) to control consciously many of their physiological processes. Green has found that these individuals are able to change at will their respiration, skin resistance, heart rate, blood flow, body temperature, and electrical brain activity. All of these processes are normally regulated automatically, but these individuals (and others) have learned how to override the automatic controls with their minds.

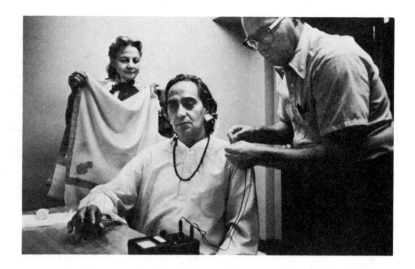

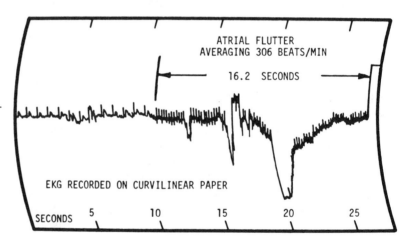

Figure 3-7
Physiological tests of a practiced meditator, Swami Rama, show that he is able to exert great voluntary mental control over several physiological functions.
The EKG tracing shows how Swami Rama is able to radically alter his heartbeat. (Photo courtesy the Menninger Foundation; EKG tracing from *Beyond Biofeedback*.)

Green (1972) and his associates measured the changes in brain activity and other physiological processes with biofeedback equipment. (A more detailed description of biofeedback and its uses is given in Chapter 10.) Thanks to these and other demonstrations carried out under laboratory conditions, we now know that the mind *can* change and influence vital physiological processes. Swami Rama was even able to demonstrate, to the consternation of the experimenters, that he could deliberately prevent his heart from pumping any blood for several seconds.

The significance of such highly proficient examples of physiological control is that they provide

evidence for what many physicians have surmised by treating and observing patients—namely, that serious diseases, including heart attacks and stroke, may be triggered by destructive thoughts and emotions. An account of one young woman who experienced many of the symptoms of a stroke without any apparent physical cause is described in Box 3-1.

Marlene Goodfriend and Edward Wolpert (1976), of the Michael Reese Hospital in Chicago, have reported an even more drastic consequence of psychological stress: the death of a woman in her twenties with no medically detectable disease. After careful analysis, they ascribed her death solely to her uncontrollable, frightening fantasies. They con-

---

BOX 3-1

THOUGHTS, FEELINGS, AND PHYSIOLOGY: ANNA T.'S CASE

The phone rang about 1 A.M. "I know it's late," the voice began, "but we think Anna's had a stroke. We're at the Student Health Clinic and Anna would like to see you."

The call was from Anna's friend Ev. Over the phone her voice was measured and careful as she tried to control her fear. "O.K.," I said, "I'll be right there."

Driving to the Student Health Clinic, I became worried. A stroke is serious. It could mean some permanent brain damage and partial paralysis for life. I thought about how scared Anna must be and realized that showing *my* anxiety would do her little good. I resolved to be supportive, calm, and positive when I saw her.

When I arrived, Anna was lying down. She was worried and frightened. She tried to tell me what happened—how she had come back from an exercise class and had lost control of her movements, finally crashing to the floor. Anna, normally very articulate, now spoke with slurred speech, and she had difficulty finding words to express herself. She could hardly move her right arm and hand and seemed to have lost some feeling in the right side of her body.

Anna was a doctoral student in her early thirties whom I knew both as her teacher and as her friend. She had been under considerable strain lately from the combined pressures of study,

motherhood (she had an infant son), and worry about getting a job when she finished her thesis and research. I reminded Anna of some of the pressures she had been under lately, and I suggested that stress might be related to this incident. Pondering that idea for a while, she began to feel better and even regained some movement in her hand.

The clinic transferred Anna to a nearby hospital where all the necessary tests could be done to determine the extent of blood vessel damage in her brain. By the time we got to the hospital, she felt worse and was again frightened.

The next day Anna underwent an extensive (and expensive) series of tests, including an arteriography and a CAT scan. Arteriography involves threading a tube from a blood vessel in the thigh all the way through the body into the brain so that a dye can be injected into the brain and the blood vessels in the brain photographed to detect possible damage. The CAT (computerized axial tomography) scan involves multiple x-ray exposures of the brain, which are integrated by a computer to form a composite image that doctors can study. All of Anna's medical tests were negative.

Anna returned home, and over the next few days all of her symptoms vanished completely. After two weeks she was com-

pletely back to normal. Prior to her "stroke," Anna had suffered from migraine headaches. Migraines are caused by blood vessels in the brain overreacting to nervous stimuli by contracting and dilating abnormally. Excessive stress might cause a blood vessel in the brain to rupture, thus producing temporary symptoms of a stroke.

About a month later Anna went to her doctor for a follow-up examination. He found her to be medically well and physically fit. She was surprised when he told her that *half* of all the people he saw with symptoms of stroke had no detectable organic blood vessel problems. However, he added that he believed that there was an organic basis to the symptoms—that there must be something wrong—perhaps only temporarily—with the blood vessels but that the tests were not sensitive enough to detect any abnormality.

After doing some reading and thinking on her own, Anna decided that symptoms like hers can be due solely to psychological stress without any underlying organic damage in brain blood vessels. She prefers now to describe her "stroke" as a message her body gave her to make some changes in her lifestyle and to reduce some of its stresses.

Case taken from authors' files.

> The man who fears suffering
> is already suffering from what he fears.
> **Montaigne**

cluded from the medical evidence that "the patient experienced anxiety of such an overwhelming nature that it set off a physiological reaction leading to death."

Medical evidence of this sort also provides an explanation for deaths precipitated by voodoo or other phenomena involving superstition. If a person believes strongly enough that pins stuck into a doll can injure or kill him, then his mind may in fact be able to produce physiological changes that *can* lead to death.

Fear and anxiety can destroy health. Fright can be an exhilarating experience for many people, especially young people—witness the popularity of horror movies and roller coasters—but *really* being scared is no fun at all, and it is destructive to health. Children in particular become easily frightened because there are so many experiences that they simply don't understand. It is one thing to know that a monster is just a friend dressed in a costume and quite another thing to *believe* that the monster is real and going to attack. This sort of fear is physiologically destructive and detrimental to health.

All fear tends to imbalance homeostasis and is therefore destructive to well-being. The more you understand of the world you live in and of how your mind functions, the less you have to fear and the more control you have over your physiology.

Pain and Its Control

One of the most common complaints that cause people to seek medical attention is the sensation of pain. Pain is a symptom; it is the body's way of informing the brain that something is physiologically malfunctioning. Persistent pain is a signal that should never be ignored; every effort should be made to determine its cause. Quite often, however, exhaustive medical tests fail to uncover any organic or physical explanation for a pain. That does not mean that the pain is imaginary or that the person does not *feel* the pain—it may be that certain thoughts and feelings are causing it.

Although people differ greatly in their ability to tolerate pain, many can learn to control pain. Hypnosis has been used for centuries to help people become insensitive or oblivious to extreme pain. More than a century ago, James Esdaile, a British surgeon, performed more than 200 operations using only **hypnoanesthesia**—hypnosis as an anesthetic—to make his patients completely insensitive to pain. (Chemical anesthetics such as chloroform and ether had not yet been discovered.) Esdaile's patients had a remarkable rate of recovery in an era when as many as four out of ten patients died from surgery or from postoperative infections. One of Esdaile's operations is described in Box 3-2.

BOX 3-2

THE PATIENT FELT NO PAIN: HYPNOSIS AS ANESTHETIC

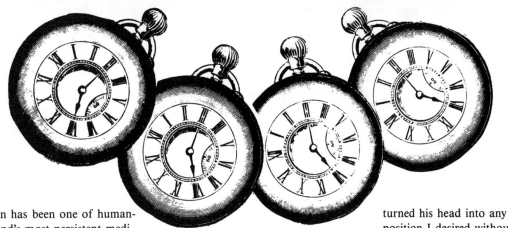

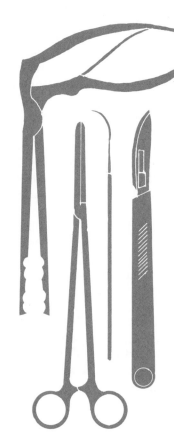

Pain has been one of humankind's most persistent medical complaints and one of its most unpleasant symptoms. Severe pain causes great suffering and is often incapacitating. Yet even severe pain—such as might be experienced during surgery performed without any anesthetic—can be controlled and prevented solely within a person's mind.

In the 1840s—years before the discovery of anesthetics or pain-killing drugs—James Esdaile, a British surgeon stationed in India, performed hundreds of major operations on patients who experienced no pain during the surgery. Esdaile and his assistants induced a state of hypnotic coma—known as mesmerism in those days—in which the patient became insensitive to pain. Here, in Esdaile's own words, is a description of one of his operations:

> I put a long knife in at the corner of his mouth, and brought the point out over the cheekbone and dissected the cheek back to the nose. The tumor extended as far as my fingers could reach and passed into the gullet. I turned his head into any position I desired without resistance, and there it remained till I wished to move it again. I threw back his head, and passed my fingers into his throat to detach the mass. He was laid on the floor to have his face sewed up, and while this was doing, he for the first time opened his eyes. (Kroger, 1977)

Although such surgery without pain seems astonishing, in recent years surgeons have performed major operations using only hypnoanesthesia—the prevention of pain by hypnosis. Babies have been delivered by cesarean section using only hypnosis—the mother required no anesthetic whatsoever during the incision and removal of the baby.

These cases are described not to suggest that you undergo surgery without an anesthetic but to emphasize that pain can be controlled by your mind. If you can learn such control, you may not need drugs for minor pain and you might find that you require less medication if you should undergo an operation.

> Many people think of hypnosis as hocus-pocus.
> That is a prejudice of many parents and health
> professionals. Hypnosis is an incredibly safe
> and useful tool.
>
> **Candace Erickson, M.D.**
> **Columbia-Presbyterian Hospital**

The work of Esdaile and others has provided dramatic evidence of the human mind's ability to control pain and to heal tissue. Even today some surgeons occasionally perform operations (including delivery of babies by cesarean section) using only hypnoanesthesia. Their patients are carefully selected and counseled, however, because the patient must have complete confidence in the physician to ensure success.

Why use hypnosis rather than chemical anesthetics and analgesics, such as ether or one of the various pain-killing drugs? The main reason is that virtually all general anesthetics and many pain-relieving drugs are toxic to human cells — particularly brain cells. Studies reported by the National Institutes of Health, for example, indicate that newborn babies may suffer brain damage from drugs given to their mothers during delivery.

Although medical science cannot fully explain the biological and chemical mechanisms that produce pain, recent experiments have shown that cells of the human brain and other parts of the nervous system normally produce molecules that act like morphine — that is, like pain-killing drugs. These pain-relieving substances are called **endorphins.** Smaller molecules that can also relieve pain, called **enkephalins,** are derived from the endorphins. Both substances are synthesized in the hypothalamus, the pituitary gland, and probably other parts of the nervous system.

The degree to which we feel pain in certain circumstances is related to the amount of endorphins and enkephalins secreted by the brain. It may be that various relaxation methods and mental techniques can stimulate the production of these pain-relieving substances. It is thought, for example, that acupuncture anesthesia is mediated through the release of endorphins and enkephalins. It is likely that hypnoanesthesia, too, leads to increased release of endorphins and enkephalins.

Everyone can learn to control and even eliminate pain — or at least the pain resulting from minor injuries (burns, cuts, bruises) and from minor medical or dental procedures. One useful hint is to think of unpleasant physical sensations as *discomforting* rather than as painful. Most people can accept the idea that they can control discomfort, but they may have trouble convincing themselves that they can control pain. Self-induced deep relaxation and positive mental imagery can be used effectively by most people, not only for controlling pain but also for helping to heal various other ailments. One middle-aged woman who became acquainted with the ideas and techniques discussed here and in Chapter 2 described her experience of applying them to a pain situation:

> Just two days ago before going for extraction of a molar, I relaxed and imagined a painless, bloodless surgery. It came to pass just as I had programmed it. No bleeding and no pain, in spite of having the bone scraped and the gum stitched. The prescription given me for codeine was not necessary.

> Pain has an element of blank;
> It cannot recollect
> When it began, or if there were
> A day when it was not.
> **Emily Dickinson**

Prior to my recent understanding, my threshold for pain was practically nonexistent. For years I bled excessively at the dentist's or while having minor surgery. Now I am no longer a "bleeder," but a "believer." Almost all my ailments, i.e.: tinnitus, lipoma, elevated blood pressure, psoriasis, etc., have been improved by relaxation and positive thinking. My psoriasis is clearing without the aid of sunshine. My blood pressure is back to what it was when I was 20 and I have learned to control the ringing in my ears.

Recent experiments have shown that people whose pain was relieved by administration of a placebo (they were told that the pill they were given contained a potent pain-relieving drug) actually increased production of endorphins or enkephalins in their brains (Levine, Gordon, and Fields, 1978). Thus, the *belief* that a pain-relieving drug had been ingested was, in itself, enough to cause the brain to synthesize more of these morphinelike, pain-relieving substances.

These examples are provided to encourage you to rely more on your mind's ability to control pain and help cure other ailments. Scientists are discovering more and more psychochemicals that are produced in the brain, including some that may be responsible for psychotic disorders as well as for some neurological and physical diseases. It is increasingly evident that people change the production of their brain chemicals continually by what they think, feel, and imagine. The belief that one will experience no discomfort and that one's body is being healed may possibly induce the appropriate chemical changes that facilitate the disappearance of symptoms and the curing of illness.

Psychoneuroimmunology

Over the past few years scientists have begun to understand how the mind—whether stimulated by hypnosis, placebo, imagery, or faith—can change the body's physiology for better or worse. Until recently it was thought that the human nervous and immune systems functioned independently of one another. However, experiments now show that the nervous, endocrine, and immune systems are intimately interconnected. It has become increasingly well documented that thoughts and emotions *can* alter not only hormone levels in a person's body but functions of their immune systems as well.

For example, recent experiments show that grieving widowers have a reduced lymphocyte (white blood cell) response. People who are depressed or unable to cope with stress also show a reduced lymphocyte response, which means that these individuals are more susceptible to infections and other kinds of disease. Blood samples taken from medical students over the course of the school year show changes in their lymphocytes during exam

> Holistic medicine is becoming respectable
> now that chemical and neurological
> links have been found between the brain
> and the immune system.
> *Discover* magazine

periods. It is becoming increasingly well established that stress and negative emotional states alter the body's immune system and may increase disease susceptibility. The title of a book by Kenneth Pelletier (1977), *Mind as Healer, Mind as Slayer,* takes on added significance now that scientists are beginning to understand the power of the mind in preventing or causing disease.

The new branch of science that studies the interaction of the mind and the immune system is called **psychoneuroimmunology.** In many respects there is nothing new or startling about psychoneuroimmunology since, in the past, healers, priests, shamans, and even ordinary people have acted from their beliefs that the mind affects health and healing. What *is* new is that we now have the technical expertise to measure and study changes in the specialized cells of the immune system such as macrophages, B-cells, helper T-cells, suppressor T-cells, and killer T-cells (see Chapter 9) as a function of different mental states.

It is now known that certain kinds of lymphocytes have cell-surface receptors for hormones and neurotransmitters, which explains how immune system cells can respond to changes in thoughts or feelings that cause changes in hormone levels. As a result of these new findings, a comprehensive new model of disease is beginning to emerge that provides strong support for many aspects of holistic health that previously had to be accepted on faith — the most significant concept being that the mind's state affects the body's functions. It is now possi-

ble to explain, in general terms if not in detail, how the environment, which includes both physical and emotional stressors, can directly affect a person's health (see Figure 3-8). In this scheme, what a person experiences in his or her environment will produce thoughts and feelings that can be either beneficial or detrimental to health. What you experience can make you happy or sad, angry or elated, depressed or ecstatic. These emotions, in turn, produce chemical changes in your nervous and endocrine systems and cellular changes in the immune system. Ultimately, emotions may determine whether you are more or less resistant to disease or how fast you will recover from illness.

No one can predict how an individual will respond to emotional distress. One person may break out in hives (an allergic reaction); another may come down with a cold or pneumonia (viral or bacterial infections); still another might experience an attack of arthritis (an autoimmune reaction). These are all examples of the negative effects of thoughts and feelings. Although the evidence that positive mental attitudes and emotions can increase the functions of the immune system is less well documented, this seems quite likely to be the case. While we cannot eliminate worries and problems completely from our lives, it surely does not make sense to make yourself "sick from worrying." The message from psychoneuroimmunology is that taking responsibility for your mental health is just as important in preventing disease — possibly even more so — as taking responsibility for good nutrition and exercise.

> A man is never so happy as when
> his mind, his senses, and his heart
> are all working harmoniously
> together.
> **Seneca**
> **Roman philosopher**

Programming Your Mind

Your beliefs greatly affect your emotions, attitudes, thoughts, and personality. Because your belief system plays such an important part in determining your health and how you deal with illness, it is worth examining how beliefs and the behaviors they engender are acquired by the mind (see Box 3-3).

One highly useful way to interpret the workings of the mind is to consider it as a highly complex computer—a biocomputer. The usefulness of this analogy stems from the fact that computers operate by means of programs, which are sets of instructions they receive from computer operators. The instructions tell the computer what to do with the data given to it. The human mind can be likened to a computer because values, beliefs, and attitudes are like programs—they govern how you think, feel, and behave in certain situations.

The noted neurophysiologist and communications expert John C. Lilly (1974) stated: "All human beings, all persons who reach adulthood in the world today, are programmed biocomputers. No one can escape one's own nature as a programmable entity. Literally each of us may be his programs, nothing more, nothing less." What Lilly means is that from the moment you are born—and even from before birth, since the brain and nervous system are formed in the first few months—everything you experience influences your mind in some way. Your experiences create programs or alter programs already part of your mind. Everything that you are taught or told,

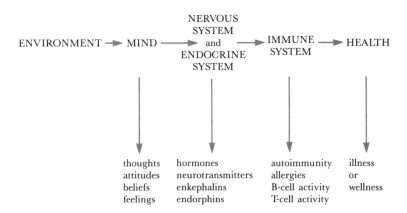

Figure 3-8
The basic model of psychoneuroimmunology. The diagram shows how the mind can alter functions of the nervous, endocrine, and immune systems, thus helping to determine whether a person is well or ill.

BOX 3-3

EXAM ANXIETY IS LEARNED BEHAVIOR

Most people in this country spend anywhere from 12 to 25 years in educational environments of one sort or another. Successful progress in the American educational system is keyed to performance on quizzes, midterms, final exams, aptitude tests, and entrance and placement exams. Students feel—justifiably so—that grades and exam scores will determine how successful their lives will be, both from their own viewpoint and that of society. People in American society equate educational success, academic degrees, and professional licenses with the attainment of important life goals, particularly financial ones. As a consequence, competition among students in the classroom has become increasingly intense.

Because of school pressures and exam anxiety, students' health often suffers. Students suffer from tension and migraine headaches, stomach upsets, frequent infections, and a host of other mental and physical symptoms that are brought on or made worse by stress. The solution to health problems associated with serious exam anxiety and physical symptoms lies with personal change, not with forcing the educational system to change, desirable as that might be. Each of us can *choose* how to react to personal pressures and how to accommodate educational goals to personal goals and desires.

The first thing to realize is that exam anxiety is learned behavior and that it probably began quite early in your life. (You may be able to recall the first time you experienced exam anxiety in school.) Like any learned behavior that is undesirable or harmful,

exam anxiety can be unlearned or the response to it can be changed, given sufficient motivation. There is absolutely nothing frightening or dangerous in exams themselves; exams are not loaded guns. Rather, the anxiety you experience is directly related to the importance you attach to your success on the exam relative to all the other people taking it. Obviously if you feel that your whole life and future hinge on how well you score on an exam, you are constructing a situation that can cause severe anxiety and such physical symptoms as headaches and diarrhea.

Image visualization can be a powerful technique for reducing the mental panic and physical symptoms of exam anxiety. By using image visualization prior to an exam, you can teach your mind and body how to relax. Find a comfortable place in your house or apartment and a time when it is quiet. Pick an environment in which you feel secure and where there are no disturbing distractions. Sit in a comfortable chair or lie down on a couch, bed, or floor. The main thing is to get physically comfortable. If music helps you relax, you can play some of your favorite instrumental music, but it should not be so loud that it becomes intrusive.

Next, close your eyes and ask your mind to recall a place where you felt content and happy. Let it be a place where you had the kind of positive feeling that you wish you had all the time. Use your imagination to reconstruct the scene or place where you felt comfortable and happy. It might be a vacation spot or a time when you were lying on a beach or hiking in the mountains. The main thing is to let your mind freely choose a

place or memory that feels the most comfortable and to let yourself become totally involved in that scene. It's like having a daydream except that you are constructing your own dream. While your mind is engaged in this pleasurable memory, your body automatically relaxes.

After your mind and body have become comfortable and relaxed, you can refocus your attention on an upcoming exam. You can visualize in your mind taking the exam while remaining relaxed and confident. Because your mind and body have already been relaxed and because you are secure and comfortable in your own environment, your mind will associate these positive feelings with the inner visualization of the exam. Use your imagination to project your mind into the future when you are taking the exam, being calm and confident as you write down the answers to the questions or write your essay.

Let your imagination construct all of the details of the exam situation. Visualize the exam room and where you are sitting; notice that you can read and understand the questions without any effort. Pay attention to how you feel as you take the exam and note the absence of anxiety and the absence of uncomfortable physical symptoms. Continue with the visualization until you feel comfortable with the experience and with the exam. Repeat this exercise for several days prior to the actual exam. When you take the exam you will be surprised at the absence of nervousness or anxiety; you will be even more surprised and pleased at the improvement in your grades.

> You should ask yourself every day
> why you're doing what you're doing.
>
> **Robert Arneson**
> **Sculptor**

the ways your behaviors are rewarded or punished, the things that frighten or please you—all are recorded by the conscious as well as unconscious parts of your mind. The language you speak, the foods you enjoy eating, the clothes you choose to wear, the cars and cosmetics you buy, the kinds of books you prefer to read, and the work you do are all determined by experiences that program the brain—the human biocomputer.

Many health habits are the result of programs that develop from early learning experiences. For example, a mother who feeds candy to her children to soothe angry and upset feelings establishes the program that sweet foods ease angry or upset feelings. A child who is told repeatedly that he or she is weak, clumsy, dumb, sickly, stupid, ugly, or undesirable is being filled with destructive and potentially harmful programs. As Lilly points out, no one can escape being programmed while growing up. What you can do *now*, however, is examine your programs and work to rid yourself of ones that make you uncomfortable and that are destructive to your health. By learning more about how your mind functions and by becoming aware of the beliefs and programs that help make you feel fully alive and well, you assist your mind in promoting health.

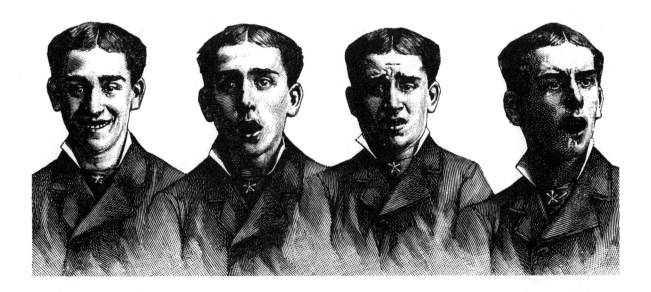

Supplemental Readings

Ader, R., ed. *Psychoneuroimmunology.* New York: Academic Press, 1981. Scientific articles describing experiments in psychoneuroimmunology.

Frank, J. D. "Mind-Body Relationships in Illness and Healing." *Journal of the International Academy of Preventive Medicine,* 2 (1975), 46–59. An excellent review of some of the ideas discussed in Chapters 2 and 3.

Gentry, W. D., ed. *Handbook of Behavioral Medicine.* New York: The Guilford Press, 1985. Contains scientific articles discussing the relation between the mind and disease.

Locke, S. *The Healer Within: The New Medicine of Mind and Body.* New York: E. P. Dutton, 1986. A physician discusses the evidence showing that the mind and body are intimately connected.

Marx, Jean L. "The Immune System 'Belongs in the Body.'" *Science,* March 8, 1985. A reporter discusses what was presented at a conference on psychoneuroimmunology.

"A User's Guide to Hormones." *Newsweek,* January 12, 1987, 50. A breezy but generally accurate account of modern research on hormones and their effects on health and behaviors.

Summary

The human mind can cause changes in body chemistry and physiology. Thoughts and feelings can have a positive or negative effect on the organs and cells of the body by altering electrical and chemical signals in the nervous and endocrine systems. The brain converts the information picked up by the senses into appropriate physiological responses by synthesizing and releasing neurotransmitters and certain hormones, which are in turn transported to the various regions of the body, where they regulate the physiological processes of their "target" organs, tissues, and cells—and thereby affect your health.

The autonomic nervous system (ANS) regulates vital body processes and helps maintain homeostasis without conscious control. But conscious thoughts and images, stress, and fear all influence how well homeostasis is maintained or how far from normal functioning body physiology will deviate. Harmonious interaction of all parts of the brain and body help to maintain optimal well-being. Psychoneuroimmunology is the branch of medicine that studies how the mind affects functions of the immune system, which helps determine susceptibility to disease.

You can learn to gain conscious control over almost any body function that you choose. It is possible to control pain through hypnoanesthesia or to communicate with a single nerve cell with the mind. You should learn to communicate with your body and to direct loving, positive thoughts to those areas that hurt or need healing. It would also be beneficial to your well-being for you to become more aware of self-destructive programming in your biocomputer (brain) and to ask your mind to erase or reevaluate experiences that cause fear or anxiety.

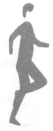

FOR YOUR HEALTH

Reprogramming the Mind

Many health behaviors are reflections of beliefs and attitudes that operate beneath the level of conscious awareness. Because these beliefs and attitudes in the mind are similar to programs in a computer, they *can* be changed. Your mind can create new, health-promoting programs to replace old, health-destroying ones.

Health problems often arise from destructive mental programs that have their origins in frightening life experiences, especially ones encountered early in life. If you can become aware of how such frightening experiences have programmed your mind and have thereby influenced your subsequent behavior, you can take steps to reprogram your mind and eliminate both the fear and the unwanted behavior.

Make a list of any fears you have, such as fear of new social situations, fear of being left alone, fear of crowds, fear of not succeeding, and so on. Then sit or lie down in a quiet, comfortable place and allow your mind to recall experiences that may have caused one of your present fears—perhaps the one that bothers you the most. Allow yourself to relax your mind and body as much as possible, then let the images just freely enter your mind. When you encounter a frightening situation, *imagine* it taking place in a manner that is *not* frightening—in your mind, any scene can be changed so that you feel safe and comfortable. Let the situation resolve itself in a positive way. Remember, since everything is going on in your mind, you have complete control of all actions and events in your imagined scene. Practice this positive imagery until you feel that your fear is less intense.

How Do You Affect Others?

You can influence how others feel simply by your words and actions. When you sincerely say to someone, "You look terrific," you make that person feel good, thereby initiating a series of psychophysiological processes that begin in the mind and affect hormonal and nervous regulation of the body in such a way that his or her wellness is enhanced. On the other hand, when you say to someone, "You look terrible," you can initiate physiological responses that are correspondingly negative.

For one week keep a record of the remarks you make to others that may affect their health and well-being, either positively or negatively. For example:

To John: "I liked the way you handled your anger in that situation. How'd you do it?"

To Sue (who is overweight):
"You sure do pack away the food. I don't see where you put it all."

Try do avoid remarks that can hurt a person's feelings or make them feel bad. Say positive things to the people you interact with. Tell others how well they look and how good they are doing things. Show them that you care how they feel. As people around you feel better, so will you.

Does Your Mind Affect Your Health?

Try to record all the times you feel sick or need medical attention. As soon as you feel ill try to remember what your state of mind was like in the recent past.

CHAPTER FOUR

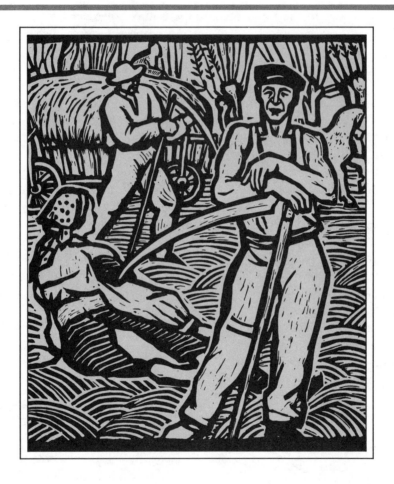

Knowing which nutrients the body
needs leads to health and wellness.

Nutrition
and Health

A man is satisfied not by the quantity of food but by the absence of greed.

Gurdjieff

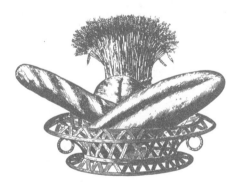

O f the many things you can do to enhance your state of health, none is more important than maintaining proper nutrition. The mind and body cannot function optimally without the proper supply of nutrients and energy obtained from food.

Many factors influence decision making regarding diet and nutrition, the foremost being availability of and access to food. In the United States and other industrialized countries of the world, food is generally plentiful and distribution of food is efficient, except to individuals whose incomes are below the poverty level.

Assuming that food is readily available and that individuals have access to it, people decide what to eat according to a variety of personal and social factors. These include dietary preferences and habits that reflect the patterns of food selection, preparation, and consumption established in one's family and associated with one's ethnic or cultural group. Social factors include income, which determines what kinds of foods are purchased (often not the most nutritious ones), social pressure (everybody eats pizza), the current food fads, and the advertising of foods, by which companies attempt to influence people's dietary decisions.

Because most of us have a great freedom of choice over our diets, we need to become aware of what constitutes a nutritious diet and how to select foods and maintain a diet that will promote health and well-being. This chapter discusses the basic principles of human nutrition and the next chapter presents guidelines for constructing a healthy diet.

> And God said, Behold, I have given you every herb bearing seed, which is upon the face of the earth, and every tree, in which is the fruit of a tree yielding seed; to you it shall be for meat.
>
> **Genesis 1:29**

Good Nutrition: Striking the Right Balance

Every person's body has a unique chemical and physical composition that corresponds to a state of optimal wellness, because the human body is constructed of atoms and molecules that are arranged in particular combinations and proportions that are unique to each person. Your body contains few of the same atoms and molecules it had even a few weeks ago, because its chemical constituents are continually replaced by different atoms and molecules acquired from the food you eat. There are about forty known essential nutrients (see Table 4-1), and perhaps others not yet identified, that must be continually resupplied to the body. Failure to obtain enough of one or more of the essential nutrients can result in a **nutritional deficiency disease,** such as **goiter** (enlarged thyroid gland), which may be caused by too little iodine; **beri-beri,** a disease characterized by weakness and wasting away that is caused by too little thiamine (vitamin B_1); **anemia** (too few red blood cells) from insufficient iron; and blindness from vitamin A deficiency, the most common cause of blindness in children worldwide. And

Table 4-1
The Essential Nutrients*

Amino acids	Fats	Vitamins	Minerals
Isoleucine	Linoleic acid	Ascorbic acid (vitamin C)	Calcium
Leucine		Biotin	Chlorine
Lysine	**Water**	Cobalamin (vitamin B_{12})	Chromium
Methionine		Folic acid	Cobalt
Phenylalanine		Niacin (vitamin B_3)	Copper
Threonine		Pantothenic acid	Iodine
Tryptophan		Pyridoxine (vitamin B_6)	Iron
Valine		Riboflavin (vitamin B_2)	Magnesium
Arginine†		Thiamine (vitamin B_1)	Manganese
Histidine†		Vitamin A	Molybdenum
		Vitamin D	Phosphorus
		Vitamin E	Potassium
		Vitamin K	Selenium
			Sodium
*Must be obtained from food.			Sulfur
†Not essential for adults; needed for growth of children.			Zinc

> Every package of sugar-sweetened life-savers,
> cough drops, breath mints, candies, chewing gum,
> and soft drinks should be labeled with a
> statement warning that excessive frequent use of
> these products can produce significant amounts
> of dental plaque and dental decay.
>
> **Abraham Nizel**
> **Professor of Oral Health**
> **Tufts University**

since all nutrients act in concert, a deficiency of one may impair the utilization of others even if the others are acquired in adequate amounts. Thus, a proper nutritional state is a matter of maintaining a complex balance of the essential nutrients.

In the industrialized countries of North America and northern Europe, clinically identifiable deficiency diseases resulting from undernourishment are not very common. However, people who restrict their diets to only a few kinds of foods may be ingesting less than the optimal levels of some essential nutrients. As a result, they may develop illnesses not directly related to diet and nutrition, they may become more susceptible to minor illnesses, including colds and various other infections, and they may not be functioning at their highest physical, mental, and emotional levels.

Poor health may also result from eating *too much* of certain kinds of food or from eating too much in general. For example, overeating is the principal cause of obesity, which contributes to the development of such serious diseases as high blood pressure, stroke, diabetes, and some forms of cancer. Cancer of the colon may be related to eating too much meat and processed foods and not getting enough fiber or roughage that may be essential to maintain a healthy colon. High salt intake is related to high blood pressure, and high sugar intake is related to tooth decay (the most prevalent disease in the industrialized world). Much tooth decay could be prevented if people followed the simple rules presented in Box 4-1.

Americans are fortunate that foods capable of supplying basic nutritional needs are readily available. We can, without too much trouble, choose an adequate diet. If we do so—that is, if we take in all the essential nutrients in optimum amounts (neither too little nor too much)—we can expect to realize the fullest expression of our biological potential and to be as healthy and energetic as we can be.

Digestion of Nutrients

Food provides us with important chemicals needed by the body and also supplies us with energy. Food is composed of six basic types of chemical substances: **proteins, carbohydrates, lipids** (fats), **vitamins, minerals,** and **water.** Proteins, most carbohydrates, and most lipids cannot be used by the body until they are broken down into smaller chemical units. Vitamins, minerals, and water need not be broken down; they are absorbed into the body as is.

The breakdown of food substances and the absorption of nutrients is called digestion. This is the function of the **digestive system** (see Figure 4-1). The digestive system, also known as the **gastrointestinal tract,** or **GI tract,** is a long tube that begins at the mouth and ends at the anus. Digestion begins in the mouth, as food is broken down into smaller pieces by chewing and saliva. The food passes to the stomach and intestines, where the

---

BOX 4-1

TOOTH DECAY AND HOW TO FIGHT IT

Tooth decay, also known as dental caries, is the most common disease in the United States and other industrialized countries. It is estimated that 95 percent of all Americans suffer from it—even though it is largely controllable.

Tooth decay is caused by the action of certain bacteria that live on the teeth. These bacteria produce acids by breaking down the sugar we eat, and the acids attack the hard surface enamel of the teeth. Some of these bacteria convert sugars and some of the material in saliva into a gelatinous substance called **dental plaque** that sticks to the teeth and fosters even more bacterial growth.

Dental caries could be prevented (1) if the bacteria responsible for it could be removed from the mouth, (2) if the sugars and other substances bacteria use to produce acids and plaque could be removed from the mouth, or (3) if teeth were protected from the attack of bacterial acids.

It is not yet possible to keep all decay-causing bacteria out of the oral cavity or to render them harmless to teeth in some way. So

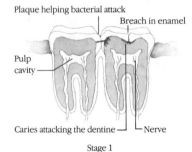

Plaque helping bacterial attack
Breach in enamel
Pulp cavity
Caries attacking the dentine
Nerve
Stage 1

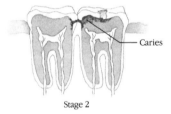

Caries
Stage 2

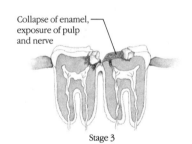

Collapse of enamel, exposure of pulp and nerve
Stage 3

efforts to prevent tooth decay must focus on keeping the mouth as free as possible of plaque and sugar. The incorporation of fluoride into tooth enamel, which occurs most rapidly when teeth are forming in early life and more slowly after teeth have erupted, greatly increases their resistance to decay. The following recommendations for the prevention of dental caries take these facts into account (Finn and Glass, 1975):

1. Don't eat sugar and sugar-containing products between meals.

2. Given a choice between sweets in liquid or in solid form, choose the liquid.

3. Avoid sticky or slow-dissolving sweets.

4. Brush and floss your teeth after each meal.

5. If you can't brush your teeth after eating, rinse out your mouth with warm water.

6. Support community and school water-fluoridation programs.

7. See your dentist regularly.

---

digestible parts are broken down into their various chemical constituents and absorbed into the blood. What is not digestible is passed out of the body in feces.

Material absorbed into the body through the walls of the intestines passes into a special network of blood vessels that flows directly to the liver, which means that the liver is the first organ that digested material encounters. Acting like a traffic cop, the liver regulates the flow of nutrients into the blood,

determining whether some nutrients are to be stored or are to be transported immediately to other organs and cells of the body. The liver also converts many of the chemicals, drugs, and pollutants that are ingested into forms that the body can excrete readily.

Once the nutrients are released into the bloodstream, they are transported to the body's billions of cells, where they are used for the assembly of cellular material and for the production of energy.

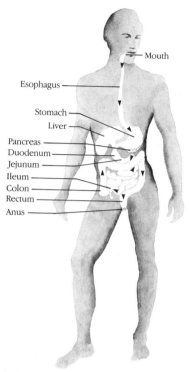

Figure 4-1
The human digestive system. Teeth and glandular secretions in the mouth help break up food, which the esophagus then transports to the stomach. The stomach breaks down some of the molecules in the food and passes it to the rest of the digestive tube: the duodenum, the jejunum, the ileum, the colon, and the rectum. Undigested material is eliminated from the body at the anus. The pancreas secretes enzymes and fluid into the duodenum to help the digestive process. The liver controls the release of absorbed nutrients into the body.

Proteins

Next to water, which makes up about 60 percent of the body mass, proteins are the most abundant substances in the body. About 20 percent of body mass is protein. The thousands of enzymes that help carry out and control all biochemical reactions are proteins. Other important protein molecules include antibodies, which help defend the body against foreign substances; hemoglobin, the oxygen-carrying molecule of the blood; and some hormones (see Figure 4-2).

Amino Acids

Proteins are large molecules that are made up of smaller units called **amino acids.** Twenty different amino acids are found in animal tissues (see Table 4-2). Every protein consists of a specific number and combination of amino acids linked together like beads on a string. As a protein is synthesized (manufactured) inside a cell, amino acids are gathered together at specific intracellular sites and chemically joined together in a genetically predetermined sequence to form the amino acid chain characteristic of that protein. If one or more of the amino acids needed for the synthesis of a particular protein is not available, however, that protein cannot be synthesized and the physiological activity that depends on that protein will be adversely affected. If one amino acid is absent, or if it is present in insufficient

Figure 4-2
The functions of proteins.

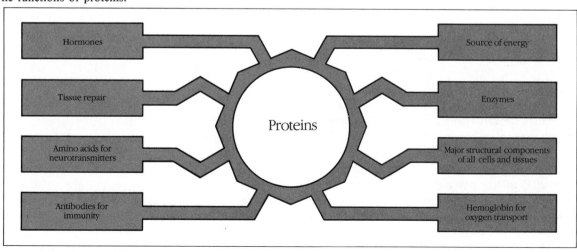

Table 4-2
The Twenty Amino Acids

Amino acid	Essential for humans
Alanine	
Arginine	Only during growth
Asparagine	
Aspartic acid	
Cysteine	
Glutamic acid	
Glutamine	
Glycine	
Histidine	Only during growth
Isoleucine	Yes
Leucine	Yes
Lysine	Yes
Methionine	Yes
Phenylalanine	Yes
Proline	
Serine	
Threonine	Yes
Tryptophan	Yes
Tyrosine	
Valine	Yes

amounts, it is said to be the **limiting amino acid** because it limits the body's production of proteins.

Some organisms, including yeasts and bacteria, can synthesize all twenty amino acids from simple chemical substances taken in from the environment. Humans, however, cannot manufacture all the amino acids they need. They lack the genetic and biochemical capability to make the amino acids phenylalanine, tryptophan, valine, threonine, lysine, isoleucine, leucine, and methionine. Thus, these eight are called the **essential amino acids,** and they must be obtained from food—that is, from animal and plant proteins. The amino acids histidine and arginine are not "essential," but amounts greater than those synthesized by human cells are required for normal growth, so young people need to ingest them along with the essential eight. The key to proper protein nutrition, therefore, is to eat enough protein each day to provide the required amino acids in amounts and proportions necessary for optimum cell functioning. To do so, you must pay attention to both the *quantity* (amount) and the *quality* (kind) of the protein you eat.

The quantity of protein that most adults need is about 35 to 40 grams a day. Individuals need this much in order to supply the body with sufficient amino acids—taking in much less can severely re-strict the manufacture of the body's proteins. But if that 35 to 40 grams contains all the essential amino acids needed for complete protein synthesis, then a person need not take in any more protein. Because amino acids are not stored in the body to any appreciable degree, excess amino acids are broken down—some to be converted to body fat, the rest to be excreted in urine.

The quality of protein is determined by how closely the amounts and proportions of the amino acids in a food match the body's need for the essential amino acids. Because the amino acid composition of most animal protein is very similar, people tend to acquire the essential amino acids in adequate quantities and proportions by eating fish, meat, eggs, and dairy products. Most vegetable proteins, however, are deficient in one or more of the essential amino acids. People who are strict vegetarians by choice or by necessity—that is, those who eat no meat, eggs, or milk products—must be sure to eat a variety of foods so that the amino acid deficiencies in some foods will be compensated for by the amino acid abundances in other foods. For example, wheat, rice, and oats contain very little lysine but have reasonably high amounts of methionine and tryptophan. Soybeans and other legumes are relatively high in lysine but are deficient in methionine and tryptophan. Meals consisting of both grains and legumes, therefore, are likely to supply adequate amounts of all the essential amino acids. **Protein complementarity** is achieved by combining foods so that amino acid deficiencies in one source are counterbalanced, or **complemented,** by abundances in another source. The essential amino acid and protein content of some common foods is shown in Table 4-3.

High Meat Consumption and Disease

Obtaining adequate amounts of high-quality protein—protein that supplies necessary amounts of the essential amino acids—is not a problem for most people in the industrialized world. In fact, in the United States and Canada, people consume on the average about twice the amount of protein they actually utilize. About two-thirds of that protein comes

Table 4-3
Protein Content and Relative Amino Acid Deficiencies in Some Foods

Food group	Food	Weight (grams)	Protein content (grams)	Relative amino acid deficiency
Dairy	Cheddar cheese (one piece)	100	25	None
	Cottage cheese (one tbsp.)	28	4	None
	Milk (8 oz.)	246	9	None
	Egg (whole, large)	54	7	None
Meats	Hamburger — cooked (from ¼ lb. raw)	85	22	None
	Ham — raw (3½ oz.)	100	33	None
	Chicken — raw (3½ oz.)	100	20	None
	Halibut — raw (3½ oz.)	100	21	None
Nuts and seeds	Almonds — dried (12–15 nuts)	15	3	Lysine and tryptophan
	Peanuts — raw (3½ oz.)	100	26	Lysine, methionine, tryptophan
	Peanut butter (1 tbsp.)	15	4	Lysine, methionine, tryptophan
	Sunflower seeds (3½ oz.)	100	24	Lysine
Legumes and grains	Soybeans (½ cup)	100	34	None
	Lentils (½ cup)	100	25	Methionine and tryptophan
	Wheat flour — whole (¼ cup)	100	13	Lysine
	Wheat germ (3½ oz.)	100	27	None
	Oatmeal — dry (⅓ cup)	28	4	Lysine
	Rice — white (¾ cup, cooked)	28	2	Lysine
	Spaghetti (¼ cup, dry)	38	5	Lysine
	Bread — white (1 slice)	23	2	Lysine
Vegetables	Lima beans — cooked (½ cup)	100	7	Methionine
	Spinach — cooked (½ cup)	100	3	None
	Potatoes — white (1 medium)	100	2	Methionine, lysine

Data from U.S. Department of Agriculture Handbook No. 456, *Nutritive Value of American Foods,* 1975; A. Bowes and C. Church, *Food Values of Portions Commonly Used* (Philadelphia: J. B. Lippincott, 1975); F. M. Lappe, *Diet for a Small Planet* (New York: Ballentine, 1971).

In 1986 Salmonella bacteria (one cause of food poisoning) were found in 37 percent of supermarket chickens, 5 percent of ground meat, and 12 percent of pork sausage.

USDA Food Safety Service

Table 4-4
Fat Content of Various Meats

Food	Fat content (percent)
Beef	
T-bone steak	43.2
Chuck steak	36.7
Sirloin steak	32.0
Round steak	14.9
Lamb	
Shoulder	26.9
Leg	21.2
Pork products	
Bacon	49.0
Sausage	32.5
Bologna	27.5
Ham	22.1
Canned ham	11.3
Fish	
Herring, Atlantic	16.4
Tuna, albacore (canned, light)	6.8
Salmon, Atlantic	5.8
Rainbow trout	4.5
Haddock	0.7
Fowl	
Chicken (fryer, dark meat)	9.7
Turkey (dark meat)	5.3
Chicken (fryer, light meat)	3.5
Turkey (light meat)	2.6

Data from U.S. Senate Select Committee on Nutrition and Human Needs, *Dietary Goals for the United States* (Washington, D.C.: U.S. Government Printing Office, 1977).

from animal sources and the rest comes from grain products and vegetables.

Many physicians and nutritionists believe that there may be some health risks associated with consuming large amounts of meat. Because meat contains fat as well as protein, eating a lot of meat may contribute to fat-related diseases such as atherosclerosis (discussed in Chapter 16) and obesity. As much as 40 percent of hamburger is fat; steak may be 30 percent fat. (Table 4-4 lists the fat content of various meats.) Trimming as much fat as possible from meat before it is cooked and eating more poultry (with drippings and skin removed) and fish, which have proportionately less fat than do red meats, is probably advisable.

Another health risk associated with high meat consumption is cancer of the colon and other diseases of the GI tract. Countries that have the highest per capita meat consumption—including New Zealand, Canada, and the United States—also have the highest rates of colon cancer. The reasons for the association of colon cancer with high meat consumption are unknown. One hypothesis holds that since most meats are commercial products, they may contain nonfood chemicals that are added during their production and packaging. These chemicals include pesticide residues (DDT), industrial chemicals (PCBs), hormone growth promoters (DES), dyes for color enhancement, and preservatives such as ni-

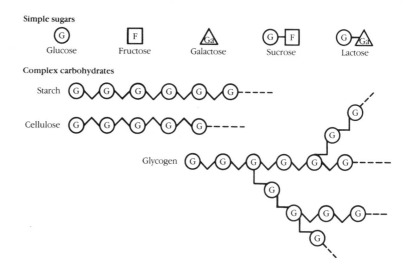

Figure 4-3
Types of carbohydrates. The dashes at the right of the carbohydrate chains indicate that the chains contain more glucose units—in some cases thousands more—than shown here. Chemical bonds connecting glucose molecules in cellulose cannot be broken by human enzymes.

trates and nitrites. Another possibility is that certain bacteria in the colon convert substances necessary for the digestion of fats (bile acids) into cancer-causing agents.

In recent years consumers have become increasingly aware of the risks associated with high meat consumption and are eating more fish and poultry. Meat producers have tried to stop this trend by lobbying government agencies to restrict the amount of information linking meat consumption with disease. They have also launched massive advertising campaigns that encourage the eating of meat and meat products.

The fact that some health risks are associated with high meat consumption does not mean that people must stop eating meat altogether in order to be healthy. As with so many other aspects of nutrition, it does mean that people need to be aware of what is in the foods they ingest and to eat a variety of foods in moderation. With regard to meat consumption, a wise course is to adopt a "prudent diet"—one that is low in environmental pollutants and animal fat.

Carbohydrates

Carbohydrates are the principal source of the body's energy. Almost all of the body's cells can break down carbohydrate molecules and make available the energy stored in their chemical bonds. Carbohydrates are also used in the synthesis of some cell components, such as the hereditary material, DNA.

The human body can manufacture carbohydrate molecules needed for energy production and cellular components from other kinds of molecules, including amino acids. This is why carbohydrates are absent from Table 4-1, "The Essential Nutrients." In theory, then, people need not eat any carbohydrates, and some ill-conceived reducing diets even recommend that no carbohydrates be eaten in order to drastically reduce the intake of calories. Nutritionists believe, however, that some carbohydrates are needed in the diet even if one is trying to lose weight. Otherwise, the body may break down muscle and other tissues to derive energy from amino acids.

There are two principal types of carbohydrates: **simple sugars,** which are found predominantly in fruit, and **complex carbohydrates,** found in grains, fruit, and the stems, leaves, and roots of vegetables. Simple sugars are made up of one molecule of sugar or two sugar molecules linked together, whereas complex carbohydrates consist of as many as several thousand of the same kinds of sugar molecules linked together in long chainlike arrays (see Figure 4-3). Studies indicate that about half the food eaten by most Americans consists of simple sugars and complex carbohydrates.

Simple Sugars

Our diets contain several kinds of simple sugars. The most common is **glucose** (also called dextrose). Glucose molecules are found in virtually all cells; they are the principal source of cellular energy. Ultimately, all sugars are converted to glucose in the body's cells. Glucose is sweet, and glucose derived from corn is frequently added to manufactured foods as "corn sugar" or "corn sweeteners."

Fructose is very similar to glucose chemically. It is found in fruits and honey along with glucose; honey, for example, contains about equal amounts of fructose and glucose. Fructose is one of the sweetest sugars, which means you can eat less fructose than other simple sugars and obtain an equivalent amount of sweetness.

Sucrose, or common table sugar, consists of a molecule of glucose and a molecule of fructose chemically linked together. Sucrose is digested by breaking this linkage and liberating the glucose and fructose portions. Sucrose is found in many plants. It is harvested from sugar cane and sugar beets to produce table sugar and the "refined" sugar that food manufacturers add to a large number of packaged foods (see Box 4-2). Because fructose is sweeter than sucrose, people who want to reduce the amount of sugar in their diets without entirely cutting out sweet tastes can replace pastries with fresh fruit and can replace table sugar with honey. In doing so, they will also be gaining other nutrients in the fruit and honey that are not present in the pure, refined sucrose.

Lactose, found almost exclusively in milk and milk products, consists of a molecule of the sugar galactose linked to glucose. When lactose is digested, the galactose and glucose are chemically separated and the galactose is converted to glucose. Whereas almost all babies have the capacity to utilize lactose (found in mother's milk), many older children and adults do not, because they lack the enzyme that splits the lactose molecule into glucose and galactose. For some reason, perhaps having a genetic basis, during the process of maturation the body's cells stop making this lactose-splitting enzyme. The wide variation in **lactose intolerance** among human populations is shown in Figure 4-4. Many black and Chinese adults lack this enzyme and cannot safely drink milk. If they do drink it, they may suffer gastrointestinal upset, diarrhea, and occasionally severe illness. Milk products in which lactose has previously been broken down by bacteria, such as cheese or yogurt, can be eaten safely by people with this enzyme deficiency.

Complex Carbohydrates

The complex carbohydrates in the diets of most Americans come principally from grains, such as wheat, rice, corn, oats, and barley; from legumes, such as peas and various kinds of beans; from the leaves, stems, and roots of plants, which make up the vast array of vegetables; and from some animal tissues. There are two major classes of complex car-

Figure 4-4
Lactose intolerance in different populations. Most Thais and Ibos (an African people) are lactose-intolerant, whereas few Swiss and Swedes are.

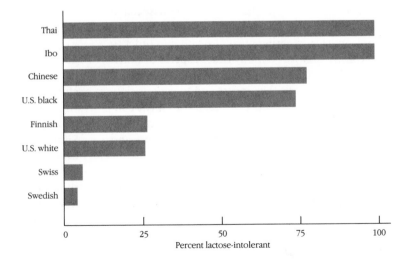

Percent lactose-intolerant

BOX 4-2

COMMERCIAL FOODS: SUGAR, SUGAR EVERYWHERE

The food manufacturing industry is capable of producing foods in astonishing quantity and variety. People should not forget, however, that food manufacturers are in business to make money and not necessarily to enhance health. Food companies generally add sugars and other sweeteners to their products to make them "taste better" (see table).

Most animals have a "sweet tooth" and humans are no exception. However, not only do people rarely need the energy from the added sugar, but it's better to obtain that energy from more nutritious foods. Because added sugar provides calories but no essential nutrients, sugar is usually described as contributing "empty calories" to the diet. Excess calories from added sugar are converted to fat, which in some cases may contribute to overweight problems. Populations that consume large amounts of sucrose (refined beet or cane sugar) exhibit high rates of heart disease, obesity, diabetes, and dental caries.

In the mid-1980s sugar consumption in the United States averaged about 127 pounds per person per year, up from 118 pounds a decade before. Sucrose, corn syrup, and a manufactured sweetener made from corn syrup, called high-fructose corn syrup, are the major types of sugar added to sweetened products.

Sugar Added to Commercial Food Products

Product	Amount	Added sugar (grams)	Added calories
Coca-Cola	12 oz.	47	190
Pepsi-Cola	12 oz.	50	200
Carnation Slender	10 oz.	32	125
Tang	8 oz.	38	150
Gatorade	8 oz.	18	70
Candy bar	1 oz.	17	56
Jell-O	½ cup	21	84
Pork and beans	½ cup	12	48
Canned peaches	½ cup	15	60
Low-fat yogurt with fruit	8 oz.	45	180
Peanut butter	1 oz.	7	35

Data from Center for Science in the Public Interest.

bohydrates: **starch,** which is digestible and is utilized to supply molecules for energy production and cell components, and **fiber,** which is nondigestible but is nevertheless important for proper gastrointestinal functioning.

Starch, which consists of many glucose molecules linked together, is used to store energy in both plants and animals. In plants, starch is usually contained in granules within seeds, pods, or roots. When the plant needs the chemical energy in the glucose molecules, it breaks down the starch, freeing the glucose to provide the cells of a sprouting seedling or an adult plant with energy. The animal form of starch, called **glycogen,** is found in muscle and liver. When energy is needed, the glycogen breaks down and its constituent glucose molecules become available to the body for energy production. Long-distance runners sometimes eat large amounts of

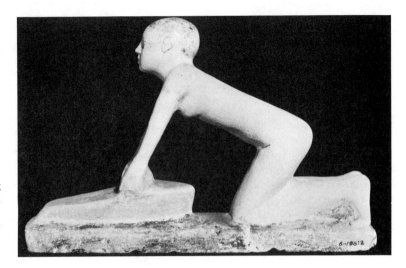

Figure 4-5
A 2000-year-old Egyptian statue from the Giza tomb. The woman is grinding wheat between stones. Wheat has been a staple in the diets of cultures since the dawn of time. (Courtesy the Lowie Museum of Anthropology, University of California, Berkeley.)

carbohydrates on the day before an important race in order to build up their supply of glycogen.

Much of the starch in people's diets comes from foods made from wheat flour, such as bread, pas-

Figure 4-6
Percentages of nutrients remaining in flour after milling to 70 percent extraction.

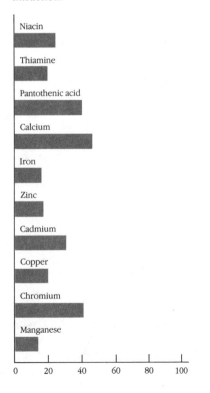

tries, and noodles. The flour is derived from the crushed grain of wheat plants. The harvested grain is crushed between large stone or steel rollers. This process separates the outer husk of the grain or seed, called the **bran,** the middle starch-containing layer, called the **endosperm,** and the inner **germ.** Variations in the crushing and separation of the parts of the grain produce different kinds of flour. The white flour commonly used in baking is referred to as "70 percent extraction," which means that 70 percent of the original grain remains after the milling is complete. This flour is almost entirely endosperm; the bran and the germ are removed in the milling process—the reason 70 percent extraction is called "refined flour." A "whole-grain flour" is produced by a 90 percent extraction of grain, from which only the coarsest particles of bran have been removed.

In the milling of 70 percent extraction flour, many of the nutrients in the wheat grain— particularly in the germ, which contains many vitamins—are removed (see Figure 4-6). So flour manufacturers and bakers add certain vitamins and minerals to their refined flour, thus producing "enriched flour." Whole-wheat flour contains nearly all of the wheat grain and does not have to be "enriched." Because not all of the nutrients that are removed in the milling of 70 percent extraction flour are replaced by the manufacturer, enriched white flour is nutritionally inferior to whole-wheat flour. For most people, the difference is probably not significant; whatever nutrients may be missing from refined flour products are likely to be obtained from

What the processed-food industry does to a grain
of wheat is awesome. Basically they take out
everything that is good for you and leave
an absolutely bland, easily digestible
white powder. . . .

Richard Watson
The Philosopher's Diet

other foods in a reasonably varied diet. However, those who wish to obtain all the nutrients in wheat may want to use whole-wheat flour.

Bread made with whole-wheat flour is brown, but not all brown bread is made with whole-wheat flour. Some bread manufacturers add molasses or honey to dough made from enriched white flour to give it a brown color. Therefore, it is always wise to read the package label to determine what kinds of flour are used in the bread.

Potatoes are starchy vegetables that have the undeserved reputation of being fattening and therefore undesirable as food. Actually, potatoes themselves are no more "fattening" than any other starchy food, unless they are cooked in large amounts of fat or oil (as in the making of french fries) or are eaten with a lot of butter or fat-containing sauces (see Table 4-5). One large potato has only about 100 calories—less than a medium-size soft drink. And unlike the soft drink, which has no essential nutrients (other than water), the potato contains some proteins, vitamin C, iron, calcium, and niacin.

The other major form of complex carbohydrate in diets is cellulose, which is obtained from the nondigestible vegetable matter called fiber, or **roughage.** Cellulose is the main constituent of all plant material and makes up more than 50 percent of the organic matter in the world. Cellulose, like starch, consists of glucose molecules. But in cellulose these molecules are chemically linked together in such a way that the human digestive system cannot break them apart. Thus, people cannot digest cellulose.

This does not mean, however, that cellulose and other nondigestible matter are not important in the diet. Studies indicate that cellulose and such other nondigestible plant materials as bran and lignin facilitate digestion and prevent several disorders of the gastrointestinal tract. Fiber adds bulk to the feces, thereby preventing constipation and related disorders such as **hemorrhoids** and **hiatus hernia,** which result from prolonged increases in pressure while defecating. Fiber also decreases the time it takes for material to pass through the GI tract and be eliminated. The longer waste material and bacteria remain in the GI tract, the greater the risk of appendicitis, diverticular disease (outpocketings in the wall of the lower intestine), and cancer of the colon and rectum.

Nutritionists recommend that individuals consume 20 to 35 grams of fiber daily. The best source

Table 4-5
Calories in Potatoes Prepared in Various Ways

Baked (medium)	75
Baked with 1 pat of butter	125
Baked with 1 pat of butter and 1 oz. of sour cream	160
French fries, 20 pieces	275
Hash browns	268
Mashed with milk and margarine	94
Potato chips, 10 chips	115

Data from A. Bowes and C. Church, *Food Values of Portions Commonly Used* (Philadelphia: J. B. Lippincott, 1975).

Table 4-6
Fiber Content of Various Foods

Food	Amount	Fiber (grams)
Whole-wheat bread	1 slice	1.6
Rye bread	1 slice	1.0
White bread	1 slice	0.6
Brown rice (cooked)	½ cup	2.4
White rice (cooked)	½ cup	0.1
Spaghetti (cooked)	½ cup	0.8
Kidney beans (cooked)	½ cup	5.8
Lima beans (cooked)	½ cup	4.9
Potato (baked)	medium	3.8
Corn	½ cup	3.9
Spinach	½ cup	2.0
Lettuce	½ cup	0.3
Strawberries	¾ cup	2.0
Banana	medium	2.0
Apple (with skin)	medium	2.6
Orange	small	1.2

of fiber is in food; high-fiber foods include legumes, vegetables, whole grains, and fruits (Table 4-6).

Lipids (Fats)

Lipids are a group of diverse chemical substances that have the common property of being relatively insoluble in water. Perhaps the most familiar lipid is **triglyceride,** otherwise known as body fat. Excess calories, whether obtained from too much sugar or too much fat, are converted by the liver into triglycerides, which are stored in all too obvious places in the body.

Other lipids, such as cholesterol and lecithin, are essential constituents of cell membranes. The steroid hormones produced by the reproductive organs and adrenal glands are lipids; vitamins A, D, E, and K are lipids; and substances in liver bile that help digest fats, the bile acids, are lipids.

Dietary lipid comes in three principal forms: cholesterol, saturated fat, and unsaturated fat. Saturated fat differs from unsaturated fat by having more hydrogen atoms in each fat molecule. Saturated fats tend to be solid at room temperature, whereas unsaturated fats tend to be liquid.

The amounts of cholesterol, saturated fat, and unsaturated fat taken into the body depend on what kinds of foods are eaten. Some foods, such as egg yolk, contain large amounts of cholesterol, whereas others, such as vegetable oils, are high in unsaturated fat and contain no cholesterol (see Table 4-7). There is considerable controversy about the health effects of eating high amounts of certain kinds of fats, although the present consensus among nutritionists and medical researchers seems to be that diets containing more than 600 milligrams per day of cholesterol and 50 grams per day of saturated fat may contribute to heart and blood vessel disease (this issue is discussed in more detail in Chapter 16). Many studies have shown a relationship between dietary fat consumption and cancer of the breast, colon, and prostate gland (Palmer, 1985).

Table 4-7
Cholesterol and Fat Content of Some Common Foods

Food	Amount	Percent fat	Cholesterol (milligrams)	Saturated fat (milligrams)	Unsaturated fat (milligrams)
Butter	1 tbsp. (14 g)	80	35	700	3,640
Mayonnaise	1 tbsp. (14 g)	78	17	2,000	8,000
Ground beef	1 oz. (28 g)	37	20	4,280	5,320
Cheddar cheese	1 oz. (28 g)	33	28	616	3,000
Egg	1 medium (48 g)	11	225	1,800	3,000
Whole milk	8 oz. (244 g)	3.5	34	4,700	3,000
Shrimp	1 oz. (28 g)	1.2	43	56	196
Corn oil	1 tbsp. (14 g)	100	0	1,780	11,650
Safflower oil	1 tbsp. (14 g)	100	0	1,320	13,500

Data from U.S. Department of Agriculture Handbook No. 456, *Nutritive Value of American Foods,* 1975; U.S. Senate Select Committee on Nutrition and Human Needs, *Dietary Goals for the United States* (Washington, D.C.: U.S. Government Printing Office, 1977).

BOX 4-3

BREAKFAST CEREALS: DON'T BELIEVE THE ADVERTISING

For thousands of years cereal grains—wheat, oats, corn, rice, rye, and barley—have been the principal components of the breakfast meal, and they still are today. Whereas the centuries-old way of ingesting cereals had been to cook the raw grain into porridge or gruel, beginning in the twentieth century American food manufacturers produced ready-to-eat "cold" cereals, which are now the primary way cereal grains are consumed at breakfast. In 1985 North American households consumed more than a million tons of breakfast cereals, which translates into $4.5 billion in sales (*Consumer Reports,* 1986).

In order to capture health-conscious individuals as consumers of breakfast cereals, manufacturers have produced a slew of "high-fiber" products, frequently with the word "fiber" or "bran" in the name. Most of these products contain a substantial amount of fiber, usually between 5 and 10 grams per ounce of dry cereal.

Although fiber and bran may be beneficial for health, they are not very tasty, and most consumers buy according to taste. So, manufacturers often add large amounts of sugar and salt to increase a product's taste appeal. And whereas the packaging and advertising may proclaim the virtues of the cereal because of its fiber content, they do not advertise the added substances. Consumers of ready-to-eat cereals must use the information on product labels to determine what has been added.

For years children have been the largest market for ready-to-eat breakfast cereals and manufacturers advertise heavily on cartoon shows. Many children's cereals consist of 40 to 50 percent sugar. Kellogg's "Tony the Tiger" has been pitching Frosted Flakes, currently 39 percent sugar, to kids for almost four decades. Aware that parents may object to such sugary breakfast fare, manufacturers have changed the names of some cereals to give the appearance of having less sugar without actually changing the cereal's contents. For example, Kellogg's "Sugar Frosted Flakes" was changed to simply "Frosted Flakes"; Post's "Super Sugar Crisp" became "Super Golden Crisp." Furthermore, cereal advertising usually emphasizes a health-related virtue, such as "fortified with vitamins" or "no preservatives," which can divert the buyer's attention from the fact that the product may contain other chemical additives besides added sugar.

The body requires one type of unsaturated fat, **linoleic acid;** not getting enough of it may lead to a deficiency disease characterized primarily by skin lesions. For this reason, you should not attempt to eliminate all lipids from your diet. Furthermore, fats provide energy. If you were to eliminate nearly all fat from your diet and not compensate with increased amounts of carbohydrate or protein, your body would break down its protein to supply itself with energy.

A few years ago researchers discovered that populations such as Greenland Eskimos and Japanese fishermen whose diets contain a considerable amount of cold-water fish (cod, salmon, sardines, herring, mackerel) tended to have a lower risk for heart disease (Kromhut et al., 1985). Further research implicated certain unsaturated fatty acids known as **omega-3 fatty acids** (FFAs) as at least partly responsible for the reduced risk of heart disease. The omega-3 FFAs are found in the body oils of the fish. Apparently the omega-3 FFAs (specifically **eicosapentaneoic acid,** EPA, and **docosahexanoic acid,** DHA) lower the levels of triglyceride and cholesterol in the blood and also reduce the chances that platelet cells will clot and cause a heart attack. Although more research is required to verify the potential beneficial effects of omega-3 FFAs, many nutritionists are now recommending that cold-water fish be included regularly in the diet (not only for the omega-3 FFAs, but also because fish contains less cholesterol and saturated fat than meat). Omega-3 FFAs can also be obtained by fish oil supplements such as cod liver oil or fish oil capsules, although one must be aware that fish liver oils contain vitamins A and D, which can be toxic in large amounts. Vegetable sources of omega-3 FFAs include purslane, walnuts, wheat germ oil, and soybean products such as tofu.

Table 4-8
Essential Minerals

Mineral	Major body functions	Dietary sources	Consequences of deficiency
Calcium	Bone and tooth formation Blood clotting Nerve transmission	Milk, cheese, dark green vegetables, dried legumes	Stunted growth Rickets, osteoporosis Convulsions
Chlorine	Formation of gastric juice Acid-base balance	Common salt	Muscle cramps Mental apathy Reduced appetite
Chromium	Glucose and energy metabolism	Fats, vegetable oils, meats	Impaired ability to metabolize glucose
Cobalt	Constituent of vitamin B_{12}	Organ and muscle meats	Not reported in man
Copper	Constituent of enzymes of iron metabolism	Meats, drinking water	Anemia (rare)
Iodine	Constituent of thyroid hormones	Marine fish and shellfish, dairy products, many vegetables	Goiter (enlarged thyroid)
Iron	Constituent of hemoglobin and enzymes of energy metabolism	Eggs, lean meats, legumes, whole grains, green leafy vegetables	Iron-deficiency anemia (weakness, reduced resistance to infection)
Magnesium	Activates enzymes Involved in protein synthesis	Whole grains, green leafy vegetables	Growth failure Behavioral disturbances Weakness, spasms
Manganese	Constituent of enzymes involved in fat synthesis	Widely distributed in foods	In animals: disturbances of nervous system, reproductive abnormalities
Molybdenum	Constituent of some enzymes	Legumes, cereals, organ meats	Not reported in man
Phosphorus	Bone and tooth formation Acid-base balance	Milk, cheese, meat, poultry, grains	Weakness, demineralization of bone
Potassium	Acid-base balance Body water balance Nerve function	Meats, milk, many fruits	Muscular weakness Paralysis
Selenium	Functions in close association with vitamin E	Seafood, meat, grains	Anemia (rare)
Sodium	Acid-base balance Body water balance Nerve function	Common salt	Muscle cramps Mental apathy Reduced appetite
Sulfur	Constituent of active tissue compounds, cartilage, and tendon	Sulfur amino acids (methionine and cysteine) in dietary proteins	Related to intake and deficiency of sulfur amino acids
Zinc	Constituent of enzymes involved in digestion	Widely distributed in foods	Growth failure Small sex glands

Minerals

Many body functions require the presence of certain chemical elements besides those that make up the organic molecules (hydrogen, carbon, oxygen, nitrogen, phosphorus, and sulfur). Sodium, potassium, and chlorine, for example, are essential for a variety of body functions, including the maintenance of cell membranes, the conduction of nerve impulses, and muscle contraction (see Table 4-8). Magnesium, zinc, copper, and cobalt facilitate certain biochemical reactions; iron is essential to the oxygen-carrying function of hemoglobin; iodine is needed by the thyroid gland to manufacture the hormone thyroxin; and calcium and phosphorus are needed to manufacture bones and teeth. These and other nutritionally essential elements make up the dietary minerals.

Minerals are found in virtually everything you eat, and most people can acquire sufficient quantities of the essential minerals simply by eating a variety of foods, especially fresh fruits and vegetables. Women and rapidly growing young people are susceptible to iron deficiency, so they must be sure to eat some iron-rich foods, such as eggs, lean meats, beans, prunes, whole grains, and green leafy vegetables. (A few people have an unusually high requirement for a particular mineral and must obtain it by dietary supplement.)

Many people take in too much sodium, which may contribute to high blood pressure (this issue is discussed in Chapters 5 and 16). The amounts of sodium naturally present in almost every kind of food pose no problems; the excess sodium in diets comes from the use of table salt (sodium chloride) and from manufactured and restaurant food, to which salt is often added to increase flavor and sales (see Table 4-9). Because the amounts of salt in commercially prepared foods are not usually stated on package labels or restaurant menus, some people consume as much as 20 grams of sodium each day, which is far in excess of the approximately 2 grams per day the body needs.

Vitamins

Vitamins are small biological molecules that, like the various minerals, are essential for certain biochemical processes. Unlike minerals, however, vitamins are not found outside of living things; they are made by the cells of various organisms. There are two major classes of vitamins: the **water-soluble vitamins** and the **fat-soluble vitamins.** They are listed in Table 4-10, along with their major functions, their sources, and the illnesses that result from their deficiencies. The fat-soluble vitamins can cause illness when taken in excess, for they may accumulate in the body until their concentration becomes toxic.

Table 4-9
Sodium Content of Some Commercially Prepared Foods

Food	Sodium content (milligrams)
Table salt (1 packet)	400
Frankfurters (2)	1100
Instant mashed potatoes (100 g)	256
English muffin	215
Kellogg's Corn Flakes (30 g)	282
Kellogg's Rice Krispies (30 g)	267
Bottled salad dressing (1 tsp.)	315
McDonald's Big Mac	1510
Instant pudding (1/2 cup)	404
Canned tuna (100 g)	800

Data from U.S. Senate Select Committee on Nutrition and Human Needs, *Dietary Goals for the United States* (Washington, D.C.: U.S. Government Printing Office, 1977); "Salt and High Blood Pressure," *Consumer Reports,* March 1979, p. 147.

Table 4-10
Water-Soluble Vitamins and Fat-Soluble Vitamins

Water-Soluble Vitamin	Major body functions	Dietary sources	Consequences of deficiency
Ascorbic acid (vitamin C)	Tooth and bone formation; production of connective tissue; promotion of wound healing; may enhance immunity	Citrus fruits, tomatoes, peppers, cabbage, potatoes, melons	Scurvy (degeneration of bones, teeth, and gums)
Biotin	Involved in fat and amino acid synthesis and breakdown	Yeast, liver, milk, most vegetables, bananas, grapefruit	Skin problems; fatigue; muscle pains; nausea
Cobalamin (vitamin B_{12})	Involved in single carbon atom transfers; essential for DNA synthesis	Muscle meats, eggs, milk and dairy products (not in vegetables)	Pernicious anemia; nervous system malfunctions
Folacin (folic acid)	Essential for synthesis of DNA and other molecules	Green leafy vegetables, organ meats, whole-wheat products	Anemia; diarrhea and other gastrointestinal problems
Niacin	Involved in energy production and synthesis of cell molecules	Grains, meats, legumes	Pellagra (skin, gastrointestinal, and mental disorders)
Pantothenic acid	Involved in energy production and synthesis and breakdown of many biological molecules	Yeast, meats and fish, nearly all vegetables and fruits	Vomiting; abdominal cramps; malaise; insomnia
Pyridoxine (vitamin B_6)	Essential for synthesis and breakdown of amino acids and manufacture of unsaturated fats from saturated fats	Meats, whole grains, most vegetables	Weakness; irritability; trouble sleeping and walking; skin problems
Riboflavin (vitamin B_2)	Involved in energy production; important for health of the eyes	Milk and dairy foods, meats, eggs, vegetables, grains	Eye and skin problems
Thiamine (vitamin B_1)	Essential for breakdown of food molecules and production of energy	Meats, legumes, grains, some vegetables	Beri-beri (nerve damage, weakness, heart failure)

Fat-Soluble Vitamin	Major body functions	Dietary sources	Consequences of deficiency or excess
Vitamin A (retinol)	Essential for maintenance of eyes and skin; influences bone and tooth formation	Liver, kidney, yellow and dark leafy vegetables, apricots	Deficiency: night blindness; eye damage; skin dryness. Excess: loss of appetite; skin problems; swelling of ankles and feet
Vitamin D (calciferol)	Regulates calcium metabolism; important for growth of bones and teeth	Cod-liver oil, dairy products, eggs	Deficiency: rickets (bone deformities) in children; bone destruction in adults. Excess: thirst; nausea; weight loss; kidney damage
Vitamin E (tocopherol)	Prevents damage to cells from oxidation; prevents red blood cell destruction	Wheat germ, vegetable oils, vegetables, egg yolk, nuts	Deficiency: anemia, possibly nerve cell destruction
Vitamin K (phylloquinone)	Helps with blood clotting	Liver, vegetable oils, green leafy vegetables, tomatoes	Deficiency: severe bleeding

> The use of sulfites to preserve raw fruits and vegetables served in restaurant salad bars was banned in 1986.
>
> **Food and Drug Administration**

Are Dietary Supplements Necessary?

At the present time there is controversy about whether people need to supplement their usual diet with minerals and vitamins. Because plants contain considerable quantities of the minerals and vitamins people require, a diet made up of a variety of fresh fruits and vegetables is likely to provide most people with the minerals and vitamins they need. The one known exception is vitamin B_{12}, which is required for certain metabolic functions and is found primarily in animal tissues and products, such as eggs, milk, and meat. Therefore, strict vegetarians must acquire vitamin B_{12} in supplements. Supplementation might also become necessary for people who eat primarily manufactured foods from which minerals and vitamins have been removed during the manufacturing process or for people who have a biological need for an unusually high amount of a particular substance.

People usually take vitamin and mineral supplements as a form of "dietary insurance"—to provide one or more essential nutrients just in case they are deficient in the diet. However, in the doses provided by manufacturers, dietary supplements, especially "multiple vitamins" or "stress-formulas," are usually superfluous, and for some individuals they may actually have negative effects. Just because vitamins and minerals are essential nutrients does not mean that "more is better." In massive doses (so-called "megadoses") some vitamins, minerals, and amino acids can be harmful. As mentioned earlier, excess consumption of fat-soluble vitamins A and D can have toxic effects (see Table 4-10). For many years it was thought that large doses of the water-soluble vitamins and minerals posed no health risk because excess amounts of these vitamins would simply be excreted by the body. There are instances, however, in which megadoses of some water-soluble nutrients are toxic. For example, some individuals may experience transient changes in heart and circulatory function after ingesting more than 2000 mg daily of niacin (vitamin B_3). More than 2000 mg daily of pyridoxine (vitamin B_6), taken by many women to relieve menstrual distress or to build up the body, can produce a numbing in the hands and feet and a temporary loss of fine motor control.

One must remember that the body has hundreds of regulatory mechanisms that maintain homeostasis and that these evolved to regulate a certain limited range of nutrients. The science of nutrition has not yet been able to define the optimum amount of nutrients for all people in all circumstances (see Chapter 5). Thus, it is possible that ingesting excessively large doses of normal and necessary nutrients can stress the body's self-regulating systems and produce symptoms of physiological imbalance.

When vitamins, minerals, or other nutrients are taken in massive doses and for therapeutic reasons, they are no longer considered nutrients. They are drugs and can be misused just like any other drug (see Chapter 13). This point is rarely mentioned by proponents of megadosing, sometimes out of a

> Natural vitamins are no
> better than synthetic vitamins.
> They have exactly the same atoms
> in their molecules, arranged in exactly
> the same way. A vitamin is a vitamin
> is a vitamin.
>
> **Jean Mayer**
> **President, Tufts University**

desire to help and other times out of a desire to increase sales and profits. We do not insist that megadosing is always harmful. We do suggest, however, that everyone be cautious in supplementing the diet with excess doses of nutrients.

Once a person has chosen to use a mineral or vitamin supplement, it makes no difference chemically if the supplement is "natural" or "synthetic." If the label on the bottle indicates that a particular substance is inside, the contents of bottles of "natural" substance and "synthetic" substance are identical, although the source of the material may be different. There may be a difference, however, in the purity of a supplement depending on the process used in its preparation. Also, many supplemental materials are compressed into pills that may contain an "inert" filler to maintain the pill's shape.

Therefore, when choosing a dietary supplement, you must know more about its manufacture than simply whether it is "natural" or "synthetic." This is yet another reason why many nutritionists recommend that minerals and vitamins be acquired in food and not pills.

It should be noted that dietary supplements containing proteins and nucleic acids (DNA or RNA) are not absorbed intact from the gastrointestinal tract. These molecules are broken down into their constituent amino acids or nucleosides by digestive processes. Therefore, claims by manufacturers, advertisers, and journalists about the health benefits derived from ingesting these substances are most likely attributable to placebo effects, as the proteins and nucleic acids themselves cannot be directly utilized.

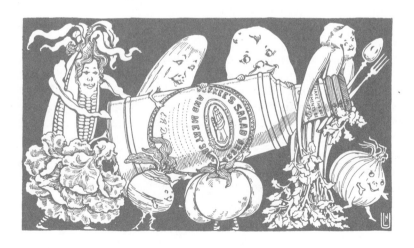

> Americans will have to change their lifestyle—their beliefs, attitudes, and practices regarding eating and exercise—if we are to solve the problem of obesity.
>
> **National Institutes of Health**

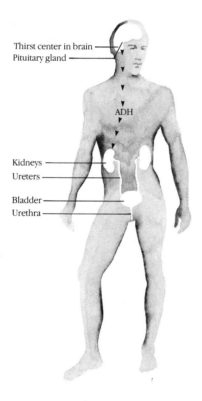

Figure 4-7
Maintaining water balance. Waste products, small molecules, and water are removed from the blood by the urinary system: the kidneys filter the blood to produce urine, which is transported to the bladder by the ureters. Urine in the bladder is eliminated from the body via the urethra. **Antidiuretic hormone** (ADH) from the posterior part of the pituitary gland controls the amount of water in urine. When body water is low, "thirst centers" in the brain motivate drinking.

Water

Water is also an essential nutrient. The human body is about 60 percent to 70 percent water by weight. Water is the principal constituent of the blood and is the major component of all cells, providing the medium in which all the cell's activities take place.

Body water is maintained at a relatively constant level by sophisticated control mechanisms involving the nervous and endocrine systems and the kidneys (see Figure 4-7). If body water is low, a person experiences thirst, which motivates drinking. Low body water also activates a hormonal mechanism that reduces the production of urine. If you have taken in a large amount of fluid, certain hormones will induce your kidneys to form large amounts of urine in order to reduce the total amount of body water.

The mechanisms that control the amount of body water are highly efficient. Unless you are ill or are in an unusually harsh environment, you needn't be much concerned about the amount of water in your body. If the amount is too low, you will know because you will feel thirsty. If your body water is excessive, you will restore your natural balance by excreting the excess.

The popular maxim that you should drink eight glasses of water a day is partially correct. The average adult loses about that much body water each day through urine, sweat, moisture in expired air, and feces. This water loss is partially offset by drinking pure water, but water is also ingested in other fluids and in foods.

> One out of four Americans are overweight.
> Thirty-seven percent of adults are on diets but
> only three percent manage to lose weight and
> keep it off.
>
> **National Center for Health Statistics**
> **1985**

Food for Energy

In addition to supplying the basic materials for the body's cells, tissues, and organs, food is the source of energy for life. All living things need a continuous supply of energy to live and to be well. The ultimate source of energy for all complex organisms on earth is sunlight, which is captured by green plants and used to manufacture plant material. Plants transform solar energy into chemical energy that is stored in the plants' molecules. When humans eat plant material or when they eat an animal that has eaten plant material, the chemical energy becomes available to them.

Energy transformations in living things are discussed in terms of calories. A **calorie** is defined as the amount of heat energy necessary to raise one gram of water from 14.5° Celsius to 15.5° Celsius. A **nutritional calorie,** or kilocalorie, which is what weight watchers watch, is defined as 1000 calories and is often written with a capital "C." In this book when we speak of "calories" what we are actually referring to is kilocalories.

Animals, including human beings, derive their energy from the breakdown of carbohydrates, fats, and proteins. Carbohydrates and proteins supply approximately 4 calories per gram, and fats supply approximately 9 calories per gram. Virtually every cell in the body is capable of the series of chemical transformations necessary to extract chemical energy from these nutrient molecules. The process of breaking down molecules to derive energy and to obtain material for synthesis of cellular molecules is called **metabolism.**

Energy from nutrient molecules is derived most efficiently when liberated in the presence of oxygen, which is one reason why you breathe. In the presence of oxygen, energy in the nutrient molecules is released, and in the process the nutrient molecules are broken down into carbon dioxide and water, which are eliminated from the body in expired air, urine, and sweat.

Energy is needed to support three major processes: **basal metabolism,** which is the minimum energy required to keep the body alive; physical activity (the things you do when you're not completely at rest); and growth. The energy to support basal metabolism keeps cells functioning, maintains the body temperature within its normal limits, and keeps the heart, lungs, kidneys, and other internal organs functioning. The basal energy usage for adults, which is called the **basal metabolic rate** (BMR), is about 1100 calories per day for women and 1300 for men.

Because muscle tissue requires more maintenance energy at rest than fat tissue does, lean people usually have a higher BMR than fat people. The BMR is greatest in infancy when the body is growing rapidly and tends to decline as you get older. This means that even if you maintain the same food intake and expend the same number of calories in physical activities each day throughout adulthood, you may develop an overweight problem in middle age because of the decrease in your BMR.

In addition to the energy you need for basal metabolism, you use energy in physical activity: walking, talking, working, and so on. The amount of energy expended for these activities depends on how strenuous the activity is, how long it is engaged in, the body's size, and the environmental temperature. It takes more energy to be active in hot weather than in moderate temperatures, and it takes more energy to maintain body temperature when the weather is cold.

Energy is also needed whenever the body produces more cells than are needed to replace ones that periodically die. Thus, all young people need additional energy for growth and physical activity. Energy is also needed to produce new cells to repair injuries.

Because the total daily energy needs of a particular person vary a great deal depending on his or her level of physical activity, it is virtually impossible—without first doing sophisticated scientific tests—to tell people what their energy intake each day should be. Fortunately, people do not need a

scientific determination of their personal energy needs. Their bodies do this for them. You know your energy needs are being met if you feel alert and healthy and if you are not overweight or underweight (the control of body weight is discussed in Chapter 7).

Nutrition and the Brain

The brain, like all other organs in the body, requires a balanced supply of nutrients in order to function properly. Because the brain controls moods, thoughts, and behaviors, your emotions and mental abilities are likely to be affected by what you eat. Studies have shown that the levels of certain neurotransmitters (discussed in Chapter 3) in the brain are modified by the ingestion of certain nutrients (Wurtman, 1982). For example, the amount of the neurotransmitter serotonin in the brain is influenced by the blood levels of the amino acid tryptophan and by the relative proportions of carbohydrate recently eaten. A meal containing tryptophan (derived from dietary protein) and high in carbohydrate causes an increase in the synthesis of serotonin. Brain levels of the amino acid tyrosine, the precursor for the synthesis of the neurotransmitters dopa-

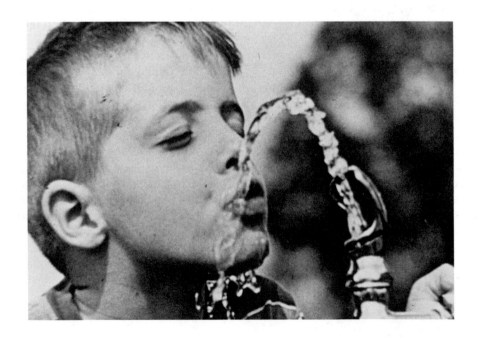

> He who doesn't mind his belly
> will hardly mind anything else.
> **Samuel Johnson**

mine, norepinephrine, and epinephrine, increase after the ingestion of protein (see Figure 3-4). Ingesting choline, a component of the dietary substance lecithin (found in egg yolk, liver, and soybeans) increases the level of the neurotransmitter acetylcholine.

It may be that moods, feelings, level of vitality, and sleep depend—at least to some degree—on the amounts of neurotransmitter precursor molecules eaten in meals. It is also possible that the administration of tryptophan, tyrosine, and choline (or lecithin) can be used therapeutically to treat certain mental disorders. Some preliminary experiments indicate that tryptophan may help induce sleep or relieve pain, that tyrosine may help relieve depression, and that choline may modify certain postural and motor disturbances.

Food can also affect thoughts and feelings through the body's response to carbohydrates—particularly to simple sugars such as sucrose, which is added to many cereals and "junk foods." The reactions people may experience include anxiety, trembling, fatigue, weakness, depression, and the inability to concentrate. Such symptoms usually occur within an hour after consuming high-sugar foods. This response is called **reactive hypoglycemia** or **idiopathic postprandial syndrome.** The cure is to avoid high-sugar junk foods.

The body has several homeostatic mechanisms that regulate the level of glucose in the blood. One of these mechanisms is the secretion of the hormone insulin from the pancreas whenever the blood level of glucose rises. When a person eats sucrose (and other carbohydrates), the sugar molecules absorbed through the intestines enter the blood. If the amount of sugar is high, the pancreas will secrete a large amount of insulin to restore the blood glucose to normal levels. Sometimes the burst of insulin released after ingestion of a lot of sugar (such as after a breakfast consisting of a couple of doughnuts and coffee with sugar) can be so potent that the blood sugar will rapidly drop far below its normal level.

It is known that very low blood sugar can produce feelings of fatigue, lassitude, irritability, grumpiness, and even mild depression. The cause of these feelings is simply that the brain is not getting enough energy-producing sugars from the blood. If these feelings appear within an hour or two after you eat foods high in simple sugars, it may be that you're one of the people whose insulin response to a sugar challenge is very strong. By cutting down on the amount of sugar-containing foods you eat at any one time, you may find yourself less bothered by highs and lows in your energy and moods.

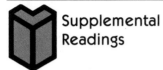

Supplemental Readings

"America's Sweet Tooth." *Newsweek,* August 26, 1985, 50. An analysis of the role of sugar in human health and disease and the risks and benefits of sugar substitutes.

Consumers Union. "The Vitamin Pushers." *Consumer Reports,* March 1986, 170. An analysis of the hype and marketing of vitamins, most of which are not needed by people with an adequate diet.

Erlichman, James. *Gluttons for Punishment.* Great Britain: Penguin Books, 1986. An American journalist who lives in London discusses and documents the health hazards of the foods we buy and eat.

Jacobson, Michael F. *Nutrition Scoreboard.* New York: Avon, 1975. A do-it-yourself guide to better eating and to evaluating foods for their nutritional value.

Lappe, Frances Moore. *Diet for a Small Planet.* New York: Ballentine, 1971. An excellent discussion of protein nutrition and methods of combining protein foods for optimal nutrition.

Nestle, Marion. *Nutrition in Clinical Practice.* Greenbrae, CA: Jones Medical Publications, 1985. A succinct and readable account of all aspects of human nutrition and its relation to health and disease.

Robertson, Laurel; Flinders, Carol; and **Godfrey, Bronwen,** *Laurel's Kitchen.* New York: Bantam, 1976. A nonfaddish guide to nutrition and diet with emphasis on whole fresh foods and vegetarianism.

Summary

In order to be healthy and well, people must obtain approximately forty essential nutrients in the proper amounts and proportions from food. These essential nutrients include eight amino acids: phenylalanine, tryptophan, valine, threonine, lysine, isoleucine, leucine, and methionine—which come from dietary sources of protein (meat, fish, eggs, dairy products, and grains and legumes). Linoleic acid, a lipid (fat) is also an essential nutrient, as are several kinds of minerals and vitamins.

Food also provides the energy for life. Food energy, measured in calories, comes principally from carbohydrates (sugars) and triglyceride, a type of fat.

Water is also an essential nutrient. The body has sophisticated mechanisms to regulate the amount of water in the body.

Thoughts and feelings can be affected by the kind of food that is ingested. The levels of certain neurotransmitters rise after their precursor molecules are ingested, which may affect brain functioning. Some people experience a mood change or feelings of fatigue or lassitude after eating a meal high in refined sugar. This occurs because the large dose of sugar produces a lowering of blood sugar (reactive hypoglycemia).

> We know more about what goes into a
> pair of socks than about what goes
> into our food.
>
> **Jonathan Aitken**
> **Member, British Parliament**

FOR YOUR HEALTH

Keep a Food Diary

Take the first step in assessing the nutritional adequacy of your diet by keeping a food diary. For at least four consecutive days, faithfully record *everything* you eat as well as the circumstances of your eating behavior. Construct and use a food data chart like the accompanying sample to record your data each day. Carry the chart with you wherever you go, so that you can make entries through the day. To use the food data chart:

1. Record every type of food eaten.
2. List amounts as weight, number of items, or volume.
3. Obtain the number of calories for each food from any calorie-counting guide or nutritional handbook.
4. Record the time of day each food item is eaten.
5. Note whether the food item is eaten as part of a meal or as a snack.
6. Record the exact locale in which each food item is eaten.
7. Note whether you eat alone, with your family, with co-workers, or with any specific individuals outside the family.

8. Note whether you are hungry when you eat. You can record the degree of hunger by using entries such as "very," "so-so," "a little," or "no."
9. Record any feelings other than hunger you experience before eating each food item. Are you depressed, bored, nervous, angry, happy, fidgety, deep in thought, lonely, tired, irritable, "blah," fine?

Analyze Your Diet

1. Using the data from your food diary, make a list of the foods that add calories to your diet but little nutrition. For most people these foods include sugar, cookies, candy, cake, ice cream, butter, soft drinks, potato chips, crackers, and alcoholic beverages.
2. How many foods do you eat that contribute fiber to your diet?
3. Do you usually eat some amount of complete protein at each meal?
4. What is the daily average of servings of fresh fruit and vegetables you eat?
5. What is your daily average intake of calories?

(Continued on next page.)

FOR YOUR HEALTH

Daily Food Record

Food	Amount	Calories	Time	Meal or snack	Where	With whom	Hungry?	Feelings

CHAPTER FIVE

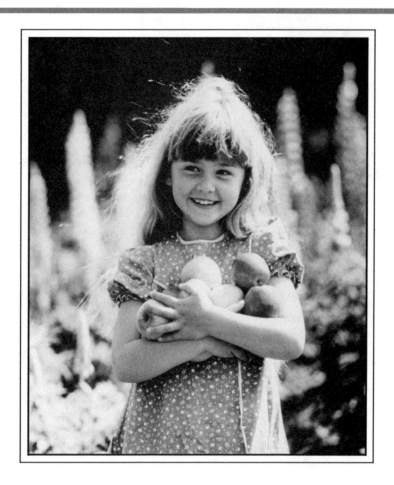

How to select a personal diet plan
that leads to optimum health

Choosing a Healthy Diet

The fact that man and all other surviving animal species continue to inhabit the earth is the clearest proof that, during the whole of their tens of millions of years of evolution they and their ancestors have selected foods that have supplied their nutritional needs.

John Yudkin
Emeritus Professor of Nutrition
University of London

We are fortunate to live in a country where good, nutritious food is abundant. For most of us, good nutrition is a matter of informed choice and not a fantasy made unrealizable by harsh environmental and economic circumstances. Unfortunately, this is not the case for people in many other parts of the world, where low personal incomes or limited food resources make obtaining adequate amounts of the essential nutrients and calories to provide energy for healthy and fulfilled living one of life's constant problems.

To someone from one of the many countries where food resources are severely limited, a walk through the aisles of one of our supermarkets would surely create wonderment that we have any nutritional problems at all. But as we indicated in Chapter 4, the American diet is associated with a high incidence of heart disease, high blood pressure, diabetes, tooth decay, obesity, and cancer of various organs. Many studies show that certain all-too-common dietary habits are related to the development of disease and other manifestations of ill health. These unhealthful dietary habits include consuming too much cholesterol, saturated fat, refined sugar, and salt; eating too few complex carbohydrates; and eating more calories than one expends.

The reason that so many people do not take full advantage of our nutritional resources to produce optimum health, and in some cases harm themselves with the foods they eat, is that most people do not plan their diets. As D. M. Hegsted (1977), former professor of nutrition at the Harvard School of Public Health, has noted, "the diet we eat today was not planned or developed for any particular purpose. It is a happenstance related to our affluence, the productivity of our farmers, and the activities of our food industry."

And those who might like to plan their diets carefully are often uncertain about how best to do so. They distrust food faddists who insist in the virtues of one strict diet or another. And they do not know what to make of the often conflicting information from hundreds of nutrition "experts" who promote particular theories about nutrition on TV, in magazine articles, and in books. If any of the dozens of diet books that have their day on the best-seller list were truly helpful, they would not be replaced by the steady stream of books with the "latest" information.

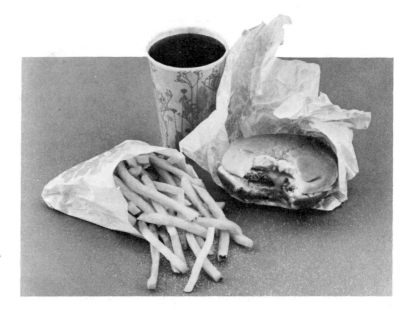

Figure 5-1
A favorite American fast-food meal.
There is nothing wrong with eating
like this once in a while. But fast
foods tend to be high in calories, fats,
salt, and sugar, making them too
unbalanced to serve as a normal
healthy diet.

Most of the essential nutrients are known, as are the potential roles of certain foods in disease development or prevention. Thus, a healthy diet includes providing the essential nutrients in amounts consistent with personal needs, obtaining only the calories needed to maintain normal weight, and choosing to eat a variety of foods so that taking in too much of one substance or too little of another is avoided. This chapter offers some guidelines for formulating a personal diet plan that accomplishes these nutritional goals.

Dietary Requirements: The RDA

In Chapter 4 we pointed out that humans require about 40 essential nutrients—certain amino acids, a lipid (linoleic acid), vitamins, and minerals—and a supply of energy (calories), all of which must be obtained from the environment in the form of food. To help determine the amounts of these nutrients that promote health, the Food and Nutrition Board of the National Research Council, a committee of the National Academy of Sciences, periodically sets forth recommendations for the nutritional requirements of Americans. These recommendations, which are based on the most recent research data, are known as the **Recommended Dietary Allowances** or RDA (see Table 5-1). The World Health Organization (WHO) also produces a set of dietary standards that differs only slightly from the RDA.

One kind of research study on which the RDA is based is called a **balance study,** which involves the controlled elimination of a particular nutrient from the diets of volunteer test subjects followed by the gradual replacement of that nutrient. The amount above which the nutrient is not utilized by the body and is broken down and excreted is monitored and recorded. When the body cannot utilize additional amounts of the nutrient being supplied, the nutrient is said to be in balance.

Because all people are genetically different, their requirements for a given nutrient are usually different, reflecting their differing biochemical makeups (see Figure 5-3). Often the results of research investigations report the *average* amount of the nutrient under study necessary for balance, although no person in the test group may actually require that specific amount. Some may need more and some less. There is nothing sacred about an average value; it is simply a convenient way to analyze several different, although related, numbers.

Realizing that many people have a greater-than-average requirement for any given nutrient, the National Research Council sets the RDA about 30 percent higher than the average, which, on a statistical basis, should accommodate virtually all healthy individuals in the population, although it may leave out a few.

Of the approximately 40 essential nutrients, the RDA lists values for protein, ten vitamins, and six minerals. It is assumed that if the nutrients listed in the RDA are acquired in the diet in the recom-

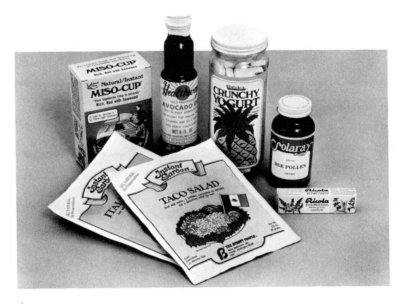

Figure 5-2
Food faddists often rely on diets made up solely of items purchased in health food stores. Not only has it *not* been scientifically proven that such foods are nutritionally superior to supermarket varieties, but they tend to be much more costly.

mended amounts, all other nutrients will also be acquired in the diet. The Recommended Dietary Allowance for protein assumes a diet containing a reasonable amount of animal protein (meat, fish, eggs, milk, and cheese) to provide the eight essential amino acids. If we were a country of vegetarians whose main source of protein is corn, the protein requirements in the RDA would be higher to account for the fact that corn is deficient in several of the amino acids essential for humans.

The RDA is designed for people who are in reasonably good health — that is, people who are not suffering from any obvious clinical disease and who are not under an unusual amount of stress. The RDA also lists nutrient requirements for children and for pregnant and lactating women.

By eating reasonable quantities of a variety of foods, almost all healthy people can acquire the essential nutrients in amounts suggested by the RDA. Many people, however, do not plan their diets carefully and, as food-consumption surveys show, do not acquire the RDA of certain nutrients. You can determine whether your diet contains the amounts of nutrients listed in the RDA by consulting summaries of the nutrient composition of foods in food tables (USDA Handbook No. 8; Bowes and Church, 1980). These summaries list the essential amino acids, carbohydrates, fats, and many minerals and vitamins in portions of foods in common use.

Diet surveys show that most Americans consume less calcium than is needed to build and maintain strong bones. Before the age of about 40, less-than-adequate calcium intake rarely produces symptoms, but in later life, inadequate calcium increases the risk of weak bones, a condition called **osteoporosis** (see Box 24-2). Each year in the U.S.

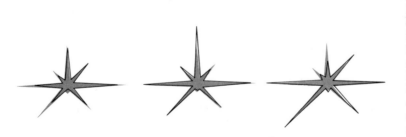

Figure 5-3
Biochemical individuality. These drawings represent the biochemical individuality for three different people. Each point in a star represents the amount of a particular nutrient needed by that individual for nutritional balance. Notice that each individual differs from the hypothetical "average" shown in color. For each person the amount of some nutrients needed for balance is greater than the average, and the amount needed for other nutrients is less than the average.

Table 5-1
Recommended Daily Dietary Allowances, Revised 1980*

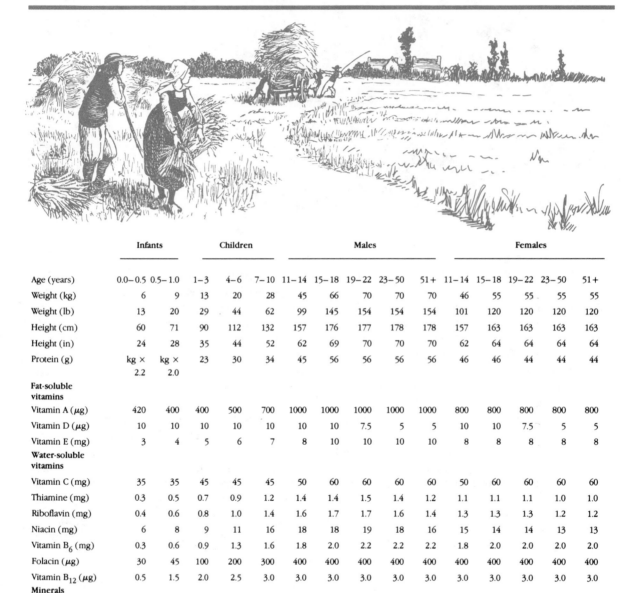

	Infants		Children			Males					Females				
Age (years)	0.0–0.5	0.5–1.0	1–3	4–6	7–10	11–14	15–18	19–22	23–50	51+	11–14	15–18	19–22	23–50	51+
Weight (kg)	6	9	13	20	28	45	66	70	70	70	46	55	55	55	55
Weight (lb)	13	20	29	44	62	99	145	154	154	154	101	120	120	120	120
Height (cm)	60	71	90	112	132	157	176	177	178	178	157	163	163	163	163
Height (in)	24	28	35	44	52	62	69	70	70	70	62	64	64	64	64
Protein (g)	kg × 2.2	kg × 2.0	23	30	34	45	56	56	56	56	46	46	44	44	44
Fat-soluble vitamins															
Vitamin A (μg)	420	400	400	500	700	1000	1000	1000	1000	1000	800	800	800	800	800
Vitamin D (μg)	10	10	10	10	10	10	10	7.5	5	5	10	10	7.5	5	5
Vitamin E (mg)	3	4	5	6	7	8	10	10	10	10	8	8	8	8	8
Water-soluble vitamins															
Vitamin C (mg)	35	35	45	45	45	50	60	60	60	60	50	60	60	60	60
Thiamine (mg)	0.3	0.5	0.7	0.9	1.2	1.4	1.4	1.5	1.4	1.2	1.1	1.1	1.1	1.0	1.0
Riboflavin (mg)	0.4	0.6	0.8	1.0	1.4	1.6	1.7	1.7	1.6	1.4	1.3	1.3	1.3	1.2	1.2
Niacin (mg)	6	8	9	11	16	18	18	19	18	16	15	14	14	13	13
Vitamin B_6 (mg)	0.3	0.6	0.9	1.3	1.6	1.8	2.0	2.2	2.2	2.2	1.8	2.0	2.0	2.0	2.0
Folacin (μg)	30	45	100	200	300	400	400	400	400	400	400	400	400	400	400
Vitamin B_{12} (μg)	0.5	1.5	2.0	2.5	3.0	3.0	3.0	3.0	3.0	3.0	3.0	3.0	3.0	3.0	3.0
Minerals															
Calcium (mg)	360	540	800	800	800	1200	1200	800	800	800	1200	1200	800	800	800
Phosphorus (mg)	240	360	800	800	800	1200	1200	800	800	800	1200	1200	800	800	800
Magnesium (mg)	50	70	150	200	250	350	400	350	350	350	300	300	300	300	300
Iron (mg)	10	15	15	10	10	18	18	10	10	10	18	18	18[†]	18[†]	10
Zinc (mg)	3	5	10	10	10	15	15	15	15	15	15	15	15	15	15
Iodine (μg)	40	50	70	90	120	150	150	150	150	150	150	150	150	150	150

*The allowances are intended to provide for individual variations among most normal persons as they live in the United States under usual environmental stresses. Diets should be based on a variety of common foods in order to provide other nutrients for which human requirements have been less well defined.

†The amount of iron needed by pregnant and lactating women must sometimes be met by supplementation with 30–60 mg iron daily.
Data from the Food and Nutrition Board, National Academy of Sciences National Research Council.

> From birth, human beings are
> highly distinctive in both
> microscopic and gross anatomy,
> in the functioning of their organs,
> in the composition of body fluids,
> and in their nutritional
> requirements.
> **Roger J. Williams**

osteoporosis is associated with about 1 to 2 million bone fractures among elderly people.

The keys to building and maintaining strong bones are eating foods that contain adequate amounts of calcium, exercising regularly, limiting alcohol consumption (it blocks absorption of calcium), and avoiding smoking. Good sources of dietary calcium are dairy products and green leafy vegetables such as spinach.

Because nutritional requirement studies are usually carried out over a short period and on a reasonably young and healthy middle-class population (American college students), the RDA is often criticized as being an inadequate standard for the nation. For example, one of the major criticisms of the RDA is that it only provides levels needed to avoid clinically obvious deficiency conditions and may not reflect the amounts needed to achieve a state of optimum health and well-being or to protect against infection or illness.

The controversy over the optimum dietary amount of vitamin C provides a good example. In the nineteenth century the British navy ordered that all of its seamen receive a daily ration of citrus juice (hence the nickname "limeys") in order to prevent scurvy, a debilitating disease that frequently resulted in death. In the twentieth century it was discovered that the "antiscurvy factor" was ascorbic acid, otherwise known as vitamin C, and nutritionists came to recognize that a certain amount of vitamin C is necessary in the diet each day to prevent scurvy. For most Americans that level is about 10 mg a day; the RDA for vitamin C is 60 mg.

In recent years serious question has been raised about whether 60 mg of vitamin C per day is adequate for optimum health, especially when a person is under stress. Certainly it is enough to prevent scurvy, but some scientists suggest that the optimum level of vitamin C might be closer to 1000–2000 mg per day (Williams, 1977). They support their ideas with several arguments:

1. In the course of evolution humans have lost the capacity to manufacture vitamin C; hence they are totally dependent on food for it. Animals, such as dogs and sheep, that manufacture their own vitamin C make, on an equivalent body weight basis with humans, 1000–10,000 mg of vitamin C per day. Although it is not always correct to extrapolate research findings in other animals to humans, these data nonetheless are suggestive.

2. In his book *Vitamin C and the Common Cold,* Linus Pauling (1970) points out that only recently in human history have people become primarily meat eaters and consumers of refined sugar and flour. He estimates that in earlier times, when people consumed more fresh vegetables and fruit, their diet contained levels of vitamin C in the 1000-mg range.

3. Some clinical studies support the idea that doses of vitamin C of 1000 mg per day are

able to reduce the severity of colds in human test groups (Truswell, 1986).

4. There are thousands of people who take 1000 mg or more of vitamin C per day and who experience beneficial effects, such as a noticeable reduction in the frequency or severity of colds and a general feeling of being invigorated—although it may be that these are placebo effects.

The RDA may be an insufficient guide for yet another reason: namely, that some people, probably a small percentage of the population, require as much as 10 to 100 times the RDA of a particular vitamin, mineral, or amino acid because of an unusually high genetically determined biochemical need for that substance. For example, there are several rare diseases, called **vitamin dependency illnesses,** that are relieved by the ingestion of high amounts of certain vitamins. If people with vitamin dependency illnesses do not receive the amounts of the nutrients they need, they suffer from illnesses that may range from mild to severe, depending on the nutrient and their individual biochemical makeup.

It is possible that some forms of mental illness might be related to vitamin dependency illnesses (Pauling, 1968). For example, some people who suffer the abnormal mental symptoms diagnosed as schizophrenia have been helped with massive doses (as much as 3000–6000 mg per day) of niacin (vitamin B_3). The RDA for niacin is 18 mg per day. Such results suggest that the aberrations in thought and behavior that led to these people being classified as schizophrenic were the result of a niacin deficiency. For some genetic/biochemical reason, a few individuals may have requirements for niacin that are much greater than those of most other people, and without increased niacin they suffer dire consequences. That does not mean that everyone with the diagnosis of schizophrenia suffers from niacin deficiency. But it *is* evidence that not everyone's unique biochemical needs may be adequately met by the levels of nutrients suggested by the RDA. It is possible, for example, that some individuals might benefit from an increased intake of niacin, ascorbic acid, or other nutrients in ways that would not be detected clinically. They might just "feel better."

It should be noted that very large doses of vitamins—especially vitamins A and D, niacin, and vitamin B_6 for some people—can be dangerously toxic (Rudman and Williams, 1983). Moreover, some people experience gastrointestinal upset and diarrhea when they take massive doses of vitamin C, although there is no evidence that large doses of vitamin C (1000–10,000 mg daily) cause harm.

In 1985 the Food and Nutrition Board of the National Research Council of the National Academy of Sciences announced that it would be unable to issue the tenth edition of the RDAs as scheduled because of "persistent difficulty in resolving scientific differences of opinion about the interpretation of data on certain nutrients and consequently on the RDAs for those nutrients." Some of the FNB's scientific considerations included whether to define the RDA in terms of preventing clinically identifiable deficiency diseases or in terms of promoting optimal health, and various methodological issues related to the gathering of nutritional data. The FNB specifically cited the need to resolve issues for several

```
NUTRITION INFORMATION
PER SERVING
SERVING SIZE: 1 OZ.
   (ABOUT ¼ CUP)
SERVINGS PER PACKAGE: 24
                                    WITH
                                    ½ CUP
                                    VITAMIN D
                                    FORTIFIED
                           CEREAL   WHOLE
                           ALONE    MILK
CALORIES          100      180
PROTEIN           3 G.     7 G.
CARBOHYDRATE      23 G.    29 G.
FAT               0        4 G.
PERCENTAGES OF U.S. RECOM-
MENDED DAILY ALLOWANCES
(U.S. RDA)
PROTEIN           4%       10%
VITAMIN A         25%      30%
VITAMIN C         *        *
THIAMINE          25%      30%
RIBOFLAVIN        25%      35%
NIACIN            25%      25%
CALCIUM           *        15%
IRON              4%       4%
VITAMIN D         10%      25%
VITAMIN B₆        25%      30%
FOLIC ACID        25%      25%
VITAMIN B₁₂       25%      30%
PHOSPHORUS        6%       15%
*CONTAINS LESS THAN 2% OF
THE U.S. RDA OF THESE NU-
TRIENTS.
```

Figure 5-4A
The product labels of many foods list the percentages of dietary requirements in a measured serving of the product. The standards used for product labeling, known as the U.S. Recommended *Daily* Allowances, are set by the U.S. Food and Drug Administration and are based on the U.S. Recommended *Dietary* Allowances established by the Food and Nutrition Board of the National Academy of Sciences.

Vegetable protein, onion, cornflour, leek, tomato, carrot, salt, beef fat, edible starch, guar gum, autolysed yeast, hydrolysed protein, monosodium glutamate, wheatflour, tricalcium phosphate, sugar, caramel, ascorbic acid, flavour, emulsifier, nicotinic acid, reduced iron, antioxidant, retinyl palmitate, thiamine hydrochloride, riboflavin and cholecalciferol.

Ingredients in a commercial "beef" casserole

nutrients including carbohydrates; saturated fat; cholesterol; vitamins A, B_6, and C; and the minerals calcium, iron, magnesium, zinc, selenium, and copper. Until the scientific issues are resolved the 1980 RDAs remain the most useful guideline.

In Search of the "Right" Diet: Orthomolecular Nutrition

Unfortunately, at the present time there is no way to determine for any individual what an optimum diet should be. Perhaps some day there will be an inexpensive set of physiological and biochemical tests that can be administered to people to determine their precise nutritional needs for optimum health. It would then be possible to design a diet that provides all the nutrients a person needs.

The idea of providing every person with an individually tailored chemically perfect diet is expressed by the term **orthomolecular nutrition.** "Ortho" is a Greek word meaning "right." In the words of Arthur B. Robinson (1974), former director of the Linus Pauling Institute of Science and Medicine, orthomolecular nutrition

would measure the amounts of all the chemical substances normally present in the body, decide what amounts of each of those substances would be consistent with optimum health, and then adjust the concentrations in the body to be those consistent with optimum health. This process of measurement,

evaluation and adjustment would comprise orthomolecular diagnosis and therapy. This does not mean that the [approach] could give the person optimum happiness, but could provide the person with a chemical environment best suited to individual needs.

The orthomolecular approach to preventing or reversing illness is termed **orthomolecular medicine,** or in the case of behavioral illness, **orthomolecular psychiatry.** Research is being carried out to try to develop the techniques by which orthomolecular nutrition can be practiced. Until more is known, however, people will have to adjust their diets by trial and error, using as guides the RDA and what nutritionist Roger Williams (1977) calls "body wisdom"—awareness of how the body reacts to what it is fed.

INGREDIENTS: Wheat bran, milled yellow corn, sugar, malted cereal syrup, salt, coconut oil, sodium ascorbate (vitamin C), niacinamide, reduced iron, pyridoxine hydrochloride (vitamin B_6), thiamine mononitrate (vitamin B_1), BHA (a preservative), folic acid, and vitamin B_{12}, BHT added to packaging material to help preserve freshness.

Figure 5–4B
Many labels list the ingredients in a product by weight, from greatest to least. The label below shows that wheat bran is the greatest constituent of this product, but note that the third and fourth substances listed are sugars. This product is probably relatively high in sugar content.

> The clue to a good diet is variation; use different foods, change brands frequently, and never use the same recipe twice. . . . Minimize the intake of packaged foods since they contain additives of unknown toxicity.
>
> **Harold Morowitz**

Planning a Healthy Diet

In 1977 the U.S. Senate Select Committee on Nutrition and Human Needs, now the Senate Agricultural Subcommittee on Nutrition, proposed a set of dietary guidelines intended to improve "the health and quality of life of the American people." It was the committee's belief that

> demands for better nutrition could bring a halt to the expansion and/or use of less nutritious or so-called "empty calorie" or "junk" foods in the American diet, as well as make nutrition the rallying point of public demands for *better* health, as opposed to *more* medical care. Most importantly, nutrition knowledge will become a means by which Americans can begin to take responsibility for maintaining their health and reducing their risk of illness.

In setting dietary goals for the country, the committee established guidelines intended to meet the RDA, as well as to focus on specific dietary practices that would likely lead to improved health and reduce the frequency of illness (see Figure 5-5). The committee's recommendations can be summarized as follows:

1. To avoid becoming overweight, consume only as much energy (calories) as you expend. If you are overweight, decrease your energy intake and increase your energy expenditure (see Chapter 7).

2. Eat enough complex carbohydrates and "naturally occurring" sugars to account for about 48 percent of your energy intake. To do so, eat fresh fruits, vegetables, whole grains, and products made with stone-ground flour (sufficient heat is generated in steel-rolled flour to destroy many of the B vitamins and vitamin E); restrict the intake of refined sugars and foods that contain sucrose, corn sugar, and corn syrup to about 10 percent of your energy intake.

3. Limit your overall fat consumption to approximately 30 percent of your energy intake. Restrict your consumption of saturated fats, whether obtained from animal or vegetable sources, to about 10 percent of your total energy intake, and ingest polyunsaturated fats to account for about 20 percent energy intake. To do so, choose meats, poultry, fish, and dairy products that are low in saturated fat.

4. Maintain your cholesterol consumption at about 300 mg per day. You can do so by controlling the amount obtained from milk products, eggs, butterfat, and other high-cholesterol sources (see Table 4-7).

5. Limit your intake of sodium to less than 5 g per day by controlling your consumption of salt and processed foods high in salt (see Table 4-9).

6. Reduce your consumption of artificial colorings, artificial flavorings, thickeners, preservatives, and other food additives.

The diet of the average
person is between 60
percent and 70 percent
fat and sugar.
Rudolph Ballentine, M.D.

Some critics of the Senate committee's dietary goals argue that they are based on probable, rather than proven, relationships between diet and disease. They also argue that even if research proved a relationship between certain dietary habits and some diseases, any suggested dietary changes should come only after scientific studies indicate that the changes prevent the occurrence of the diseases and bring about the betterment of health. These criticisms have merit. They do not, however, alter the fact that the Senate committee's dietary goals are important. Nutritionists D. M. Hegsted (1977) answers the critics with this counter-argument:

The diet has become increasingly rich — rich in meat, other sources of saturated fat and cholesterol, and sugar. It should be emphasized that this diet which affluent people generally consume everywhere is associated with a similar disease pattern — high rates of ischemic heart disease, certain forms of cancer, diabetes, and obesity . . . The risks associated with eating this diet are demonstrably large. The question to be asked, therefore, is not why should we change our diet but why not? What are the risks associated with eating less meat, less fat, less

Figure 5-5
Dietary goals for individuals recommended by the Senate Select Committee on Nutrition and Human Needs. These goals are compared to present and past consumption.

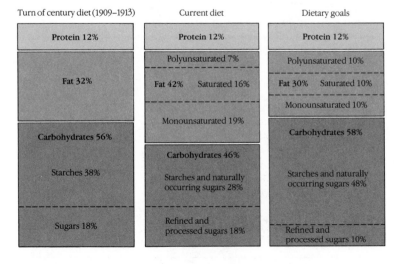

> **Many people have difficulty understanding that the same substance can be both "toxic" and "safe," depending on how much is used and how it is used. Especially, they do not recognize the biological truth that there is no substance so toxic that the body cannot manage some tiny amount of it harmlessly; and there is none so safe that a great enough excess will not do injury.**
>
> **Ronald S. Deutsch, *Realities of Nutrition***

saturated fat, less cholesterol, less sugar, less salt, and more fruits, vegetables, unsaturated fat and cereal products—especially whole grain cereals? There are none that can be identified and important benefits can be expected.

A dietary plan that meets the goals set forth by the Senate Select Committee (see Table 5-2) emphasizes the consumption of lean meat, fish, and poultry for protein, and fresh fruits and vegetables as sources of carbohydrates. Required fats are obtained from vegetable sources and from low-fat dairy products. This is a hypothetical plan; it is not intended to prescribe the one and only diet for optimum health. There are many possible diets that fulfill the body's needs for the essential nutrients and other food substances, including fiber, which appear to contribute to good health.

A series of dietary guidelines have been issued jointly by the Department of Agriculture and the Department of Health and Human Services (see Box 5-1). These guidelines are much like those suggested by the Senate Select Committee in 1977. Unlike the Select Committee's, however, they contain no specific quantities for any nutrients.

The National Academy of Sciences and the National Cancer Institute have issued reports recommending certain dietary guidelines that might help to prevent cancer. These guidelines are discussed in Chapter 17 and listed in Table 17-4.

Table 5-2
Daily Diet Based on Goals Set Forth by U.S. Senate Select Committee on Nutrition and Human Needs*

Food and portion	Child 6–8 years	Woman 20–54 years	Man 20–54 years
Eggs (each)	0.4	0.8	0.4
Nonfat milk (cups)	2.9	1.2	1.7
Lean meat, boned and cooked (oz.)	1.3	1.6	2.7
Poultry and fish, cooked and boned (oz.)	1.1	1.6	2.3
Mature beans or peas, cooked (tbsp.)	1.9	1.8	2.0
Bread or equivalent in bakery products (slices)	7.8	8.0	12.9
Cereal or pasta (oz.)	2.9	3.5	2.7
Vegetables and fruit (cups)	2.0	2.5	2.6
Margarine, oil (tbsp.)	3.4	2.9	3.6
Sugar, sweets (tsp.)	6.0	4.7	6.7

*This suggested diet meets the RDA for energy (calories), vitamin A, thiamine, riboflavin, niacin, vitamin C, calcium, and iron.
Data from B. B. Peterkin, R. L. Kerr, and C. J. Shore, "Diets That Meet Dietary Goals," *Journal of Nutrition Education,* 10 (1978), 15.

BOX 5-1

SUMMARY OF U.S. DEPARTMENT OF AGRICULTURE/HEW DIETARY GUIDELINES FOR AMERICANS

1 Eat a variety of foods daily including selections of fruits; vegetables; whole grain and enriched breads, cereals, and grain products; milk, cheese, and yogurt; meats, poultry, fish, and eggs; and legumes (dry peas and beans).

2 Maintain acceptable body weight by losing excess body weight and improving eating habits.

To Lose Weight

- Increase physical activity
- Eat less fat and fatty foods
- Eat less sugar and sweets
- Avoid too much alcohol

To Improve Eating Habits

- Eat slowly
- Prepare smaller portions
- Avoid "seconds"

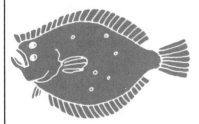

3 Avoid too much fat, saturated fat, and cholesterol.

- Choose lean meat, fish, poultry, dry beans and peas as your protein sources
- Moderate your use of eggs and organ meats (such as liver)

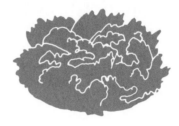

- Limit your intake of butter, cream, hydrogenated margarines, shortenings and coconut oil, and foods made from such products
- Trim excess fat off meats
- Broil, bake, or boil rather than fry
- Read labels carefully to determine both amount and types of fat contained in foods

4 Eat foods with adequate starch and fiber.

- Substitute starches for fats and sugars
- Select foods that are good sources of fiber and starch, such as whole-grain breads and cereals, fruits and vegetables, beans, peas, and nuts

5 Avoid too much sugar.

- Use less of all sugars, including white sugar, brown sugar, raw sugar, honey, and syrups
- Eat less of foods containing these sugars, such as candy, soft drinks, ice cream, cakes and cookies
- Select fresh fruits or fruits canned without sugar or light syrup rather than heavy syrup
- Read food labels for clues on sugar content—if the names sucrose, glucose, maltose, dextrose, lactose, fructose, or syrups appear first, then there is a large amount of sugar
- Remember, how often you eat sugar is as important as how much sugar you eat

6 Avoid too much sodium.

- Learn to enjoy the unsalted flavors of foods
- Cook with only small amounts of added salt
- Add little or no salt to food at the table
- Limit your intake of salty foods, such as potato chips, pretzels, salted nuts and popcorn, condiments (soy sauce, steak sauce, garlic salt), cheese, pickled foods, and cured meats
- Read food labels carefully to determine the amounts of sodium in processed foods and snack items

7 If you drink alcohol, do so in moderation.

- Refrain from sustained or heavy drinking (more than two drinks per day).

> Last year each of us, on average, swallowed three pounds of flavorings, coloring, preservatives, glazes, antispattering agents, emulsifiers, bleaches, and other additives with our food.
>
> **Joan Morgan, M.D.**

The Vegetarian Option

Properly planned vegetarian diets can meet the body's nutritional needs. There are several kinds of vegetarian diets. **Lacto-ovovegan** diets include both dairy products and eggs; **lactovegan** diets include dairy products but no eggs; **ovovegan** diets include eggs but no dairy products; and **vegan** diets include neither dairy products nor eggs and are therefore composed solely of grains, legumes, nuts, seeds, fruits, and vegetables.

People choose to be vegetarians for various reasons. Among them are:

1. To avoid killing animals—either killing them oneself or killing by others. Some people who have a strong affection for other animals, and feel a certain biological and spiritual kinship with them, object to killing them for food.

2. To contribute to the more efficient utilization of world protein supplies. It takes approximately 10 pounds of livestock feed, usually corn or soybeans, to produce 1 pound of meat. Obviously the 10 pounds of corn or soybeans could feed more people than 1 pound of meat can. With the population of the earth doubling about every 30 years, some people feel a moral obligation to avoid overconsuming food resources in the hope

that ways will be found to distribute the world food supply more equitably.

3. To contribute to a more healthy personal life. Avoiding meat eliminates whatever health risks may be associated with excessive meat eating (and it does appear that there are some, as discussed earlier). Also, eating more grains and vegetables reduces the risks associated with low-fiber diets.

Vegetarians must plan their meals carefully, however, to be sure that protein sources are complemented to provide adequate amounts of the essential amino acids (protein complementarity was discussed in Chapter 4). Strict vegetarians (vegans), who eat neither dairy products nor eggs, may not acquire any vitamin B_{12} (cobalamin), so they should supplement their diets with this vitamin.

Coping with Food Additives

Most foods today are produced by a manufacturing technology that adds chemicals to them in order to produce texture, stability, flavor, color, longer shelf life, and sales appeal. At present, there are several thousand food additives approved by the federal government's Food and Drug Administration (FDA) for use in processed and manufactured foods, and it is estimated that the U.S. per capita consump-

Table 5-3
Seven Food Dyes That Remain in Use in American Foods
All of these dyes have been banned in one or more countries in Europe.

Dye	Uses	Pounds used (1984)	Toxicity
Red 3	Candy, pastries	241,265	Thyroid tumors
Red 40	Candy, pastries, drinks, pet foods	2,630,578	Lymphomas
Blue 1	Candy, pastries, drinks	260,417	Chromosomal damage
Blue 2	Candy, drinks, pet foods	101,223	Brain tumors
Green 3	Candy, drinks	3,597	Bladder tumors
Yellow 5	Drinks, pastries, pet foods	1,620,540	Tumors, allergies
Yellow 6	Drinks, pastries, candy	1,530,050	Tumors, allergies

tion of chemical additives is about 5 pounds a year. Besides these additives, large amounts of sugar and salt are added to many canned, packaged, and frozen foods (see Chapter 4).

Some additives are useful. Without certain preservatives, many foods would quickly spoil; it is estimated that about 20 percent of the world's food supply is lost to spoilage each year. However, many chemical additives in our food are nutritionally unnecessary, and some may adversely affect health. Also, unnecessary sugar and salt are added to many food products to enhance taste and to increase sales. The food dyes currently approved for use in the U.S. have been banned in European countries because they have been implicated in human cancers and allergies (see Table 5-3). The Food and Drug Administration estimates that as many as 100,000 Americans are intolerant to the chemical additive tartrazine, a yellow dye added to hundreds of commercially packaged foods. People intolerant to tartrazine may develop skin rashes and symptoms of hay fever or asthma. Labels on commercial foods note the presence of tartrazine by the phrase "FD&C yellow No. 5."

Food Preservation

Most packaged foods are preserved with one or a combination of chemicals. A nonchemical method of preserving food is exposure to relatively high levels of gamma irradiation. The gamma rays penetrate the food substance — milk, chicken, fruits, grains, vegetables — and destroy the parasites, fungi, bacteria, and viruses that may cause spoilage or produce harmful toxins. The use of irradiation to destroy harmful microorganisms in food is analogous to the therapeutic use of radiation to destroy cancer cells in the body.

Preservation of spices by gamma irradiation has been in use in the United States for many years. However, in 1986 the Food and Drug Administration (FDA) approved its use on fruits and vegetables, white potatoes, wheat, and wheat flour. (Irradiation of pork was approved earlier.) Doses of up to 100,000 rads can be used to preserve these foods (3 million rads is approved for use on spices). Under the new FDA regulations products must be labeled "treated by irradiation," which is more accurate and informative than the term "picowaved," which was preferred by food manufacturers. However, in the future the labeling will change, and only a small, flower-like symbol need be used to show that the product was irradiated.

Those who oppose the use of irradiation to preserve foods argue that its safety is not proven (Fraser, 1986). Opponents are concerned that the irradiation may produce carcinogenic or toxic byproducts in some foods. There is also some evidence that irradiation increases the likelihood of bacterial and fungal contamination of food by radiation-resistant strains. The loss of nutrients, particularly vitamins, is increased by irradiation. Like most controversies in nutrition, there are valid arguments for and against the use of irradiation to preserve foods (Urbain, 1986; Goldbaum, 1986).

You can determine which of the foods you normally eat have chemical additives by reading the product label. Food manufacturers must list all the chemicals they add to their products. They do not, as yet, have to list the amounts of these additives, but they must list the ingredients in the order of their relative proportions in the food. You cannot assume that foods labeled "natural" or "organic" or "health foods" are free from additives, extra sugar, salt, or pesticide residues. The only sure way to ascertain the contents of a food is to know how it was grown or produced (ask your grocer), or to grow it yourself (see Figure 5-6).

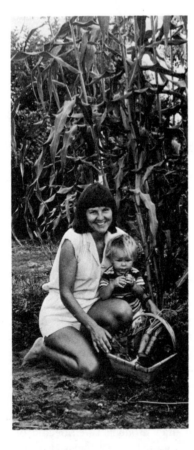

Figure 5-6
Home vegetable gardening is becoming increasingly popular as people become more aware of the health benefits, economy, and satisfaction that come from "growing your own."

Artificial Sweeteners

Artificial sweeteners are probably the most common of all food additives. As a presumed ally in what seems to be a continual battle against overweight, and as a theoretical help to diabetics, these substances are used as sugar substitutes in packaged cereal, powdered drinks, candies, and other foods. By far their widest use is in "diet" soft drinks. It is estimated that 50 to 70 million Americans are regular users of artificial sweeteners in one form or another.

The three major artificial sweeteners that have been used in recent years—cyclamate, saccharin, and aspartame ("NutraSweet")—have all been implicated as health risks. In fact, in 1970 cyclamates were banned by the Food and Drug Administration because studies showed that they could cause cancer in experimental animals. (Ironically, the FDA is now considering reversing the ban because the earlier decision may have been based on faulty data.) In 1977 saccharin, too, was banned after tests showed that it could cause bladder cancer in experimental animals. However, so great was the public outcry that the FDA has not enforced the ban and saccharin is still added to foods and beverages.

Aspartame is the latest in the parade of artificial sweeteners. This substance is a combination of the natural amino acids aspartic acid (in a chemically modified form) and phenylalanine. Unlike saccarin, which is synthesized from petroleum products and has no caloric content, aspartame contains 4 calories per gram. Aspartame is 180 times as sweet as sucrose; thus, minute quantities can be used to sweeten foods. Because of the possible health risks associated with saccharin and because aspartame leaves no aftertaste, soft drink manufacturers are eager to use the new sweetener.

However, after investigating consumers' complaints associated with aspartame ingestion, government agencies have recommended continued study of aspartame-associated mood changes, insomnia, and seizures in certain individuals. As yet, a safe amount of aspartame has not been determined, but it is assumed that most adults are unlikely to consume sufficient aspartame in a day to be harmed. Growing children, on the other hand, because they consume large amounts of soft drinks, breakfast cereals, chewing gum, candies, and other products containing aspartame, may suffer adverse effects. It is also possible that aspartame consumption during pregnancy could harm the developing embryo. Consumers of NutraSweet should not be misled by enthusiastic advertisers proclaiming it to be a "natural sweetener" and therefore completely safe. Questions regarding its safety in the diet remain (Pardridge, 1986).

It needs to be emphasized that no artificial sweetener has ever been shown to help people lose or control their weight or shown to help diabetics, yet millions of people buy "diet" drinks and use artificial sweeteners. Most studies show that people compensate for the sugar missing in artificially sweetened foods by eating foods that contain sugar. Finally, there is no evidence that using artificial sweeteners reduces the incidence of tooth decay.

So why are artificial sweeteners used in such enormous quantities and why does their use generate such controversy? Sales of soft drinks constitute a $25 billion market, and "diet" drinks are a sizable portion of that market. It is estimated that sales of aspartame could reach $600 million a year if it were used by all soft drink companies. As with many health issues, decisions on whether to use artificial sweeteners have become a matter of dollars and sense (see Figure 5-8).

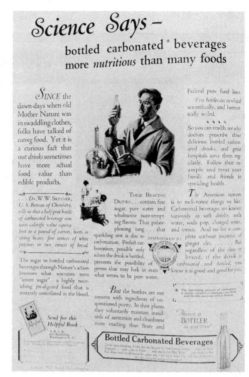

Figure 5-7
A 1927 advertisement for soft drinks. Manufacturers of sugary, carbonated drinks have been pushing their products for 60 years.

Figure 5-8
Soft drink consumption in the U.S. has tripled since 1960. The average American consumes 40 gallons of soft drinks yearly. This provides about 8 percent of the daily calories. A can of Coke contains 9.2 teaspoons of sugar.

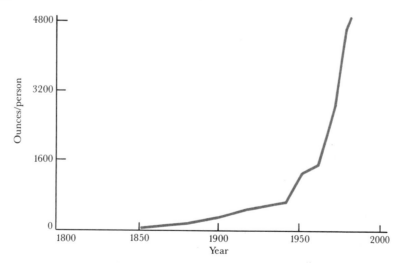

BOX 5-2

EATING ON THE RUN

Grabbing a meal in a fast-food restaurant is an ever-increasing trend in eating behavior. There are about 140,000 fast-food outlets in the United States and thousands more throughout the industrialized world, and it is estimated that about one-quarter of the adult population of the industrialized countries eats in fast-food places each day (*Consumer Reports,* September 1979).

The Consumers Union has prepared an analysis of the nutrients in many kinds of fast foods, a summary of which is presented in Table 5A. The analysis shows that most fast-food entrées contain hundreds of calories, lots of protein, little complex carbohydrate, and large amounts of fat and salt. The fast-food entrées are not nutritionally worthless, however. Nearly all supply large percentages of the RDA for certain vitamins and minerals as well as for protein.

Note: Foods were analyzed in 1979. Since formulations may have changed, Consumers Union cannot be sure that the analyses are still applicable.

Table 5A. Nutrient Levels in Certain Fast Foods

	Serving Size	Calories	Fat	Carbohydrates	Total sugars	Sodium	Protein*	Vitamin A*	Thiamine*	Riboflavin*	Vitamin B$_6$*	Vitamin B$_{12}$*	Niacin*	Calcium*	Phosphorus*	Iron*
Hamburgers																
Burger King Whopper	9 oz.	660	41 g	49 g	9 g	1083 mg	57%	12%	51%	30%	19%	67%	55%	9%	29%	26%
Jack-in-the-Box Jumbo Jack	8¼	538	28	44	7	1007	61	9	56	41	13	70	57	13	29	24
McDonald's Big Mac	7½	591	33	46	6	963	59	5	52	33	13	63	55	23	44	23
Wendy's Old-Fashioned	6½	413	22	29	5	708	62	8	36	26	13	83	45	8	24	27
Sandwiches																
Roy Roger's Roast Beef Sandwich	5½	356	12	34	0	610	63	5	38	29	16	37	60	2	28	23
Burger King Chopped-Beef Steak Sandwich	6¼	445	13	50	0.7	966	67	5	48	34	25	40	66	15	37	30
Hardee's Roast Beef Sandwich	4½	351	17	32	3	765	41	4	36	22	10	47	42	8	29	17
Arby's Roast Beef Sandwich	5¼	370	15	36	1	869	52	4	36	21	10	53	56	5	35	20
Fish																
Long John Silver's	7½	483	27	27	0.1	1333	72	5	17	12	16	133	24	3	46	3
Arthur Treacher's Original	5¼	439	27	27	0.3	421	46	3	11	6	10	27	18	2	32	3
McDonald's Filet-O-Fish	4½	383	18	38	3	613	35	3	39	19	6	23	25	14	27	9
Burger King Whaler	7	584	34	50	5	968	48	3	38	20	7	60	31	8	50	12
Chicken																
Kentucky Fried Chicken Snack Box	6¾	405	21	16	0	728	78	4	21	25	19	40	72	6	35	14
Arthur Treacher's Original Chicken	5½	409	23	25	0	580	57	3	12	10	24	10	87	2	33	4
Specialty entrées																
Wendy's Chili	10	266	9	29	9	1190	50	51	20	169	18	47	8	9	27	27
Pizza Hut Pizza Supreme (½ 10 in. pizza)	7¾	506	15	64	6	1281	61	36	59	40	17	43	49	41	46	24
Jack-in-the-Box Tacos (2)	5½	429	26	34	3	926	35	25	16	13	15	27	18	20	33	12

*Recommended Daily Allowance for an adult woman as set by the National Academy of Sciences National Research Council.

> Thirty percent of the products in grocery stores today could be thrown out and nobody would be the worse.
>
> **D. Mark Hegsted**
> **Professor of Nutrition**
> **Harvard University**

Formulating Your Diet Plan: Some General Recommendations

Just about every week the best-seller lists include at least one book about health and nutrition. The steady popularity of such books reflects widespread concern about what to eat and how to design a healthful diet. With so many kinds of foods available and with so many extraneous factors — colorful packaging, enticing supermarket displays, television advertising, and so on — influencing the choice of foods, it is no wonder that many people are confused about nutrition and seek guidance in making their dietary choices.

In Chapter 4 we discussed the basic nutrition groups (proteins, carbohydrates, fats, minerals, vitamins, and water) and the role of these substances in the maintenance of health and the development of disease. What follows are guidelines for formulating a personal diet plan that take into account the nutritional principles and recommendations presented in this chapter and Chapter 4. Keep in mind that there is no "one and only" healthy diet.

1. Become aware of the foods you regularly eat that provide you with little nutritional benefit and those that may actually harm you. These include foods high in simple sugars, such as snack foods and soft drinks, foods high in animal fat, such as red meats, and manufactured foods containing large amounts of salt. Once you are aware of what you are eating, you can make beneficial changes.

2. Begin to substitute nutritious (and tasty) foods for less nutritious ones. For example, you can substitute: whole-wheat bread for bread made of refined flour, fresh vegetables for canned and frozen ones, low-fat dairy products for those high in fat, lean meats for meats with large amounts of fat, fish for red meats, fruit for candies or cookies, and fruit juice for soft drinks.

3. Be sure your diet gives you the RDA for protein and at least the following eight nutrients: vitamin A, thiamine, riboflavin, niacin, vitamin C, vitamin B_{12}, calcium, and iron. Such a diet is likely to provide the RDA for the other essential nutrients as well. Remember that for some of the nutrients in the RDA, more is not always better. If you consume more calories than you expend, you will gain weight. If you eat too much protein, the excess will be converted to body fat. And if you take in much more than the RDA of vitamin A, you may damage your liver.

> As a nation
> we commit over 224 million tons
> of food and drink to our garbage dumps
> and sewers over the course
> of a year.
>
> **Anita Borghese**

4. Construct your diet so that most of the carbohydrates you ingest are complex carbohydrates found in fresh fruits, vegetables, beans, and whole grains. By eating these foods, you will avoid constipation, reduce the risk of large bowel cancer and other gastrointestinal diseases, and reduce the risk of tooth decay, because you will be consuming proportionately less simple sugar. You will also obtain other nutrients (vitamins and minerals) that are refined or processed out of manufactured food.

5. Begin each day with a breakfast that provides approximately one-third of your daily protein and calorie requirement. This practice will keep you from feeling tired in midmorning and is also likely to promote regular eating habits and less between-meal snacking. Studies show that people with regular eating habits are healthier than people who eat irregularly.

6. Choose foods that are as close to the natural state as possible. This will help you avoid being influenced by advertisers, whose primary motivation is not the promotion of your health (how often do you see ads for fresh fruit and vegetables?). Remember that simply because a product label says "natural" or "organic" does not assure that the product is free of nutritionally worthless or potentially harmful additives. Read the product label to determine the ingredients; check with the supplier or producer if you are unsure of anything, and whenever possible, select fresh, unprocessed foods. Many different combinations of foods can supply the essential nutrients and calories you need for good health.

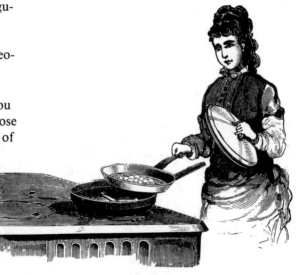

> After dinner sit awhile,
> after supper walk a mile.
> **English proverb**

BOX 5-3

WHAT ABOUT FASTING?

There is little scientific evidence to support the contention of some diet enthusiasts that fasting is physiologically beneficial. Nevertheless, people who regularly go on periodic short-term fasts usually claim that the fast has made them "feel better." There is little scientific information to guide anyone wishing to experiment with fasting. But if at the end of the fast the individual feels better, it may well be that the body has cleansed itself of accumulated tissue, debris, food additives, and environmental pollutants, just as the proponents of fasting claim.

Most fasting regimens call for 1-day or 3-day fasts, during which time the only material ingested is water, or, in the case of 3-day fasts, occasionally fruit juice. Longer fasts of as many as 7 or 10 days are less common, and it is usually recommended that they be monitored by a person experienced with helping in lengthy fasts.

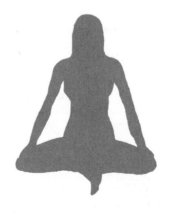

Guidelines for breaking a fast of any length include consuming at first only juice and then small portions of soft, palatable foods. The usual diet is resumed only after a day or two of careful eating.

The experience of fasting is often accompanied by a certain pattern of changes in feelings. Not long after beginning a fast, the person may feel hungry, but after a time the hunger feelings subside. About 5 hours after having passed up the usual first meal of the day, the person may feel tired and even irritable. This phase eventually passes, however, and the faster experiences a renewed feeling of energy and a coincident loss of interest in eating. This usually happens at the end of a 1-day fast. If the fast is carried on for additional days, similar cycles in feeling may occur, but often the time spent in the "down" phase becomes progressively less and the time of feeling energetic becomes progressively greater as the fast continues.

Experienced fasters usually feel refreshed and invigorated after their fasts, and many also claim increased feelings of harmony with their environment and their spiritual selves. This is one reason that fasting has been used for thousands of years by many religious persons as a way to purify the spirit.

The Heimlich Maneuver is a technique for saving the life of a person choking on food or another object. It consists of external compression of the air in the lungs in order to provide a flow of air from the larynx sufficient to expel the obstructing object.

Henry Heimlich, M.D.

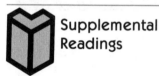

Supplemental Readings

Breneman, James C. *Basics of Food Allergy.* 2nd ed. Springfield, IL: Charles Thomas, 1986. Everything you want to know about food allergies. Authoritative and readable.

Eaton, S. Boyd, and **Konner, Melvin.** "Paleolithic Nutrition." *New England Journal of Medicine,* 312 (1985), 283–289. An excellent analysis of the evolution of human nutrition and diet, and how modern diets deviate from the evolutionary trend.

"Fad Diets: Unqualified Hunger for Miracles."*Medical World News,* August 11, 1986, 44. Explains why fad diets cannot work.

Fraser, L. "Food Irradiation— Zapping What You Eat." *Science for the People Magazine,* March/ April 1986.

Goldbaum, E. "Irradiation Prompts Food for Thought." *Industrial Chemical News,* August 1986.

Pauling, Linus. *How to Live Longer and Feel Better.* New York: W. H. Freeman, 1986. As Nobel prize winner Pauling approaches a healthy and active 90, he is worth reading whether you agree with all of his ideas or not.

Peterkin, Betty; Kerr, Richard L.; and **Shore, Carole J.** "Diets That Meet Dietary Goals." *Journal of Nutrition Education,* 10 (1978), 15–18. Healthy dietary plans designed by U.S. Department of Agriculture nutritionists.

Urbain, W. M. *Food Irradiation.* New York: Academic Press, 1986.

U.S. Senate Select Committee on Nutrition and Human Needs. *Dietary Goals for the United States.* Washington, D.C.: U.S. Government Printing Office, 1977. Suggestions for individuals on how to improve their diets for maximum health.

Summary

In our country we have thousands of food items to choose from. Thus, for most of us good nutrition is a matter of informed choice.

The research of nutritionists and other scientists has produced a set of dietary recommendations, called the Recommended Dietary Allowances, or RDA, which specify amounts of certain nutrients to be ingested each day for adequate nutritional status. The RDA lists values for calories, protein, and many vitamins and minerals. Using compilations of the nutrient values of foods, people can determine the adequacy of their diets by comparing the amount of the nutrients in their foods with the recommended intakes set forth by the RDA. Many food products list the percentage of the RDA in a given portion of the food directly on the product label. Some people may feel the need to take in certain vitamins and minerals in excess of the amounts listed in the RDA for optimum health and vigor.

A committee of the U.S. Senate has formulated a set of dietary guidelines in addition to those in the RDA. They include maintaining a proper body weight by consuming only the necessary amount of calories, eating proportionately more complex carbohydrates and less sugar, and reducing the intake of saturated fat, cholesterol, and salt. People should also try to limit their consumption of nonfood substances such as food additives. The key to good nutrition is to eat a variety of fresh, natural foods in moderate amounts.

FOR YOUR HEALTH

Refer to your food diary (see FOR YOUR HEALTH at the end of Chapter 4) and do the following:

1. Determine what percentage of your daily calorie intake comes from complete meals and what percentage comes from between-meal snacks.

2. Discover whether you have any habitual snacking patterns, such as taking coffee breaks, buying food from vending machines, or eating before bedtime.

3. Develop a strategy for replacing foods that add calories without nutrients to your diet with more nutritious foods.

4. For one of the days that is representative of your usual diet, determine the amounts of calcium, iron, thiamine, and vitamin C you ingest (use a food composition handbook to determine the amounts of these nutrients in your food). Then compare your results with the RDA for these nutrients.

5. On your next visit to the supermarket, take notice of the ways commercial foods are packaged. Observe how brightly colored the packages are. Also notice the many "junk food" displays located at the front of the store and near the checkout counter, placed there to tempt the impulsive shopper.

CHAPTER SIX

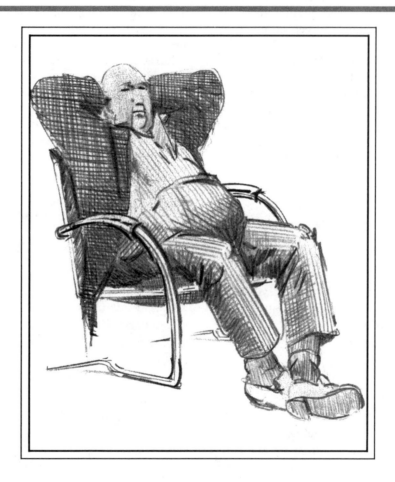

How movement and exercise lead to
physical, mental, and emotional
harmony.

Physical Activity

Frank is a graduate student who took up jogging about a year ago because so many of his friends were runners, including his fiancée, Susan. Although he wasn't overweight, Frank nevertheless thought he could stand to have firmer muscles, especially in his thighs and abdomen. He began to run with Susan on the college track several times a week.

At first, Frank found running to be very hard. He had never before been physically active. In fact, he had always hated sports because of bad experiences in high school physical education classes. Also, he smoked about a pack of cigarettes a day, which severely limited his breathing ability. On the first day he could barely run one lap of the track—one-fourth of a mile—and without Susan's encouragement he probably would have quit right then. She agreed that one lap wasn't very far, but she reminded Frank that it would take time to undo the years of inactivity and smoking, and that he should have patience. Frank decided to give his new routine time to work, and set the goal of running one mile by the end of one month's running.

Frank's graduate work is very demanding, so it was hard for him to keep his schedule organized so he could meet Susan for their appointed running times. Learning to say "no" to work was probably one of the hardest parts of the running program. Susan is a law student, and learning to say "no" to excessive studying had been one of the hardest things for her as well. Susan had learned, though, that having the discipline to follow through on the commitment to "feeling better" led to a stronger sense of accomplishment, independence, and control over life than anything she had ever done before. She insisted that they promise not to be late or to miss a run.

Frank is very stubborn, and once he took up the challenge, he progressed rapidly. He completed his goal of running one mile by the end of the third week, and within three months he and Susan were running three miles, four days a week. Occasionally, Susan talks of entering a "fun run," a locally sponsored race for amateur runners. She likes the idea of competing once in a while. She says the goal of doing well in a race gives her daily running more meaning. Frank, however, is content with their private runs. He is satisfied that his commitment to running helped him stop smoking, after many previously unsuccessful tries, and that he feels stronger and healthier. He also likes the privacy that his running affords; he says he gets his best ideas after about a half hour of running, when his breathing becomes regular. At that point he says he has "run away" from a lot of the extraneous thoughts that accumulate during the day, and he feels his mind and body have achieved a harmonious rhythm.

Frank and Susan are among the millions of people who schedule time in their lives for **body work,** some kind of regularly practiced physical activity, whether it be a sport, a special type of exercise program, a hobby that involves movement, or simply walking. According to the National Center for Health Statistics, only about 15 percent of the 90 million American adults who exercise regularly are Frank's and Susan's fellow joggers.

The idea of body work is to put into life the good feelings and health benefits that come from movement. Research has shown that being physically active is related to better health and well-being. The studies have found that people who often take part in such recreational activities as active sports, exercises, and gardening are significantly healthier than those who do not. In this chapter we discuss the many ways regularly practiced physical activity— body work—can bring about increased health and well-being.

Physiological Benefits of Physical Activity

Our industrial society depends on an enormous variety of machines that free people from an equally enormous number of physical tasks. Some of these tasks, such as heavy construction work or large-scale farming, would be well-nigh impossible without the help of machines. Others, such as traveling to work or school, getting to the seventh floor of a building, or washing clothes, could be accomplished without the aid of machines (and some people argue they ought to be), but few of us are likely to give up the use of cars, elevators, and washers. They simply make the tasks of daily living easier. As a result, few people do much moving around under their own muscular power. That is, many of us get little exercise.

According to William B. Kannel and Paul Sorlie (1979) who have studied the effects of lifestyle on the occurrence of heart disease:

> Over the past quarter of a century, there has evolved a growing suspicion that the transformation of man by modern technology from a physically active agrarian creature to a sedentary industrial one has exacted a toll in ill health. The evidence on which this is based comes from epidemiological studies, clinical observation, and the work physiologist. Most of the attention has been focused on the possible contribution of physical indolence to the development of cardiovascular disease, the chief health hazard of affluent societies and their leading cause of death.

It is unlikely that physical activity can, by itself, prevent the occurrence of heart disease (see Box 6-1). But much evidence indicates that regular physical activity, whether it be work-related or recreational, dramatically lowers the risk of disability and death from heart disease (Simonelli and Eaton, 1978). One classic study showed that conductors on

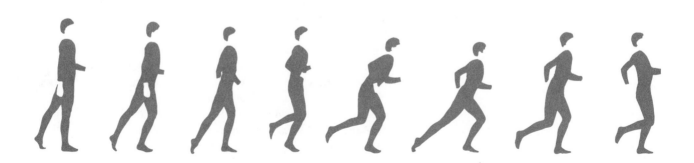

BOX 6-1

JAMES FIXX (1931–1984), AUTHOR AND AVID RUNNER

Perhaps more than any other person, James Fixx was responsible for encouraging Americans' passion for running. After the publication of his best-selling book, *The Complete Book of Running,* Fixx's name became synonymous with the sport. He made numerous guest appearances on television and radio, wrote many articles and books, and was considered the spokesperson for amateur running in the United States.

Then, in the summer of 1984, at the age of 53, Jim Fixx died of a sudden heart attack while running in Vermont. The world of amateur sports was shocked, and many people were dismayed. If running is supposed to be so good for you, they wondered, why did Jim Fixx, the runner's runner, die at such an early age of a heart attack?

Although there are no conclusive answers, there are some ideas. First, before reaching the age of 40 Fixx had many of the risk factors associated with heart disease. He smoked, he was overweight, and he was overstressed at work. Also, his family had a history of heart disease. It is likely that his conversion to running was partly a response to his awareness of the health dangers of his former lifestyle. There is no telling, however, how much irreversible damage his cardiovascular system may have suffered before he began running.

Second, in the weeks preceding his death, Fixx complained of tightness in the throat and chest, which at the time were dismissed by Fixx and his family as insignificant because he thought he was healthy and fit. After his death, cardiologists pointed out that such symptoms are suggestive of heart trouble and should have been heeded. Was Fixx so arrogant about his state of health that he consciously ignored the warning signs? Were the symptoms not severe enough to alarm him? Did he ignore the message his body was giving him because he feared the truth? No one will ever know. It is evident, however, that Fixx's attitude contributed to his death.

Sports physicians point out that Jim Fixx's death does not mean that running or any other form of exercise is likely to lead to an early death. In fact, considerable research demonstrates that the opposite is more likely. However, no one can expect to live forever just because of superior physical fitness. Every body has its limits, and the wise athlete learns to pay attention to the body's signals.

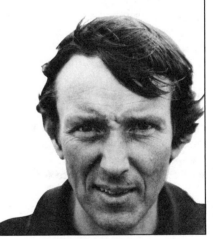

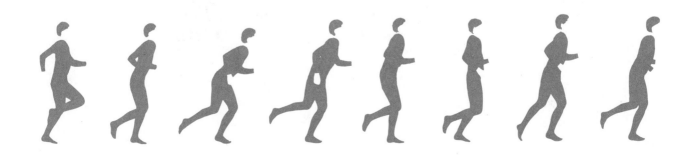

> If we buy into the demands to conform physically to some fashionable image of someone else, that's getting on a treadmill of anxiety that I personally have been victimized by.
>
> **Jane Fonda**

London's double-decker buses had about 30 percent less heart disease than their co-workers who drove the buses (Morris et al., 1953). The proposed reason for this difference is that the conductors were much more active than the drivers because they continually moved between the decks of the buses taking passengers' tickets. A more recent survey of over 16,000 men showed that those who exercised regularly (expending more than 2000 calories a week by walking, climbing stairs, or sports activity) had a much lower risk than nonexercisers of developing cardiovascular disease or experiencing a heart attack (Paffenbarger et al., 1984; 1986). A summary of the mechanisms by which physical activity may reduce the occurrence or severity of coronary artery disease is presented in Figure 6-1.

In addition to contributing to the health of the heart and blood vessels, regular physical activity has been shown to have other benefits (Lamb, 1978; Pollock, Wilmore, and Fox, 1978):

1. Maintenance of normal blood pressure and reduction in blood pressure in people with hypertension.
2. Maintenance of body weight within generally accepted normal limits.
3. Prevention and alleviation of chronic low-back pain.
4. Improved sleep.
5. Greater energy reserve for work and recreation.
6. Improved posture, which leads to improved physical appearance and the ability to withstand fatigue.
7. Greater ability of the body to cope with illness or accidents.

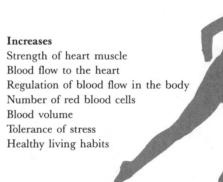

Increases
Strength of heart muscle
Blood flow to the heart
Regulation of blood flow in the body
Number of red blood cells
Blood volume
Tolerance of stress
Healthy living habits

Decreases
Amount of
fat in blood
Amount of body fat
Blood pressure
Heart rate
Vulnerability to
irregular heartbeat

Figure 6-1
How physical activity may reduce the occurrence or severity of coronary artery disease.

Psychological Benefits of Physical Activity

In addition to the physiological benefits, regular physical activity has psychological and spiritual benefits as well. For example, studies indicate that regular exercise reduces anxiety, tension, and fatigue, and enhances vigor and the ability to deal with the negative aspects of stress (Blumenthal et al., 1982; Roth and Holmes, 1985). Exercise may also help to alleviate or even prevent depression. In addition, regular exercisers report an improved self-image and self-esteem (Callen, 1983).

One of the principal psychological benefits that can come from regular body work is experiencing periods of relaxed concentration, characterized by reduction in physical and psychic tensions, regular breathing rhythms, and increased self-awareness. This experience is often compared to meditation. Tennis instructor Tim Gallwey (1976) describes four stages for obtaining a state of relaxed concentration through body work. The first stage, "paying attention," occurs at the beginning of a body work session and involves riveting your concentration on your body work and excluding all other thoughts. The stage of paying attention requires a certain degree of self-discipline — the desire and ability to say "no" to other demands on your time and energies and to say "yes" to yourself.

The second stage, that of "interested attention," is a time when you no longer have to concentrate hard on eliminating distractions and are able to flow with your activity. By the third stage, "absorbed attention," you are so absorbed in what you are doing that it is almost impossible for your attention to be distracted by what is going on around you. This stage is often accompanied by altered perceptions of space and time, and the mind moves to thoughts and images seemingly without your direction. The experience is almost dream-like, except that you are entirely conscious.

The final stage of relaxed concentration is that of "merging," when you no longer seem to be aware of the separation between yourself and what you are doing. It is transcendent experience, often referred to as the "runner's high" (see Figure 6-2), although it can be experienced in any form of body work. Tennis pro Billie Jean King (1974) describes "merging" as happening

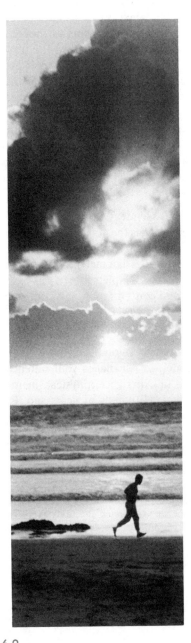

Figure 6-2

Confession of an inveterate runner: "Running makes me feel real good. It is a daily achievement; a source of satisfaction. It's usually difficult to start a day's run, but once you're into it, it's great. And when you finish, there's no feeling quite like it. My mind is clear; I smile more. I'm more relaxed. I don't think the metaphysical experiences of running are deeply religious, but they are soothing, quieting times when you're aware of your mind and body and unaware of the work of running."

on one of those days when everything is just right, . . . when my concentration is so perfect that it almost seems as though I'm able to transport myself beyond the turmoil on the court to some place of total peace and calm. I've got perfect control of the match, my rhythm and movements are excellent, and everything's just in total balance. . . . It's a perfect combination of violent action taking place in an atmosphere of total tranquility. My heart pounds, my eyes get damp, and my ears feel like they're wiggling, but it's also just totally peaceful.

The transcendent experience achieved in the stage of merging is the aim of all Eastern body work activities, including Hatha yoga, t'ai chi ch'uan, and several forms of Asian martial arts. These activities strive for nearly complete loss of self-consciousness through total concentration on various body movements (see Figure 6-3). Yoga instructor Lilias Folan (1972) explains:

Yoga means union . . . union with all that you are . . . All that is your potential—total union in experience: physical, mental, and spiritual. Hundreds of years ago, Patanjali, a Yogi of great wisdom, formulated a scientific system of spiritual exercises . . . for the totally committed with an unquenchable thirst for God. To know God . . . the body and mind were made fit and healthy for that great task. It was difficult to search for God if the body was full of aches, pains, and stiffness, and the mind ridden with erratic thoughts and desires.

The ancient men of wisdom evolved this scientific system of exercises called Hatha Yoga to promote a physical fitness and mental well-being.

Folan's comments are echoed by t'ai chi ch'uan instructor Sophia Delza (1961):

The goal of t'ai chi ch'uan is the achievement of health and tranquility by means of a "way of movement," characterized by a technique of moving slowly and continuously, without strain, through a varied sequence of contrasting forms that create stable vitality with calmness, balanced strength with flexibility, controlled energy with awareness.

T'ai chi ch'uan is an art in the deepest sense of the word. Aesthetically it can be

Figure 6-3

The sun salute, a Hatha yoga exercise, is a series of twelve postures or asanas, intended to be done in one flowing routine. Each of the twelve postures is held 3 seconds. The entire routine should be done at least twice in succession, alternating the legs. The sun salute is an excellent way to stretch the body every morning or any time you may need to relax tense muscles and restore deep regular breathing.

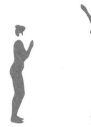 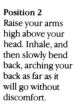   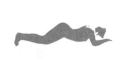

Position 1
Stand erect with your palms together in front of your chest. Inhale and exhale slowly and calmly.

Position 2
Raise your arms high above your head. Inhale, and then slowly bend back, arching your back as far as it will go without discomfort.

Position 3
Bend forward from the waist, keeping your arms extended and your head between them. Keep your legs straight, but relax your head, neck, shoulders, and arms. Exhale.

Position 4
Bend both knees and place your palms flat on the floor by the outer sides of your feet. Move your right leg back, touching the knee to the floor. Stretch your chin up toward the ceiling. Inhale.

Position 5
Place both legs back, holding your body straight, supported only by your hands and toes. Continue to hold the breath taken at position 4.

Position 6
Place your knees, chest, and forehead on the floor, but hold your abdomen up. Exhale.

compared to a composition by Bach or a Shakespearean sonnet. However, t'ai chi ch'uan is not an art directed out toward an audience. It is an art-in-action for the doer; the observer, moved by its beauty, can only surmise its content. The *experience* of the form in process of change is an art for the self.

The calmness that comes from harmonious physical activity and mental perception, and the composure that comes from deep feeling and comprehension are the very heart of this exercise.

Frequently a commitment to an exercise program of any kind brings about the adoption of behaviors that lead to positive wellness. For example, many people who become physically active pay more attention to proper nutrition, drink less alcohol, and stop smoking (Surgeon General, 1979a). There are several possible reasons for this. One is that people do not want to undo the many benefits of physical activity by engaging in some harmful behavior. It may also be that people simply lose or reduce their desire for junk food, regular heavy alcohol drinking, or cigarettes. Perhaps the tensions from life's stresses are reduced by physical activity so that other stress-reduction methods are no longer needed. By becoming interested in some kind of regularly practiced body work, people are able to "let go" of certain cravings. This demonstrates the phenomenon of **positive addiction**—the compelling desire to engage in a health-promoting behavior instead of a health-harming one (Glasser, 1976).

Yet another benefit of regularly practiced physical activity comes simply from setting aside time from life's other activities and responsibilities in order to devote yourself to something you enjoy doing. For many people, demands made by school, jobs, family responsibilities, and the like can sometimes seem unending. The few hours a week given to body work are times when your attention is diverted from your responsibilities, giving you the opportunity to relax, reflect, indulge your creative imagination, and assess your life situation and your life goals.

Several hypotheses have been offered to account for the psychological benefits of exercise:

1. Exercise becomes a means for autohypnosis, which increases the tendency for creative visualization.
2. Exercise increases the body's output of epinephrine, which produces feelings of euphoria.
3. Exercise changes the pattern of the secretion of brain neurotransmitters, particularly norepinephrine, which produces changes in mood.
4. Exercise increases the secretion of the brain's natural opiatelike substances, endorphins and enkephalins.

Figure 6-3 *(continued)*

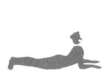   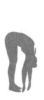 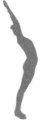 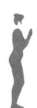

Position 7
Drop your hips to the floor and slowly raise your head and chest to arch the spine, supporting yourself on bent elbows. Point your chin to the ceiling while inhaling.

Position 8
Jackknife your hips toward the ceiling, keeping your legs straight and your heels on the floor. Exhale.

Position 9
Bring your left leg up between your hands while dropping the right knee to the floor. Raise your chin toward the ceiling and inhale.

Position 10
Bring your right foot forward so that both feet are together. Bend forward from the waist, keeping your legs straight and upper body relaxed. Try to touch your head to your knees. Exhale.

Position 11
Slowly straighten your body with arms extended over your head. When your arms are parallel to the floor, stretch toward the wall and slowly inhale. Straighten, then bend backward, arching your back.

Position 12
Exhale while bringing your hands together in front of you. Close your eyes and reflect on the sensations in your body.

> If a person died during exercise, he or she
> did not die *from* exercise.
>
> **Ernst Joki**

Fitness and Conditioning

It is generally recognized that a major outcome of regular physical activity is **fitness.** However, fitness is an elusive concept, not easily defined. For some, fitness means a lean, svelte, muscular body. For others, fitness means "being in top shape" — having the capacity to engage in strenuous exercise, such as hiking, swimming, running, or skiing long distances. But a lean, muscular body or exceptional physical endurance probably represents the extreme of the concept of fitness. Most people do not have the time, physiological capacity, or desire to become models of fitness, however experts define it. Fortunately, nearly everyone can reach a level of fitness that is commensurate with good health, with their life goals, and with their individual capabilities. Sports physiologists usually define fitness as (1) having adequate muscular strength and endurance to accomplish one's individual goals, (2) having reasonable joint flexibility, (3) having an efficient cardiovascular system, and (4) having a body composition that falls within the normal range of body weight and percent body fat (Katch and McArdle, 1983).

Because modern lifestyles do not require a lot of physical movement, few adults in North America and northern Europe are naturally fit. Rather, being fit requires a commitment of time and energy to activities other than school, work (particularly sedentary work), and family responsibilities. To be fit, one must engage in activities that challenge the mind and body to perform beyond what is required by a sedentary lifestyle. Furthermore, one must regularly engage in activities that improve fitness; otherwise the beneficial effects are quickly lost.

Activities to improve fitness are referred to as conditioning programs or training regimens. A wide variety of fitness programs are possible, but they tend to fall into two major categories: **aerobic training,** which increases the body's abilities to utilize oxygen and improves endurance, and **strength training,** which enhances the size and strength of particular muscles and body regions.

Aerobic Training

Aerobic training, or **aerobic exercise,** is described by Kenneth Cooper, a pioneer developer of aerobic exercise programs, as exercise that

> stimulates heart and lung activity for a time period sufficiently long enough to produce beneficial changes in the body. Running, swimming, cycling, jogging — these are typical aerobic exercises. There are many others. The main objective of an aerobic exercise program is to increase the maximum amount of oxygen that the body can process within a given time. This is called your *aerobic capacity.* It is dependent on an ability to (1) rapidly breathe large amounts of air, (2) forcefully deliver large volumes of blood, and (3) effectively deliver oxygen to all parts of the body. In short, it depends upon efficient lungs, a powerful heart, and a good vascular system.

Table 6-1
Fitness Points for Various Aerobic Activities

Exercise	Amount	Duration	Points
Cycling	6 mi.	less than 18 min.	9
Rope skipping		30 min.	9
Rowing	20 strokes/min.	36 min.	8
Running in place	100–110 steps/min.	15–17 min.	9
Swimming	1,000 yd.	17–25 min.	10½
Walking/running	1.5 mi.	under 9 min.	10
	3.0 mi.	30-36 min.	11

Data from K. Cooper, *The New Aerobics* (New York: Bantam Books, 1970).

Changes in physiology resulting from aerobic exercise are collectively called the **training effect.** If a person does not exercise vigorously or long enough, no training effect will take place; hence, little benefit will be derived. Cooper has developed a system for measuring the training effect of any exercise program. The system assigns "fitness points" to various exercises, depending on how strenuously and how frequently they are engaged in. Cooper's recommended standard of fitness is an accumulation of at least 30 fitness points a week for men and 24 points for women. This total can usually be derived from 15 to 30 minutes of strenuous exercise three times a week (see Table 6-1).

Intense exercise is the key to effective aerobic conditioning. One must move vigorously enough to challenge the cardiovascular system. One way to be sure that the level of exercise is sufficient to induce a training effect is to increase the heart rate during exercise to more than 70 percent of the theoretical maximum heart rate. For college-age individuals,

that corresponds to an exercising heart rate of about 130 to 140 beats per minute. Figure 6-4 shows the training zone for exercising heart rate for people of various ages. During exercise, the heart rate should exceed the threshold level of 70 percent of the maximum heart rate but should not exceed 90 percent of the maximum. The exercise period should begin with several minutes of warm-up and stretching, should continue with at least 15 minutes of exercise that gets the heart beating beyond the 70 percent of maximum level, and should finish with several minutes of cooling down (see Appendix C).

Three days per week of aerobic conditioning is sufficient to produce a training effect. For people who are already in relatively good condition, two days a week may suffice. However, one day of aerobic exercise per week does very little to increase one's aerobic capacity, while more than three days a week does not further increase aerobic capacity. Additional exercise helps use up calories, but excessive exercise also makes one more susceptible to injuries.

Figure 6-4
Training zone for exercising heart rate for people of various ages.

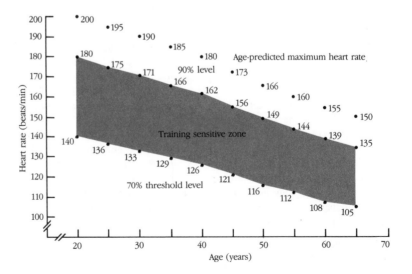

Bicycling at 10 miles per hour uses the equivalent
in food energy of 1.4 ounces of gasoline.
That means that the human body gets about
914 miles per gallon.

Strength Training

Strength training involves repetitively moving muscles against resistance in order to strengthen them. The most common forms of strength training utilize weights—barbells, dumbbells, and exercise machines—to supply resistance. Another form of strength training, called **isometric training,** involves pushing against an immovable object.

People undertake strength training for a variety of reasons. Strengthening various muscles can improve performance and reduce the likelihood of injury in almost any sport. Specific strength training regimens have been developed for nearly every major athletic activity (Sprague, 1979). Becoming stronger can also enhance one's self-esteem and sense of accomplishment, which can make one feel more confident in other life endeavors. In addition, many people are drawn to strength training for cosmetic reasons, since it develops the size and shape of the muscles. Well-developed muscles give the body a trim, muscular appearance that is currently in vogue as a symbol of health, vigor, and physical and sexual attractiveness.

BOX 6-2

THE LIQUID ATHLETE

The food industry has created a new glamour drink that is associated with the image of the successful athlete. So-called "sports performance drinks" are typified by Gatorade, the biggest seller. Today the market for these products exceeds $200 million annually.

Whereas these products are promoted as beneficial to sports performance, the only essential ingredient that they contain is water. Studies have shown that the sugars and salts that are added to these drinks, presumably to replace what is lost in physical activity, in fact may actually *retard* recovery from physical exertion since they tend to block absorption of water from the intestines.

As with many other aspects of nutrition and physical activity, the use of sports performance beverages benefits the manufacturers and advertisers of these products much more than athletes.

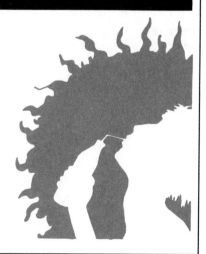

> A muscle can carry
> an emotional charge or tension,
> held over from
> past fears or angers.
> **Ursula Hodge Casper**

Compared to most aerobic exercises, strength training produces only a modest improvement in cardiovascular fitness. Although the exercises increase strength, the actual time spent exercising is insufficient to increase the heart rate for a time long enough to induce a training effect. Furthermore, the energy expenditure during strength training is about 4 calories per minute, about the same as for walking or swimming at a comfortable pace. Therefore, strength training alone is not very helpful for losing weight.

Putting Physical Activity into Your Life

For many people, the mere mention of physical activity conjures up unpleasant images of painfully boring exercises or rough competitive sports whose proposed beneficial effects on health and character development rarely seem to meet the promises made by enthusiastic players and coaches.

Fortunately for most of us, physical activity need not be so narrowly defined. Physical activity is anything you do when you are not sitting or lying down. Walking is a form of physical activity. So is dancing. So is gardening. Part of the idea of body work is to incorporate a playful or joyful activity into your life for its own sake. That kind of feeling also promotes health and is an added benefit. Americans are highly product-oriented; we tend to value what we do on the basis of outcome. With body work, the **process of doing** is itself the reward. So choose activities that you will enjoy. If you

like to be around people, join a class or organize some friends to work out with you. After you have accomplished a difficult task, reward yourself with praise. And remember, body work, even active sports, does not have to involve competition unless you want it to.

Some guidelines to keep in mind when incorporating any kind of body work into your life include (Cooper, 1970; Pollock, Wilmore, and Fox, 1978):

1. *Have a plan.* Before beginning any body work program, you need to develop a plan and to commit yourself to it for some reasonable amount of time. To make a body work plan that will help you achieve your personal goals, you can consult a high school or college coach, attend a class at a YMCA or similar organization, or follow the plan in one of the "how to" books that have been written for almost every body work activity. One of the best body work plans designed to increase cardiovascular fitness is the aerobics program developed by Kenneth Cooper (1970, 1973, 1977).

2. *Get a physical checkup.* If you have been inactive for many months or have concerns about your body's ability to perform at the level you would like, you may want to have a physician check you over.

3. *Accomplish goals.* The goal of any body work program is attainment of complete mind-body harmony. This can be done by progressively attaining higher and higher

Physical fitness is the ability to carry out daily tasks with vigor and alertness, without undue fatigue, and with ample energy to enjoy leisure time pursuits and to meet unforeseen emergencies.

President's Council on Physical Fitness

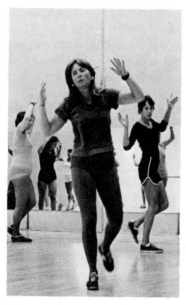

Figure 6-5
Confession of an active dancer: "Why dancing? I know four good reasons. The first is to have fun. That way you want to keep doing it, which is the most important thing about any exercise—to keep doing it. The second is to improve cardiovascular fitness. The third is to increase flexibility. And the fourth is to firm muscles. It's a total fitness activity. It's impossible to be depressed when you're dancing. You get into the music and you get to do beautiful movements. Imagine a whole room full of people doing beautiful movements! It's like a real chorus line."

goals. It is customary in our culture to measure progress by "how far" and "how fast." Such goals might be suitable for competitive athletes, but they are unsuitable for people who engage in body work activities for the purpose of receiving greater enjoyment from living. For most of us, personal goals based on such questions as "Does this level of activity make me feel good?" or "Does this help me toward my goal of losing weight?" make more sense than blind adherence to a stopwatch.

4. *Progress slowly.* Slow, deliberate progress gives you the opportunity to integrate your body work activity into your normal life routine. Don't impulsively try to run a long distance the first day. That could be so unpleasant that you may never want to run again. It could also injure you: suddenly engaging in some sort of vigorous physical activity after months or years of relative inactivity could damage a muscle, a ligament, a tendon, or a joint. If you have done little or no body work for a long time, begin by setting a goal of jogging or swimming (or whatever you choose to do) for only a minute. Then progress to two minutes when you are physically and mentally ready to undertake the challenge. That may be in a day or it may be in a week. Take your time, use common sense, and progress in moderation.

5. *Warm up and cool down.* All body work activity should be preceded by a brief period

of stretching, breathing, and relaxation to prepare your mind and body to receive the utmost benefit and pleasure from body work. This is a good time to focus attention on how your body feels. You can do this with a simple body awareness exercise (see Box 6-4). Some useful warm-up exercises are presented in Figure 6-6. When you have finished your body work activity, it is a good idea to let your body cool down slowly. If you have been involved in strenuous aerobic exercise, slowly reduce the pace of your activity until your heart rate and breathing return to almost normal. By slowly reducing your activity level you also help prevent muscle cramps that sometimes occur when strenuous activity is suddenly stopped. You can prevent later muscle stiffness by doing a few stretching exercises to loosen the muscles that have worked hard during exercise. While cooling down, try to focus your attention on the sensations that your body work has brought you. Notice

any special feelings of warmth or an increased sense of mind-body harmony and inner peace.

Exercise Abuse

In recent years it's become fashionable to be svelte, strong, and physically fit, presumably for health reasons but also to be socially desirable. Although few would argue that being healthy and attractive are desirable goals, many people are so zealous in the pursuit of those goals that they harm themselves. For example, some individuals place a higher priority on running or some other fitness activity than they do on work, family, interpersonal relationships, and even their own health, as evidenced by their unwillingness to stop exercising (even for a day!) to attend to other matters in life or to allow an exercise injury to heal properly (Dishman, 1985). In their attempts to attain the "perfect body," a large number of women exercise and lose weight to such extremes that they stop menstruation (**athletic amenorrhea**). The menstrual irregularities cease when exercise is

---

BOX 6-3

DRUGS AND ATHLETIC TRAINING

A storm of controversy has arisen around the use of certain drugs—principally anabolic steroids (testosterone and testosterone-like substances) and growth hormone—by athletes in training. Athletes take these drugs to increase muscle mass and stamina, usually because of a fanatical dedication to athletic achievement or to the pursuit of an ideal body shape.

Among American amateur athletes, the use of anabolic steroids is rarely supervised by qualified medical experts, and athletes frequently take dangerously large doses. Such large doses can lead (in both women and men) to a deepening of the voice, an al-

tered pattern of hair growth, hair loss, liver damage, and infertility. Similarly, abuse of growth hormone can cause disturbances in

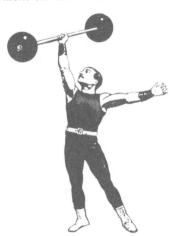

metabolism and aberrations in bone structure.

Both amateur and professional athletes are susceptible to the idea of using drugs in their pursuit of athletic prowess and athletic success. Because international sports competition has become highly politicized, amateur athletes may even be encouraged by official sports organizations and coaches to abuse their bodies with these drugs. However, standards of athletic excellence, health, and physical attractiveness should never include the taking of drugs to accomplish goals. And no athletes, especially young persons, should ever be encouraged to use such drugs.

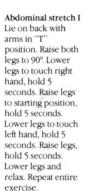

Abdominal stretch I
Lie on back with arms in "T" position. Raise both legs to 90°. Lower legs to touch right hand, hold 5 seconds. Raise legs to starting position, hold 5 seconds. Lower legs to touch left hand, hold 5 seconds. Raise legs, hold 5 seconds. Lower legs and relax. Repeat entire exercise.

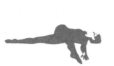

Abdominal stretch II
Lie on back with arms in "T" position. Raise left leg to 90°, keeping knee straight. Lower left leg across the body to touch right hand; hold 5 seconds. Raise leg to 90° position, then relax. Repeat for right leg, crossing over to touch the left hand. Do exercise twice.

Gastrocnemius stretch
Lean against a wall at an angle of between 45° and 60°. Keeping heels on the floor, lean closer to the wall. Hold 15 seconds. Relax.

Groin stretch
Assume stretch position and pull ankles toward the body to increase the stretch on groin muscles.

Abductor stretch
Lift leg to the point of resistance, hold 30 seconds; relax.

Push-ups
Do at least 30.

Figure 6-6
Flexibility exercises. A good flexibility program for running is: (1) walk or run easily for one quarter of a mile, (2) hamstring stretch I, (3) abdominal stretch I, (4) abductor stretch, (5) groin stretch, (6) hamstring stretch II, (7) push-ups, (8) hurdle stretch, (9) gastrocnemius stretch. A good flexibility program for tennis and other racket sports is: (1) trunk circling, (2) hamstring stretch II, (3) groin stretch, (4) abdominal stretch II, (5) push-ups, (6) gastrocnemius stretch, (7) ski stretch, (8) run in place for 1 minute, (9) jump in place for 1 minute, (10) practice strokes—10 each of forehand, backhand, and overhead.

reduced and the ratio of body fat to body weight returns to a normal level.

The most common form of exercise abuse is exercising a body part or the entire body beyond its biological limit to the point of injury. Such injuries are referred to as **overuse syndromes.** It is estimated that between 25 and 50 percent of athletes visiting sports medicine clinics have sustained an overuse injury (Peterson and Rehnstrom, 1986). Commonly, overuse injuries affect the muscles, tendons, ligaments, joints, and skin, which are constructed of fibrous bands of protein (see Table 6-2). These fibers can be torn if they are overloaded, as when lifting a heavy weight or running at top speed, or when forced to perform when fatigued. Damage can also occur by repeated small injuries that lead over time to a more serious problem. The common causes of overuse injuries are excessive exercising, faulty technique, and poor equipment.

Table 6-2
Common Overuse Injuries

STRAIN	Commonly referred to as "pulled muscles" or "pulled tendons." Caused by overstretching, tearing, or ripping of a muscle and/or its tendon
TENDONITIS	Inflammation of a tendon caused by chronic, low-grade strain of a muscle-tendon unit
BURSITIS	Inflammation of the lubricating sac that surrounds a joint (*bursa*) caused by repeated low-grade strain of the joint's supporting tissues
SPRAIN	Overstretching or tearing of ligaments
BLISTERS	Fluid-filled swellings on the skin caused by undue friction from the rubbing of skin against shoes, clothing, and equipment

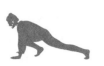

Ski stretch
Hold 30 seconds.

Hurdle stretch
Keep knee straight.
Hold 30 seconds.

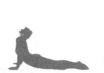

Trunk circling
Take 5 seconds to
circle clockwise;
relax. Repeat in
counterclockwise
direction. Do each
direction at
least twice.

Cobra posture
Lie face down with
hands under
shoulders. With
forehead on floor,
slowly raise
forehead, then nose,
then chin, then
shoulders, upper
and middle back.
Take 10 seconds to
complete extension;
hold extension 5
seconds. Relax.

Hamstring stretch I
Slowly raise one leg
to an angle of 90°,
keeping the knee as
straight as possible.
Grasp the raised
ankle with both
hands and gently
increase the stretch.
Hold 5 seconds;
relax. Repeat for
other leg. Do each
leg twice.

Hamstring stretch II
Bend at the waist
holding onto toes or
ankles. Attempt to
place head on
knees, hold 30 or 60
seconds.

All bodies are not anatomically capable of the same degree of physical exertion, especially the high performance exhibited by marathon runners or triathletes. The architecture of the body, the alignment of the legs, the capacity of the lungs, the size and strength of the bones and muscles, and other anatomical factors set limits on an individual's physical ability. Few people have the biological endowment to perform at championship levels. Physical activity can be much more enjoyable when you respect, accept, and appreciate your body's biological limits.

Don't ask your muscles to do more than they are capable of. Relishing the pain of overexertion — "going for the burn" — is dangerous. The pain of overexertion is the body's message that something is wrong, not that the exerciser is lazy and must exceed the pain threshold. If you want to increase your performance, build muscle strength slowly, following a supervised regime. Also, pre- and post-activity stretching helps to prevent damage to muscles and joints. Injuries are more likely if equipment such as special shoes, weights, and various kinds of apparatus are improperly used, are worn out, or are in disrepair.

Most people participate in physical activity because (1) they want to have fun, (2) they want to do something well so that they can gain a sense of accomplishment, and (3) they want to feel physically and psychologically better. And while pursuing these goals, no one wants to be hurt. It turns out that maximizing the have fun/do well/feel good aspects of exercise and minimizing the potential for injury go together. Physical activity is most satisfying when you are totally absorbed in it, when your body responds readily to your commands, when you run or play with confidence, and when your equipment and conditions are best. Take sports seriously enough to get enjoyment, but minimize the likelihood of injuries.

Walking and Health

If jogging, swimming, cycling, aerobic dancing, and other strenuous activities aren't for you, try walking. Walking as a form of regular exercise contributes many of the health benefits that other activities do, including strengthening muscles, increasing aerobic capacity, clearing the mind, reducing stress, and expending calories. And walking has advantages that other activities do not: other than appropriate walking shoes, no special clothing or equipment is required and walking can be fit easily into a busy schedule.

Walking contributes the most to health when it is done on a regular basis (about four times a week) for about an hour each time. How strenuous the walk should be depends on the desires and physical abilities of the walker. Most of the benefits can be derived by walking between 2 and 4 miles per hour. Aerobic capacity can be increased by walking briskly enough to increase the heart rate (see Figure 6-4).

BOX 6-4

A BODY AWARENESS EXERCISE

Choose a quiet place where you can lie down and stretch out comfortably. Most people find that it's easiest to lie on a pad or blanket, on a carpeted floor, or on a flat lawn. Lie on your back with your arms at your sides, palms turned upward, and feet spread slightly (about 12 inches apart). For those who know Hatha yoga, this is **savasana** — the relaxation pose, or sponge position. Be sure your shoulders are relaxed; let them drop. Once you've assumed the relaxation pose, close your eyes and take a deep breath by inhaling slowly to the count of 8. Hold the air in your lungs for a count of 3 and slowly exhale to a count of 8. Is your breathing smooth and regular? It should be. Take three breaths in this manner.

After taking the deep breaths, become aware of any regions of your body that seem unusually tense to you, and use autosuggestion to relax those regions while breathing normally. To do so, you may want to create a mental image of that body region and concentrate on the feelings of relaxation; or you can actually "talk" to the regions of tension as if they were good friends, gently exhorting them to relax and therefore feel better.

When you feel relaxed and ready to begin the exercise itself, focus your attention on your left foot. Visualize it in your mind's eye if you like (image visualization is described in Chapter 2). Now ask yourself about your left foot. How does it feel? Is it tired, sore, full of energy, or neutral? Wiggle your toes. In doing so, you're unconsciously sending nervous impulses from the brain down through your spinal cord, along nerves that course through the left leg and terminate on the muscles of the foot and lower leg, and that control the movement of the toes. As you wiggle your toes, with eyes closed, imagine a flow of energy or electricity going from your brain down your back through your leg, providing the impulses that say "move toes." Now do the same with the other foot.

When you've finished your toe wiggling, focus your attention on your ankles and lower legs — first the left, then the right. As with your feet, try to get a sense of how they feel. Then slowly focus your attention on the rest of your body, one region at a time, first the left side, and then the right — the upper left leg, the upper right leg, the genital region, the buttocks, the pelvis, the abdo-

men, the chest, the back, the shoulders, the upper arms, the forearms and wrists, the hands, and the fingers. All the while, keep your eyes closed, breathe naturally, give relaxing suggestions to particularly tense regions of your body, and be aware of how the various body regions feel. As you turn your awareness to a particular part of the body region, try to visualize the organs *inside* that body region.

Now focus your awareness on your face, eyes, ears, and nose. Focus your attention on the top of your nose and be aware of the air going in and out for a few breaths. Is the air predominantly moving through one nostril or both? Focus your attention on your brain. How does it feel? How do you feel?

When you've completed the mental excursion of your various body regions, relax and visualize your entire body. Imagine blood pulsating throughout all your arteries and veins and the power of the electrical energy of the transmission of thousands of nervous impulses. Then spend a few minutes in quiet relaxation, breathing normally and allowing your mind to be free of plans, thoughts, problems, and worries.

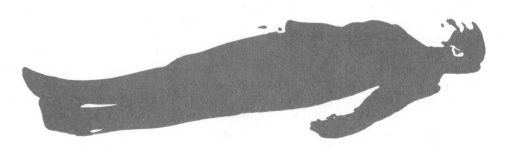

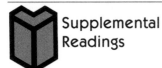

Supplemental Readings

Alter, Judy. *Stretch and Strengthen.* Boston: Houghton Mifflin, 1986. A safe, comprehensive exercise program to balance strength and flexibility.

Bailey, Covert. *Fit or Fat?* Boston: Houghton Mifflin, 1978. An easy-to-understand guide for improving fitness and maintaining body weight.

Cooper, Kenneth. *The New Aerobics.* New York: Bantam, 1970. A complete plan for physical fitness.

Hodge, Ursula. *Joy and Comfort Through Stretching and Relaxing.* New York: Seabury Press, 1982. An exercise and stretching guide for people who are unable to engage in vigorous exercise.

Perry, Paul. "Are We Having Fun Yet?" *American Health,* March 1987, 58–63. A summary of the philosophy of exercise and how to make it enjoyable.

Sprague, Ken. *The Gold's Gym Book of Strength Training.* Los Angeles: J. P. Tarcher, 1979. A complete guide to all forms of strength training, with regimens for strength training for nearly all major sports.

Ullyot, Joan. *Women's Running.* Los Altos, Calif.: World Publications, 1974. A thorough guide to running for women *and* men.

Summary

Many people spend much of their waking hours in sedentary activities that may contribute to being overweight and that sometimes produce muscular and mental tension. By incorporating regular physical activity into their lives, they can stretch stiff unused muscles and joints, restore natural deep-breathing rhythms, get rid of a lot of tension, clear their heads of daily worries, and reestablish a sense of mental and physical harmony. If people choose body work activities they enjoy, not only will they feel better, but they will have fun as well.

Many people who decide to incorporate some kind of body work activity into their lives find that the physical benefits they derive from their activities give rise to psychic benefits that are also rewarding and meaningful. Although they may have taken up jogging, swimming, or Hatha yoga to lose weight, firm sagging muscles and skin, or prevent heart disease, they find that regular physical exercise gives them more self-reliance, an improved self-image and greater emotional stability.

FOR YOUR HEALTH

Enhancing Your Body Awareness

Set aside at least 30 minutes per day for a two-week period to enhance your body awareness. Spend the first ten minutes of that time being alone and quiet. It is best to sit or lie quietly on your back, although you may walk if you prefer. During the next ten minutes do the body-awareness exercise described in Box 6-4. Be particularly mindful to take three deep breaths. End the session with a good stretch, such as the "Salutation to the Sun," or a combination of some other stretching exercises.

Improving Your Physical Fitness

Take the step test (Appendix C) to determine your fitness index. Then design and undertake a fitness program and chart your progress in a journal or with the help of a fitness program chart, such as the one below.

Fitness Progress Chart

Date	Activity	Time or amount of activity	Body weight	Resting heart rate	Maximum heart rate	Describe changes in sleep, appetite, and food

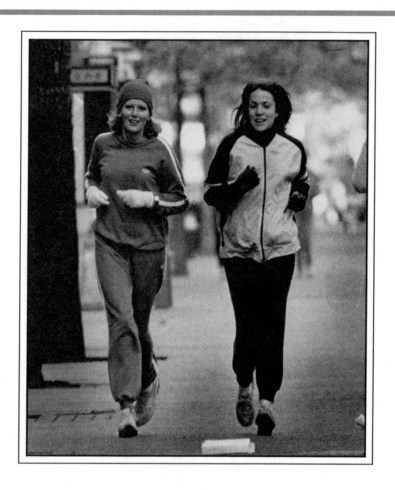

CHAPTER SEVEN

Mind-body harmony can help
maintain healthy body weight.

Weight Control

The deli case is not the only place to find "lite" baloney.
Business Week Magazine

Judging from the number of books and magazine articles extolling various "surefire" weight loss programs and the popularity of "lite" foods and beverages (see Box 7-1), it would appear that the American national pastime is dieting, not baseball. Indeed, almost everyone is somewhat calorie-conscious, particularly since current standards of social attractiveness dictate that people be slim and athletic.

Data from national nutritional surveys indicate that 14 percent of men and 24 percent of women between the ages of 20 and 74 weigh at least 20 percent more than the weight recommended by nutritionists (see Figure 7-1). Because overweight is associated with a number of illnesses, such as heart disease, diabetes, and high blood pressure, many overweight people would probably improve their health if they were to lose weight. To maintain the recommended weight does not mean, however, to be as thin as possible, since being very much underweight also carries health risks.

It is important to remember that body fat is not an enemy. Body fat represents stored energy essential for life, and the capacity to store energy as body fat is a normal physiological function. In the modern era, the abundance of food and a relatively sedentary lifestyle make storing energy less vital than it was for our more active ancestors, but the many adaptive and complex mechanisms that contribute to body fat production and storage are still a part of human biology. Health issues related to body weight, therefore, must be considered not as problems in the normal fat-control mechanisms but rather as problems in excess food consumption and reduced energy expenditure. In this chapter we discuss both strategies for weight control and eating disorders that involve excessive calorie restrictions.

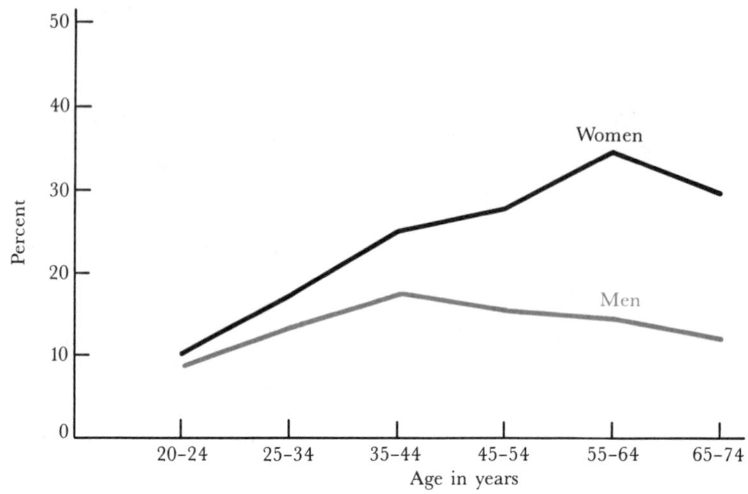

Figure 7-1

Percentage of U.S. men and women who weigh at least 20 percent more than recommended weight. (Data from the National Center for Health Statistics.)

The Definition of Overweight

In most instances, concerns about being *overweight* are really concerns about being *overfat*. There is a difference. Some professional male athletes, for example, weigh much more than the recommended weight standards for the normal population. Yet as little as 1 percent of their body weight may be fat. The major proportion of the body weight of a well-conditioned athlete is muscle and bone.

When considering issues of body weight and body fatness, it is useful to think of the body as being composed of two distinct parts, **lean body mass** and **body fat**. Lean body mass is made up of the structural and functional elements in cells, body water, muscle, and bone. Body fat is composed of two parts: **essential fat**—that which is necessary

for normal physiological functioning, such as nerve conduction—and **storage fat**. Essential fat composes about 3 to 7 percent of the body weight in men and about 15 percent of the total body weight in women. This sex difference, which is presumably caused by sex hormones, is due to the deposition of greater amounts of fat on the hips, thighs, and breasts in females. Female body builders, who are the leanest of all female athletes, have about 8 to 13 percent of their total body weight as fat, which is nearly all essential fat. This probably represents the lower limit of fat for a healthy woman. Storage fat, also called depot fat, constitutes only a few percent of the total body weight of lean individuals and 5 to 25 percent of the body weight of the majority of the population (see Figure 7-2). However, depot fat can account for 40 to 50 percent of the body weight of clinically obese persons.

Figure 7-2

Percent of total body weight as body fat, for men and women, by age.

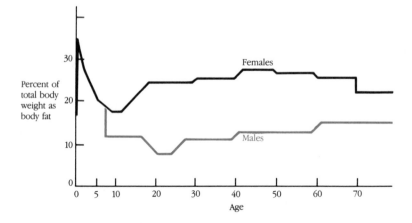

BOX 7-1

THE "LITE" HYPE

The atmosphere was electric at the advertising firm of Smith, Cram, Abernathy, and Moss because the company had just been awarded the account for Moonlight Bakery's new product, Lite Cookies. SCAM's top executives were gathered to map out the advertising strategy for their new client. The meeting was in chaos because much money was involved (full-color magazine spreads, national TV advertising) and no one could agree on a plan.

SMITH: I still say we need a beautiful, slim model in a bikini. Those football fanatics will certainly pay attention to that. And we'll convey that the cookie is non-fattening, too. The women will love it!

CRAM: No good, Smith. It's not a low-cal cookie. The name comes from its color; it's a lighter shade than their regular cookie. If we say its nonfattening, the FTC will be down on us.

SMITH: We won't actually say it's nonfattening. Show the model, give the product's name, and let the viewer's imagination do the rest.

ABERNATHY: I still think we should go with the wrestler. Look what he did for the sales of Lean Burgers. That guy could sell shoes to snakes.

MOSS: I think we should focus on getting "lite" beer drinkers to switch to the "lite" cookie.

SMITH: Maybe get that TV actor who plays the doctor, ah . . . what's his name, to say that our cookie has no more calories than the average "lite" beer . . .

The executives at SCAM are working hard, for they know that products called "lite" (and also "lean") sell. Diet foods, which include low-calorie, low-fat, and low-salt products, cost more than the regular products. Advertisers also are aware that there are no standards to define "lite" and "lean," so just about any product can carry such a label with no regard to its actual calorie, fat, or salt content.

Some "Lean Cuisine" frozen dinner entrées have the same amount of calories on an ounce-for-ounce basis as regular frozen dinners. What makes them "lean" is that they have smaller portions. Van de Kamp's "Light Flounder" is lighter in color yet has more calories than the traditional product. "Fritos Lights" became "Crisp 'N Thins" when consumers complained that the product actually contained more calories than regular Fritos.

Consumer outrage at the blatant misrepresentation by the use of the words "lite" and "lean" may one day bring about laws that set labeling standards for the food industry. Even with labeling standards, however, consumers would be wise to remember that no scientific evidence shows that the consumption of low-calorie, low-fat, and low-salt packaged foods provides health benefits. Moderate consumption of natural, unprocessed foods is still the best diet. Let the advertisers and manufacturers of "lite" and "lean" products eat their words.

As yet there are no universally accepted standards for the most "desirable" or "ideal" body weight or body composition (percentage fatness). One reason is that social and psychological factors, as well as health considerations, influence what is considered desirable. For example, fatness, particularly in women and children, is prized in some cultures. In these cultures, women who have a significant proportion of their body weight as storage fat are considered physically attractive and sexually desirable, and fatness in children is considered a sign of robust health. In our culture, attitudes about desirable body configuration tend to fluctuate and are often keyed to fashion trends. During the 1950s, for

> As it was co-opted by fashion, the "bean-lean" body became, arbitrarily, a mark of status, sexual competitiveness, and self-mastery.
>
> **William Bennett, M.D., and Joel Gurin**

example, a large body size, characterized by "full-figured" women and "he-men," was considered desirable, whereas today it seems that thin is "in."

A health-related index of desirable body weight is given in tables of "ideal weight-for-height" issued by insurance companies and based on actuarial statistics for longevity. These tables are based on total body weight and not body fatness and therefore do not take into account that some people, particularly the athletically active or those with physically demanding occupations, may be heavy by the standards in the tables but nevertheless rather lean. Also, the insurance company tables do not take into account any statistical correlation between body weight or body fatness and either good health or poor health.

Despite these drawbacks, it appears that the insurance company weight-for-height tables give a reasonable approximation of a healthful weight for most people. Several studies indicate that good health is associated with weighing no more than 5 percent below the standards and no more than 20 to 30 percent above the standards (Belloc and Breslow, 1972; Metzner, Carmen, and House, 1982). In particular, significant overweight carries a risk to health. For men, that level is about 20 percent above the weight-for-height standard; for women, it is 30 percent. Beyond these threshold levels, people have an increased risk for diabetes, gallstone and gallbladder disease, varicose veins, arthritis, heart disease, stroke, high blood pressure, difficulty breathing, and accident proneness (due to having a large body). Greatly overweight people often face social costs as well, such as job discrimination, lower social acceptability, and lower self-esteem.

The Causes of Overweight/Overfatness

There is no doubt that the principal cause of being overfat is consuming more calories in the diet than are expended overall. Too often it is assumed that overfatness is solely due to eating too much and overfat people are chided for being undisciplined eaters. Whereas this may be true for some people, for others overfatness may be due to low (relative to caloric intake) energy expenditure.

A number of factors may contribute to being overfat. Some are internal and involve how efficiently the body processes food. Others involve lifestyle—what one eats, how often one eats, how much one eats, and how one expends energy.

Physiological Factors

In some individuals overfatness may be related to a malfunction in the physiological regulation of appetite and eating behavior. A region of the hypothalamus located in the brain, called the body's **appestat,** is responsible for controlling appetite and eating behavior. The appestat is sensitive to certain physiological conditions, such as the level of glucose in the blood, and it responds to situations that signal that the body is in need of food by activating the sense of hunger and motivating eating behavior. Besides blood glucose level, the appestat monitors and responds to the state of the digestive system. When the digestive tract is distended, signals from the digestive tract to the appestat produce a decrease in appetite and eating behavior. When

---

BOX 7-2

ARE YOU OVERWEIGHT?

Most people can tell if they are overweight or obese simply by looking at themselves in the mirror or by discovering that clothes no longer fit. In case there is any doubt, and also to provide some scientific definition of overweight and obesity, there are two standard methods by which a more objective measure can be made.

The first of these standards is the table of suggested weights for heights (see accompanying tables). These tables list the desirable range of weights for small, medium, and large body frames for each sex. The listed weights assume that individuals are wearing indoor clothing; the men's heights assume 1 inch for shoes while the women's assume 2 inches.

Another determination of overweight is the skin fold measurement. If possible, such a measurement is made with calipers, a device whose jaws are calibrated to measure the distance between them. Skin fold measurements are usually made on the triceps at the exact midpoint of the back of the upper arm; they may also be made on the abdomen in men and on the hip in women. Without the accuracy of calipers, skin fold measurements can be approximated by simply measuring the thickness of the folded skin pinched between your thumb and forefinger. For men, a triceps or abdominal skin fold thickness of more than 16 mm (5/8 in.) indicates excess fat. The value for excess fat in women is 20 mm (7/8 in.).

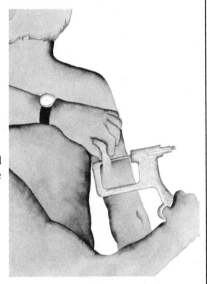

Measuring the amount of fat under the skin with skin fold calipers.

Desirable Weights for Women (with clothing)

Height (with shoes, 2-inch heels)	Small frame	Medium frame	Large frame
4′10″	92–98	96–107	104–119
4′11″	94–101	98–110	106–122
5′0″	96–104	101–113	109–125
1″	99–107	104–116	112–128
2″	102–110	107–119	115–131
3″	105–113	110–122	118–134
4″	108–116	113–126	121–138
5″	111–119	116–130	125–142
6″	114–123	120–135	129–146
7″	118–127	124–139	133–150
8″	122–131	128–143	137–154
9″	126–135	132–147	141–158
10″	130–140	136–151	145–163
11″	134–144	140–155	149–168
6′0″	138–148	144–159	153–173

Data from Metropolitan Life Insurance Company. Used by permission.

Desirable Weights for Men (with clothing)

Height (with shoes 1 inch heels)	Small frame	Medium frame	Large frame
5′2″	112–120	118–129	126–141
3″	115–123	121–133	129–144
4″	118–126	124–136	142–148
5″	121–129	127–139	135–152
6″	124–133	130–143	138–156
7″	128–137	134–147	142–161
8″	132–141	138–152	147–166
9″	136–145	142–156	151–170
10″	140–150	146–160	155–174
11″	144–154	150–165	159–179
6′0″	148–158	154–170	164–184
1″	152–162	158–175	168–189
2″	156–167	162–180	173–194
3″	160–171	167–185	178–199
4″	164–175	172–190	182–204

Data from Metropolitan Life Insurance Company. Used by permission.

> **It is clear from reading magazines or watching television that public derision and condemnation of fat people is one of the few remaining sanctioned social prejudices in this nation.**
> Faith T. Fitzgerald, M.D.

the stomach is empty, contractions of that organ ("stomach growls," "hunger pangs," or "hunger contractions") stimulate the appestat.

Some researchers suggest that the appestat has an internal set point, much like the temperature set point on a thermostat, that controls the amount of body fatness within certain limits. Evidence for the possibility of an appestat set point comes from experiments with animals and humans in which, after having been force-fed, subjects ate less than usual until their bodies returned to the pre-experiment size.

If further research confirms the appestat set-point hypothesis, it is possible that some cases of overfatness can be explained in terms of a higher-than-normal set point in the person's appestat. This high set point might cause the individual to feel hungry and to eat in excess of what is considered normal. The opposite would be true for some lean, underweight individuals. A lower-than-normal set point might produce a weak appetite and, consequently, a minimal amount of body fat.

Because the hypothalamus can be influenced by a variety of biological, hormonal, and psychological factors, it is possible that a higher- (or lower-) than-normal set point in the appestat could be caused by genetic abnormalities, by metabolic disturbances, or by stress and emotional upset, which can change hormone levels.

Another possible mechanism to account for aberrations in the set point of the appestat is the amount of body fat itself. The **lipostatic hypothesis** suggests that neural and hormonal signals from depots of storage fat in the body are relayed to the brain, signaling the relative size of these fat storage depots. This hypothesis presumes that there is a

physiological set point for a certain amount of total body fat, so that if storage fat falls below the norm established by the set point an individual will feel hungry and eat until the set point level of body fat is reached. The lipostatic hypothesis is often used to explain why overfat people who are highly motivated to lose weight have tremendous difficulty maintaining a reduced body size on a long-term basis.

Storage fat, called triglyceride (see Chapter 4), is deposited in cells called **adipocytes.** Throughout the adult years the number of adipocytes typically remains fairly constant, and the fat that is stored in the body is stuffed into preexisting adipocytes. Hence, gains and losses in body fat are accompanied by increases and decreases in the relative size of the body's adipocytes, not by an increase or decrease in their numbers. There are times in life, however, when the number of adipocytes does increase. These are the last three months of fetal development, between the ages of 12 and 18 months, and in early adolescence. Some investigators suggest that the increase in adipocyte number during these stages of life can be influenced by the amount of body fat at that time: the more fat, the greater the number of fat cells that develop.

Another idea regarding the control of body fat suggests that it is the *number* of adipocytes, and not the total volume of body fat, that controls the body's set point for fatness. If this hypothesis is confirmed, it would indicate that the amount of body fat in early childhood and adolescence should be controlled in order to prevent a large increase in the number of fat cells and the ensuing propensity for overfatness in adulthood.

> For fast acting relief,
> try slowing down.
> **Lily Tomlin**

Behavioral Factors

Many people overeat and are overfat not because they are continually hungry as a result of a malfunction in the body's appetite control mechanisms but because their eating behavior is improperly triggered by external stimuli and is unrelated to feelings of hunger or satiety. Everyone is susceptible to environmental cues that stimulate eating behavior and appetite regardless of actual hunger feelings. A good example is eating at predetermined times each day regardless of whether or not we are hungry. Regular mealtimes are a form of social programming, and in many cases social interaction (for example, among family members) or a break from work is the primary reason for the meal, not the need for food or nutrients. In addition, the design of the menu and the proportions of food served are often based on family custom and economic factors rather than on nutritional or energy needs.

Some people are "recreational" overeaters, meaning that their principal forms of recreation include the ingestion of food—again, not because of hunger but because it is part of the ritual surrounding that form of recreation. Snacking while watching television is a common form of recreational overeating, and television advertisers know this. That is the reason so many TV commercials advertise soft drinks, beer, and snack foods. Another form of recreational overeating is drinking alcoholic

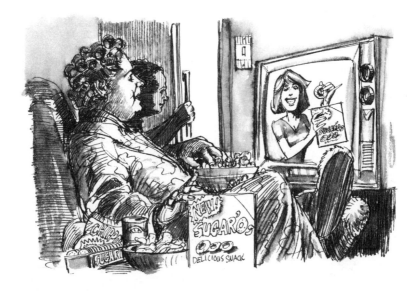

beverages. A primary form of socializing in some communities and groups is to gather at a local restaurant, tavern, or bar, where social interactions are combined with drinking alcohol. Since alcohol contains the energy equivalent of 7 calories per gram (50 percent more than sugar), a few beers or mixed drinks several evenings a week can lead to a fatness problem rather quickly.

Frequently, people with a weight problem are unaware of the many environmental cues that trigger their eating behavior. When they pass by a refrigerator or a soft drink machine, they may habitually succumb to the lure of eating or drinking something. Studies show that overfat people who have free access to food tend to eat more than normal-weight people, irrespective of feelings of hunger (Schacter and Rodin, 1974). Apparently, the sight and smell of food stimulates its consumption.

Psychologists have observed that stress, anxiety, and feeling lonely, bored, or angry can stimulate eating. Many people derive emotional comfort from ingesting food. One possible explanation is that as children most people learn to associate eating (particularly nursing as infants) with receiving love, affection, and comfort. This association persists throughout life, so that overeating becomes a generalized behavioral pattern for dealing with psychological distress.

A final behavioral source of overweight is lack of activity. In fact, the overwhelming majority of overweight people are so because their level of physical activity is too low to match the calories they consume (see Figure 7-3). Because machines do a lot of our work for us, and because many occupations (including going to school) involve many hours of sitting, it is easy for most individuals to ingest more calories than they expend. Moreover, the ready availability of food, especially high-calorie snack foods such as potato chips, candy, and the like, makes it even easier to acquire needless calories and excess pounds.

The energy equivalent of 1 pound of body fat is 3500 calories. That means that if you ingest 120 calories a day more than you use up in various activities, you will have gained a little over a pound of fat in the course of a month. This daily 120 calories can be accounted for by two large (3 in.) oatmeal cookies, a small milkshake or soft drink, a glass of lemonade, a scotch and soda, a glass of beer, two slices of bread, ten pretzels, ten potato chips, or a very small piece of pizza. This number of calories can be used up by walking for 20 minutes, bicycling for 15 minutes, running for 6 minutes, or walking up five flights of stairs twice a day. In other words, to maintain a state of energy balance, all you have to do is compensate for every cookie by a short walk or run (see Table 7-1).

Sensible Weight Reduction

If you want to adopt a weight-reducing program that results in a loss of 1 pound a month, you can easily plan your dietary and physical activities so you can produce a net daily deficit of 120 calories. All you would have to do is to walk a little more each day or to cut out a soft drink or a couple of cookies.

Figure 7-3
People whose occupations involve physical activity tend to have lower body weight than those in sedentary occupations. (Data from Mayer and Bullen, 1960. Used by permission.)

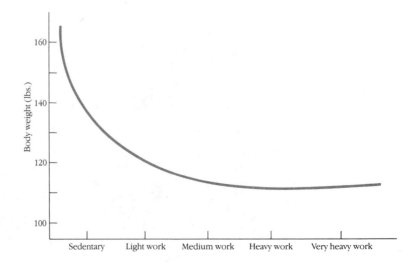

Table 7-1
Activity Equivalents of Some Foods (in minutes)

Food	Walking	Cycling	Swimming	Running	Yoga
Apple	20	12	9	5	20
Can of beer	30	18	13	8	30
Piece of cake	70	45	35	20	70
Two cookies	20	12	9	5	20
One doughnut	30	18	13	8	30
Double-scoop ice cream cone	40	25	18	11	40
Piece of pie	70	45	35	20	70
Piece of pizza	35	22	16	10	35
Twenty french fries	60	40	30	17	60
Ten potato chips	20	12	9	5	20
8 oz. soft drink	25	15	11	7	25
Hamburger	70	45	35	20	70

Data from F. Konishi, *Exercise Equivalents of Foods*
(Carbondale, Ill.: Southern Illinois University Press), 1973.

Of course, most people who want to lose weight want to lose it faster than a pound a month. Many are impatient for results and try all sorts of special diets and other rapid-weight-loss programs. Such programs plunge people into unusual and sometimes bizarre exercise and eating behaviors that may produce temporary weight loss but that, because they are so unusual, cannot be sustained. People become impatient with time-consuming exercises and become bored with restricted diets; soon they give up and return to their former lifestyles and habits. In order to achieve permanent weight loss and energy balance at a desired weight, overweight people have to change their long-term eating behaviors and their levels of physical activity. In short, successful weight loss and permanent weight control require a lifestyle change.

A weight-loss plan that has proved successful for many people is to reduce the number of calories ingested each day and increase the number of calories expended each day, for a net deficit of 500 calories per day. This program will produce a loss of 1 pound a week. Studies have shown that when a person loses 1 pound per week, the weight loss is likely to be permanent (Stuart and Davis, 1972).

Many studies indicate that overeating involves behavior that is independent of feeling hungry (Stuart and Davis, 1972). For whatever motivating reasons, whether boredom, fear, stress, or anxiety, many people overeat because various stimuli in their environments trigger eating behavior whether or not

they are hungry. Apparently, for them eating has become a habit that fulfills an emotional need—a need unrelated to the need to eat for physical survival. Therefore, successful weight loss involves first determining where nonessential calories are coming from in the diet and *why* they are ingested.

To plan a net 500-calorie-per-day deficit, you must determine the kinds of foods that can be safely reduced or eliminated from your diet. One way to do so is to keep a diary of everything you eat during four consecutive days and record the circumstances associated with each individual food intake (consult the FOR YOUR HEALTH section of Chapter 4 for a sample food diary). *Everything* in your diet must be recorded, from a carrot stick to a five-course meal. You can consult tables that list the caloric contents of various foods to determine the number of calories in each item.

Once you know the sources of your nonessential calories and the reasons you eat what you do, it becomes a matter of informed choice as to how to reduce the number of calories in your diet. A number of weight-control suggestions are presented in Box 7-3. By eliminating that daily soft drink, candy bar, beer, or bag of french fries, you can cut 200 calories out of your diet. Thus, to reach your goal of a net 500-calorie-per-day deficit, you need only expend 300 calories a day more than usual. This can be done in various ways (see Table 7-2).

Some people have the mistaken idea that if they increase their level of physical activity their appetite will increase proportionately and they will not lose weight. As shown in Figure 7-4, however, a person's appetite is likely to *decrease* if physical activity increases within reasonable limits. Appetite will increase along with the level of physical activity only when abnormally large numbers of calories are expended in vigorous work or play.

Weight-Control Fads and Fallacies

"Lose weight effortlessly, even as you sleep!" "New diet discovery lets you lose excess pounds in just one week!" So claim the advertisements for products and eating regimens that are directed to chronic dieters and others who are concerned about being overfat. Because the current social custom calls for the "slim and fit" look, the weight control industry is bigger than ever, with annual sales over $220 million.

Unfortunately for consumers, nearly all of the claims made by the heavily advertised weight control regimens and products are exaggerated and misleading. By themselves, these programs are not likely to produce a significant reduction in body fat on any long-term basis. Whatever weight loss they do bring about is usually a reduction in lean body tissue or in body water. The only proven way to reduce body fat and to maintain normal body weight is a lifestyle change that includes changing eating behaviors and increasing the level of physical activity.

Table 7-2
Approximate Energy Expenditures During Various Activities

Light exercise
(4 calories per minute)

Cycling 5 mph	Softball
Walking 3 mph	Golf
Canoeing	Ping pong
Housecleaning	Yoga
Slow dancing	T'ai chi ch'uan
Volleyball	

Moderate exercise
(7 calories per minute)

Tennis	Heavy gardening
Fast dancing	Snowshoeing
Cycling 9 mph	Walking 4.5 mph
Basketball	Roller skating
Swimming 30 meters/min.	

Heavy exercise
(10 calories per minute)

Jogging	Cycling 12 mph
Climbing stairs	Handball & racquetball
Football	Skiing
Mountain climbing	Ice skating

Three major faddish, and generally ineffective, weight control products or schemes are (1) body wraps, (2) diet pills (including vitamins), and (3) special diets.

Figure 7-4
Caloric intake as a function of physical activity. (Data from Mayer and Bullen, 1960. Used by permission.)

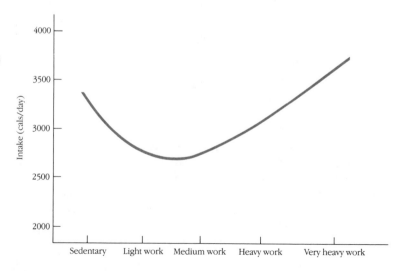

BOX 7-3

WEIGHT-CONTROL SUGGESTIONS

Control your home environment in these ways:
1. Do all at-home eating at the kitchen or dining room table.
2. Eat without reading or watching TV.
3. Keep tempting foods out of sight, hard to reach, and bothersome to prepare.
4. If you must snack, have low-calorie foods accessible, visible, easy to reach, and ready to eat.
5. Store tempting foods in containers that are opaque or difficult to open.
6. Give other family members their own snack food storage areas.
7. Don't do non-food-related activities in the kitchen; stay out of the kitchen as much as possible.

Manage your daily food sources:
1. Do not shop when hungry.
2. Shop from a list prepared beforehand.
3. Shop quickly.
4. Avoid buying large sizes of hard-to-resist high-calorie foods.
5. Prepare foods during periods when your control is highest.
6. Try to prepare several meals at once (lunches with dinners).
7. Remove leftovers from sight as soon after mealtime as possible (use opaque storage devices).

Eat slowly:
1. Put down the eating utensil, sandwich, drink, or chicken leg between bites.
2. Swallow what is in your mouth before preparing the next bite.
3. Cut food as it is needed rather than all at once.
4. Stop eating a few times during the meal to control your eating rhythm.
5. Make each second serving only half as large as the usual amount.

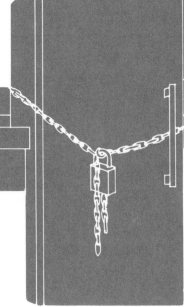
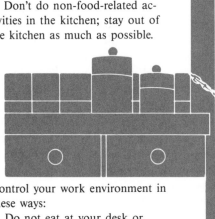

Control your work environment in these ways:
1. Do not eat at your desk or while working. Eat at some place designated (by you) for eating only.
2. Do not keep tempting food near your workplace.
3. Prepackage low-calorie snacks and take them with you to work.
4. Carry no change to use at vending machines.
5. Use exercise instead of food when you need to take a break from work.
6. If you eat in a cafeteria, plan your order in advance and bring only enough money to cover your order.

Control your mealtime environment:
1. Do not keep serving bowls at the table.
2. Use smaller plates, bowls, glasses, and serving spoons.
3. Remove the plate from the table as soon as you finish eating.
4. Practice polite refusal when extra food is offered to you.

Control snacking:
1. Instead of snacking, do an activity incompatible with eating.
2. Instead of snacking, do something you like to do, or a small task around the house or office.
3. Instead of snacking, do a short burst of intense activity or a relaxation exercise.
4. Brush your teeth or use mouthwash to curb the urge to eat.
5. Make snacks difficult to get.
6. Drink a large glass of water before snacking.
7. Have low-calorie snack foods on hand rather than high-calorie foods.

Data from J. Waltz, *Food Habit Management* (Seattle, Wash.: Northwest Learning Associates, Inc.), 1978.

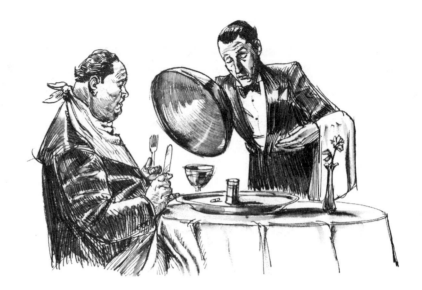

Body Wraps

Body wraps are plastic or rubber garments, ranging from waist belts to entire body suits, that are worn during exercise, routine daily activity, or sleep in order to produce weight loss. A wrap designed for just one part of the body (such as the waist or hips) is supposed to reduce the size of just that body region ("spot reducing").

Body wraps do produce weight loss and a reduction in body size. The catch is that the lost weight is body water and not body fat. These garments increase perspiration; they do not diminish the body's fat stores. The lost body water is quickly regained and so is the lost body weight. Because these products cause a loss of body water, they make dehydration a potential, although not very likely, danger associated with their use.

The appeal of body wraps stems from the common misconception that fat can be eliminated from the body by heat. The phrase "burning off fat" is part of the professional physiologist's jargon and contributes to this false notion. The process by which body fat is reduced does not involve heat. (Human body temperature is uniformly maintained at 37°C.) The "burning" that physiologists speak of is a chemical breakdown of fat molecules requiring oxygen, not the liquefaction and evaporation that one would expect from high temperatures. Hence, the claim that body wraps reduce body size by "melting away fat" is quite misleading.

Diet Pills

A number of products that contain drugs and "natural" substances are sold as weight-loss remedies. Quite often these products are used in conjunction with dieting, modification in eating behavior, and exercise programs, so they appear effective to the naive consumer. However, no single product by itself has been shown to reduce weight.

Amphetamines and amphetaminelike drugs have been used for years as appetite suppressants. However, there is considerable debate as to the wisdom of using amphetamines for weight loss—or of using any other drug for that matter (see Chapter 13)—because of the lack of proven efficacy and because of the potential for drug abuse and dependence.

Phenylpropanolamine (PPA), is an amphetaminelike substance that is the principal ingredient in several weight loss products sold over the counter (Dexatrim, Appedrine, Control, Dietac). PPA is thought to be an appetite suppressant, but the doses recommended in commercial preparations are probably not effective, and higher doses (greater than 75 mg per day) are likely to cause nervousness, nausea, insomnia, headaches, and elevated blood pressure.

Benzocaine, an anesthetic, is found in candies, lozenges, and chewing gums sold as aids to weight reduction. Benzocaine is supposed to help produce

No diet book can supply you with the will power that nature forgot. Diet books, like Broadway and Hollywood, are selling dreams.

Jon Carroll

weight loss by numbing the sense of taste and thereby reducing the desire for food. There is no scientific evidence, however, that temporarily reducing the sense of taste leads to weight loss. Because benzocaine is intended as a topical anesthetic, these products are useful (if at all) only if they are not swallowed.

Bulk-producing agents, such as methylcellulose, psyllium, and agar, are supposed to produce a sense of fullness in the gastrointestinal tract, thus suppressing appetite. These agents swell when mixed with water and are much more effective as laxatives than as weight reducers. Glucomannan, a bulk-producing starch derived from konjac tubers, is often touted by health food enthusiasts as a "natural" weight loss method. There is no evidence that glucomannan or any other bulk producer reduces appetite and produces weight loss.

Hormones, such as human chorionic gonadotropin (HCG) and thyroid hormone, are occasionally offered by unscrupulous clinics as aids for weight loss. Neither of these hormones is effective as a weight reducer. Moreover, because hormones are regulators of the body's homeostatic mechanisms, it is never wise to take them unless the effects of supplementation are monitored closely by a well-trained clinician.

Vitamins, minerals and some amino acids (including arginine, ornithine, tryptophan, and phenylalanine) are occasionally sold as agents for weight

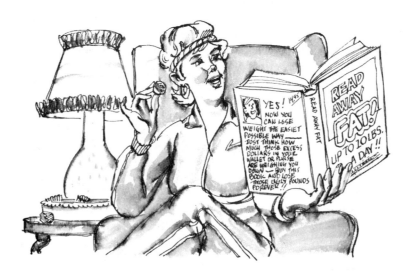

> If your stomach disputes you, lie down and pacify
> it with cool thoughts.
> **Leroy "Satchel" Paige**

loss. For example, Spirulina, a product made from blue-green algae, is claimed to be effective in reducing weight because it contains the amino acid phenylalanine, which supposedly regulates the body's appestat. Vitamins, minerals, and amino acids have not been shown to be effective in producing weight loss. And in very high doses, some of these substances, although "natural," can be harmful.

Fad Diets

If you want to make some money, get involved in the publishing of a book that describes a "revolutionary" new diet for weight loss. So many people make a hobby of trying fad diets that the book is virtually guaranteed to sell a large number of copies. Be sure that the diet you invent requires no exercise, is based on some "new" dietary or nutritional discovery, carries an air of authoritativeness, and promises a rapid reduction in body weight, although not necessarily a reduction in body fat. It doesn't matter a bit if the lost weight is regained in a short time. In fact, it's probably better for the weight loss industry if your diet does not produce permanent weight loss, since that would reduce the sales of the next crop of diet books.

Many of the weight loss diets that have come and gone have been based on altering the usual proportions of the three basic types of foods— protein, fat, and carbohydrate. Hence, the high-fat, low-fat, high-carbohydrate, low-carbohydrate, high-protein, and low-protein diets have all had their day and made their proponents wealthy. Occasionally diet regimens require the ingestion of only certain kinds of foods, such as fruits (grapefruit or papaya), cottage cheese, or steak. Fortunately, most of these unusual diets are too expensive, too boring, or too fatiguing to maintain for long, and people give them up before the nutritional deficiencies they can produce cause irreparable harm. Unfortunately, that is not always the case, and a few people have died from unsound dieting practices (such as stringent macrobiotic diets).

A relative newcomer among unusual weight loss regimens is the low-calorie all-protein diet. This diet is based on the theory that restricting the intake of calories in the form of dietary carbohydrate and fat but supplying the body's requirements for essential amino acids, minerals, and vitamins will produce the desired reduction of body fat while sparing the loss of lean body tissue. During the 1970s several deaths were associated with such high-protein diets, primarily because the ingested material was a liquid hydrolysate of a nutritionally low-quality protein. Products on today's market contain high-quality protein (often egg albumin) and a supply of essential vitamins and minerals. Nevertheless, the safety of even these dietary regimens is questionable (Felig, 1984).

Eating Disorders

Today virtually everyone wants to be thin. Best-selling books, films, TV shows, and most of the popular magazines (especially women's magazines) are replete with examples and messages that our society holds the thin body in high esteem and the corpulent body in some degree of contempt.

The current emphasis on slimness is partly a fad — there have been times (and they probably will return) when thinness was associated with being sickly and a full body was a sign of robust health and sexual attractiveness. The desire for slimness today is a reflection of the widespread concern with being healthy and physically fit. For both women and men, a lean body carries with it high status, sexual attractiveness, the aura of youthfulness, and a demonstration of the personal power to be trim and fit in a culture in which sedentary habits and overeating are prominent. For women, a slim body reflects the current trend toward sexual equality (androgyny); it represents a rejection of the traditional woman's role as homemaker and child-bearer and emphasizes a new femininity characterized by individualism, athleticism, and nonreproductive sexuality.

Whereas freedom from traditional sex-role behavior may be praiseworthy, using slimness as a measure of social achievement has become an oppressive standard for many, particularly for young people. In some instances, individuals develop such a morbid fear of becoming fat that they adopt unusual (and very unhealthy) eating behaviors. For example, a group of otherwise healthy adolescents were found to have severely restricted their intake of food simply because they feared becoming obese (Pugliese et al., 1983). Counseling that included dietary information, reassurance that obesity would not occur under professional supervision, and resolution of family conflicts was sufficient to restore normal eating behavior.

Young athletes, who are often obsessed with high achievement in sports, may also be susceptible to an inordinate fear of fatness. Most serious athletes are encouraged to be as lean as possible, and some overreact to the expectations of parents and coaches by restricting their food intake to excessively low amounts. This behavior, called **anorexia athletica,** affects both males and females. According to Nathan J. Smith, an expert in sports medicine, "Losing fat becomes a challenge in which the athlete promises himself uncompromised success. Hunger pains become gratifying signals of accomplishment, and food becomes the opponent in a contest that he is dedicated to win by an overwhelming score" (Smith, 1980). Counseling and reassurance that athletic goals can be met without such drastic eating behavior usually alleviate the condition.

Although abnormal eating behavior can be caused solely by the fear of becoming obese, there are instances when a compulsive desire to be slim is a manifestation of more complex psychological stress. Increasing demands on school health services for help with abnormal eating behavior indi-

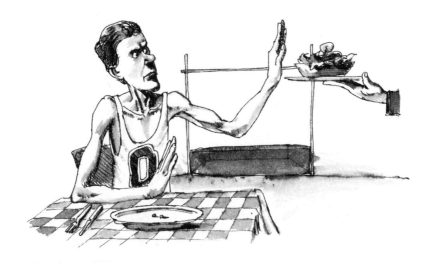

cate that a large number of young people, especially young women, have problems associated with eating. Two of the most common eating disorders are **anorexia nervosa,** a voluntary refusal to eat, and **bulimia,** characterized by binge eating and immediate purging of the ingested food either by vomiting or by using laxatives.

Anorexia Nervosa

Anorexia nervosa, which means lack of appetite for psychological reasons, is a condition characterized by progressive weight loss and metabolic disturbances caused by refusal to eat. About 95 percent of anorectics are women and nearly all are adolescents or young adults. Anorexia is not caused by any known physical agent, but the self-induced starvation can result in disturbances in thought, mood, and perception, loss of normal menstrual function (amenorrhea), and heart problems that could lead to death.

Elizabeth Barrett Browning (1806–1861), one of England's most famed poets is thought to have suffered from anorexia nervosa. As a teenager, Elizabeth was nagged by her parents to eat and gain weight, yet she stubbornly refused to eat much more than toast. When she met her future husband, poet Robert Browning, she weighed merely 87 pounds. Apparently, the Barrett family possessed characteristics found in other families with an anorectic member: overprotectiveness, overinvolvement with each other, and inability to express or resolve intrafamilial conflict.

Stubbornness and irony are characteristic of anorexia nervosa. For example, a person with anorexia nervosa is likely to vehemently defend his or her emaciated appearance as normal and will insist that *any* weight gain makes her or him feel fat. Besides such distortions in normal body image, anorectics tend to have a fanatical preoccupation with food. They may spend an inordinate amount of time planning and preparing elaborate meals for others, while they themselves eat only a few bites and claim to be full. Often they will not eat in the presence of others, and when they do eat, they frequently dawdle over their food for an hour or two. Some anorectics resort to self-induced vomiting or diuretic or laxative abuse to reduce their body weight. These practices may lead to a severe depletion of body minerals, which can precipitate abnormal heart rhythms and even cardiac arrest. Despite the low intake of calories, anorectics are remarkably energetic and tend to be hyperactive.

Another characteristic of anorexia nervosa is a paralyzing sense of ineffectiveness. The anorectic sees herself or himself as responding to demands of others rather than taking initiative in life. As children, anorectics were obedient, dutiful, helpful, and excellent students. Some psychologists interpret the intense preoccupation with weight loss as an expression of an underlying fear of incompetence. Control of eating and body weight becomes one way of demonstrating control and competence.

No one really knows what causes anorexia nervosa, although there are several theories. One theory holds that the preoccupation with weight loss

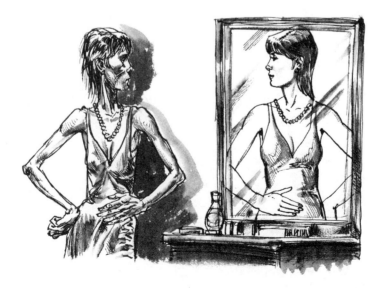

> The primary function
> of fasting is to allow
> the gastrointestinal tract to rest.
> **Rudolph Ballentine, M.D.**

is an attempt to avoid adolescence and adulthood and to remain a child who is cared for and fed by others, who can be stubborn and obstinate, and who has no sexual identity or inclinations. Another theory suggests that anorexia is the manifestation of a struggle for a sense of identity and personal effectiveness through controlling the environment; the resulting stubborn, rejecting behavior then becomes reinforced by the attention received from others. Yet another theory sees anorexia as a manifestation of impaired family interaction. The family of the anorectic becomes so engrossed with the anorectic's symptoms that they avoid attending to conflicts among family members.

Three goals characterize the treatment of anorexia nervosa: (1) weight gain, (2) a change in attitude toward food and eating, and (3) a resolution of the underlying personal and family conflicts. Unfortunately, therapeutic intervention is not always successful and the condition may persist for years. Anorexia nervosa has a 15 to 20 percent mortality rate.

Bulimia

Bulimia is characterized by a voluntary restriction of food intake that is usually followed by episodes of extreme overeating, usually of high-calorie junk foods, immediately followed by self-induced vomiting or use of diuretics and laxatives. Like anorexia nervosa, bulimia occurs primarily in young women with a morbid fear of becoming fat, and who pursue thinness relentlessly. Some surveys indicate that on college campuses as many as 20 percent of the female students are bulimic (Hawkins and Clement, 1980). Most bulimics are model individuals—good students, athletes, extremely sociable and pleasant. Fearing discovery of their bulimic behavior, they frequently carry out their binge-purge episodes in private. Usually bulimics are aware that their eating/vomiting behavior is abnormal; however, they are unable to control it. Many feel guilty and depressed about their problem. Bulimia can pose a serious risk to health for many of the same reasons that anorexia is dangerous.

Theories have also been proposed to account for bulimia. One is that bulimia is a response to psychological stress: abnormal eating behavior may be a maladaptive way of dealing with anxiety, loneliness, and anger. Another theory suggests that bulimia is a manifestation of the drive to become the "ideal" woman, which in our society has come to mean slim and trim. Bulimics tend to have low self-esteem and a weak sense of identity. The pursuit of thinness may reflect a passive dependency and the need for approval. Many bulimics are extremely uncomfortable dealing with close personal relationships, either with family or with peers.

Recovering from bulimia includes stopping the binge-purge cycle and regaining control over eating behavior. It is also necessary for the bulimic to establish more appropriate ways to handle unpleasant feelings and discomfort with close relationships. The bulimic's self-esteem must also be improved. Many colleges now have programs to help people with eating disorders. The National Association of Anorexia Nervosa and Associated Disorders (Box 271, Highland Park, IL 60035) provides information and help nationwide for persons with eating disorders.

Supplemental Readings

Ballentine, Carol L. "Hunger Is More Than an Empty Stomach." *FDA Consumer,* February 1984. An article explaining the many physiological factors that affect the regulation of appetite.

Bruch, Hilde. *Eating Disorders.* New York: Basic Books, 1973. A complete treatise describing anorexia nervosa, bulimia, and other eating disorders.

Sarker, Ira M., and **Zimmer, Marc A.** *Dying to Be Thin.* New York: Warren, 1987. Explains in full detail the causes and symptoms of bulimia and anorexia nervosa and how and where to find help.

Stuart, Richard B., and **Davis, Barbara.** *Slim Chance in a Fat World.* Champaign, Ill.: Research Press, 1972. A thorough explanation of the factors leading to overweight and how those factors can be changed.

Waltz, Julie. *Food Habit Management.* Seattle, Wash.: Northwest Learning Associates, 1978. An individualized workbook that teaches the reader how to manage eating behavior.

Summary

Approximately 60 million Americans weigh more than 15 percent over what is considered normal weight for height. A weight problem is caused by the accumulation of body fat in the fat-storing regions of the body. Body fat is stored rather than "burned" because more calories are ingested than are used up in basal metabolism and in providing energy for physical activity.

One cause of being overfat may be a malfunction in the body's regulation of appetite. Also, people can become overfat because they eat for reasons other than satisfying hunger. Food-and-drink-centered social activities, food-associated habits, and psychological stress contribute significantly to the overconsumption of food in our society.

The principal reason that people are overfat is that their lifestyles do not include sufficient physical activity to use up the calories ingested in food.

Many people live sedentary, inactive lives, which contribute to overfatness.

Successful weight control involves reducing one's intake of calories (often by recognizing the social and psychological reasons that cause one to overeat) and by increasing one's level of physical activity. Heavily advertised reducing schemes such as body wraps, diet pills, and fad diets are almost totally ineffective in producing permanent fat reduction and weight loss.

Because our society has placed a high value on thinness, many people, particularly adolescents and young adults, adopt unusual eating behaviors in an attempt to become slim, fashionable, and sexually desirable. Anorexia nervosa and bulimia are two extreme eating disorders; both are manifestations of psychological stress and maladaptive behaviors that must be managed in a more appropriate way.

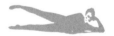

FOR YOUR HEALTH

Watching Your Weight

Refer to your food diary (see FOR YOUR HEALTH at the end of Chapter 4) in order to complete the following assessment:

1. List all the feelings other than hunger that are associated with your eating behavior. Does one feeling predominate?
2. Make a list of activities that you can do instead of eating when you are not hungry.

Slimming Down

If you are overweight, design a weight loss program for yourself. Make the goal of your plan the loss of 1 pound a week, which means expending 500 calories a day more than you ingest. Your plan should include increasing your level of physical activity and eliminating unnecessary calories from your diet.

Body Image

How do you feel about the appearance of these regions of your body?

	Quite satisfied	Somewhat satisfied	Somewhat dissatisfied	Very dissatisfied
Hair	☐	☐	☐	☐
Arms	☐	☐	☐	☐
Hands	☐	☐	☐	☐
Feet	☐	☐	☐	☐
Waist	☐	☐	☐	☐
Buttocks	☐	☐	☐	☐
Hips	☐	☐	☐	☐
Legs and ankles	☐	☐	☐	☐
Thighs	☐	☐	☐	☐
Chest/breasts	☐	☐	☐	☐
Posture	☐	☐	☐	☐
General attractiveness	☐	☐	☐	☐

Which of your regular thoughts and actions enhance your body image? Which of your regular thoughts and actions are likely to be detrimental to your body image? What could you do to become more satisfied with your body image?

UNIT TWO

Illness

CHAPTER EIGHT

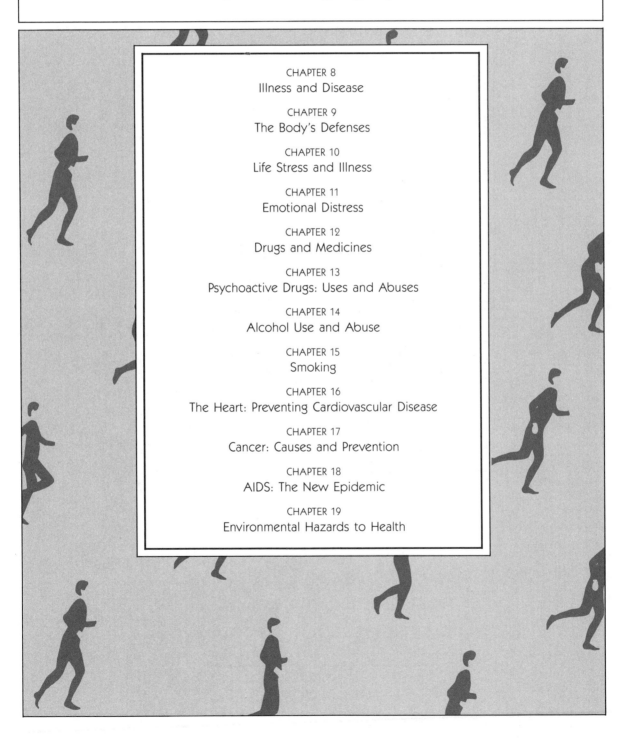

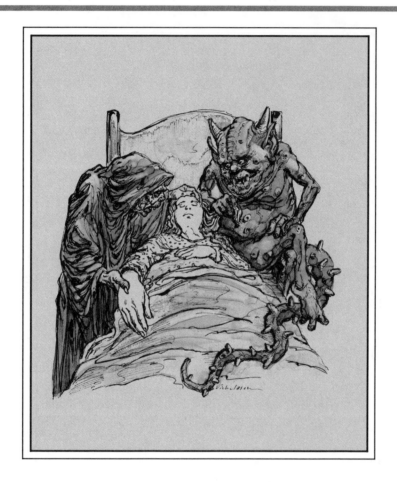

Knowing what produces illness is the
first step in prevention.

Illness and Disease

For most people, life consists of extended periods of wellness punctuated by occasional times of illness. While the purpose of this book is to help you achieve maximum wellness and enjoyment of life, it would be foolish to pretend that you will never become sick or that diseases do not exist. Health and wellness are achieved not only by preventing illnesses but by having a positive healing attitude during times of sickness and injury.

Your **attitudes** toward illness are very important. Anger and frustration are common responses to sickness or injury. Some people become angry at their bodies for failing to carry out their accustomed functions or they become frustrated that they are unable to do all the things they want to do. But there are other, more positive ways to deal with disease and illness. One way is to regard times of sickness as unavoidable parts of living. Another way is to recognize that sickness or injury can be your body's way of telling you that you need rest—that perhaps you have been pushing yourself too hard in your studies or in your job. Yet another positive way is to use periods of illness to reexamine the stresses and habits that may contribute to disease susceptibility. Viewed positively, many illnesses may become more tolerable. And by reducing anger, frustration, and worry, you can speed the body's natural healing processes.

In this chapter we define what we mean by illness and disease and describe some of the major categories of disease. Understanding something about illness and disease processes can help you achieve optimal wellness, because each of you can do a great deal to prevent diseases and help cure them. Understanding something about the mechanisms of disease processes also enables you to be a more intelligent consumer of medical care. You will know what questions to ask the health practitioners you consult, and you will have a better understanding of how to cooperate with them to reestablish wellness.

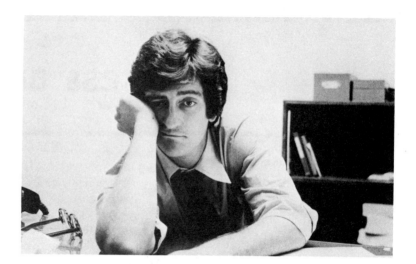

Figure 8-1
Illness and disease are not the same thing. Illness is a person's experience of feeling unwell; disease is abnormal body functioning revealed by medical diagnosis. (Photo courtesy CRM-McGraw Hill Films.)

Distinguishing Between Illness and Disease

There are a number of important distinctions between illness and disease. It is useful to make such distinctions because you are responsible for dealing with your feelings of being ill. Basically, **illness** is something experienced by an unwell person, whereas **disease** is what is diagnosed by the physician if some tangible evidence for abnormal body functioning can be found. A person may "feel ill" without a disease being evident or diagnosed; likewise, a person may have a disease without experiencing any illness or suffering. For example, millions of Americans have high blood pressure, which may be symptomless until a heart attack occurs. Another common example of "illness in search of a disease" is low back pain. About 5 percent of working Americans suffer from low back pain and about two out of every hundred of those are disabled by the persistent pain (Williams and Hadler, 1983). Doctors are rarely able to diagnose any disease or identify a medical problem that could be causing the pain. The treatment most commonly recommended is aspirin for pain relief and bed rest to allow the lesion to heal. Recent studies show that "more than 80 percent of patients will be well or much better within two weeks" (Hadler, 1986).

Anthony Reading (1977), professor of psychiatry at the University of South Florida College of Medicine, describes the distinction between illness and disease:

Illness tends to be used to refer to what is wrong with the patient, disease to what is wrong with his body. Illness is what the patient suffers from, what troubles him, what he complains of, and what prompts him to seek medical attention. Illness refers to the patient's experience of ill-health. It comprises his impaired sense of well-being, his perception that something is wrong with his body, and his various symptoms of pain, distress, and disablement. Disease, on the other hand, refers to various structural disorders of the individual's tissues and organs that give rise to the signs of ill health.

The onset and severity of any illness can be affected by the ways in which a person deals with it. If you become angry or depressed at being sick or excessively concerned about the outcome of the illness, you can interfere with the body's natural ability to heal itself. Disturbed emotional states may lower resistance to disease by reducing the immunological responsiveness of the body (see Chapter 3). Stress and worry can also produce physiological changes that not only may interfere with the natural healing mechanisms of the body but may contribute to illness and disease. As Lewis Thomas (1979), former president of Memorial Sloan-Kettering Cancer Center, suggests, worrying about health is not healthy:

Far from being ineptly put together, [people] are amazingly tough, durable organisms, full of health, ready for most contingencies. The

> ### Disease is only a failure of bodily function to adjust itself to the environment, and crime a similar failure in behavior.
> **J. B. S. Haldane**

new danger to our well-being . . . is in becoming a nation of healthy hypochondriacs, living gingerly, worrying ourselves half to death.

Optimism and a positive attitude can not only reduce the severity of illness and disease but also reduce one's susceptibility to becoming sick.

Causes of Disease

Traditionally, medical practitioners refer to diseases as resulting from specific causes. The cause of a disease is called its *etiology*. For example, specific bacteria are said to cause pneumonia or gonorrhea; certain viruses are said to cause measles, mumps, and hepatitis; a broken leg may have been caused by a fall.

Few diseases, however, actually have a single cause. Whether or not a person gets sick depends on a wide range of modifying factors (see Figure 8-2). The noted microbiologist René Dubos (1968) points out that

all manifestations of human disease are the consequence of the interplay between body, mind and environment. This situation creates a difficult dilemma for physicians and medical scientists. They recognize that the analytic breakdown of the problems of disease into their component parts never results in a true picture; yet they know from practical experience that the artificial reduction of these problems into their constituent parts, or their conversion into simpler models, is an absolute necessity for scientific progress.

The common cold, for example, one of the most widespread human diseases, involves infection of the upper respiratory tract (nose and throat) by any one of hundreds of different cold viruses (see Box 8-1).

Figure 8-2
Various internal and external factors determine whether or not disease results from infections by viruses, bacteria, fungi, worms, protozoa, and other kinds of infectious agents.

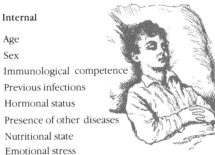

Internal

Age

Sex

Immunological competence

Previous infections

Hormonal status

Presence of other diseases

Nutritional state

Emotional stress

External

Infections in the community

Season of the year

Hygiene and sanitation

Drugs and medications being used

Environmental pollution

BOX 8-1

THE COMMON COLD

Virtually everybody catches a cold sometime or other. Schoolchildren may contract as many as a dozen different colds a year. It is estimated that 100 million serious colds occur each year in the U.S., causing 30 million days lost at school and work. Sales of over-the-counter cold remedies (which do not cure colds but may relieve symptoms) amount to about $1 billion annually. The common cold is clearly something that everyone prefers not to catch or to suffer from.

In 1914 a German scientist, W. Von Kause, first proposed that colds are caused by viruses. However, an actual cold virus (adenovirus R-167) wasn't isolated until 1953. Finally, in 1985, a detailed three-dimensional picture of a cold virus was obtained by using high-energy x-rays. Despite these major advances in cold virus research, a cure for the common cold is still not in sight. Even the development of a vaccine that would effectively prevent colds is doubtful due to the large number of different viruses that can cause colds and the ease with which

cold viruses change their antigenic properties.

Six major classes of cold viruses—rhinoviruses, coronaviruses, adenoviruses, myxoviruses, paramyxoviruses, and coxsackieviruses—have been identified. And within the rhinovirus class alone more than 120 different types have been observed. To prevent infection by all of these 120 different rhinoviruses, many different vaccines would have to be developed and administered. Scientists hope to find some common feature shared by most of the different cold viruses so that a single vaccine could be used to prevent most colds. However, such a prospect is still quite remote and may not even be possible.

New evidence shows that most colds are not transmitted through the air by sneezing or coughing but by hand-to-hand contact. The infected persons have viruses on their hands either from blowing or touching their nose and can then transfer viruses to others simply by hand-to-hand contact. The second person becomes infected by touching his or her nose with a hand or contam-

inated object. Frequent washing of your hands when you are around people with colds may reduce your chance of catching a cold.

The idea that cold, damp weather or drafts predispose people to catching cold has been disproved in numerous experiments. Volunteers who are deliberately infected with cold viruses and then placed in a cold damp room for two to three hours did not catch cold more easily than a control group. Recent experiments show that a nasal spray containing alpha-interferon (see Figure 9-4) can reduce the chances of catching a cold if the nasal spray is used just prior to virus exposure. The problem with using interferon is that it is a potent drug and its safety has not been demonstrated, especially in children. And for the drug to be effective you would have to spray interferon into your nose daily since you never know when or where you may become exposed to cold viruses.

The unfortunate conclusion from all the studies is that a cure for the common cold is still uncertain and certainly lies years into the future.

Yet the mere presence of a virus does not always cause a cold. In experiments with volunteer subjects in which suspensions of cold virus were sprayed into the nose and throat, not everyone in the study developed symptoms. For a variety of reasons some persons were more resistant to developing a cold than others.

Similarly, the cause of tuberculosis is not simply the presence of the infecting organism, a bacterium called *Mycobacterium tuberculosis*. Tuberculosis was one of the leading causes of death in the United States at the turn of the century, but today few deaths are attributed to tuberculosis even though the infecting bacterium has not disappeared from the environment. Robert Koch, a famous microbiologist of the nineteenth century, called TB "the disease of poverty" because it tended to be associated with squalor, overcrowding, poor nutrition, and poor sanitation. Many persons today have small tubercular lesions in their lungs, yet they never ex-

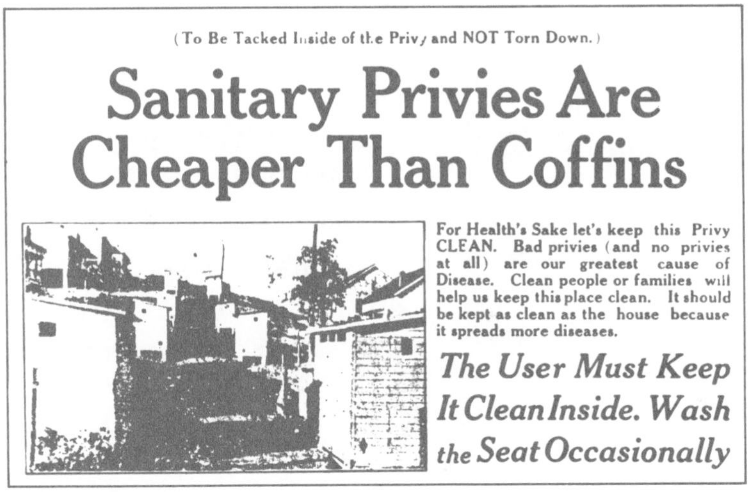

(To Be Tacked Inside of the Privy and NOT Torn Down.)

Sanitary Privies Are Cheaper Than Coffins

For Health's Sake let's keep this Privy CLEAN. Bad privies (and no privies at all) are our greatest cause of Disease. Clean people or families will help us keep this place clean. It should be kept as clean as the house because it spreads more diseases.

The User Must Keep It Clean Inside. Wash the Seat Occasionally

Figure 8-3
A poster circulated in the 1930s to alert people to the importance of sanitation in eliminating infectious diseases.

perience any symptoms of illness. Thus, poverty, poor nutrition, and stressful environments are as much the "causes" of TB as are the infectious bacteria.

Discussing a disease in terms of a single cause is mostly a matter of convenience. In reality, many factors contribute to the initiation and course of a disease. It is possible, however, to classify diseases according to the *principal* factor causing them. The principal factors accounting for nearly all disease are (1) heredity, (2) infectious organisms, (3) lifestyle and personal habits, (4) accidents, and (5) poisons and toxic chemicals. In this chapter we will discuss the first three factors; accidents and toxic substances are discussed in Chapter 19.

Keep in mind that, with rare exceptions, anyone can influence the development of a disease — for better or worse. Disease disrupts a person's balance of body, mind, and spirit and his or her interactions with other people. Whatever can be done to restore mind-body harmony can help cure most diseases and reestablish health.

Inherited (Genetic) Diseases

About 5 percent of all human beings are born with hereditary defects that result in anatomical or physiological abnormalities; these inherited abnormalities are called **genetic diseases.** They result from permanent changes in the physical structure of a person's chromosomes, the microscopic structures

that contain all the hereditary material (DNA). Changes in the genetic material result from **mutations;** many environmental substances, such as chemicals, x-rays, and atomic radiation can increase the chance that mutations will occur (see Chapter 19).

Altogether, about 3000 human genetic diseases resulting from single gene defects have been identified, most of which, fortunately, are quite rare. Some of the better-known ones are listed in Table 8-1. The more serious genetic defects often do not permit the fetus to survive to birth and are the cause of as many as half of all spontaneous abortions (miscarriages).

In order to assign unambiguously a disease or defect to genetic causes, at least one of three criteria must be met: (1) the disease must show a pattern of inheritance from generation to generation that obeys the laws of inheritance discovered by the founder of genetics, Gregor Mendel, (2) the chromosomes of cells in affected individuals must show some observable abnormality, and (3) a basic biochemical defect, such as the loss of an essential enzyme, must be demonstrated in cells of the affected individual.

Sometimes a particular disease is said to "run in the family." This means that there is a higher frequency of that disease among closely related persons than there is in the general population. This clustering of individuals with the same disease is called a **familial pattern.** Such diseases are not necessarily due to genetic or hereditary changes; they may be due to some factor in the family's common environment. This is an exceedingly important point

> In nature there's no
> blemish but the mind.
> None can be called
> deformed but the
> unkind.
>
> **William Shakespeare**
> *Twelfth Night*

to remember. People who are told that a disease is familial and believe that it is inherited often feel they are doomed to get it even though they may have no symptoms; believing that a disease is genetic can lead to unnecessary feelings of hopelessness and worry that can undermine one's health.

Unfortunately, many common diseases in our society are regarded as being hereditary or as having a strong genetic basis even though the disease does not clearly follow any of the three rules for inheritance. Examples of diseases with familial patterns are allergies, alcoholism, schizophrenia, diabetes, rheumatoid arthritis, hypertension, and even some rare forms of cancer, but it is incorrect to regard these as genetic diseases in the same sense

as those listed in Table 8-1. These diseases are caused by complex interactions of the genes with the environment, and they can be started and affected by nutrition, stress, emotions, hormones, drugs, and other environmental interactions. From the standpoint of personal health, it is advisable not to accept a genetic explanation for a disease unless the scientific evidence is unambiguous.

Doctors and other medical scientists sometimes refer to a person's **genetic susceptibility,** meaning that one's overall genetic make-up may make one more prone to developing a particular disease than another person with a different genetic make-up. In some respects the use of the term genetic susceptibility can lead to confusion in the mind of the per-

Table 8-1
Some Relatively Frequent Human Genetic Diseases

Genetic Disease	Major Consequences	Genetic Disease	Major Consequences
Albinism	Disturbed vision	Hemophilia	Bleeding — blood does not clot
Phenylketonuria	Mental retardation	Lesch-Nyhan syndrome	Mental retardation, self-mutilation
Alkaptonuria	Arthritis	Cystic fibrosis	Respiratory disorders
Galactosemia	Cataracts, mental retardation	Pituitary dwarfism	Short stature
Porphyria	Abdominal pain, psychosis	Hurler's syndrome	Coarse facial features, mental
Homocystinuria	Mental retardation		retardation
Down's syndrome (mongolism)	Mental retardation	Xeroderma pigmentosum	Skin cancers
		Agammaglobulinemia	Defective immune response
Tay-Sachs disease	Neurological deterioration	Myotonic dystrophy	Progressive muscular weakening
Retinoblastoma	Blindness	Turner's syndrome	Sterility
Sickle-cell anemia	Blood disorder	Klinefelter's syndrome	Sterility

> Wherever there is gold
> there is a chain, you know,
> and if your chain is gold
> so much the worse
> for you.
> **Alice Walker**

son so labeled, since he or she may believe that a genetic disease is involved. Many people think of diseases in absolute terms—either one's genes or the environment is at fault. However, the expression of genes is always influenced by both internal and external environments to some degree.

For example, not everyone who smokes two to three packs of cigarettes a day for many years will die of lung cancer. From this fact, some people (especially those who are employed by tobacco companies) would like to argue that cigarette smoking is a relatively harmless habit and that those persons who do contract lung cancer were genetically susceptible to the effects of cigarette smoke in the first place. A similar deceptive and false argument has been used to support the notion that exposure to radiation and radioactivity is safer for some people than for others because people vary genetically in their ability to repair radiation-damaged cells. To push this kind of argument into absurdity, one could argue that people over 7 feet tall are genetically defective and prone to head injury since they are more likely to hit their heads on doorways and low-hanging objects.

The point to realize in all of these examples is that some element of the environment is hazardous, whether it is cigarette smoke, radiation, or low doorways. The fact that people respond differently to these environments does not mean that they are genetically handicapped in any way. Each of us can choose and change our environments; we cannot choose or change our genes.

Treatment of Genetic Diseases

People often feel helpless and fatalistic when told they have a genetic disorder because they assume that "genetic" means incurable and irreversible. Although this is true for some hereditary diseases, it should be remembered that all genes function by interaction with the environment. The symptoms of **phenylketonuria** (PKU), a genetically determined defect of metabolism, can be controlled by maintaining the appropriate diet, provided the disorder is diagnosed early enough, as can a number of other inherited metabolic disorders. **Hemophilia,** a well-understood genetic disease that causes excessive bleeding because of the inability of the blood to clot, can be controlled by transfusions, by administration of the purified clotting factor, and in some cases by autosuggestion. Wallace LaBaw has conducted a clinic for children with hemophilia at the University of Colorado Medical Center. He has been successful in teaching some of the children how to control their bleeding using self-hypnosis. This ability to control bleeding resulting from a genetic defect demonstrates once again that the mind can influence the body's physiology in dramatic ways.

Huntington's chorea, a hereditary disease that killed the famous folk singer Woodie Guthrie, causes degeneration of certain nerve cells. Symptoms usually do not appear until midlife. Studies of related individuals who are known to carry the genetic defect reveal an interesting fact. Some persons begin to show symptoms of the disease in their

30s, while others are symptom-free into their 60s or even 70s. Many factors can influence how the genetic information is expressed in an individual.

Prenatal Detection of Hereditary Defects

Prevention of hereditary diseases and prenatal detection of genetic defects are important goals of modern medicine. Genetic counseling of parents who are at risk for bearing a child with a hereditary disease can help them reduce their chances of having a genetically handicapped child. Already several hundred hereditary human diseases can be detected by **amniocentesis** and more are being added yearly (see Figure 8-4). This prenatal diagnostic procedure is used to test for genetic and developmental defects in the fetus. Around the fifteenth week of pregnancy, a sample of amniotic fluid is removed; fetal cells cultured from this fluid are then subjected to various genetic tests, including visual examination (karyotyping) of the chromosomes. Amniocentesis also determines the sex of the fetus, although it is never performed solely for this purpose.

Inserting a needle into the amniotic sac to remove fluid entails a small but finite risk to the fetus; therefore, amniocentesis is generally recommended only in the following situations: (1) The pregnant women is age 35 or older or the father is over age 50, (2) the couple have had a previous child with a chromosomal abnormality or neural tube defect, (3) the pregnant woman is suspected of being a carrier of a deleterious X-linked trait, (4) both parents are known to be carriers of recessive genes that cause a hereditary disease or one parent is a carrier of an abnormal dominant gene.

The most frequent chromosomal abnormality detected by amniocentesis is **Down's syndrome,** a hereditary disorder that affects about 5000 children born in the United States annually (see Figure 8-5). Down's syndrome results from an extra chromosome (number 21) that is present in all of the individual's cells. Persons with Down's syndrome are severely mentally retarded and require special care and attention through their lives. Most individuals with Down's syndrome now live 40 to 50 years or longer. Many families are drained both emotionally and financially in caring for Down's syndrome children, and most affected individuals are eventually placed in institutions when they reach adulthood.

Amniocentesis is used to detect serious genetic defects in the fetus early enough so that the pregnancy can be terminated if that is the parents' decision after the results of the test are known. Because the fetus must have been developed for four to five months before the test can be given, development of tests that would permit an earlier diagnosis is desirable. One new test, called **chorionic villi sampling,** can be performed as early as 8 weeks after conception; however, the safety and reliability of this procedure remain to be proven. Early results with a small sample indicate that the fetal loss rate is un-

Figure 8-4
In the diagnostic procedure called amniocentesis, a sample of the fluid that surrounds the developing fetus is collected. Both the fluid sample and the fetal cells it contains are then analyzed for biochemical or chromosomal defects. Amniocentesis is performed early in pregnancy, whenever possible, so that the parents can decide whether to continue the pregnancy or abort the fetus. The decision is generally made after discussion and counseling with their physician.

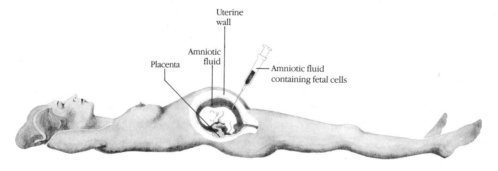

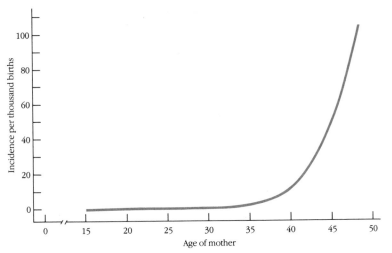

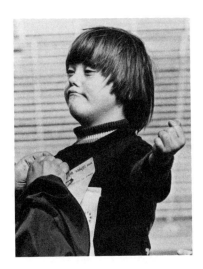

Figure 8-5
Frequencies of children born with Down's syndrome (mongolism) in relation to the age of the mother at the time of birth. At around age 35 the risk of this particular chromosomal defect begins to rise sharply. (Data from E. B. Hook, 1977; photo © Cheryl A. Traendly.)

acceptably high and that chorionic villi sampling is therefore not as safe as amniocentesis (Hecht et al., 1984).

One of the medical advances that has contributed to the safety of amniocentesis is the use of **ultrasound scanning,** an accepted and (presumably) safe technique for visualizing the fetus. Ultrasound scanning, or **sonography** as it is sometimes called, involves the use of high-frequency sound waves to outline the structural features of the fetus's body (see Figure 8-6). The sound waves penetrate the womb and are reflected differently from embryonic tissues that differ in composition and density. The reflected sound waves are displayed on a screen, and the pattern is interpreted by the doctor.

Ultrasound scans can be used to detect multiple fetuses and to determine the orientation of the fetus in the womb. They can also ascertain the location of the placenta, which is particularly important if amniocentesis is to be performed. They can also be used to gauge the fetus's head size, thereby providing an independent means of determining the age of the fetus and of ascertaining normal or abnormal brain development. Despite the apparent safety of ultrasound scans, pregnant women are advised to expose their fetus only if it is clear that the health of the mother or the fetus is in jeopardy (Williams, 1983).

Congenital Defects

Any abnormality that is present at birth is called a **congenital defect.** Some congenital defects are due to genetic changes and are hereditary. However, many others result from abnormal development of the fetus during pregnancy and are not hereditary. Developmental defects in the fetus can be due to injury, exposure to harmful chemicals, nutritional deficiencies, hormone imbalances, virus infections, and even severe stress.

In recent decades there have been a number of tragic occurrences of congenital defects that were caused by drugs prescribed for women during early stages of pregnancy. **Thalidomide,** a sedative taken as a sleeping pill, interferes with the development of the bones of the arms and legs of the fetus. Between 1960 and 1962 several thousand babies were born in Europe and Asia with deformed arms and legs before the effects of the drug were discovered. Fortunately for Americans, the drug was not distributed in this country, mainly because of the efforts of physicians Frances O. Kelsey and Helen B. Taussig.

In the 1950s and 1960s, the synthetic hormone **DES** (diethylstilbestrol) was prescribed as a fertility drug in women and also as a "morning after" birth control pill. Many daughters of women who took

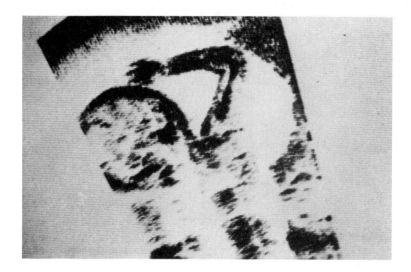

Figure 8-6
Image of a fetus obtained by ultrasound scanning. Such ultrasound scans reveal the position of the fetus and may also indicate cetain physical abnormalities. (Courtesy of Willard Centerwall, University of California, Davis, Medical Center.)

DES before or during pregnancy are now discovering that they have abnormalities in their reproductive organs. The daughters of women who took this drug also have a higher risk of developing vaginal cancer. It is not yet clear what effects, if any, the drug has had on male offspring.

The congenital defects caused by these drugs are *not* hereditary. Offspring of the people with congenital defects will not necessarily have the same defects. The important lesson from these cases is that during pregnancy—especially during the first few months—extra care should be taken and *no* drugs should be ingested, not even caffeine, aspirin, or alcohol if they can be avoided.

Infectious Diseases

A remarkable variety of organisms, ranging from viruses to worms, can infect the human body and, under certain conditions, can cause disease and suffering. Diseases caused by such organisms are called **infectious diseases**. Any organism that can produce a disease in an animal is called a **pathogen;** the major kinds of pathogens are illustrated in Figure 8-7. Most of the organisms in Figure 8-7 can be transmitted from person to person, and so the diseases they cause are called **communicable diseases.** Colds, measles, mumps, and gonorrhea are all examples of communicable diseases. Pathogenic organisms may also be transferred to people from other animals, in which case the animal is

referred to as the **vector,** or carrier of the disease. For example, malaria is caused by parasitic protozoa. These microscopic organisms are transmitted to people by mosquitoes that are infected by the protozoa; the mosquito is the malarial vector. Rabies is caused by a virus that can be transmitted to people who are bitten by infected dogs, bats, or other animals. The particular animal then becomes the vector for rabies infections in people.

Infectious Diseases in Human History

Throughout human history, infectious diseases have killed hundreds of millions of people. To appreciate how your health has benefited from the eradication of many infectious diseases, it is worth briefly reviewing some of that history. Keep in mind that while each disease is causally associated with a particular organism, the epidemics, deaths, and human suffering of the past were also the result of ignorance, poor sanitation, absence of sterile techniques, malnutrition, and other factors.

During the Middle Ages, **plague** repeatedly decimated Europe's population. This disease is estimated to have killed more than 150 million persons in past centuries. Caused by the bacterium **Pasteurella pestis,** plague is primarily a disease of rats and is transmitted to humans by fleas. If populations of rats or other rodents are kept from flourishing, there is no reservoir of the bacterium and people do not become infected—the reason that

> In nature
> there are neither rewards nor punishments—
> only consequences.
>
> **Robert G. Ingersoll**

rodent control measures are vital to health. Plague is not completely eradicated; there are still occasional small outbreaks in the United States and other countries. But diligent control measures have kept these outbreaks under control; cases rarely exceed a handful, and fatalities are even rarer.

In 1703, in Philadelphia, 5000 people died from **yellow fever.** At that time no one even suspected that the disease was caused by a virus transmitted to people by mosquitoes (viruses were unknown). Now, with control of the mosquito population, yellow fever has virtually disappeared from most sections of the United States.

In the sixteenth century, the Spanish brought **smallpox** with them to the American continent. It is estimated that half of the entire North and South American Indian population was killed by this viral disease; the epidemic greatly facilitated the Spanish conquests. Smallpox is the first human infectious disease believed to be completely eradicated from the world. As a result of a massive worldwide vaccination program carried out by the World Health Organization (WHO), it now seems that there is not a single person left who is infected with smallpox virus. The exciting story of smallpox eradication is summarized in Box 8-2.

Figure 8-7
Different kinds of disease-causing organisms.

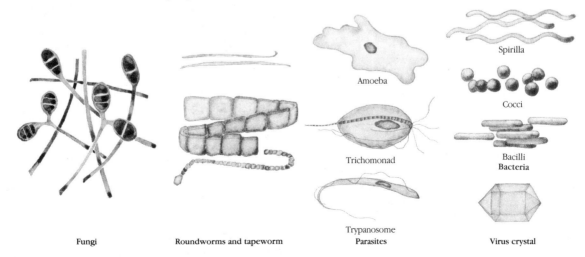

Fungi Roundworms and tapeworm Trichomonad Trypanosome Parasites Amoeba Spirilla Cocci Bacilli Bacteria Virus crystal

Following the Russian Revolution in 1917, 3 million Russians died of **typhus,** a disease caused by the microorganism *Rickettsia prowazekii.* Typhus is transmitted from person to person by body lice; in this instance poor santitation and personal hygiene were responsible for the typhus epidemic. In 1918, a worldwide influenza epidemic swept the globe, including the United States, killing more than 20 million people. Every few years a new strain of "flu bug" (influenza virus) appears, and carried from country to country by travelers, it causes outbreaks of influenza that often reach major epidemic proportions. Until early in this century, the principal causes of human sickness and suffering were infectious diseases. Since then, the death rates for many infectious diseases — especially those likely to strike in infancy and childhood, such as tuberculosis and typhoid fever — have fallen sharply.

Today, most life-threatening infectious diseases are no longer a serious health problem in the United States. Unfortunately, this is not the case in many other areas of the world, where hundreds of millions of people still suffer and die from infectious diseases. Various kinds of worms (roundworm, pinworm, hookworm, and tapeworm) infect about 1 billion persons worldwide; another 200 million people are debilitated by the water-borne parasite that causes the disease **schistosomiasis** (Anderson and May, 1982). Malaria still attacks as many as 300 million people each year and accounts for at least a million deaths annually in Africa. Even more serious as a cause of disease and death are the episodes of acute diarrhea in children under 5 years of age. Most surveys show that about a billion children suffer from diarrheal attacks in Asia, Africa, and Latin America, and approximately 5 million of them die each year (Holmgren, 1981).

Clearly, infectious diseases are still a major source of human suffering and death in many parts of the world. Hygienic measures such as clean water supplies and safe disposal of human wastes and sewage would dramatically reduce the number of deaths and cases of infectious and diarrheal disease. However, many countries do not have the capacity to introduce such life-saving public health measures. Americans are fortunate that sanitary and nutritional measures have largely eliminated these kinds of infectious diseases in this country. However, these statistics do show why it is essential that U.S. citizens take health precautions when traveling to other areas of the world, where they can become exposed to unfamiliar infectious organisms.

Table 8-2
Some Types of *Herpes* Viruses Remain in the Body for Life Once Individuals Are Infected

Type	Symptoms	Spread by:	Remains in:
Herpes simplex I	Cold sores on lips or in mouth	Direct contact; most infectious when lesions are present	Nerve cells
Herpes simplex II	Painful blisters on genital organs	Direct contact; oral-genital sex can transmit type I or II to mouth or genital area	Nerve cells
Cytomegalovirus (CMV)	No symptoms in most children and adults; CMV can cause stillbirth and mental retardation in fetuses	Body fluids: blood, urine, saliva	White blood cells
Varicella-Zoster virus	Chicken pox in children; shingles in adults	Close contact	Nerve cells
Epstern-Barr virus (EBV)	Mononucleosis	Saliva (kissing)	Lymph glands

---

BOX 8-2

THE CONQUEST OF SMALLPOX

Smallpox is an ancient disease. The earliest direct evidence of it is found on the mummy of Pharoah Ramses V, who died around 1160 B.C. Written records from China and India indicate that the scourge of smallpox was known even earlier. Apparently, a form of vaccination was practiced by the Chinese and Indians thousands of years ago: the inhalation of dried material from pox sores. The drying probably killed the virus without destroying its capacity to stimulate the body's production of antibodies (see Chapter 9), which provided immunity.

However, it was not until the eighteenth century that vaccination against smallpox became widespread. You may have heard the expression "A complexion as clear as a milkmaid's." Edward Jenner, an English physician, noticed that milkmaids almost never contracted smallpox. He reasoned that they escaped smallpox because most of them had been infected with the similar, but much milder, disease of cows called

cowpox, which somehow made them resistant to the more serious disease. In 1796, Jenner exposed an 8-year-old boy, James Phipps, to cowpox and subsequently to smallpox. The boy survived. Within a few years vaccination became widespread.

Despite massive vaccination programs, by 1967 smallpox was still endemic in thirty-three countries, and there were 10–15 million

cases worldwide. Three facts led the World Health Organization to attempt total eradication of the disease: (1) there are no animal carriers, (2) there is no human chronic carrier state, and (3) there exists a safe, effective vaccine. In October 1977, what is regarded as perhaps the last naturally occurring case of smallpox in the world was found in Somalia. No cases have been reported since then.

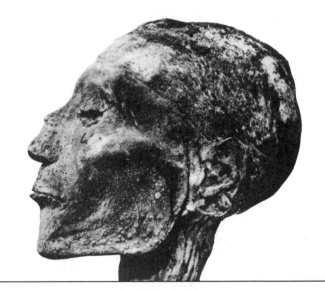

Fighting Infectious Diseases

Although the great French scientist Louis Pasteur established the germ theory of disease in the late nineteenth century, the medical profession was slow to accept his novel idea that "germs" (microorganisms) were the cause of diseases. Pasteur aroused the anger of many doctors when, in 1874, he advocated sterile surgical techniques:

> If I had the honor of being a surgeon, I would never introduce into the human body an instrument without having passed it

through boiling water or, better still, through a flame and rapidly cooled right before the operation. (Quoted in Bender, 1966)

The use of antiseptic (sterile) techniques to reduce infections in hospitals was slow to be adopted even though Joseph Lister had successfully applied Pasteur's ideas in his hospital ward as early as 1865. Until that time, a broken arm or leg often meant death, as a consequence of the infection that usually followed. It wasn't until the late nineteenth and early twentieth centuries, when the ideas of Pasteur and Lister were manifested in large-scale sanitation and

> The object of preventive medicine is to enable
> people to die young as old as possible.
>
> **Ernst L. Wynder**

public health programs, that the incidence of infectious diseases such as tuberculosis, plague, cholera, and diphtheria declined dramatically.

In the late 1940s another highly effective method for dealing with infectious diseases was discovered in the form of the antibiotic penicillin, which itself is produced by certain species of the mold *Penicillium*. Nowadays, hundreds of different antibiotics are available to combat infections from all kinds of microoganisms — with the general exception of viruses. Antibiotics interfere with functions in living cells. Those used medically are chosen for their **selective** interference; that is, for their ability to kill infectious organisms while doing little or no harm to the patient's own body cells. Because viruses are not cells, they are not directly affected by antibiotics. However, antibiotics are often prescribed to control a bacterial infection that might follow a viral infection. For example, lung cells frequently are so weakened after a bout with a flu virus that potentially fatal bacterial pneumonia may develop. The administration of an antibiotic to prevent growth of the pneumonia bacterium is often an appropriate measure.

Here are the essential points to remember about infectious diseases:

1. All infections require the presence of a pathogenic organism (virus, bacterium, or parasite). But development of disease and its symptoms depends greatly on one's mental, emotional, immunological, and nutritional state.

2. A healthy environment, adequate nourishment, personal cleanliness, and appropriate immunizations can prevent most infections.

3. Antibiotics are justifiably called "miracle drugs" and are often appropriate treatments, if and when serious infections develop.

4. The body's healing process usually can be helped by a "get-well" attitude and positive mental images of health and healing.

Infections Acquired in Hospitals

We usually do not think of hospitals as environments that are dangerous to health or as sources of infectious diseases. We tend to view the hospital as a hygienic, sterile environment where we go to be treated for some disease or disability. Unfortunately, the modern hospital, despite recent advances in medical technology and enforcement of strict hygienic measures, has become a place that increasingly endangers the health of patients. It has become a primary source of serious infectious disease. Surveys conducted by the Centers for Disease Control in Atlanta indicate that 5 percent of all hospital patients contract an infectious disease while hospitalized for some unrelated problem. Even more disturbing are data showing that 3 percent of those who do become infected in the hospital actually die from the hospital-acquired infection.

BOX 8-3

LEGIONNAIRES' DISEASE: A NEW BACTERIUM IDENTIFIED

In the summer of 1976, over 200 persons became ill during and following the fifty-eighth annual convention of the Pennsylvania American Legion branch in Philadelphia. Ultimately, 34 persons died of pneumonia-like symptoms. This mysterious epidemic was dubbed "Legionnaires' disease" by the press; months of investigation finally culminated in identifying a new bacterium, *Legionella pneumophilia,* as the cause of the disease and deaths.

Because of the organism's unusual growth requirements and failure to respond to conventional bacterial staining techniques, its discovery required months of experiments and tests by scientists at the Centers for Disease Control of the U.S. Public Health Service in Atlanta, Georgia. The Center is responsible for investigating unusual disease outbreaks in the United States. Once the disease-causing organism had been isolated, blood serum — previously taken from the sick Legionnaires and frozen — could be tested for the presence of antibodies to the newly discovered bacterium. More than 90 percent of the blood samples tested positively, demonstrating that those persons had been infected by these bacteria at the time of their illness.

It is now known that previous outbreaks of pneumonia and deaths in the United States were also due to this previously unidentified bacterium. It is estimated that more than 20,000 cases occur each year in the United States. Fortunately, most people who are exposed to the bacterium do not become ill; those who do usually respond to antibiotic treatment. The interesting story of Legionnaires' disease shows that there are still things to be learned about the causes of human infectious diseases.

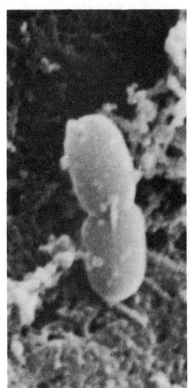

Scanning electronmicrograph showing Legionnaires' bacteria.

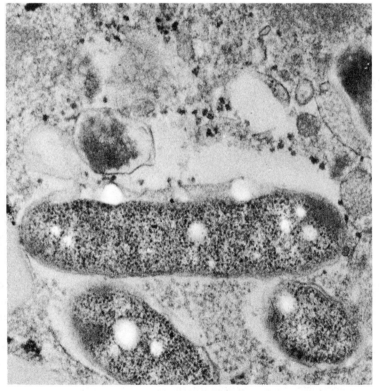

Higher magnification of a section of lung tissue infected with Legionnaires' bacteria. (Photos courtesy of Dr. Chao N. Sun, Veterans Administration Medical Center, Little Rock, Arkansas.)

From the beginnings of life
it has been the thousands of single-
celled microbes—always there
trying to destroy us everywhere along our way—
more than any cataclysm of nature,
that have been our real opponents
in the long struggle
for existence.

Ronald J. Glasser
The Body Is the Hero

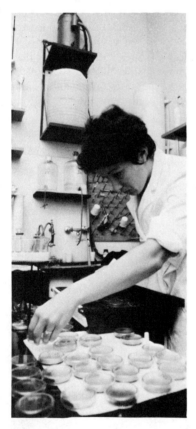

Figure 8-8
Testing for infectious organisms. The
kind of bacteria that are causing a
disease can be determined by culturing
a fluid sample from an infected
individual. Other tests can determine
the antibiotic sensitivity of the bacteria
so that the most effective drug can be
administered.

Hospital-acquired diseases are called
nosocomial diseases and are mainly caused by
bacteria. A few years ago the Centers for Disease
Control recognized the seriousness of the problem
and established a hospital infections program that
monitors outbreaks of nosocomial diseases. For
example, approximately 7.5 million Americans undergo bladder catheterization in hospitals every year,
usually because they are immobilized and are unable to urinate normally. About half a million of
these individuals develop urinary tract infections and
are also three times more likely to die as a result than
are catheterized patients who do not develop infections (Platt et al., 1982). Furthermore, nosocomial
infections invariably prolong the duration of the patient's stay in the hospital, and they contribute significantly to higher hospital costs.

The two bacteria mainly responsible for
nosocomial infections are *Escherichia coli* and
Staphylococcus aureus. Ironically, these bacteria are
normal inhabitants of the body, and when restricted
to their usual locations in healthy individuals do not
cause any disease. In hospital patients, however,
these bacteria often invade areas of the body where
they are not normally found and, in so doing, cause
infections and disease. Moreover, the particular infectious bacterial strains in hospitals are often resistant to many of the most effective antibiotics,
making nosocomial infections difficult to treat.

The dramatic increase in antibiotic-resistant
pathogenic bacteria in hospitals (as well as in the
environment outside hospitals) is due largely to the
enormous increase in the production and use of antibiotics over the past 20 years. At present more than

> Two million patients acquire infections in hospitals each year. The infections cause 20,000 deaths, contribute to an additional 60,000 deaths and add $2.5 billion a year to the nation's health care costs.
>
> **U.S. Public Health Service**

9 million pounds of penicillin are produced in the United States annually, and somewhat lesser amounts of other antibiotics, such as tetracycline, aureomycin, and ampicillin, are produced. The primary use of antibiotics is not as a treatment for infectious diseases in people but as a routine additive to animal feed used in raising chickens, pigs, cows, and other animals. The widespread dissemination of millions of pounds of antibiotics in the soil and water has resulted in the selection of bacteria that have been resistant to some or all of the commonly used antibiotics, and these antibiotic-resistant bacteria eventually wind up in people. While many scientists have been concerned about the dramatic increase in antibiotic-resistant bacteria and nosocomial infections, the problem of antibiotics overuse has only recently received serious public attention (Schell, 1984).

What is the message in all this as far as personal health is concerned? First, realize that hospitalization is a serious matter and that hospitals should be used only for serious illness. If a choice exists between treatment in a hospital or outside, it may be wiser to choose the outside treatment. You can also ask your doctor or hospital administrator what the hospital's record is when it comes to nosocomial infections.

Lifestyle Diseases

So far we have primarily discussed diseases of genetic and environmental etiology. However, the majority of diseases that afflict Americans today, such as diabetes, most arthritis, cardiovascular diseases, allergies, ulcers, colitis, and even cancer, have no single principal environmental or genetic cause and are increasingly regarded as **diseases of lifestyle**. This means that there are a multitude of factors in our daily lives that contribute to the development and progression of each of these diseases. These factors include stress, poor nutrition, weakened immunological defenses, destructive habits such as smoking cigarettes or drinking alcohol, being overweight, and probably many more. Medical science is becoming increasingly aware of the multifactorial nature of many diseases. As Lewis Thomas (1978) puts it:

> The new theory is that most of today's human illnesses, the infectious aside, are multifactorial in nature, caused by two great arrays of causative mechanisms: the influence of things in the environment; and one's personal lifestyle. For medicine to become effective in dealing with such diseases, it has become common belief that the environment will have to be changed, and personal ways of living will also have to be transformed, and radically.

Fundamentally, most diseases can be regarded as the failure of a biological process, a failure of an organism to adapt to its natural, cultural, and social environments. Furthermore, most lifestyle diseases, once they have occurred, cannot be cured; at most the doctor and medicines can relieve suffering and alleviate symptoms. Herbert Weiner (1978), professor of psychiatry and neuroscience at Albert

> If the health of man is to become fully manifest it
> must prevail not only in the individual but in
> mankind as well.
> Health is wholeness and sickness implies
> impairment of parts of the whole.
>
> **Jonas Salk**

Einstein College of Medicine, points out some of the factors of living that increase a person's risk for developing a variety of diseases:

> The stress of being an air-traffic controller is associated with an increased incidence of elevated blood pressure, peptic duodenal ulcer, and sometimes, diabetes mellitus. Bereavement that is not coped with and produces the "giving-up, given-up" complex has been estimated to precede different diseases. Bereavement plays an important role in many, if not all, patients with "psychosomatic" diseases. Real or threatened loss has often been cited as a factor contibuting to the initiation of other diseases as well: cancer, tuberculosis, diabetes mellitus, lymphomas and leukemias, juvenile diabetes mellitus, and heart failure. Depressive moods, the attitude of giving up, and the loss of all hope also adversely affect the outcome of surgical operations.

Diabetes Mellitus: A "Typical" Lifestyle Disease

Diabetes mellitus, called **diabetes** for short, is a disease worth examining in some detail because in many respects it typifies a disease of lifestyle.

Diabetes is one of the ten leading causes of death in the United States. It is estimated that as many as 10 million Americans may have some form of diabetes, and perhaps half of those do not know that they have it. The more severe form is called **Type I,** or **insulin-dependent, diabetes** since insulin is required to control the symptoms. Type I diabetes was formerly called "juvenile onset" since most of the cases are observed in children or adolescents. The majority of diabetics (about 90 percent) have **Type II diabetes,** which is noninsulin-dependent and often can be controlled by diet, exercise, or drugs other than insulin. Type II diabetes was formerly called "maturity onset" since most of the cases occur in adults and older people.

Diabetes is a metabolic disorder in which the body is unable to regulate the level of sugar (glucose) in the blood. Normal blood sugar levels range between 50 and 100 mg of glucose per 100 ml of blood. If a person's blood sugar level is persistently too high (or too low), serious symptoms may develop. Diabetes is diagnosed by measuring the rate at which glucose is metabolized by an individual, but it is now recognized that glucose intolerance can be caused by at least thirty different disorders. Consequently, the disease referred to as diabetes is actually a heterogeneous group of diseases (Jarrett, 1982).

Blood sugar level is regulated by a hormone, **insulin,** that is manufactured by special cells of the pancreas. To avoid serious illness, persons with diabetes must carefully control the amount of sugar in their diets and may also require daily insulin injections.

While there is usually no family history of diabetes in Type I diabetes, there is often a familial pattern in Type II that contributes to the belief that diabetes is mainly a genetic disease. However, studies

Recent studies have shown that most diabetics receive inadequate dietary advice and counseling. . . . It is worth reevaluating the role of diet in the management of diabetes.

A. Chait
E. L. Bierman

by James V. Neel, professor of human genetics at the University of Michigan Medical School, led him to conclude that "Diabetes mellitus is in many respects a geneticist's nightmare. As a disease, it presents almost every impediment to a proper genetic study which can be recognized" (Neel et al., 1965).

Abner L. Notkins (1979), a diabetes researcher at the National Institute of Dental Research, asserts that recent research

> has supported the contention that diabetes is a heterogeneous group of diseases rather than a single one. This work has also indicated that diabetes arises from a complex interaction between the genetic constitution of the individual and specific environmental factors. . . . Since family members share the same diet and environment, a high incidence of diabetes in a given family does not necessarily prove that genetic factors are involved.

Frequently, Type II diabetes is associated with overweight. For every 20 percent increase in overweight, the chance of diabetes doubles. Many times weight loss cures such a diabetic condition. Infection of the pancreas by certain viruses may be responsible for many cases of Type I diabetes and perhaps contributes to cases of Type II diabetes. It is likely that some persons are more susceptible to pancreatic infections and hence have a higher risk of developing a diabetic condition. It is also possible that a deficiency of chromium, a trace mineral essential for normal sugar metabolism, may be

responsible for some cases of Type II diabetes (Underwood, 1977).

For more than a hundred years, scientists and doctors have noted that stress and emotional upset can bring about symptoms of diabetes and can change blood sugar levels. In a review of the psychological factors in diabetes, Donald E. Greydanus and Adele D. Hofmann (1979) conclude that

> there is a notable degree to which psychological factors seem to influence the course of diabetes mellitus. Though it is difficult to show the role of stress in the precipitation of its onset, it is noted by many that these factors can profoundly affect the metabolic control of a diabetic.

As of 1986 the effects of stress on elevating blood glucose levels in diabetics still had not been resolved. The authors of one study concluded that psychosocial stress has no effect on the control of diabetes (Kemmer et al., 1986). However, a diabetic physician countered their conclusions with his own personal experience. He monitored his own blood glucose levels before, during, and after taking the National Medical Board exams. He reported that his blood glucose levels almost doubled during the exam as compared to levels in blood samples taken before and after the exam ordeal (Bernstein, 1986).

To test for diabetes, individuals with symptoms suggestive of diabetes are given a **glucose tolerance test.** This test measures blood sugar levels under standard conditions in which the individual fasts and then ingests a fixed amount of sugar. If the test shows blood sugar levels to be excessively high, the

> In recent years, environmental influences increasingly have been implicated in the pathogenesis of diabetes. This is particularly the case in the juvenile-onset form of the disease.
>
> **John E. Craighead, M.D.**
> **University of Vermont Medical School**

person is said to be hyperglycemic and diabetes is suspect. One should be extremely cautious in accepting a diagnosis of diabetes from a single glucose tolerance test. A diagnosis of diabetes usually is more certain after several elevated glucose tolerance tests, accompanied by other symptoms of the diabetic condition.

Preventing Diabetes and Other Lifestyle Diseases

Diabetes is a disease of lifestyle that has been increasing at a disturbing rate in recent years, although the reasons for the increase are not apparent. Some individuals may be more susceptible to diabetes because of previous infections or because of their genetic make-up. For the majority, however, the problem is lifestyle, obesity in particular. Diabetes is only one of the chronic diseases of lifestyle that afflict millions of people in this country. Many lifestyle diseases develop over a period of years as a consequence of personal habits. Improving nutrition, maintaining normal body weight, reducing stress, and avoiding exposure to harmful substances can help prevent diabetes and other lifestyle diseases. A person is never too old to experience benefit from adopting healthy living habits.

Supplemental Readings

Alper, J. "Better Weapons for Antibiotic Warfare." *High Technology,* December 1983. Discusses how antibiotics destroy bacteria and how new antibiotics are chemically constructed.

Farley, D. "Test-tube Skin and Other High-Tech Treatments for Burns." *FDA Consumer Magazine,* June 1987. Explains the remarkable advances that have been made in treating serious burns.

Fincher, J. "Notice: Sunlight May Be Necessary for Your Health." *Smithsonian,* June 1985. Describes the many effects of light on health and a possible cure for depression and disease.

Genetic Counseling. The National Foundation/March of Dimes, Box 2000, White Plains, NY 10602. A small booklet explaining what genetic diseases are and the sort of tests and medical help that are available.

Notkins, Abner L. "The Causes of Diabetes." *Scientific American,* November 1979. A clear discussion of this lifestyle disease.

"Osteoporosis Protection Plan." National Institutes of Health recommendations. *Prevention,* August 1987. Discusses how to prevent this disease from occurring later in life.

Rotter, J. I., and **Rimoin, D. L.** "The Genetics of Diabetes." *Hospital Practice,* May 15, 1987. An excellent account of the various types and causes of diabetes.

Shell, Orville. *Modern Meat.* New York: Random House, 1984. A well-written tale of the health problems associated with use of antibiotics in animal feed.

Summary

Every person becomes sick at one time or another. Illness is what a sick person experiences; disease is what a doctor can diagnose from symptoms and test results.

Few diseases have a single cause (etiology). Most are the result of the interaction of personal (both physical and emotional) and environmental factors. Even though few diseases have a single cause, it is convenient to talk about disease causation in terms of the principal factors that bring on a disease. These factors are heredity, infectious organisms, lifestyle and personal habits, accidents, and poisons and toxic chemicals.

About 5 percent of all human beings are born with a hereditary disease. Diagnosis of hereditary disease involves the application of certain rules. Even though a disease is hereditary, its course can be influenced by lifestyle and other factors.

Infectious diseases are primarily caused by pathogens, disease-causing organisms such as viruses, bacteria, and protozoa. Infectious diseases have largely been controlled through sanitation, sterile techniques, improved nutrition, immunizations, and antibiotics.

Many diseases, such as heart disease and cancer, are diseases of lifestyle. Factors related to their causation are stress, poor nutrition, weakened immunological defenses, smoking cigarettes, and being overweight. Diabetes is a typical lifestyle disease in that it has many contributing causes.

FOR YOUR HEALTH

When You're Ill

Illness is a personal experience. It's how you feel when you are sick, regardless of what particular disease process may be going on in your body. Make a list of the things that feel different when you feel ill. Do you have less energy or more? Do you feel "blue" or depressed? Do you tend to eat more or less? Do you crave certain kinds of foods?

After you have made your list, determine which of the feelings you might be able to change to hasten your recovery from illness and the return of good feelings. For example, if you become depressed when ill, simply reminding yourself that the illness and depression are related can improve your spirits, which is health promoting.

Diseases You Have Had

Knowing the diseases you have had can be helpful whenever you get sick, especially if you seek advice and treatment from medical practitioners. Make a list of all diseases you have had (or presently have). Record the name of the disease, when you had it, how it was treated, and by whom. Include your childhood diseases, such as measles and chicken pox. Also include major injuries, such as broken limbs, and any allergies. Confer with parents and family members to be sure your list is complete. A sample medical history is provided in Appendix E.

CHAPTER NINE

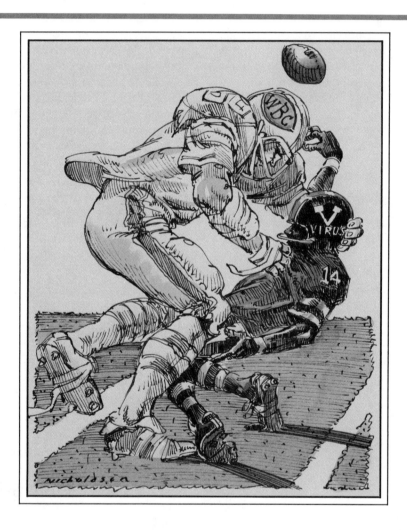

How to maintain optimal functioning
of the immune system and other
body defenses.

The Body's Defenses

Most people feel healthy and well most of the time. This is because the body contains a remarkable array of defense mechanisms that, when functioning optimally, help keep noxious substances and disease-causing organisms out of the body and also help eliminate any diseased cells and infectious organisms that are found within the body.

Your body naturally provides habitats for a variety of viruses, bacteria, and other potential pathogens. These microorganisms are always present, yet they rarely make you sick or cause disease. Every day you ingest harmful organisms and toxic substances in the food you eat, from the air you breathe, and from the water you drink. Yet your body rarely falls prey to any of these harmful substances. If you become sick, it is probably because you had excessive or prolonged exposure to a harmful substance or because you have become more susceptible to it.

This chapter discusses the body's various lines of defense and the biological mechanisms that are involved. Most of the responses of the body's defense systems, as well as the detoxification of chemicals in the liver and the repair of damage to cells and tissues, are physiological processes regulated automatically by the body itself. But these defense mechanisms can be hampered by poor nutrition, stressful environments, emotional upset, and negative mental attitudes. Understanding how the body's defense mechanisms protect you from disease will also help you understand how physical and mental well-being and harmonious interactions with the environment can keep the body's defenses functioning optimally.

> When it comes to the various kinds of artificial materials which human beings apply to their skin in the attempt to temporarily improve its appearance or to retard its aging there is little to be said. The various claims are not scientifically based, and long-term benefits have not been demonstrated.
>
> Donald M. Vickery, M.D.
> James F. Fries, M.D.

The First Line of Defense: Keeping Harmful Substances Out

The best way to prevent disease caused by foreign substances, whether they are living organisms (pathogens) or nonliving substances such as pesticides or asbestos, is to exclude them from the body. The skin prevents the entry of most microorganisms and harmful substances by functioning as a physical barrier (see Figure 9-1). In addition, the mildly acid surface of the skin provides a poor habitat for most harmful bacteria, while allowing certain beneficial bacteria to colonize the skin.

The **mucous membranes** provide another vital barrier to disease-causing substances. Our eyes, nose, throat, and breathing passages are protected by membranes that continuously produce secretions that flush away harmful particles. These membranes also secrete enzymes that degrade foreign substances. The mouth, gastrointestinal tract (digestive system), and excretory organs are similarly encased and protected by membranes that guard the body's internal cells and organs.

Tears keep the surface of the eyeball moist and also serve to wash away foreign particles that lodge in the eye. Wax secreted from the ears protects the delicate hearing apparatus. The mucous coating of the respiratory tract is sticky and provides a trap for irritating particles and organisms; microscopic

Figure 9-1
The skin provides the first line of defense in protecting the body from harmful substances. It is actually a complex tissue consisting of several layers and specialized organelles.

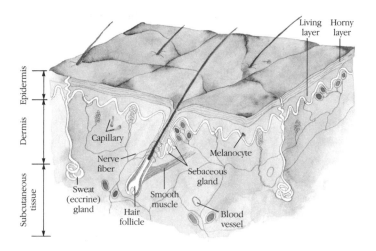

> Life is still
> what it always has been,
> a battle of molecules, of our chemistry
> against the invaders'.
>
> **Ronald J. Glasser**
> *The Body Is the Hero*

hairlike fibers called **cilia** keep the mucus of the respiratory tract moving out of the bronchial tubes so that eventually you are able to cough or spit out the foreign irritating substances. Sneezing and blowing the nose eliminate irritating particles that are inhaled.

Enzymes and substances in the blood form a clot that rapidly seals any break in the skin and thus prevents entry of harmful substances and organisms. Still other enzymes and special cells in the blood attack and kill harmful bacteria and other microorganisms that might have entered the body through the wound before it was sealed.

If a toxic chemical or pathogenic microorganism should breach these physical defenses of the body and enter the bloodstream or gastrointestinal tract, other defenses are called into action. In the stomach, strong acid secretions and special enzymes help destroy pathogenic microorganisms. For toxic chemicals, the body has a vast array of enzymes, especially those synthesized in the liver, that can **biotransform** or detoxify most harmful chemicals, thereby protecting the body from damage or disease. One form of detoxification carried out by liver enzymes is the biotransformation of alcohol, a highly toxic substance that, if allowed to accumulate in the body, may cause serious disease and even death. Enzymes convert the alcohol in the body into carbon dioxide and water. The unpleasant symptoms of alcohol intoxication are felt when the body's enzymes cannot biotransform ingested alcohol fast enough. The problems and disease that derive from alcohol abuse are discussed in Chapter 14.

Internal Defenses

White Blood Cells and Macrophages

If microorganisms or foreign particles should find their way into the blood or if they should accumulate in body tissue, they soon encounter specialized blood cells called **leukocytes.** These are the colorless **white blood cells,** so called to distinguish them from the red blood cells that transport oxygen to all the body's tissues. Leukocytes engage in a process called **phagocytosis** (eating of cells) in which foreign organisms and particles are engulfed and destroyed. Only about one cell in 700 in the blood is a leukocyte, but their number can increase dramatically in times of acute infection. That is why, for example, the blood is tested for an elevated white blood cell count when an infection is suspected; increased production of white blood cells is the body's response to the the infectious organisms proliferating in the body.

There are other kinds of specialized phagocytic cells called **macrophages** that are associated with specific organs and tissues and are vital to the body's defense mechanisms. Figure 9-2(a), shows an alveolar macrophage (a special cell that protects the air sacs in the lungs) that is about to engulf and remove some irritating fly ash particles that have entered a lung exposed to air polluted by the burning of coal. Leukocyte and macrophage cells have a relatively brief life span in the body, usually a few weeks

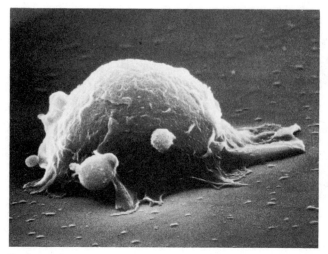

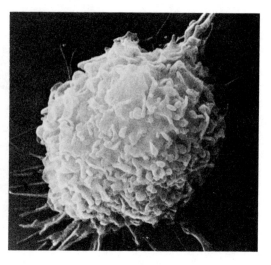

Figure 9-2

(a) An electronmicroscopic view of a lung macrophage cell about to engulf a fly ash particle. Such particles are released into the air from burning coal and are later inhaled. (Photo courtesy Lawrence Berkeley Laboratories.)

(b) A mouse macrophage cell from the stomach lining. Macrophage cells in the gut protect animals from foreign substances entering the body via the digestive system. (Photo courtesy Sloan Kettering Cancer Center.)

or months, after which they themselves are destroyed and replaced by other leukocytes and macrophages that have been newly synthesized in the bone marrow. Your health depends on the continuous monitoring and removal of foreign material and cellular debris from all regions of the body by phagocytic cells of various kinds and functions.

The ways in which the body regulates the production of essential white blood cells are not well understood. Occasionally, a person's synthesis of white blood cells goes out of control, producing too many white blood cells, which crowd out other blood substances. The result is a disease called **leukemia,** a form of cancer. Leukemia can occur in either an acute or chronic form. The acute form is characterized by rapid cell proliferation. Chronic leukemia is the more easily manageable form of the disease and generally cycles through periods of normal and abnormal production of white blood cells. The disease is said to be in **remission** when the white blood cell level is normal.

From the viewpoint of personal health it is important to remember that you may be able to influence the course of infectious diseases, and possibly even of cancer, by stimulating or retarding

the production of various white blood cells the body uses to protect tissues and combat disease. Even though all the physiological mechanisms by which the mind affects the production of white blood cells are not yet understood, a person can help healing by using the mind through relaxation and visualization techniques to positively influence the body's physiology and cellular defenses. How the mind affects the immune system is discussed later in this chapter.

Inflammation

One of the body's internal defenses is **inflammation** — a reaction of tissue to injury or the invasion of microorganisms. Inflammation stimulates a complex series of events in a wounded or diseased area. The damaged cells usually release histamine and related substances that dilate (increase the diameter of) local blood vessels. This often causes swelling and may also stimulate pain-sensitive nerve fibers to respond, thereby causing the sensation of pain. White blood cells are attracted to the wound or diseased region in large numbers to clean away the tis-

BOX 9-1

ACNE

Acne—the appearance of pimples (called whiteheads, blackheads, or "zits") on the face and occasionally on the shoulders, chest, and back—afflicts millions of people. Acne is so common among adolescents that many consider it to be "normal" for that stage of life. Few of those afflicted with acne seem to agree, however, since they spend millions of dollars on acne medications each year.

Acne comes from the blocking of oil-producing glands (sebaceous glands) in the skin. Normally, these tiny glands produce an oily substance called sebum, which drains onto the skin through a hole or pore. For reasons that are not understood, sometimes a pore becomes plugged by dead cells, bacteria, and sebum, preventing normal gland products from getting out. When all this material builds up within the gland, along with skin pigment particles (causing the blackhead) and white blood cells that get involved to "clean up" the problem, a pus-filled pimple forms.

No one know what causes the plugging of sebaceous glands in acne. Contrary to what many believe acne is not due to the over-consumption of chocolate, cola drinks, or greasy foods. Neither is it a bacterial infection of the skin, even though it may worsen because of the degradative action of certain bacteria on sebum. In some instances, acne may result from physically covering the pores of sebaceous glands. Athletes and hikers can develop acne in skin areas pressured by their gear. Wearing a hat can lead to acne on the forehead. Even resting your

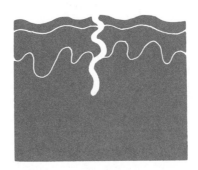

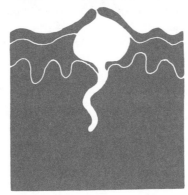

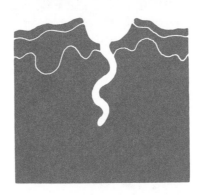

hands on your face while studying can sometimes produce a localized bout of acne. Virtually all makeups, especially the pancake type, are likely to worsen an acne condition.

Acne can be affected by hormones. Sebum production increases in response to the sex hormone testosterone. In some women, pregnancy or taking birth control pills makes acne worse, whereas in others pregnancy and oral contraceptives may clear up acne completely. Some women experience minor flare-ups of acne near the beginning of their menstrual cycle.

Because the cause of acne is unknown, there is no single way to clear it up; neither is there a simple preventive measure. Most dermatologists recommend a combination of cleanliness and certain types of medications to control acne. They especially suggest proper washing that removes surface oils and dirt but that does not irritate the skin. Medicines containing benzoyl peroxide are often useful in clearing up and preventing acne. The prescribing of antibiotics, especially tetracycline, to prevent and treat acne may not be the best course except in severe cases. Disfiguring cases of acne can be treated with a new drug, 13-cis-retinoic acid (trade name: Acutane). Although this drug is very effective, it produces a number of side effects including elevated cholesterol in the blood. This drug should only be used under close medical supervision.

For many, acne is worst in times of emotional turmoil. Some experts in psychosomatic medicine suggest that acne is a response to the anger engendered by the belief that one's sense of independence or individuality is being threatened. More than one person has had an acne condition clear up as soon as he or she moved away from home to go to college. As with many other conditions, the role of the mind in prevention and treatment of acne cannot be ignored.

sue debris and any foreign matter that has entered the body. A mixture of white blood cells and debris from damaged cells makes up pus, which sometimes accumulates in wounds and infected areas. The existence of pus tells you that your body's defenses are working and that healing is taking place.

Interferon

Humans as well as many other kinds of animals have a special internal defense mechanism that protects them from virus infections. Viruses are infectious particles consisting of genetic material (RNA or DNA) that is encapsulated in a protein shell. They can only grow and reproduce in cells that they infect; in this way more viruses are produced. Infection of even one cell in the body by a single virus can result in the rapid production of hundreds or thousands of identical new viruses by that cell. The new viruses are then released from that cell; once outside, they attack other cells. That is why viral infections spread so quickly through the body's cells and why viral diseases can make you extremely sick in a short period of time. To combat virus infections, some of the body's cells, especially certain white blood cells called **lymphocytes** (because they are found in the lymphatic system), produce a substance called **interferon** that interferes with a virus's growth and hence its ability to infect cells.

Each animal makes its own special kind of interferon, and the kind of interferon even varies from one tissue to another within the body. Nobody knows exactly how interferon inhibits viral development, but it is clear that viruses do not multiply in cells containing interferon. Even more intriguing is the observation that once interferon production has been stimulated in a cell by viral infection, that cell and others in its neighborhood become resistant to infection by many other different kinds of viruses.

Although the use of pure interferon to successfully treat certain viral diseases was predicted soon after its discovery in 1957 (see Figure 9-4), until recently it was difficult to obtain enough pure interferon to conduct clinical studies of its efficacy. Now, however, new techniques using genetically engineered organisms allow the production of large amounts of interferon, and soon more information about its potential usefulness in treating virus diseases such as herpes infections (cold sores) and the common cold will be at hand. There is also some hope that interferon will be effective in the treatment of certain kinds of cancer.

The Final Defense: Immune Responses

When foreign substances such as bacteria, viruses, pollen, cells and molecules from other organisms, and many industrial chemicals enter the body, a complex series of reactions take place that together

Figure 9-3
Penetration of the skin by any unsterile sharp object often produces an inflammation response, the regular response of the body to injury or infection.

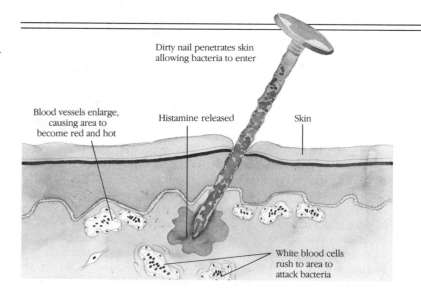

Dirty nail penetrates skin allowing bacteria to enter

Blood vessels enlarge, causing area to become red and hot

Histamine released

Skin

White blood cells rush to area to attack bacteria

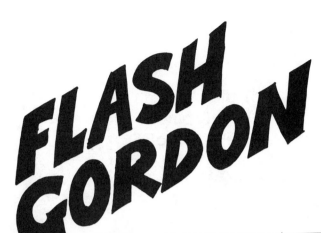

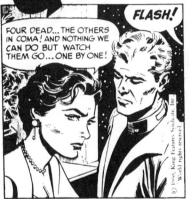

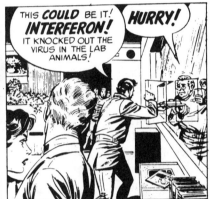

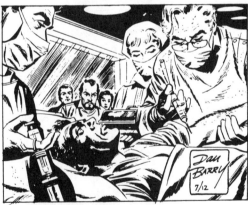

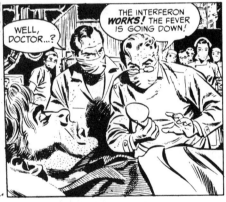

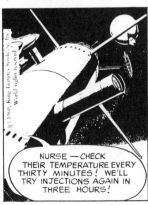

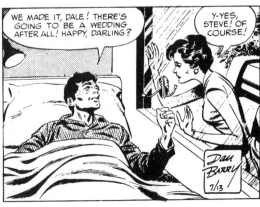

> The composition and quality of the diet can exert important influences on the development and expression of immunological functions, autoimmunities, diseases of aging, resistance to infection, and cancer.
>
> **Robert A. Good, M.D.**

are called **immune responses.** The end result of immune responses is the production of specific protein molecules, called **antibodies,** and certain kinds of blood cells, called lymphocytes, that recognize and attach to the foreign substances and begin to eliminate them from the body. Antibodies and lymphocytes inactivate the foreign material until it can be digested and removed by macrophages and phagocytic cells that are carried throughout the body in the blood. Any substance that enters the body and is capable of stimulating immune responses is called an **antigen (anti**body **gen**erator).

The immune responses provide the body's last and most effective defense against disease and they are also responsible for the lasting protection (immunity) that may follow an infection. The other defenses we have mentioned can be regarded in some respects as stopgap measures that the body uses until the immune system can produce sufficient antibodies to neutralize all the invading organisms or harmful substances. Typically it takes the body a week or more to fully develop an immune response to a particular substance. This is why other, faster-acting defense mechanisms are also needed. For healing to be complete, the body's immune system must ultimately respond to infecting organisms and destroy them all.

The Lymphatic System

The cells that are responsible for the recognition of antigens and the production of antibodies originate mainly in bone marrow and are transported to all

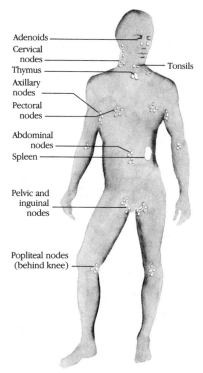

Adenoids
Cervical nodes
Thymus
Tonsils
Axillary nodes
Pectoral nodes
Abdominal nodes
Spleen
Pelvic and inguinal nodes
Popliteal nodes (behind knee)

Figure 9-5
The body's lymphatic system. The principal lymph nodes and other organs of the immune system are shown. The lymphatic system performs many functions in protecting the body from disease.

parts of the body through a series of special vessels called the **lymphatic system** (see Figure 9-5). The lymphatic vessels contain a circulating fluid called **lymph,** and located at various intervals along the lymphatic vessels are masses of specialized tissue called **lymph nodes.** Lymph nodes filter out bac-

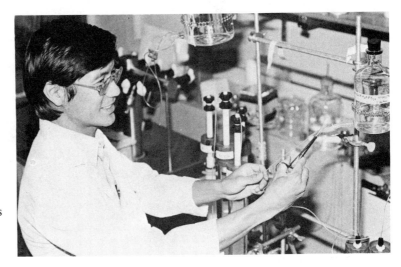

Figure 9-6
Leo Lin, a research scientist at Cetus Corporation, Berkeley, isolates proteins of the immune system, that may be useful in treating cancer and other diseases.

teria and other foreign particles from the lymph, and they also manufacture antibody producing cells (lymphocytes). The "swollen glands" that people have in the neck or under the arms when they have a bad cold or other infection are enlarged lymph nodes engaged in the removal of the invading organisms from the body.

The tonsils, adenoids, spleen, and thymus gland are also organs of the immune system. They carry out several functions in maintaining an effective immune response as well as produce active lymphocytes. Until recently it was a frequent medical practice to remove tonsils (tonsillectomy) or adenoids (adenoidectomy) if they became inflamed in the course of their normal role in fighting an infection, and sometimes when no infection was present,

on the theory that if those organs were removed they could not become inflamed. Today, however, the importance of these organs to the overall immune defenses of the body is widely recognized, and most health care practitioners agree that no child or adult should have these operations performed unless there is compelling medical reason to do so.

The specialized lymphatic cells involved in immune responses are called **B-lymphocytes** and **T-lymphocytes.** The B-lymphocytes eventually change into cells that produce specific antibodies (the protein molecules that attach to particular antigens), whereas the T-lymphocytes are ready to attack foreign substances at once by recognizing the "foreignness" of specific antigens on the surfaces of viruses, bacteria, or even other cells (see Figure 9-7).

Figure 9-7
The synthesis of all immune system cells begins in bone marrow. Precursor cells are processed in various parts of the body and acquire their specialized functions. Mature T-lymphocytes attack and destroy invading microorganisms directly. Mature B-lymphocytes manufacture antibody proteins (immunoglobulins) that bind to antigens and inactivate foreign organisms and toxins.

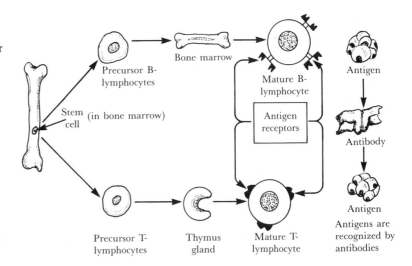

Penicillin and streptomycin may kill the majority of bacteria in an infected wound, but it is the body itself that must go after and destroy the last resistant microbe.

Ronald J. Glasser
The Body Is the Hero

It is thought that the T-lymphocytes play a crucial role in the detection of cancer cells and other abnormal cells that arise in the body. Most scientists now believe that cancer cells develop in the body throughout our lives but that their number is small and when they do arise, the cancer cells are recognized as foreign and are destroyed by vigilant T-lymphocytes circulating in the blood. If this hypothesis is correct, then lifelong health is highly dependent on the activeness of the immune responses.

Recognition of "Self"

So far we have described the ability of the immune system to recognize and destroy virtually any substance or organism that is foreign to the body. What prevents the immune system from reacting to your own tissues and cells? In some mysterious fashion, by mechanisms that have yet to be discovered, the immune system is able to distinguish between all the molecules and cells of the body that are recognized as "self," and all other substances that are "not self." It is thought that during embryonic development, as body tissues are being formed, all the antibody-producing cells that could eventually produce antibodies directed against any of the body's normal cellular components are destroyed or inactivated. Scientists do not yet know how these particular antibody-producing cells are eliminated before they can react and damage the body's own tissues.

During fetal development, before the child's own immunological system is functional, he or she receives antibodies from the mother that pass from her blood across the placenta into the fetus's blood. In this way the newborn infant is protected from infections and foreign substances for several months after birth. Antibodies are also passed to the child in the mother's milk, which is one reason that breast-feeding is so beneficial. Eventually the child's own immune system becomes activated and capable of producing antibodies against harmful organisms and substances that he or she encounters.

One of the principal causes of diseases in infants and young children is malnutrition or starvation, either of which results in the immune system's inability to produce the lymphocytes and antibodies that are necessary to ward off disease. This explains why malnutrition increases the chances of infectious diseases and also their severity. Poor nutrition and pathogenic organisms are both responsible for disease and childhood mortality in much of the world's undernourished populations (Rosenberg, Solomans, and Levin, 1976).

Autoimmune Diseases

You can appreciate the precision with which the immune system must function in order to distinguish "self" from "nonself," because any mistake that resulted in antibodies attacking the body's own cells could result in serious disease or death. Unfortunately such diseases do exist; they are called **autoimmune diseases.** Some genetic disorders, fortunately quite rare, may result in loss of immune responsiveness or in a breakdown in the mechanisms responsible for "self" recognition. Other autoimmune disorders may or may not have a genetic basis but still cause serious diseases and even death.

Lupus erythematosus is an autoimmune disorder that mainly affects women ages 18 to 35. In this disease, for reasons still unknown, autoantibodies are synthesized and directed against the person's own DNA and cell nuclei. Many organs of the body may be affected, and the symptoms — rashes, pain, and anemia — usually flare up and fade away throughout life.

Another serious disease partly caused by an autoimmune response — one that affects millions of people — is **rheumatoid arthritis.** In this disease autoantibodies are directed primarily against the body's joints, producing inflammation, pain, and suffering. We described arthritis (in Chapter 8) as a disease of lifestyle since there are no known genetic or environmental causes. There is also evidence that in some people the symptoms of arthritis can be arrested or reversed by nutritional changes or by changes in mental state. (Later in this chapter we discuss how nutrition and emotions affect the immune responses.) Unfortunately, there is no single nutritional or mental change — or medical treatment — that has been scientifically demonstrated to lead to a cure or to permanent remission of the painful symptoms of this suspected autoimmune disease.

An autoimmune disease that affects the central nervous system is **multiple sclerosis,** more commonly known as MS. Recent research suggests that MS may be initiated by a viral infection that somehow triggers the immune system to produce antibodies directed against myelin, a substance that sheaths and insulates nerve fibers in the brain and spinal cord. Interferon is one of the experimental drugs being tested in patients with MS to see whether it will reduce or eliminate the MS attacks and symptoms.

Some rare immune deficiency disorders such as **agammaglobulinemia** have a genetic basis and result in an inability of the immune system to produce any cells capable of making antibodies. When the mother's antibodies begin to disappear from the newborn's blood, it suffers from recurrent infections. The child's survival depends on antibiotic therapy, injections of antibodies, and, for a few such children, living in an isolated germ-free environment. The most famous case of agammaglobulinemia is David, who was delivered under sterile conditions and kept in a germ-free environment for 12 years in a Texas hospital (see Figure 9-8). David was born without a thymus gland, lymph nodes, or tonsils, and he lacked the ability to make any antibodies. Shortly before his twelfth birthday, David's physicians along with David and his family decided to attempt a bone-marrow transplant from his sister, in order to provide him with cells capable of producing antibodies. Unfortunately, the transplanted tissue was rejected, and David died in 1984.

Blood Transfusions and Rh Factors

Today people are concerned about blood transfusions because of possible contamination with the AIDS virus (see Chapter 18). In the early part of this century a blood transfusion often led to the patient's death. That's because the patient's immune

Figure 9-8
A photo of David on his eleventh birthday, September 21, 1982, in his germ-free "bubble chamber" room. (Courtesy of Baylor College of Medicine.)

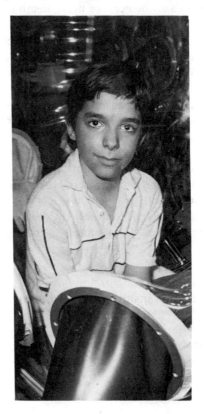

> The remarkable capacity of the
> immune system to respond to many
> thousands of different substances
> with exquisite specificity saves us all
> from certain death by infection.
> **Martin C. Roff**

system recognized the donor's blood cells as being "foreign" and attacked them with both phagocytic cells and antibodies. The antibodies caused clumps of blood cells to form in the veins and arteries, impeding the flow of blood and oxygen to, and waste products from, the body's tissues. If oxygen and nutrients are prevented from reaching essential tissues such as the heart or brain, death may occur from a heart attack or stroke.

Your red blood cells have many different potential antigens on their cell surfaces, each of which can evoke an antibody response when recognized as "not self." However, as we have pointed out, you do not make antibodies against your own antigens. The two most important groups of human red blood cell antigens are the ABO and Rh-positive/Rh-negative groups. There are actually many other groups of antigens on red blood cells, but these are by far the most important ones in terms of evoking an immune response that can endanger health. Table 9-1 shows the pattern of donor-recipient ABO blood types that must be matched for a successful transfusion.

People with type O blood have neither the A nor B antigens on their red blood cells, so their immune system makes A and B antibodies early in life because these antigens are also prevalent in bacteria and plants that people eat. People with type O blood are *universal donors;* their blood cells will not stimulate an antibody response in the recipient, no matter what his or her blood type. People with type AB blood have both antigens present on their red blood cells and do not synthesize A or B antibodies, because these antigens are recognized as "self" and those antibody-producing cells are destroyed in the embryo. People with type AB blood are **universal recipients;** they can accept blood from any of the four groups.

The Rh-positive antigen and the antibody that reacts against it cause problems primarily in pregnancy. A woman is termed Rh-negative if her red blood cells do not contain any of this antigen. If the red blood cells of a developing fetus have the Rh-positive antigen (inherited from the father), and if any of the fetus's red blood cells enter the mother's

Table 9-1
How Blood Transfusions Are Determined According to ABO Blood Groups

Blood group	Genotype	Antigens on red blood cells	Transfusions cannot be accepted from	Transfusions are accepted from
O (universal donor)	OO	none	A, B, AB	O
A	AA, AO	A	B, AB	A, O
B	BB, BO	B	A, AB	B, O
AB (universal recipient)	AB	A, B	none	A, B, AB, O

> Autoimmune disease can be regarded
> as evidence of a partial
> breakdown of the homeostatic
> and self-monitoring quality of the immune system.
>
> **Sir F. M. Burnet**

blood supply , production of anti-Rh antibodies can be stimulated by her immune system, which recognizes the fetal cells as foreign. This usually does not cause any difficulty during the first pregnancy and might even go unnoticed until the woman became pregnant again.

Now, if the second fetus is also Rh-positive, the Rh-positive antibodies (synthesized during the first pregnancy) in the mother's blood will attack the developing infant's red blood cells, resulting in anemia, brain damage, or even death. Fortunately, doctors can manage this problem safely and effectively. At the time the first child is delivered, the mother is given an injection of anti-Rh antibodies that destroy any fetal blood cells that might have entered her blood. In this way her immune system is prevented from responding to the fetal antigen and producing Rh-positive antibodies that might endanger the fetus during a subsequent pregnancy.

Tissue Transplants and Immune Responses

Can you recall when heart transplants made headlines? Although organ transplants make exciting headlines, the fact is that many transplant operations are only marginally successful. A few of the more than 10,000 kidney transplants have lasted as long as ten years, but the average time before the transplanted kidney is rejected is about three years. Heart transplants have proven to be even less successful, and only a few carefully selected individuals with heart disease receive transplants nowadays.

Like blood cells, all body cells have potential antigens on their surfaces that are different for everyone (except in the case of identical twins), just as everyone's fingerprints are different. If foreign tissue or organs are grafted onto your body, your immune system produces antibodies to the foreign cell antigens, causing destruction of the cells and rejection of the transplanted organs.

The body's normal immune response can be controlled to some degree with **immunosupressive drugs** (corticosteroids, cyclosporin); however, treatment with these drugs lessens resistance to infections and sometimes enhances development of other diseases. The long-term use of immunosuppressive drug therapy itself results in increased susceptibility to cancer. In terms of health, then, it makes more sense to seek ways to prevent the kidney and heart diseases, so that surgical transplants would become less needed.

The more alike two persons are genetically, the more likely it is that the transplanted tissue will be accepted by the body. Identical twins are genetically identical; this is why tissue transplants between identical twins have the greatest chance of success. Brothers and sisters are only 50 percent genetically identical. To minimize the risk of rejection of transplanted tissues, the **histocompatibility** (similarity of cell surface antigenic) between the donor and recipient is determined by immunological tests. Just as red blood cells have particular groups of antigenic proteins on their cell surfaces, other cells in the body also have groups of antigenic proteins called **HLA** (human leukocyte antigens) that are crucial in de-

> To see a world in a grain of sand,
> And Heaven in a wildflower,
> Hold infinity in the palm of your hand,
> And eternity in an hour.
>
> **William Blake**

termining whether a transplant will be accepted or rejected (see Figure 9-9). It has been shown that the greater the similarity in HLA antigens or leukocytes between donor and recipient, the greater the chance that the tissue will be accepted and function normally in its new host. From the number of HLA antigens already determined, calculations show that there are so many different HLA antigen combinations that each person is immunologically unique.

One surprising research finding is that certain HLA antigens appear much more frequently than one would expect by chance in people with particular diseases. The most dramatic observation to date has been the association of one specific HLA antigen, HLA-B27, in about 90 percent of persons with the disease **ankylosing spondylitis,** a degenerative, slowly crippling, rheumatoid-like condition of the spine. Different HLA antigens are associated with muscular dystrophy, arthritis, and about forty other immunological disorders.

Although scientists do not believe that these HLA antigens are directly responsible for the diseases, the particular pattern of HLA antigens a person has might afford a means of identifying people "at risk" for certain diseases. In the same way that knowing the ABO blood type of a person permits a doctor to predict which transfusions are safe, it may be possible in the future for a doctor, knowing a person's histocompatibility (HLA) type, to suggest preventive health measures to individuals at risk *before* a disease develops. This might be an important step in the reorientation of medical care toward prevention of disease.

Figure 9-9
Major histocompatibility (HLA) antigens are shown here schematically. A vast array of different antigens are embedded in the outer membranes of cells, projecting beyond their surfaces. These antigens can be recognized by the body's immune cells and antibodies. Since every person's antigens are different, tissue transplanted from one person to another is usually rejected because the donor's HLA antigens are recognized as foreign by the immune response of the recipient.

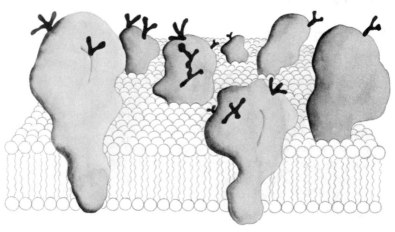

> The liver cell of your brother,
> even though it does the same thing
> for him that your liver cell does for you,
> has markers on its walls which are
> different from yours, and the same
> holds true for the cells
> that make up the tissues of your kidneys
> and your heart, pancreas,
> muscles, and lungs.
>
> **Ronald J. Glasser**
> *The Body Is the Hero*

Vaccination: "Priming" the Immune System

One of the great achievements of modern medical science has been the development of vaccinations against a variety of serious bacterial and viral diseases, including smallpox, whooping cough, poliomyelitis, measles, diphtheria, and tetanus. Vaccination is the administration of substances called vaccines (usually by injection, which is why they are called "shots") that stimulate the immune response to combat infecting organisms if they are subsequently encountered.

When a person is vaccinated, specific antigens—from inactivated viruses, bacteria, or toxins—are injected into the body. The immune system responds with the production of lymphocytes and antibodies directed against those antigens. If the body later encounters the natural disease-causing agents, it already has an immunity and is protected. For example, the polio vaccine developed by Jonas Salk employed a chemically inactivated virus. The polio vaccine currently in use in this country, developed by Albert Sabin, uses genetically inactivated strains of polio virus that cannot cause the disease but that can stimulate long-lasting immunity. Genetic inactivation produces a strain of virus that is incapable of causing disease but that still has antigens similar to the original virus. The antibody made in response to the genetically modified virus is equally effective against the naturally occurring, disease-causing virus.

In general, vaccination is a safe, effective procedure for disease prevention, and has resulted in vastly improved human health. The reason that a single—or at most several—inoculation produces long-term immunity is that the immune system, once stimulated by a particular antigen, maintains special white blood cells that "remember" that particular antigen. If the body is again challenged by that antigen, even after many years, those "memory cells" proliferate rapidly and produce sufficient antibodies to combat the disease.

Serious diseases for which vaccines are available are listed in Table 9-2. Vaccination for milder diseases, such as influenza, is still controversial, since it is not clear that the benefits outweigh the risks for all people. Some people may respond adversely to any vaccination because of emotional anxiety or allergic reactions, or they may even contract the disease because of some unforeseen complication with their own biochemical processes. Most healthy people recover quickly from a "bout of flu" and probably don't need flu shots. Smallpox immunizations are no longer necessary or recommended; the risks of an adverse reaction from the shot far outweigh the risks of contracting smallpox, since no cases have been reported for a number of years (see Box 8-2).

The most recent addition to the list of effective immunizations is **hepatitis B** vaccine. About 200,000 cases of hepatitis B are diagnosed in the U.S. each year. Hepatitis B is a serious liver disease caused by a virus that infects liver cells and impairs liver functions. Hepatitis B vaccination is recom-

Table 9-2
Immunizations Available in the United States

Type of immunization	Effectiveness of immunization and frequency of booster doses
Cholera	Only partial immunity; recommended renewal every 6 months for duration of exposure
Diphtheria	Highly effective; recommended renewal every 10 years
Influenza	Renew every year (because viral strains change easily)
Mumps	Believed to confer lifetime immunity
Plague	Incomplete protection; boosters necessary every 3 to 6 months
Polio	Long-lasting immunity; no booster necessary unless exposure anticipated
Rabies	A vaccination each day for 14 to 21 days beginning soon after the bite
German measles	Highly effective; need for boosters not established
Measles	Highly effective; usually produces lifelong immunity
Smallpox	Immunization no longer required
Spotted fever	Effectiveness not established
Tetanus	Very effective; renew every 10 years or when treated for a contaminated wound if more than 5 years have elapsed since last booster
Tuberculosis	Highly effective
Typhoid fever	About 80 percent effective
Typhus	Renew every year (if exposed)
Whooping cough	Highly effective
Yellow fever	Highly effective; provides long-lasting immunity
Hepatitis B	Effective; only for individuals at risk

mended for particular groups that are at high risk for becoming infected—health care workers who are exposed to the disease, heroin addicts, male homosexuals, and sexually promiscuous persons. The original vaccine was made from the blood of human carriers of the virus, but an equally effective vaccine produced by genetic engineering techniques should be available within a few years.

Allergies

Allergies are some of the less desirable responses of the immune system to foreign substances called **allergens** (substances that produce an allergic response). Pollens, grasses, grains, molds, dust, animal hair, foods, and drugs contain allergy-causing antigens. Almost anything containing a foreign substance can be an allergen. The allergic response is due to synthesis in the body of a particular class of antibodies that are different from the ones that recognize and inactivate bacteria, viruses, and cells. No one is really sure what benefit accrues

from our being able to synthesize this special class of allergy-related antibodies (called immunoglobulin E), but millions of people can attest to the misery and discomfort caused by this immune response (Figure 9-10).

The allergic reaction is usually accompanied by inflammation (discussed earlier), mucus secretion, and the release of histamine, a chemical that is stored in cells that are abundant in the skin, respiratory passages, and digestive tract. Thus, it is no coincidence that many allergic reactions are associated with skin (eczema, hives, poison ivy), the respiratory tract (hay fever, asthma), and the digestive tract (vomiting, diarrhea).

Though allergies certainly involve physiological and immunological responses in the body, they are also strongly tied to a person's emotional and psychic state. Asthmatic children often become much improved when separated from their parents. Sometimes skin eruptions are a sign of "itching to get away" from something or someone. Sneezes may be seasonal or interpersonal.

Allergies are blamed on many substances, yet allergens are but one component of the complex immunological response. Allergy specialist C. W. Moorefield (1971) has successfully treated asthmatic patients using hypnosis and behavior therapy. It is his view that

> In asthma a conditioned bronchial spasm is the common pathway for a complexity of physical, allergic, and emotional mechanisms. Most studies have shown that even in the presence of allergic conditions, some emotional overlay usually triggers the attack of asthma. It is known that emotional influences are activated through the autonomic nervous system. It is quite likely that emotions acting via the autonomic nervous system produce local conditions in the mucosa of the bronchial tubes, which would make the respiratory system sensitive both to infections and allergens.

Millions of allergic people receive inoculations that are supposed to desensitize them to the irritating substances to which they showed positive reactions in allergy tests. Some people do get better with the program of desensitizing shots, yet there is scant scientific evidence to substantiate the idea that "allergy shots" are beneficial. In fact, several studies have shown that placebo injections can be just as effective as the injections of allergens. One detailed study concluded:

> A five-year study has been done on children sensitive to ragweed in which a comparison was made between specific hyposensitization injections and placebo injections. Even though the allergen injections may have had some beneficial effect on some children, the amount of benefit was indistinguishable from differences likely to occur in pure randomization experiments. No justification was found for promising any greater benefit to children treated with allergens than they would obtain from placebo injections. (Fontana, Holt, and Mainland, 1966)

Allergies of all kinds can be caused and cured by a person's beliefs and by suggestion. The human skin is particularly vulnerable to disturbed emotional and mental states. Millions of people suffer from rashes, eczema, acne, and other skin disorders. Arthur Bobroff (1962), a dermatologist at the University of Washington School of Medicine, sums up his unconventional medical view of eczema in strong language:

> I now regard every new case of eczema as immediately curable with absolute certainty, provided the patient (or the parent if the patient is a child) is of average intelligence and willing to make a reasonable effort. For I now know that any eczema—regardless of extent, severity, or duration—can, without the slightest doubt, be made to disappear within two weeks by easily mastered procedures which the patient can be taught to perform for himself. At the same time the patient can be trained in the simple preventive measures that will thereafter preclude any recurrence of eczema.

Figure 9-10
Between one-third and one-half of all Americans suffer from some form of allergy.

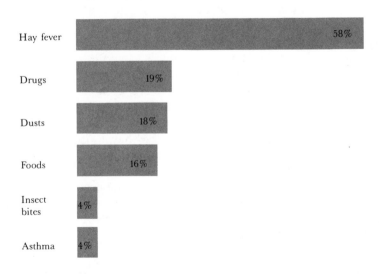

Hay fever	58%
Drugs	19%
Dusts	18%
Foods	16%
Insect bites	4%
Asthma	4%

> Negative emotions, persisting over a long period of time, can impair the immune system, thus lowering the body's defenses against disease.
>
> **Norman Cousins**

Bobroff argues that the successful treatment of eczema requires (1) elimination of itching and (2) elimination of inflammation. For many patients he recommends applying cold damp compresses for about 20 minutes several times each day. Following this regimen the skin usually clears up within a week or two.

Other patients were cured simply by wrapping the affected area for two weeks to prevent scratching and irritation. Bobroff also dealt with his patients' emotional and personal problems. Their skin eruptions were invariably associated with unresolved personal problems or relationships. Bobroff practiced holistic medicine long before the concept became widely accepted.

Allergies are real. People do not imagine that they are unable to breathe or that their skin itches. But the causes are complex and lie as much within us as in what we are exposed to in the environment. A holistic approach to coping with an allergic problem would begin by determining what has upset a person's mental and emotional tranquility. When mind-body harmony is disturbed, the immune responses are affected, and one of the undesirable responses can be allergic reactions. Box 9-2 describes an experiment performed with Japanese students in which rashes on the skin were either produced or prevented solely by the power of suggestion and the students' belief. The experiment suggests that people who suffer from poison ivy, poison oak, or other forms of rash or skin eruptions might be able to change their physiological responses by changing their mental state.

The Role of Nutrition

Finally, the effect of nutrition on the responsiveness of the immune system needs to be emphasized. It has been known for a long time that nutritional deficiency and susceptibility to disease are closely intertwined. Lack of essential nutrients impairs the body's ability to defend itself against infectious organisms.

Although few people actually starve in the United States, many people are not optimally nourished. Both undernourished and overnourished people may suffer impairment of their body's defense mechanisms, especially the ability of the immune system to protect them from infectious organisms and cancer cells. We cannot emphasize often enough that the body needs all of the essential nutrients in order to synthesize the cells and antibodies and other molecules that keep a person healthy.

What does all this mean as far as health is concerned? It means that the more positive your mental attitudes and emotional states, the less you are stressed by your environment; the more adequate your nutrition, the more responsive and functional your immune system will be. And as we have seen, a healthy immune response means that you are likely to experience fewer infections. Allergies may decrease or disappear. You may be less likely to fall victim to any of the autoimmune diseases, and you will probably be less susceptible to cancer formation.

BOX 9-2

THINKING MADE IT SO: PRODUCTION AND INHIBITION OF CONTAGIOUS DERMATITIS

Two Japanese physicians, Ikemi and Nakagawa, reported an experiment demonstrating that suggestions can exert remarkable control over skin responses. The subjects participating in the experiment were 13 high school students who were very sensitive to plants found in Japan that produce reactions resembling those produced by our poison ivy, poison oak, or poison sumac. When these students came in contact with the leaves of poisonous plants, they showed a dermatitis consisting of an abnormal redness of the skin due to congestion of the blood capillaries (erythema), small circumscribed solid elevations of the skin (papules), and small blisters (vesicles), together with edema, a burning sensation, and itching.

Five of the students were exposed to a hypnotic induction procedure; when their eyes were closed they were told they were being touched by leaves from the poisonous tree, although they were actually being touched by leaves from a harmless tree. The remaining eight subjects were assigned to a nonhypnotic treatment; when their eyes were closed they were also touched by harmless leaves, but were told they were being stimulated by the poisonous leaves. There is every reason to believe that both the hypnotic subjects and the nonhypnotic subjects could accept the suggestions as true. Both kinds of subjects had their eyes closed and could not see

what kind of leaves were being placed on their arms. Furthermore, the experimenter was a physician with high prestige, and the experiment was conducted in a highly respected medical setting. When the physician said that he was stimulating the subject's arm with the poisonous leaves, there was no reason why the subjects (high school students) should doubt the physician's statement.

Skin changes were produced by the believable suggestion that the arm was being stimulated with poisonous leaves (when it was actually stimulated by harmless leaves). When the subjects were led to believe that they were being stimulated by poisonous leaves, the *harmless* leaves produced a slight to marked degree of dermatitis (e.g., flushing, itching, erythema, and papules) in *all* of the hypnotic subjects and in *all* of the nonhypnotic subjects.

In the next part of the experiment, the subjects were told that they were being touched on the other arm with the leaves of a harmless tree; they were actually stimulated by the poisonous leaves. When thus led to believe that the poisonous leaves were harmless, four of the five hypnotic subjects and seven of the eight nonhypnotic subjects did not show the expected dermatitis.

The data presented by Ikemi and Nakagawa indicate that in individuals who show marked dermatitis when stimulated by the leaves of poison ivylike plants (1)

at least some aspects of the dermatitis can be produced by a harmless substance when the individual is led to believe it is the dermatitis-producing substance, (2) the dermatitis generally can be inhibited when the individual is led to believe that the poisonous leaves are harmless leaves, (3) formal hypnotic induction procedures are not necessary or especially useful in producing these effects, and (4) the critical variable in producing the phenomena is the subjects' belief that a harmless substance is actually a dermatitis-producing substance and, vice versa, that a dermatitis-producing substance is actually a harmless substance.

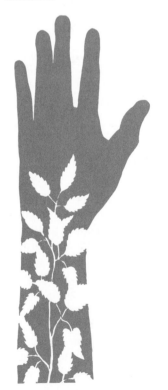

> Overnutrition as well as undernutrition can alter immune responsiveness. Thus, "optimum nutrition" is the key phrase for dietary influences to keep immune responses within normal limits.
>
> **R. K. Chandra and P. M. Newberne**

Supplemental Readings

Atkins, F. M., and **Metcalfe, D. D.** "The Diagnosis and Treatment of Food Allergy." *Annual Review of Nutrition,* 4 (1984), 233–255. A comprehensive scientific review of food allergies.

Chisholm, R. "On the Trail of the Magic Bullet." *High Technology,* January 1983. An article describing how monoclonal antibodies may be used to diagnose and treat diseases.

Hopson, J. L. "Battle at the Isle of Self." *Science 80,* March/April 1980. An article describing how autoimmune diseases occur.

Huffer, T. L.; Kanapa, D. J.; and **Stevenson, G. W.** *Introduction to Human Immunology.* Boston: Jones and Bartlett, 1986. A basic introductory text to the immune system for those who want to know more.

Jaret, P. "Our Immune System—The Wars Within." *National Geographic,* June 1986. A wonderful, up-to-date article on the immune system. Includes some remarkable photos of immune cells in action.

Rodger, J. C., and **Drake, B. L.** "The Enigma of the Fetal Graft." *American Scientist,* January/February 1987. Presents the problem of why babies should be rejected as foreign tissue and yet are not.

Summary

The human body has a variety of defense mechanisms that prevent disease and help maintain health. The skin and mucous membranes serve to prevent infectious organisms and harmful substances from entering the body. Specialized white blood cells circulate throughout the body, attacking and destroying any foreign substances that manage to enter the body's tissues. Enzymes in the liver detoxify and eliminate harmful chemicals from the body. A protein substance called interferon is synthesized by lymphocytes when viruses invade the body; as the name suggests, it interferes with virus growth.

The body's main defense is provided by the immune responses, one of which is to synthesize antibodies that can inactivate virtually any foreign substance that enters the body. If the immune system is not functioning properly, the body is susceptible to disease—not only infectious diseases but also autoimmune diseases and cancers of various kinds. Immune system malfunctions also cause allergic reactions. The immune system is regulated by the autonomic nervous system, which in turn reflects mental and emotional states. Stress and malnutrition reduce the ability of the immune system to respond to harmful organisms. Optimal health depends on the normal functioning of the immune system.

FOR YOUR HEALTH

Colds as Messengers

If you tend to get colds, flu, or sore throats frequently, your body may be telling you something about your lifestyle. For the next six months, keep a record of the times you are sick and also record your life experiences during the weeks and days prior to getting sick. Try to discern whether worry, fatigue, and stress are associated with your illnesses, and then take steps to make healthful changes.

Help Your Immune System Help You

The next time you think you are about to catch cold, or the next time you have a cold, carry out this visualization exercise to help your immune system rid your body of the cold. Imagine your cold to be caused by hundreds of tiny virus particles that have invaded your nose, throat, and anywhere else you have cold symptoms. Then imagine your antibodies and white blood cells having the capacity to destroy the virus particles in some way. Some people imagine them to be fish capable of engulfing the viruses. Others think of antibodies and white blood cells as knights with lances that pop the viruses as if they were balloons. Choose any images that suit you, and spend 10 minutes, twice a day, imagining your antibodies and white blood cells vanquishing the viruses and ridding your body of their cold-producing powers.

Help Your Skin Heal Itself

Next time you get a minor bruise, cut, or burn, try this exercise. Immediately find a quiet place. Close your eyes and visualize the wound or the part of the body as feeling and appearing completely normal and well. Continue to visualize the healing process until you feel confident that it is going to be all right. This kind of visualization exercise can help speed healing, reduce inflammation, and prevent infection of the injured area.

Your Vaccination Record

Make a record of your vaccinations using a chart like this one:

Vaccine	Years initial series completed	Years revaccinated					
Diphtheria							
Influenza							
Measles							
Mumps							
Pertussis (whooping cough)							
Polio							
German measles (rubella)							
Tetanus							
Tuberculosis							
Other							

CHAPTER TEN

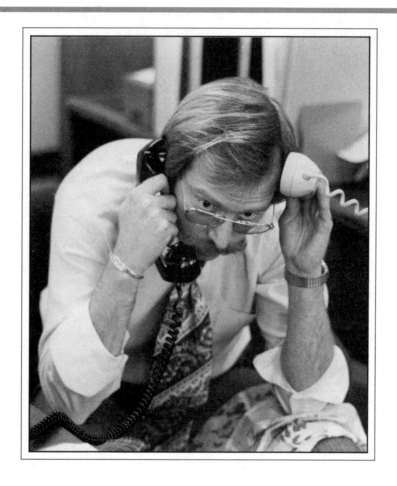

Stress-related illnesses can be reduced
by understanding their causes.

Life Stress
and Illness

L ife is filled with a never-ending array of challenges, some of which present themselves as hassles or obstacles to accomplishing necessary daily tasks or life goals. Other challenges provide opportunities for positive and unplanned changes in our lives.

When confronted with a particular challenge, whether it is achieving good grades in school, obtaining a well-paying job, becoming a parent, becoming involved in an intense love relationship, or living with an uncompromising roommate, we may experience negative feelings—anxiety, sadness, depression, anger, fear—that may cause symptoms such as sleeplessness, gastrointestinal upset, headache, or muscular tension. These symptoms signal a disruption in our state of psychobiological balance and are a response to stress. Usually this disruption is brief, for we find ways to meet the challenge and to restore our well-being. And often confronting and resolving a challenge becomes a positive growth experience. Other times, however, disruption in mindbody harmony is prolonged or severe, and we are said to be "under stress" or "stressed out." Prolonged, unresolved stress situations can contribute to the development of several kinds of **stress-related illness** (see Table 10-1).

In this chapter we discuss the various definitions of stress and how the manifestation of stress may lead to illness. We also suggest ways to reduce stress and to prevent stress-related illness.

> To most individuals, the word Buick is not a
> stress, but it is to a thief who has just stolen one.
> Seymour S. Kety, M.D.

The Definition of Stress

Although most people have had experiences that they would label as being "under stress" or "stressed out," it is important to recognize a significant difference in how the word "stress" is used in these two expressions. The phrase "under stress" refers to the *cause* of the disruption of psychological and/or physiological balance, as in the example, "She was under stress from having to take five final exams in two days." "Stressed out," on the other hand, refers to the consequences of the particular stressful situation, as in the example, "During final exams she was so stressed out that she suffered from stomach cramps, diarrhea, and insomnia."

Because it is confusing to use the word stress to represent both causes and results of challenging or disruptive life experiences, the term **stressor** will be used in this chapter to refer to circumstances and events that produce disruptions in mind-body harmony. The term **stress** will be used to refer to the symptoms resulting from stressors. More specifically, stress can be defined as "a relationship between the person and the environment that is appraised by the person as taxing or exceeding his or her resources and endangering his or her well-being" (Folkman, 1984).

Defining stress in terms of a person's response focuses attention on an individual's experience rather than on some external factor (the stressor) as being the key element in the relationship between stress and illness. Moreover, this distinction places the avoidance or prevention of stressful experiences under the control of the individual, and suggests

Table 10-1
Some Disorders That Can Be Caused or Aggravated by Stress

Gastrointestinal disorders	Skin disorders	Metabolic disorders
Constipation	Eczema	Hyperthyroidism
Diarrhea	Pruritus	Hypothyroidism
Duodenal ulcer	Urticaria	Diabetes
Anorexia nervosa (severe loss of	Psoriasis	Cardiovascular disorders
appetite)	Musculoskeletal disorders	Coronary artery disease
Obesity	Rheumatoid arthritis	Essential hypertension
Ulcerative colitis	Low back pain	Congestive heart failure
Respiratory disorders	Migraine headache	Menstrual irregularities
Asthma	Muscle tension	Cancer
Hay fever		Accident proneness
Tuberculosis		

that stress-related illnesses can be prevented by reducing stressful interactions or by coping with them in ways that do not cause a breakdown of mind-body harmony.

How Stress Contributes to Illness

Although stress has been described as a disruption of mind-body harmony, a more detailed and scientific definition of stress is required in order to understand how stress can contribute to illness. Stress-related illnesses such as high blood pressure (hypertension), asthma, arthritis, ulcers, and skin problems have traditionally been referred to as psychophysiological or psychosomatic disorders (see Chapter 2). These illnesses are not phantom problems, as the term *psychosomatic* is sometimes thought to mean, but are real physical conditions. They do not, however, necessarily stem from the direct action of some physical agent on the body. Instead, psychophysiological disorders are the result of a physical response to emotionally charged, and therefore stressful, life situations and events. The physical response is mediated by the nervous, endocrine (hormone), and immune systems, which, as discussed in Chapter 3, link the thought and feeling centers of the brain with the rest of the body.

When a person experiences stress, the feelings associated with that experience activate the nervous and endocrine systems, which in turn produce changes in body physiology (see Figure 10-1). These nervous and endocrine responses are a characteristic of normal physiology, meant to deal with immediate and short-term stressful situations. Illness arises when these stress-response mechanisms are continually activated, and overstimulated organs begin to wear down or become diseased. Stress can also impair normal functioning of the immune system. Lowered immunity is probably responsible for the increased susceptibility of stressed people to infection and perhaps even cancer (Hales, 1983).

Current theories of stress (Eisdorfer, 1985; Smith and Ascough, 1985) identify three components of the stress-illness relationship (see Figure 10-2): (1) **activators,** (2) **reactions,** and (3) **consequences.** Activators are occurrences, situations, or events which are potential stressors. They become actual stressors only when an individual reacts to

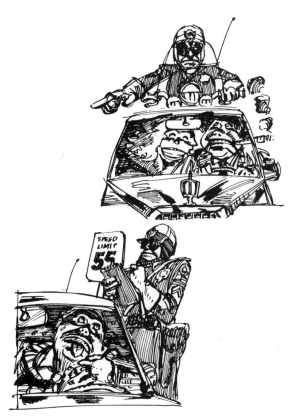

Figure 10-1
Stressful incidents produce hormonal and nervous system reactions that can lead to abnormal changes in body physiology.

them in ways that disrupt mind-body harmony. Reactions refer to an individual's physiological and psychological responses to the stressor. It is through one's reactions that a given situation is experienced as stressful; some people may react very strongly to an event while others may not take any notice. For example, if someone we are close to dies, we become emotionally upset; if we read about the death of someone we do not know in the obituary column, we do not become emotionally upset. Consequences are the effects of a reaction. When a reaction is severe and/or prolonged, a consequence may be unhealthy behaviors—increased cigarette smoking, overconsumption of alcohol, or abuse of tranquilizing drugs—to quell the upsetting emotions. Another possible consequence is the initiation of some form of illness. A study of Detroit-area residents revealed that occupational stress was associated both with health-harming behaviors such as drinking alcohol and various kinds of illnesses (House et al., 1986).

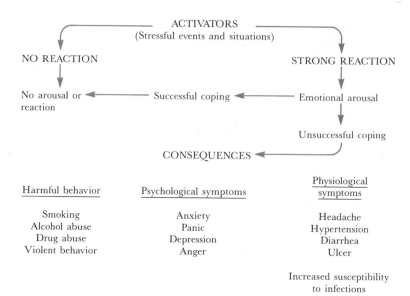

Figure 10-2
The hypothetical stress-illness
relationship.

Activators of Stress

Activators are situations that have the potential to disrupt a person's emotional or mental state. Activators or stressors can be major external events (war, flood, famine) or unpleasant interactions with people (divorce, job loss), or they may result from changes in the body, resulting from puberty, accidents, or aging. Activators can also be an unmet emotional need or even happy events such as marriage or winning a lottery.

In an attempt to identify and measure the potential for certain experiences to be activators, Thomas Holmes and Richard Rahe (1967) devised the Schedule of Recent Experience (SRE). The SRE lists common life events and for each event a corresponding number of life change units (LCUs) is assigned that measure the relative stressfulness of the event (see Table 10-2). The SRE scores the death of a spouse as requiring the most adjustment, (arbitrary numerical LCU value of 100), marriage carries a value of 50 LCUs, and a vacation has a value of 13 LCUs.

Research using the SRE has shown that the accumulation of more than 150 LCUs in a year correlates with a high probability that a person will experience a negative health change within that year or soon thereafter. The likelihood of negative health changes increases as the number of accumulated LCUs increases. The negative health changes include heart attacks, accidents, infectious diseases, worsening of a previous illness, injuries, and metabolic disease. A modified version of the SRE that is designed to assess stressors in the lives of students is given in Table 10-3. Note that both the original SRE and the student version contain positive life events such as taking a vacation or beginning a new love relationship.

Recognizing that people's reactions to various life situations may differ in intensity, Irwin Sarason and his colleagues (1985) developed the Life Experience Survey (LES). The LES lists 47 life events that are potential activators of stress (34 of which appear on the SRE) but does not assign a value of their importance. Each respondent is asked to rate the degree of distress experienced with each event. Results of research with the LES are similar to the results obtained with the SRE.

It is important to remember that surveys such as the SRE and LES are culture-bound, that is, their effectiveness in predicting health problems associated with activators depends on the similarity of the people in the group being surveyed. The potential for health changes depends on the meaning and importance people place on certain events. Because individuals from different social strata or ethnic groups have different values, beliefs, and attitudes, they will often respond differently to the same activator (see Box 10-1).

Reactions to Activators

Reactions depend largely on the individual's personality and emotional make-up and not on the nature of the activator itself. Everyone interprets the world and events differently. Each of us is born with a capacity for certain behaviors, which are greatly modified and shaped by what we learn and experience. Each of us reacts to a particular situation according to our individual values, beliefs, and attitudes.

Because of these differences, a situation that may be very stressful and upsetting to one person may not even bother another. According to stress researcher Susan Folkman (1984), experiencing stress requires that an individual interpret a given situation as significant (This situation is important to me.) and that he or she decide what to do with the situation (What can I do about it?). For most people situations that are interpreted as stressful include (1) **harm-and-loss**, (2) **threat**, and (3) **challenge**.

Harm-and-loss situations include the death of a loved one, theft or damage to one's home, physical injury or loss of an organ, physical assault, or loss of self-esteem. Harm-and-loss situations create stress because an important physical or psychological need is not satisfied. Emotions that signal harm or loss include sadness, depression, and anger. Note that eight of the first ten items on the SRE involve harm-and-loss.

Threat situations are perceived and interpreted as likely to produce harm or loss whether or not any harm or loss actually occurs. The experience is one of continually warding off demands that tax one's abilities to cope with life. Emotions associated with threat include anger, hostility, anxiety, frustration, and depression.

Challenge situations are perceived and interpreted as opportunities for growth, mastery, and gain. Very often such situations involve major life transitions such as leaving one's family to start life on one's own, graduating from college, or getting married. Even though they are interpreted as "good," life transitions can nevertheless be stressful because they require considerable psychological and physical adjustment. Often a life transition involves both sadness and excitement: sadness for the loss of what is familiar and excitement in anticipation of the new.

Besides interpreting a situation as harmful, threatening, or challenging, reacting to a situation also involves deciding what to do about it. This is referred to as **coping** (discussed in more detail in

Table 10-2
The Schedule of Recent Experience (SRE)

Rank	Event	Life change units
1	Death of spouse	100
2	Divorce	73
3	Marital separation	65
4	Jail term	63
5	Death of close family member	63
6	Personal injury or illness	53
7	Marriage	50
8	Fired from job	47
9	Marital reconciliation	45
10	Retirement	45
11	Change in health of family member	44
12	Pregnancy	40
13	Sex difficulties	39
14	Gain of new family member	39
15	Business adjustment	39
16	Change in financial state	38
17	Death of close friend	37
18	Change to different line of work	36
19	Change in number of arguments with spouse	35
20	Mortgage over $10,000	31
21	Foreclosure of mortgage or loan	30
22	Change in responsibilities at work	29
23	Son or daughter leaving home	29
24	Trouble with in-laws	29
25	Outstanding personal achievement	28
26	Wife begin or stop work	26
27	Begin or end school	26
28	Change in living conditions	25
29	Revision of personal habits	24
30	Trouble with boss	23
31	Change in work hours or conditions	20
32	Change in residence	20
33	Change in schools	20
34	Change in recreation	19
35	Change in church activities	19
36	Change in social activities	18
37	Mortgage or loan less than $10,000	17
38	Change in sleeping habits	16
39	Change in number of family get-togethers	15
40	Change in eating habits	15
41	Vacation	13
42	Christmas	12
43	Minor violations of the law	11

Chapter 11). Coping refers to efforts to manage a situation and is independent of outcome. This definition differs from the popular idea that coping with a problem necessarily means success.

Table 10-3
Stress "Units" Associated with Some Common Life Changes Experienced by Students

Event	Life change units	Event	Life change units	Event	Life change units	Event	Life change units
Death of close family member	100	Pregnancy	45	First quarter/semester in college	35	Chronic car trouble	26
		Sex problems	44			Change in number of family get-togethers	26
Death of a close friend	73	Serious argument with close friend	40	Change in living conditions	31	Too many missed classes	25
Divorce between parents	65	Change in financial status	39	Serious argument with instructor	30		
Jail term	63	Trouble with parents	39	Lower grades than expected	29	Change of college/change of work	24
Major personal injury or illness	63	Change of major	39	Change in sleeping habits	29		
Marriage	58	New girlfriend or boyfriend	38			Dropped more than one class	23
Fired from job	50			Change in social activities	29	Minor traffic violations	20
Failed important course	47	Increased workload at school	37	Change in eating habits	28		
Change in health of family member	45	Outstanding personal achievement	36				

The ability to cope often depends on a person's belief about how much control he or she has over the situation. Control, in turn, depends on how powerful the situation is perceived to be and resources that the individual can muster to meet the challenge (see Table 10-4). People who believe that they can control their environment, who perceive life changes to be opportunities for growth, who hold a personal commitment to respond to challenges, and who are optimistic about potential success have been shown to experience less stress than those who believe that they lack control, who are helpless in the face of change, who hold little hope for a positive outcome, and who seek permission from others before acting.

Consequences of Reactions

Although it is the human mind that interprets a given situation as harmful, threatening, or challenging, it is the nervous and endocrine systems, which link the brain and the rest of the body, that bring about the changes in physiology that lead to harmful behaviors or to disease. The feelings associated with stressful experiences (fear, anger, sadness, etc.) activate the nervous and endocrine systems, which in turn produce changes in the immune system and in physiology (see Chapter 3). Illnesses arise when the nervous and endocrine systems are continually activated or overstimulated. As a consequence, organs begin to wear down or become susceptible to disease.

Table 10-4
Various Kinds of Resources for Coping with Stress

PHYSICAL
  Genetic predisposition to stress and illness
  Health status
  Nutritional status
  Physical strength and endurance

PSYCHOLOGICAL
  Beliefs and attitudes about change
  Beliefs and attitudes about one's abilities and skills
  Motivation to manage challenge and change
  Previous history with managing challenge and change
  Self-esteem

SOCIAL
  Availability of other people who offer care and support
  Social climate (absence of prejudice, racism, expectations)
  Institutional support and services
  Stable social and economic environment

MATERIAL
  Income, food, shelter
  Access to information
  Access to helping services
  Access to tools and equipment

BOX 10-1

ARE YOU SUSCEPTIBLE TO STRESS?

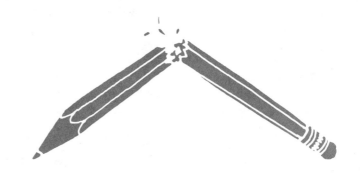

Some persons are more susceptible to the harmful effects of stress than others. The following test, developed at the Boston University Medical Center, can give you some indication of your susceptibility. Score each item from 1 (almost always) to 5 (never) as it applies to you. Any number less than 50 indicates you are not particularly vulnerable to stress. A score of 50–80 indicates moderate vulnerability, and over 80, high vulnerability.

___ 1. I eat at least one hot, nutritious meal a day.

___ 2. I get seven to eight hours sleep at least four nights a week.

___ 3. I am affectionate with others regularly.

___ 4. I have at least one relative within 50 miles on whom I can rely.

___ 5. I exercise to the point of sweating at least twice a week.

___ 6. I smoke fewer than ten cigarettes a day.

___ 7. I drink fewer than five alcoholic drinks a week.

___ 8. I am about the proper weight for my height and age.

___ 9. I have enough money to meet basic expenses and needs.

___ 10. I feel strengthened by my religious beliefs.

___ 11. I attend club or social activities on a regular basis.

___ 12. I have several close friends and acquaintances.

___ 13. I have one or more friends to confide in about personal matters.

___ 14. I am basically in good health.

___ 15. I am able to speak openly about my feelings when angry or worried.

___ 16. I discuss problems about chores, money, and daily living issues with the people I live with.

___ 17. I do something just for fun at least once a week.

___ 18. I am able to organize my time and do not feel pressured.

___ 19. I drink fewer than three cups of coffee (or tea or cola drinks) a day.

___ 20. I allow myself quiet time at least once during each day.

TOTAL ___

Adapted from a test developed by L. H. Miller and A. D. Smith.

The challenge-response systems activate the **fight or flight** response. All mammals, including humans, are capable of displaying this particular response when confronted with challenges they interpret as frightening or as a threat to survival. The response is characterized by a coordinated discharge of the sympathetic nervous system and portions of the parasympathetic nervous system and by the secretion of a number of hormones, especially epinephrine. When a person (or other animal) experiences a threatening situation, the associated emotions (usually fear or rage) that arise in the limbic system portion of the brain are translated automatically into the appropriate physiological responses through nervous and hormonal pathways mediated by the hypothalamus.

Some of the more prominent aspects of the fight or flight response are an elevation of the heart rate and high blood pressure (to provide more blood to muscles), constriction of the blood vessels of the skin (to limit bleeding if wounded), dilation of the pupil of the eye (to let in more light, thereby improving vision), increased activity in the reticular formation of the brain (to increase the alert, aroused state), and liberation of glucose and free fatty acids from storage depots (to make more stored energy available to the muscles, brain, and other tissues and organs). Figure 10-3 lists the physiological reactions of the fight or flight response.

Everyone is capable of the fight or flight response; it is part of the human biological make-up. Individuals display this reaction to some extent when they narrowly escape from a dangerous mishap or when they get angry or frustrated and lose their temper. The heart rate quickens, the person becomes more alert and tense, and he or she experiences a rush of excitement from increased secretion of epinephrine into the blood. In short, the person becomes ready to take action to deal with the situation.

In our modern civilized society, however, literally fleeing from a threatening situation or engaging in physical combat is often an inappropriate —and sometimes impossible—response. Social norms dictate that people handle many difficult situations "civilly." Moreoever, many threats are symbolic. The fear of losing a job, social status, or a lover is not the same as being confronted by a ferocious animal or thug, but the anxiety can produce similar stress-related physiological responses. Thus,

one of the consequences of having a highly evolved brain with the ability for symbolic thought and the intellectual capacity to produce a "civilized" society is the existence of social norms that make people unwilling or unable to take direct action when confronted with threatening situations. Civilized humankind has, in most situations, outgrown the original usefulness of the fight or flight reaction, which was essential to human survival in more primitive times. Unfortunately, human biological changes have not kept pace with cultural and social changes. Thus, we are left with a biological response that is inappropriate for most stressful situations that are encountered.

General Adaptation Syndrome

Hans Selye, a pioneer in researching responses to stress, found that continued physiological responding to stressors led to a characteristic response called the General Adaptation Syndrome (GAS). The GAS is characterized by a three-phase response to any stressor (see Figure 10-4). In the first phase, called the **stage of alarm,** a person's ability to withstand or resist any type of stressor is lowered by the need to deal with the stressor, whether it is a burn, a broken arm, the loss of a loved one, or the fear of losing one's job. During the second phase, the **stage of resistance,** the body adapts to the continued

Figure 10-3
The fight or flight response.

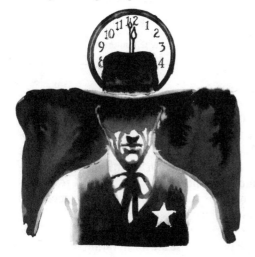

Heart
Increase in heart rate and force of contractions

Blood vessels
Constriction of abdominal viscera and dilitation in skeletal muscles

Eye
Contraction of radial muscle of iris and relaxation of ciliary muscle

Intestines
Decreased motility and relaxation of sphincters

Skin
Contraction of pilomotor muscles and contraction of sweat glands

Spleen
Contraction

Brain
Activation of reticular formation

> Without your exercising any conscious control over it, your autonomic nervous system and all your body functions react vigorously to both stress and depression.
>
> **C. Norman Shealy, M.D.**

presence of the stressor by increasing its resistance — for example, by producing more epinephrine, raising the blood pressure, activating the immune system, releasing glucose into the blood, or tensing certain muscles. If interaction with the stressor is prolonged, the ability to resist becomes depleted, and the person enters the **stage of exhaustion.** It is during the stage of exhaustion that disease may be initiated. Because many months or even years of wear and tear may be required before the body's resistance is exhausted, illness may not appear until long after the initial interaction with the stressor.

Experiments with laboratory animals performed by Selye and others have demonstrated that profound changes in vital body organs — principally the adrenal glands, the thymus gland, the lymph nodes, and the lining of the stomach — can be caused by activation of the GAS. For example, stomach ul-

cers can often result in humans or other animals from a prolonged interaction with a stressor. In a study of over a hundred air traffic controllers, more than half were found to be suffering from gastrointestinal illness. Among those who were ill, over half were diagnosed as having peptic ulcers. The constant stress from worrying about airplane crashes and collisions caused ulcers in many of the persons engaged in this kind of job (Cobb and Rose, 1973).

Animals receiving an intermittent mild electric shock tend to develop more ulcers than animals that are not shocked. More significantly, animals receiving prior warning of an impending electric shock develop fewer ulcers than do those not given a warning. Of special relevance to humans is the observation that animals given the opportunity to avoid or delay the shock develop only slightly more ulcers than do animals who receive no shock at all (Weiss, 1972). This implies that if ways are found to avoid

Figure 10-4

The three phases of the general adaptation syndrome. In the stage of alarm, the body's normal resistance to stress is lowered from the first interactions with the stressor. In the stage of resistance, the body adapts to the continued presence of the stressor and resistance increases. In the stage of exhaustion, the body loses its ability to resist the stressor any longer and becomes exhausted.

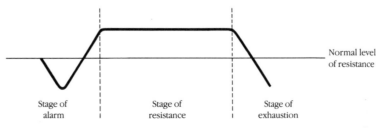

persistent stress, or at least to modify its effects, many stress-related illnesses might be avoided.

Type A Behavior and Stress

More than a decade ago physicians Meyer Friedman and Ray Rosenman proposed that some people respond to stress in a way that predisposes them to heart disease; they dubbed this response the **type A behavior pattern.** They defined type A persons as being "engaged in a relatively chronic struggle to obtain an unlimited number of poorly defined things from their environment in the shortest period of time, and, if necessary, against the opposing ef-

forts of other things or persons in the same environment." In short, the type A behavior pattern is a "hurry sickness" (see Box 10-2).

As might be expected, Friedman and Rosenman suggest that a personality type opposite that of type A—what they call type B—is associated with greater health. Their description of the type B person is someone who "is rarely harried by desires to obtain a widely increasing number of things or participate in an endlessly growing series of events in an ever-decreasing amount of time." Despite an enormous amount of research, recent evidence does *not* support the idea that type A persons are more susceptible to heart disease and heart attacks (discussed in more detail in Chapter 16).

BOX 10-2

DO YOU HAVE "HURRY SICKNESS"?

	Almost always	Only sometimes	Almost never
1. Do you interrupt other people before they have finished speaking?			
2. Are you irritated when you have to wait in line?			
3. Do you eat fast?			
4. Do you try to do more than one thing at a time?			
5. Are you annoyed if you lose at sports or games?			
6. How often do you forget what you were going to say?			
7. Do you tap your fingers or bounce your feet while sitting?			
8. Do you speed up and drive through yellow caution lights at intersections?			
9. Do you race the car engine while waiting for the signal to change?			
10. Do you fall behind in the things you need to accomplish?			

Here's how to determine your score. If you checked almost always, give yourself 3 points; if you checked only sometimes, 2 points; and for almost never, 1 point. Add up all of the points. If you scored 25–30, you probably have hurry sickness (don't worry, it's not fatal) and need to work on slowing down or relaxing more. If you scored 16–24, you have a potential for hurry syndrome. If you scored less than 16, you are probably pretty laid back.

> Since you cannot build a life completely free from stress or even distress, it is important that you develop some ways of dealing with stress.
>
> **National Institute of Mental Health**

Stress and the Immune System

Long-term activation of the nervous and endocrine systems is responsible, at least in part, for reduced functioning of the immune system, which produces increased susceptibility to infections (see Chapter 3). For example, one study showed that stress associated with taking exams can reduce the level of antibodies (in this study, immunoglobulin A) that are normally present in saliva (Jemmott et al., 1983). Samples of saliva were taken from a group of dental students at various times during their first year of dental school. Students returning from vacation had the highest levels of antibody, whereas during the exam periods the students' antibody levels were significantly lower. These data provide an explanation for the long-standing observation that colds and other infectious diseases increase in student populations during exams. If stress can interfere with immune system responses, then it also can predispose one to infections and other diseases.

Other studies have confirmed that stress can impair the functioning of the immune system. For example, one study found lower-than-normal levels of immune system cells in men whose wives had recently died (Stein and Schleifer, 1985). This finding may explain the observation that among older people a surviving spouse has a higher-than-expected risk of death during the period of bereavement. In addition to bereaved spouses, unhappily married and recently divorced people also have reduced immune system functions.

Managing Stress

We have seen that stress-related illness is the result of a chain of psychological and physiological responses that consists of (1) the appraisal of a situation as personally threatening or disruptive, (2) unsuccessful attempts to deal with the disruption, and (3) persistent activation of the nervous, hormone, and immune systems that eventually results in illness.

Because stress-related disorders depend on mental attitudes and processes, it is possible for people to exert control over the steps that may lead to illness. For example, people can change how they interact with disruptive persons and situations by disengaging from a stressful situation (change jobs, change roommates, change college major, etc.).

An individual also can try to alter her or his response to a given situation by changing beliefs and attitudes, and goals. Winning may be an athlete's highest goal, but the fear of losing may bring about an ulcer. The solution need not be to give up sports but to change one's priorities—perhaps by emphasizing one's performance and not the outcome of the competition. Another way to handle stress is to change one's usual way of coping. People who are

> I look for therapeutic techniques that help break through resistance to change while doing no harm.
>
> **Joan Nelson**
> **Psychologist**

inclined to act regardless of the situation may find that being patient and postponing action will produce greater rewards. At the other extreme, people who are inclined not to take action may find it useful to become more assertive when confronted with a stressful situation.

The key to dealing with life stress is to change some aspect of life or to change the way that situations are experienced. There is no stress-reduction pill; neither do alcohol nor tranquilizers offer any real solution to reducing stress. The taking of tranquilizers, although often prescribed by physicians to reduce stress, offers at best only limited short-term relief—and at worst, offers habituation to and even physiological dependence on a particular drug (this issue is discussed in detail in Chapter 13). The best way to deal with stress is to replace stressful ways of living with beliefs, attitudes, and behaviors that promote peace, joy, and mind-body harmony. That does not mean that you must become reclusive or try to eliminate all sources of conflict, tension, and anxiety from life. People need a certain degree of tension to overcome challenges in order to be creative and to grow psychologically and spiritually. It may mean, however, that it would be wise to change some habitual ways of being and thinking that are self-destructive.

One way to make a lifestyle change is to seek help from a teacher, counselor, psychotherapist, or coach who can offer guidelines and suggestions on how to recognize sources of stress and also ways to deal with them. With this information, a person can adjust his or her lifestyle to reduce the exposure to particular stress-producing situations.

Another way to deal with stress is to employ one of several methods of stress reduction that make use of techniques that produce a psychophysiological condition opposite to the fight or flight response. Such a condition has been termed the **relaxation response,** or **hypometabolic state,** and its use is based on the notion that continual discharge of the sympathetic nervous system and excessive secretion of adrenal hormones as a response to long-term stress ultimately leads to ill health and that reducing these psychophysiological reactions to stress can improve health. The techniques that produce the relaxation response include autogenic training, meditation, progressive relaxation, and hypnosis, all of which are discussed in Chapter 2. Apparently, the physiology of the relaxation response can be elicited by any of these techniques and is not specific to any one of them, which is why we urge everyone to learn some mental relaxation technique and to use it to reduce the physiological effects of stress.

Fortunately, nearly all stress-related illnesses are preventable by avoiding or reducing stressful life experiences and relationships. Although you cannot avoid all potentially stressful situations, you can en-

> A person has two legs and one sense of humor and if you're faced with a choice it's better to lose a leg.
>
> **Charles Lindner**

deavor to choose an occupation that is consistent with a peaceful frame of mind rather than to engage in tasks that result in continual stress. Each person has to be sure that his or her choice of a livelihood is consistent with personal life goals. For some, the tensions of air traffic control are too great and bring on illness. Clearly, these people should not continue as air traffic controllers unless their on-the-job duties change to become less stressful for them or they learn to cope with their duties more successfully. For others, the challenge of air traffic control is stimulating and they have no problems with it. The same applies to any kind of work—firefighting, law enforcement, tax accounting, or childcare. Health and wellness come from avoiding situations that are stressful to the point of causing illness.

 ## Supplemental Readings

Benson, Herbert. *The Relaxation Response.* New York: Wm. Morrow, 1975. A scientific explanation of the relaxation response and how it can be used to reduce stress.

Goleman, Daniel, and **Goleman, Tara Bennet.** *The Relaxed Body Book.* New York: Doubleday and Co., 1986. The editors of *American Health* magazine have assembled a series of simple, gentle relaxation exercises derived from a variety of techniques.

Hamberger, L. K., and **Lohr, J. M.** *Stress and Stress Management.* New York: Springer, 1984. A detailed and complete discussion of all aspects of stress research and its applications.

Pelletier, Kenneth R. *Mind as Healer, Mind as Slayer.* New York: Delta, 1977. A summary of the author's views on the role of stress in causing illness and ways to prevent stress disorders.

Schafer, W. *Stress, Distress and Growth.* Davis, Calif.: International Dialogue Press, 1978. A popular book on various aspects of stress and how to manage it.

Zales, Michael, ed. *Stress in Health and Disease.* New York: Brunner/Mazel, 1985. A compilation of articles dealing with particular aspects of stress and its effect on health.

Summary

Life presents people with innumerable situations that have the potential to disrupt mind-body harmony. Situations and events that cause such disruptions are stressors; the experience of mind-body disharmony is stress. Prolonged interaction with a stressor can impair functioning of the body's organs and/or immune system and result in illness.

Activators are situations and events that have the potential to become stressors depending on how the mind interprets the particular situation. Reactions are an individual's response to activators. The nature and degree of a person's reaction depends on how challenging and/or threatening he or she perceives the situation to be. Consequences are the psychological and physiological effects of a reaction. An appraisal of how difficult it is to deal with the situation determines how well a person is able to cope.

The onset of stress-related illness depends on several factors, including the mental interpretation of a situation as stressful, followed by the response of the body to the mind's assessment of stress via hormonal and nervous links between the brain and the rest of the body. These hormonal and nervous signals unbalance normal body physiology (homeostasis) and illness eventually results.

Stress reduction can be achieved by eliminating the stressors in the environment, by controlling your reaction to a given situation, or by reducing the magnitude of the stress on the body. Stress can also be reduced by various techniques, including meditation, autogenic training, hypnotherapy, biofeedback therapy, and just plain "taking it easy."

FOR YOUR HEALTH

What Are Your Stressors?

Situations, relationships, and ways of being are common sources of stress. Make a list of the situations, recurring events, relationships, and personal behaviors that you believe contribute stress to your life. Some common ones are job pressures, arguments with loved ones, money worries, and dislike for work, teachers, and co-workers.

What Are Your Stress Reactions?

Many people experience particular physical reactions to excessive stress. Here's a list of some common stress reactions. Which ones do you frequently experience? Can you add some reactions that are not on the list?

Headaches	Rapid heart rate
Nervous tics and twitches	Impotence
	Pelvic pain
Blurred vision	Stomachache
Dizziness	Diarrhea
Fatigue	Frequent urination
Coughing	Dermatitis (rash)
Wheezing	Hyperventilation
Backache	Irregular heart rhythm
Muscle spasms	High blood pressure
Itching	Delayed menstruation
Excessive sweating	Vaginal discharge
Palpitations	Nail biting
Constipation	Heartburn
Jaw tightening	

Keeping a Stress Journal

Recording how often you feel stressed or hassled during each day can help you begin to learn what things cause you stress and to develop ways to reduce stress in your life. Start keeping a stress journal (at least for several weeks) and respond to the following questions whenever you feel stressed:

1. What time of day did the stressful situation occur?
2. What caused the stress (if you can identify it)?
3. Did you experience any physical or emotional symptoms?
4. How long did the symptoms last?
5. Any thoughts or comments on the stressful event?

By examining your stress journal after a period of time, you may be able to identify a pattern to the stressful situations. Perhaps then you can take measures to avoid stressful situations or to manage stress better.

Calculate Your Life Change Units

Complete the Schedule of Recent Experience (see Table 10-2) and total the number of life change units (LCUs) you've accumulated in the past year. If you have accumulated more than 150 LCUs, how can you change your present lifestyle to decrease the number of changes you may encounter in the near future and thereby reduce your risk of illness?

CHAPTER ELEVEN

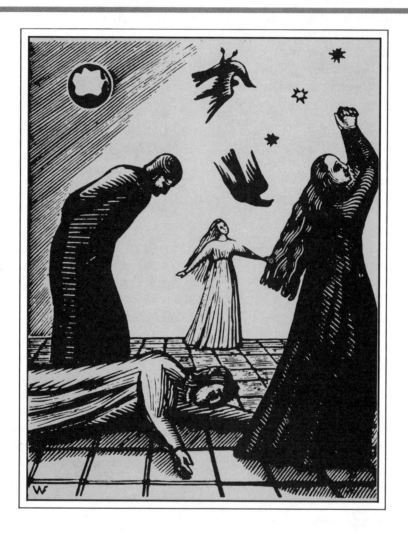

You can learn to use periods of
emotional distress as opportunities for
personal growth.

Emotional Distress

We all experience periods of emotional distress. To occasionally feel angry, anxious, blue, lonely, or depressed is a normal aspect of living.

Most of us would undoubtedly prefer always to feel happy, content, and secure. But that is not possible—neither is it even desirable. If nothing ever changed, we might escape periods of emotional distress, but such an existence would surely be incredibly boring.

Besides, humans apparently need certain kinds of stimulation because they do not tolerate long periods of isolation very well. People are creative, curious, interactive beings who induce change in their lives simply by the act of living. New situations that require adjustment arise all the time. Very often, the message that it is time for an adjustment in one's thoughts, attitudes, or behaviors is communicated by emotional distress, and failure to heed such messages may bring about a stress-related illness. Negative emotions signal that something is not altogether right with life, and they motivate individuals to seek ways of being that make them feel better. Viewed in this way, emotional distress can be seen as a stimulus for personal growth and self-improvement.

In this chapter we consider the dynamics of emotional distress and the ways in which negative feelings can be used to accomplish personal growth. Please remember that the unpleasant feelings that accompany the fears, frustrations, and sadnesses of everyday life are quite different from the severe distress that is associated with prolonged periods of abnormal thoughts, feelings, and behaviors that seriously disrupt some people's lives for months or even years. Unfortunately, many conditions that involve feeling bad are often labeled "mental illness," and carry with them the stigma of being "neurotic" or "crazy." This is not the case in some parts of the world where social customs and even employment practices recognize that everyone has occasional "blue" days and antisocial periods. We prefer to differentiate the emotional distress that accompanies problems of living from the abnormal thoughts, feelings, and behaviors that are often the result of severe abnormalities in brain physiology and biochemistry (some of which may be genetically based) or of brain injury.

> Madness is a relative state. Who can say which of us is truly insane?
>
> Woody Allen
> *The Lunatic's Tale*

Motivation, Emotion, and Emotional Distress

Psychologists tell us that much of our behavior is motivated by the desire to fulfill certain basic human needs, of which there are two general kinds: **maintenance needs,** which involve actual physical survival, and **growth needs,** sometimes called needs for **self-actualization,** which involve emotional stimulation and spiritual growth. This theory, advanced by Abraham Maslow (1970), is based on the premise that most people are unable to concentrate on philosophical or spiritual development if they are starving or sick (see Figure 11-1).

Although basic needs are intrinsic to all humans, the ways in which people satisfy them are not. Everyone may need to eat, but not everyone obtains food in the same way. Neither does everyone choose to eat the same kind of food. Similarly, people engage in a great variety of living arrangements, jobs, and recreations to find the best way to fulfill their needs for love, security, and self-esteem. The many different strategies that people employ to try to fulfill their basic needs are the most remarkable examples of human creativity.

From childhood, people are developing and refining strategies for meeting their basic needs. As infants, the repertoire of need-fulfilling abilities is very limited. A child can cry when he or she wants to be fed or receive attention. And he or she can smile to encourage touching and play, which fulfill needs for love and stimulation. As people grow into adults, they acquire a greater number of ways that can be used to fulfill their needs. Among them are a set of values, beliefs, attitudes, and behaviors that they expect will help them by producing harmonious interactions with the environment—especially with people with whom they exchange love and trust. When individuals are successful in fulfilling their needs, they experience positive emotions such as joy, happiness, and contentment. When individuals are not successful, however, they experience negative feelings, or **emotional distress.** We get hungry when we need food or thirsty when we need water. Hunger and thirst are experienced as basic discomforts that motivate us to fulfill those maintenance needs. If we are confronted with an obstacle that prevents us from attaining a certain need, we can become frustrated and angry (see Box 11-1). If our security is threatened, we can become fearful or anxious. The loss of love or self-esteem can bring about a period of depression.

Dealing with Emotional Distress

Such is the condition of human life that people never reach a state of complete satisfaction. Even if all your maintenance needs were met, and even if you lived in wonderfully harmonious family relationships and worked at a job that is meaningful and self-fulfilling, you would still probably face frustration and conflict in life because you would continue to seek new and enriching experiences to satisfy your need for self-actualization. There are times, of course, when everything seems to be going really well, and it is possible to experience reasonably long

> People who scream about others being possessed
> by the Devil are generally possessed themselves,
> and their lack of compassion comes about
> because they cannot confront the evil inside
> themselves.
>
> **William Irwin Thompson**

periods of great joy. One of the principal goals of holistic health is to maximize the time you are joyous and happy and to minimize the times of emotional distress.

The various ways people devise to solve their life problems are referred to as **coping strategies.** Coping is "any response to external life-strains that serves to prevent, avoid, or control emotional distress" (Pearlin and Schooler, 1978). There are three general ways people can cope: (1) they can try to change the situation that is causing the emotional distress, (2) they can try to alter their interpretation of the significance of the situation so it has less importance, and therefore is not as distressing, or (3) they can try to alter the negative feeling state without trying to change the situation or how they think about it.

There are many ways of changing a situation that is causing emotional distress. One way is to make a rational appraisal of the situation and then to attack the problem directly by removing or surmounting the obstacle. Another approach is to withdraw from the situation—either by avoiding it altogether or by deciding to be patient in the belief that circumstances will ultimately change. Still another way to change the situation is to adapt oneself to it. This can be done by changing habitual ways of thinking, feeling, and behaving, by modifying unrealistic assumptions about how people are supposed to act, and by increasing self-knowledge and insight.

Coping strategies that attempt to alter the significance or interpretation of a distressing situation are probably used the most often (Pearlin and

Figure 11-1
Maslow's hierarchy of human needs.

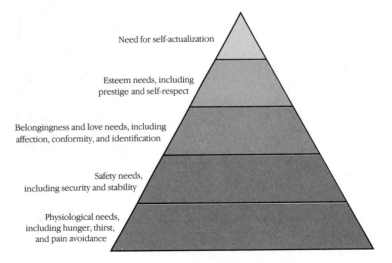

Need for self-actualization

Esteem needs, including
prestige and self-respect

Belongingness and love needs, including
affection, conformity, and identification

Safety needs,
including security and stability

Physiological needs,
including hunger, thirst,
and pain avoidance

BOX 11-1

DEALING WITH ANGER

Anger is one of the most common expressions of emotional distress. At all stages of life, from infancy to old age, people get angry if their needs are not being met. They get angry if they are cheated, lied to, hurt, punished, betrayed, or prevented from realizing their desires. People get angry when others whom they care for are being hurt in some way. And they sometimes get angry at others—as a form of self-defense—when they feel disappointed with themselves or guilty about something they did (or did not) do.

For many people anger is a difficult emotion to deal with, usually because it is difficult to express. Oftentimes, when it is directed toward an authority figure, anger can be difficult to express for fear of retaliatory punishment. Anger at a loved one is sometimes hard to express because of the risk that the other person may become angry in turn and withdraw his or her love. Some people are confused by their anger at loved ones. They see it as inconsistent with feelings of love and hence become unable to express it, even if they feel justified in doing so. Another reason anger is hard to deal with is that it is often associated with the desire to inflict physical harm.

Psychologists say that anger is the result of frustration, which is the feeling that comes when you are prevented from attaining a particular goal. Therefore, one good way to handle anger is to assess the merits of the goal you cannot attain and the strategy you've been employing to attain it. We often get angry with other people because we ask them for things that they cannot give, or because they are not providing the help we expect from them in attaining our goal. Often, however, we haven't told them what the goal is, or how we expect them to help. So it's no wonder they don't perform the way we want them to.

Before you get angry at someone or something, first ask yourself if your goal is realistically attainable. Have you expected too much of yourself? Have you expected too much of someone else? Have you tried to get what you want in the best possible way? If such self-assessment leads to the conclusion that you have set an unattainable goal for yourself, or that your strategy for attaining a goal is not well thought out, then you have no one (or nothing) to blame for your anger but yourself—and this realization usually makes angry feelings evaporate. Remember, most of the time other people don't make you angry. *You* make yourself angry. Being honest and realistic with yourself and being direct with others is one way to prevent anger from occurring, and a reassessment of your goals and strategies is one way to diffuse an anger-provoking situation.

There are times, of course, when feeling anger and expressing it toward someone else is appropriate. For example, anger is justified when someone knowingly abuses you (physically or psychologically) or someone or something you care for. Anger is also appropriate if the person abuses himself or herself. Another time that anger could be deemed appropriate is when someone breaks a promise. It's always wise to be very clear about promises. There would be a lot less anger and frustration if people promised to do only things that they knew they could follow through on.

What about dealing with someone who is angry at you? Being on the receiving end of anger often makes you want to protect yourself from the physical or psychological harm you imagine will come with hostility. And one way to protect yourself is to get angry in return. Getting angry in return, however, is rarely a good solution. It is better to realize that the angry person is frustrated, disappointed, and emotionally upset. If the angry person were wounded and bleeding, you would certainly try to help. Think of this anger as symbolic of an emotional wound. Be patient with the angry person and try to offer support for his or her feelings. This will help remove the pain of frustration and eventually the anger will subside.

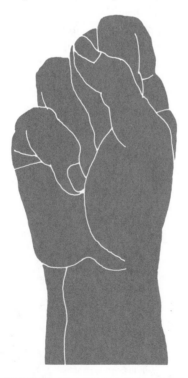

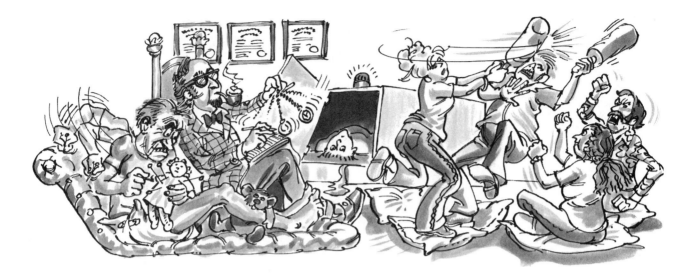

Schooler, 1978). One way people do this is to make positive comparisons, which are represented by sayings like "count your blessings," "we're all in the same boat," or "things are bound to get better." Another way is to focus on the good in a situation and try to minimize or ignore the bad. Most everyone can see the flaws in another person, but how often do we notice a person's good qualities?

It is also possible to devalue a goal that might have been important and to replace it with another. For example, one might come to believe that taking time for meditation and physical relaxation each day is preferable to a day full of tension-producing work. Another way to alter the significance of a situation is to turn awareness for a time to the inner, private, perhaps mystical nature of being rather than focus constantly on external experience and pressures. This can be done by increasing both body and mental awareness through any number of methods, such as exercise, yoga, dance, and various forms of meditation. Those who take time to expand self-awareness often claim increased self-knowledge and increased mastery over their feelings; they say that they have found a way to personal and emotional peace. In response to the charge that they are simply escaping from their problems, they answer that there is much to gain by "turning off the world" for a brief period each day. "It's still there when you turn it on again, but it usually looks a lot different . . . and better."

People can also cope with a distressing situation by trying to alter their negative feelings about it. Some people release their emotions in ways other than confronting the distressing situation. For example, they can express their anger at their boss or a family member by taking part in competitive sports or by hitting a punching bag. Some people adjust by accepting the bad feelings that accompany life difficulties, thinking that perhaps it was "meant to be" or that "you have to take the bad with the good." And some people are like the Biblical Job: they endure their emotional distress in the belief that such behavior is a virtue that will be rewarded in the hereafter. People can also try to cope by escaping into the fantasy of books, films, or television or by ingesting alcohol or drugs. Although trying to change how you feel can help reduce the intensity of a negative emotional state, it does not in itself change the situation causing the problem and in some cases may actually prolong arriving at a permanent solution.

Facilitating Coping

Although negative feelings make distressed people aware that something in their lives is not going well, it is not always possible for them to ascertain what the problem is or what might be the best way to deal with it. And even if someone does understand the problem and knows how it might be solved, he or she may still be unable to proceed because of fear and ingrained habits. Most people prefer to stick with the old ways of being, even if they produce dis-

> People through finding something beautiful
> think something else unbeautiful
> Through finding one man fit
> judge another unfit.
>
> **Lao-tzu**

comfort, because they are familiar. One of the hardest things in life is to overcome the fear of the unknown. "If I leave this person, will I ever find another to love me?" is a common fear.

When people are troubled, they need not suffer with their problems in silence for fear of being labeled "crazy." Comfort and advice are available from trusted family members and friends and from professional advisers such as clergymen, attorneys, counselors, psychotherapists, and physicians. In talking to these helpers, distressed persons may gain a new perspective on their problems from which a workable solution presents itself. Another benefit from talking to a helper is the release of what can be a great deal of controlled negative emotion. While talking to a helper, a distressed person might cry, shout, or even pound a table to relieve the intensity of feelings he or she may have been holding in.

Psychotherapists are professionals who have undergone considerable training to help people deal with emotional distress (see Box 11-2). Whether a person has feelings of inferiority, is troubled by painful dependency in a love relationship, or has some other problem that is causing distress, a therapist can facilitate change that can bring about improvement in a person's life. This change is accomplished not only by "just talking," but also by helping the distressed person feel what it is like to be different. It is one thing to intellectually know the source of personal anxiety, and even what to do about it, but it is quite another to change thoughts and actions so as to actually change the negative feelings.

The value of psychotherapy, regardless of the technique, is that the distressed person (the client) has faith in the professional healer's (therapist's) ability to help effect a change. This faith produces a situation of trust that enables the client to be honest about himself or herself—to disclose painful and unflattering thoughts and feelings that would not likely be disclosed to a friend or relative.

Depression

According to the National Institute of Mental Health, each day approximately one person in seven experiences some form of depression, characterized by such feelings as dejection, guilt, hopelessness, and self-recrimination and by some or all of the following depressive symptoms: loss of appetite, insomnia, loss of interest in sex, reduced interest in doing previously enjoyable activities, withdrawal from social contacts, inability to concentrate and to make decisions, lowered self-esteem, and a focus on negative thoughts and the bad things in life. If asked how they feel, most depressed people respond by saying something like "I've got the blues," or "Life's a drag," or "What's the use of doing anything?"

Most commonly, depression is a reaction to one of two general kinds of life event: the loss of status in the group, or the loss of love, companionship, and group belonging (Henry and Stephens, 1977). Thus, people become depressed and feel worthless and defeated when they receive criticism or experience

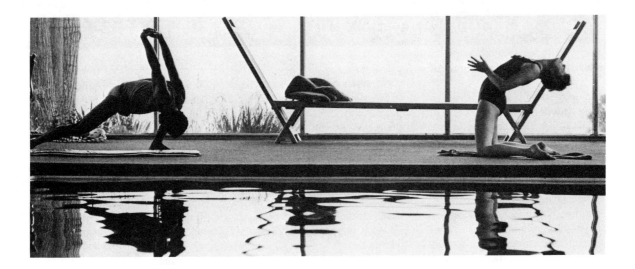

failure at a task they wanted very much to accomplish. People also feel depressed when they are lonely, and most particularly when they are experiencing discord with a marital partner. In fact, it has been estimated that nearly 70 percent of all common depression is precipitated by marital problems (McLean, 1976).

One of the characteristics of depression is that it can intensify itself, thus creating what is called the depressive cycle. The depressed person's negative thoughts, social withdrawal, the loss of interest and activity only serve to reinforce feelings of worthlessness, helplessness, gloom, and doom. The fact that depression can make itself worse means that overcoming depression often necessitates a two-pronged strategy: (1) to interrupt the depressive cycle, and (2) to correct the life situation that brought on the depression. Sometimes both goals can be accomplished simultaneously by a particular life change.

Dealing with Depression

The best way to deal with depression is to get life moving again. Little improvement can be expected unless the withdrawal/inactivity cycle is interrupted. One way to do so is to establish a simple, attainable goal and then to set out to accomplish it. It should be a concrete behavior or task that can be done in a brief period of time, and it should involve movement. That way inactivity stops and some sense of mastery over life is restored. Perhaps the reason jogging helps depressed people feel better is that it pro-

vides an attainable goal that also carries with it the value of being "good for you." When people jog, they learn that they are capable of succeeding at something that improves their lives. It might also be that jogging or any other kind of physical exercise alters the chemistry of the brain and the body and produces positive feeling states in place of negative ones.

It is also important for depressed people to increase their interaction with other people. Remaining in seclusion only reinforces feelings of loss and worthlessness. Of course, depressed people are not necessarily pleasant to be around if they dwell on their troubles during conversations. Thus, it may be preferable for depressed people to begin taking part in such social activities as going to a movie or playing tennis rather than to discuss what's wrong with them with an acquaintance. By becoming active, they will divert attention from their negative inner dialogue, and this will help break the depressive cyle.

In most cases, depression is a reaction to a particularly disturbing life event, such as the loss of a loved one. As such, it is a normal reaction. But when the severity and length of a depressive episode are excessive, or when the depression cannot be attributed to any life change that would be likely to bring about deeply depressed feelings, the cause of the depression may be an imbalance in brain biochemistry. Many authorities support the hypothesis that malfunctions in the normal processes that control the brain levels of certain neurotransmitters (see Chapter 3) can lead to the onset of depressive symptoms (Schildkraut, 1978).

BOX 11-2

A CONVERSATION WITH A PSYCHOTHERAPIST

Question: What is the purpose of psychotherapy?

Answer: To help people relieve their emotional distress. People come to see me when they're in emotional crisis—when what they usually do to cope with the world around them doesn't work very well or at all anymore. They come to me saying, in one way or another, "My life isn't working anymore." Sometimes they're crying and sometimes they're screaming and sometimes they're being very intellectual about it. The purpose of psychotherapy is to help people function in life again, and hopefully in a better way than before.

Q: What kinds of problems do people normally have? Do people have to be crazy in order to see you?

A: There's a range of problems. Some people do have a thinking process problem. They may be having delusions or hallucinations. They have a hard time telling the real from the unreal. There are others who simply aren't happy with their lives, their jobs, or their relationships. Problems with interpersonal relationships are quite common. Some people are severely depressed. Some are suicidal. The causes of these problems are varied. Some could be biological, others environmental. Overall, everyone I see professionally has problems and bad feelings about life, and sometimes those people become so distraught, they cannot function at work or at home.

Q: What does a psychotherapist do to help people with their problems?

A: First, the therapist listens. And then the therapist tries to put himself in the client's place and understand what the client's situation must feel like. The therapist helps the client define what the problem actually is, and also helps the client assess his or her strengths and resources for dealing with the problems and changing things for the better. Therapists also help people express the emotions that accompany their life problem. Most of us believe we have to be strong all the time, but we need to express our feelings if we want to deal successfully with a problem.

Q: What happens in psychotherapy?

A: At the beginning, the client and the therapist discuss the nature of the client's problem or problems. Then the client and therapist set some mutual goals for the outcome of therapy, and during the subsequent sessions how well the goals are being achieved is discussed. The idea is to focus attention on the problem, how it affects the client's life, what sort of changes the client is willing to make, and what it will take to make these changes. Talk is cheap, but personal change is hard. The object of therapy is to make changes so that the problems that bring a person into therapy don't happen over and over again.

Q: What is the difference between various psychotherapists?

A: A psychiatrist is a medical doctor who has additional years of training in psychiatry, which is essentially human psychology. Psychiatrists know about drugs that affect the mind and they prescribe medications when they are needed. The medical aspects of thought, mood, or behavior problems are their specialty. When a psychiatrist does psychotherapy, the methods are not necessarily different from other therapists. Psychologists approach psychotherapy like other psychotherapists, too, but their training helps them administer diagnostic tests. Clinical social workers tend to approach problems from a broader perspective—the family and the community. The marriage, family, and child counselors focus on those types of therapy, although they do individual psychotherapy, too. Doctors of divinity look at the spiritual aspects of life problems. In many schools and colleges there are people trained to help with educational and vocational problems.

Q: What about quacks?

A: Some people who have state licenses and other socially approved credentials aren't at all effective or helpful. Others who don't have any professional credentials but have received some training can be terrific therapists. The issue is effectiveness, not prestige.

Q: Any final messages?

A: We all have times in life when we experience some really heavy stress, and as good as we might be at coping, it's sometimes helpful to go to a psychotherapist and find out why at this particular time things are really uncomfortable and difficult. It may sometimes be quite a difficult decision—you worry that your family and friends, and even your therapist, will think you're crazy. That's a common fear, but it's unnecessary. That doesn't happen. Sometimes it's necessary to have a helper so you don't have to wrestle with a terribly overwhelming problem alone, you don't have to become physically ill, you don't have to sleep all day, or you don't have to take drugs or become an alcoholic. It also helps if people take time for themselves, whether they do it through psychotherapy or through exercise or meditation. It's important to give yourself time to release pressures, to contemplate life, and to enjoy. The best thing in life is joy.

> ## The human race consists of the dangerously insane and such as are not.
>
> ### Mark Twain

In addition to malfunctions in neurotransmitter function, other biological factors may play a role in the onset of certain depressions. We have already mentioned (see Chapter 4) that certain people may react to excessive sugar intake with a reactive surge in insulin secretion that lowers blood sugar and brings about the symptoms of mild depression. It is also possible that people with an unusually high requirement for a certain vitamin or other nutrient may suffer occasional depressions if they do not receive sufficient amounts of that nutrient. Treating these people with large doses of nutrients can sometimes completely eliminate their depressive episodes.

The helplessness and hopelessness of depression is something all of us experience at some time in our lives. (Copyright Oslo Kommunes Kunstsamlinger, Munch-Museet.)

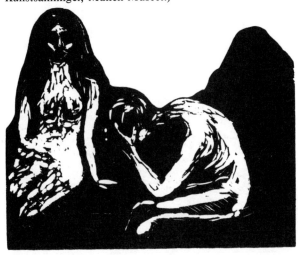

Depression and Suicide

One of the most worrisome aspects of depression is that a severely depressed person may become so dejected that the only relief thought possible is suicide. The psychological states most commonly associated with suicide are feelings of hopelessness, helplessness, and intolerable despair.

During the decade of the 1970s, the National Center for Health Statistics reported approximately 27,000 suicides per year in the United States, which ranked suicide among the ten most frequent causes of death. The number of reported suicides represents only 10–15 percent of the number of people who attempt suicide (Schneidman, 1979). Among young people, suicide ranks second to accidents and murder as a leading cause of death. And in recent years the suicide rate among young people has increased (see Figure 11-2).

Suicide is not a disease, nor is it a disorder that can be inherited. And suicides are not caused by unusual weather or by a full moon. And most important of all, many people who contemplate suicide are not psychotic. Most of the time, people consider suicide because they feel overwhelmed by some unhappy life situation, and they believe suicide to be their only remaining option in dealing with their extreme distress. Much of the time, people attempt suicide not because they really want to die but because they want to express their anger at others or to signal others for help. In such instances, suicide attempts are characterized by limited self-destructive acts, such as taking less than a lethal dose of sleeping pills or arranging that the suicide attempt will be discovered in time for them to be saved.

> The man who is unable to people his solitude
> is equally unable to be alone in a bustling crowd.
> **Charles Baudelaire**

Occasionally a person will express thoughts of suicide to a relative or a friend. This can be extremely distressing for the listener, who may react with disbelief ("You've got to be kidding"), panic ("What am I supposed to do about it?"), or avoidance ("Why tell me?"). In attempting to deal with his or her own uncomfortable feelings, a listener might say things like "Cheer up," or "You're better off than I am," or "You can't be serious." These and similar statements have the effect of denying the distressed person's feelings. According to suicidologist Louis Wekstein (1979), the best approach is to speak directly about the suicidal thoughts ("Tell me more about why you want to kill yourself"), to offer the distressed person nonjudgmental sympathy and concern, and firmly, but patiently and sym-

pathetically, to direct the distressed person to seek professional help immediately.

Oftentimes a suicidal individual will offer excuses for not seeing a professional and may even try to blackmail a friend into silence with covert threats. But the friend must hold firm and if necessary make an appointment with a counselor, psychiatrist, student health center, hospital emergency room, or suicide prevention center and deliver the distressed person there. If possible, parents or a spouse should be informed. The attempt to help a suicidally distressed person should be shared by as many concerned people as possible.

At the time a person contemplates suicide, life can seem exceedingly hopeless. But few life problems are beyond solution. Life crises do pass and distress-

Figure 11-2
Suicide rate of white and black males and females ages 15 to 24, 1950–1980. (Data from the U.S. National Center for Health Statistics.)

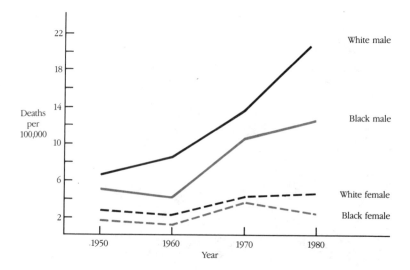

BOX 11-3

HINTS FOR EMOTIONAL WELLNESS

People Who Have a Positive Self-Image

. . . are not incapacitated by their emotions of fear, anger, love, jealousy, or guilt.

. . . can take life's disappointments in stride.

. . . have a tolerant attitude toward themselves and others; they can laugh at their shortcomings and mistakes.

. . . respect themselves and have self-confidence.

. . . are able to deal with most situations that come along.

. . . get satisfaction from simple, everyday pleasures.

People Who Feel Positive About Other People

. . . are able to give love and accept others the way they are.

. . . have personal relationships that are satisfying.

. . . expect to like and trust others and take it for granted that others will like and trust them.

. . . respect the many differences they see in people.

. . . do not need to control or push other people around.

. . . feel a sense of responsibility to friends and society.

People Who Are Able to Meet Life's Demands

. . . do something about their problems as they arise.

. . . accept their responsibilities.

. . . shape their environment whenever possible; otherwise they adjust to it.

. . . plan ahead but do not fear the future.

. . . welcome new ideas and experiences.

. . . use their natural capacities and talents.

. . . set attainable and realistic goals for themselves.

. . . get satisfaction from what they accomplish.

---

ing life situations improve; time does heal many hurts. And the experience gained by working through a distressing time of life can bring confidence, insight, and understanding. As you acquire experience and understanding, you are better able to cope with life's problems. And you are better able to help others deal with theirs.

Mental Disease

The brain, like all the other body organs, is composed of molecules and cells whose functioning is controlled by the genetic information in every cell. It is possible, therefore, for brain tissue to be affected by injury, infectious disease, chemical toxins, and inherited genetic errors, just as any other organ can be. When injury or disease occurs in the brain, a departure from what is considered normal thought, mood, or behavior can occur. Such conditions are examples of "mental illness."

A number of conditions are known to affect brain biology and lead to mental disturbances. The classic example of the biological basis for some mental illness is cerebral syphilis, which involves a deterioration of mental and emotional capabilities

during the late stages of the disease. Abnormalities in the secretion of hormones from the thyroid and adrenal glands can also lead to unusual thoughts and behavior. Deficiency in vitamin B intake can sometimes bring about bizarre thoughts and ideas. And deterioration of the brain tissue with age is yet another biological condition that can produce abnormality.

George III, King of England during the American Revolution, was judged to be "mad" by his physicians and others at court. During his severe attacks he became irrational and violent and had to be restrained. We now know that he suffered from a rare genetic disease called **porphyria**. Porphyrins are essential chemicals present in the hemoglobin of red blood cells. If the body does not properly regulate the amount of porphyrin in the body, a range of physical and mental symptoms develop, including rages, fits, and delirium. What appears as madness is due solely to a biochemical imbalance in the blood.

At the present time there is considerable investigation into the possible biological origins of schizophrenia. Many theories suggest different causes of schizophrenia, but the fact that the incidence of the condition is higher in genetically iden-

> *Psychiatrist:* Why are you waving your arms
> around like that ?
> *Patient:* To keep the wild tigers from attacking.
> *Psychiatrist:* But there aren't any tigers in here.
> *Patient:* That's right. It really works, doesn't it!

tical twins than in nonidentical (fraternal) twins, and that the often bizarre behavioral symptoms can be reduced more effectively by certain drugs than by traditional forms of learning-based psychotherapy, indicates that some kind of biological/biochemical abnormality may be involved. For the estimated 10 to 20 million Americans who are afflicted with some degree of schizophrenic symptoms, a biological explanation for their condition would be welcome, for it would lessen the stigma of being labeled crazy or psychotic.

Fears and Phobias

Everybody has been frightened by something at one time or another. We all learn to overcome common fears or else we learn to live with them. Specific things or experiences in our daily lives may cause some anxiety, but usually the fears are not severe enough to cause us any serious problems or illness. For example, a person may be somewhat anxious about encountering a snake while hiking, but this common fear does not deter the individual from the

A letter written by a psychologically disturbed man. Note the jumbled thought processes.

Michael,

My warmest appreciation for me getting anything here to san francisco. Presently I'm going after work doing illustrations. Certainly I would like more design work.

I'm happy with my work especially when a pretty girl make my day. Should there be any one around my thought is interest in their idea on how to get one to be a wife. Interestingly enough I was using most of my energies to get one until I ran out! Good luck with your pursuits and have a good day.

Kenny

BOX 11-4

IDENTIFY YOUR FEARS OR PHOBIAS

Frightening situations or objects	No fear	Mild fear	Strong fear
Airplanes			
Birds			
Bats			
Blood			
Cemeteries			
Dead animals			
Insects			
Crowds of people			
Dark places			
Dentists			
Doctors			
Hospitals			
Dirt and/or germs			
Lakes or oceans			
Dogs			
Cats			
Other animals			
Guns			
Closets or elevators			
Heights			
Public presentations			
Loud noises			
Driving in a car			
Being shouted at			
Being rejected			
Walking alone at night			
Other fears:			

enjoyment of hiking. Most of us have some mild fear that we can cope with without interfering with living.

A **phobia,** on the other hand, involves intense fear and can seriously disrupt a person's life. Between 5 and 10 percent of the general population reports a mildly disabling phobia; about one person in two hundred has a phobia of open spaces and about three persons in a hundred have phobias of illness or injury. Some of the common phobias are fear of heights (acrophobia), fear of open spaces (agoraphobia), fear of enclosed spaces (claustrophobia), fear of dirt and germs (mysophobia), fear of snakes (ophediophobia), and fear of animals (zoophobia). To check your own fears or phobias a simple quiz is provided in Box 11-4.

Phobic reactions produce severe anxiety and even panic reactions that cause marked physiological disturbances. Phobias and panic attacks are serious forms of emotional distress and should receive medical attention. Often people can learn to reduce their fears and phobias to the point where they can cope with them without undue distress. A variety of counseling strategies are available for dealing with phobias, so a person who is motivated can become free of fear.

> We do not have
> to visit a madhouse to find
> disordered minds; our planet is the
> mental institution of the universe.
>
> **Goethe**

Sleep and Dreams

Sleep and dreams are normal parts of every person's daily experiences, and they can play an important role in maintaining health. Most people do not pay much attention to how much they sleep or what they dream about. Studies indicate, however, that sleeping 6 to 8 hours a night is associated with greater health (Wiley and Camacho, 1980). And for centuries people have used dreams to help them deal with their troubles and problems in life. Virtually all modern theories of human behavior recognize that dreams have significance, and recently methods have evolved to help people use their dreams to relieve or prevent emotional distress.

Everybody dreams when asleep. Even people who deny that they dream actually do dream, but generally they cannot recall their dreams when they wake up. On the other hand, some people have vivid recall of the several dreams they have each night.

In 1952, Nathaniel Kleitman (1960) and his student Eugene Aserinsky noticed that a sleeping person's eyes move rapidly and jerkily for brief periods during the night. By awakening people during these sleep periods of **rapid eye movement (REM),** they discovered that people were invariably having a dream and that they could recount their dream material.

Many dream experiments over the years have shown that most people experience four distinct stages of sleep each night (see Figure 11-3), and that the cycle from Stage 1, light sleep, to Stage 4, deep sleep, occurs several times during the night. It is usually between Stage 4 sleep and returning to Stage

Figure 11-3

Tracings of the electrical signals (EEGs) produced during the various stages of sleep. Tiny electrodes are placed on a person's scalp and eyelids that detect electrical signals within the brain and movements of the eyes. Notice that rapid eye movement (REM) occurs during a dream period.

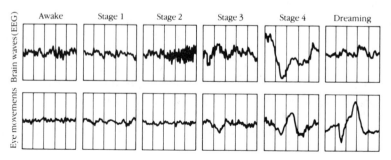

> People who
> don't have nightmares
> don't have dreams.
> **Robert Paul Smith**

1 that REM and the most vivid and detailed dreams occur. During the non-REM periods of sleep, dreams may also occur, but to a lesser degree.

People dream at every age from infancy to old age, and even other animals dream, as judged by the presence of REMs while they are asleep. Sleep and dreams must fulfill basic biological functions, although the exact nature of those functions is not yet clear. Hormone levels in the brain and body are usually quite different during sleep and during waking hours. It has been suggested that REM-dreaming states are necessary for brain growth, daily information processing, and cellular rejuvenation. Non-REM, deep-sleep states may be necessary to restore body processes and replenish physical reserves. Experimental subjects who have volunteered to go without sleep for several days usually develop bizarre behaviors and sometimes symptoms of psychosis after a period of sleep deprivation. They recover their normal behaviors after a good night's sleep, during which they have a significant increase in the amount of REM-dream sleep.

Using Your Dreams

For thousands of years dreams have been used in many cultures to restore mental and physical health. The temples of Asclepius were used by ancient Greeks for over a thousand years as places where people went for healing dreams. Belief, suggestion, dreams, and sleep were all used by the priests and priestesses to cure the disorders of those who came to the Asclepian temples.

Evidence showing that dreams can reduce emotional distress comes from studies of the Senoi, a primitive Malaysian tribe, who have come to be known as the "dream people" (Noone, 1972). The Senoi live in a nonaggressive, noncombative society. They have little desire or need for personal possessions and live communally. The most interesting fact about the Senoi, however, is that trained scientific observers have been unable to detect any signs of abnormal behavior or psychotic disorders among any members of this tribe.

One of the major factors that apparently contributes to the remarkable mental health of the Senoi is their daily ritual of attending to and interpreting their dreams. Both children and adults recount their dreams to one another, singly and in groups. According to Senoi custom, the events, anxieties, and people in a dream are considered "real" and must be acknowledged and dealt with. Such behavior is notably similar to our own custom of discussing dreams with psychotherapists or in group psychotherapy, where dreams are often discussed as symbolic representations of important emotional conflicts.

Interpreting Your Dreams

In our culture, many theories of dream interpretation have been proposed. Perhaps the most well known are those of Sigmund Freud and Carl Jung, which propose strict, universally applicable rules for uncovering the meaning of symbols and events in a person's dream. Dream researchers Calvin Hall

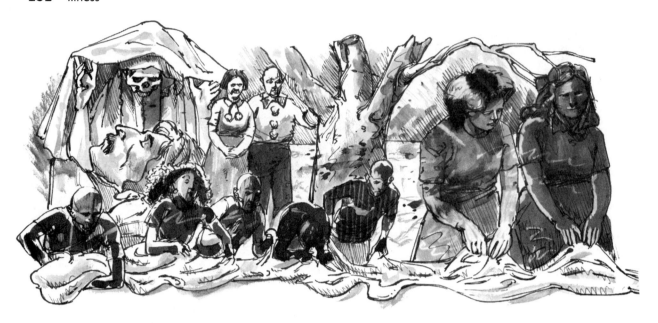

(1966) and Ann Faraday (1973), however, do not believe in universally applicable rules for dream interpretation. They and many other modern dream experts believe that the accurate interpretation of dreams can be made only by the dreamer himself or herself. According to Hall, "a dream is a personal document, a letter to oneself." Faraday's view is that "the surest guide to the meaning of a dream is the feeling and judgment of the dreamer himself, who deep down inside knows its meaning."

Dreams are private conversations with ourselves, communicated in a private language of visual images that are often dramatic and exaggerated. Much dream research suggests that dreams are reflections of recent happenings, thoughts, and feelings that are not dealt with in everyday conscious activities. Many people are too busy during the day to attend to everything that enters their experience. And even if people were free to do so, many would not, because some of their thoughts and experiences are unpleasant. In a dream, however, you "come clean" with yourself. In dreams you bring forth subtle feelings and impressions not attended to during the day. Dreams can involve your deepest and innermost thoughts and feelings about fears, worries, conflicts, and problems that you choose not to deal with while awake. Thus, many problems are presented to you in dreams, which is why paying attention to dreams and gaining insights from their interpretation can relieve emotional distress and enrich your life.

That dreams involve dramatic, sometimes humorous, and sometimes confusing symbolism is not to mask the true identities of actors in dreams or a dream's meaning, but rather to communicate intricate thoughts and feelings in a highly efficient way. As such, dreams are like movies, poems, and other works of art. According to Calvin Hall (1960): "There are symbols in dreams for the same reason that there are figures of speech in poetry and slang in everyday life. Man wants to express his thoughts as clearly as possible in objective terms. He wants to convey meaning with precision and economy."

Dream interpretation would probably be easier if a dream's meaning were communicated as straightforwardly as a computer printout, but it surely would not be as much fun.

To find the message of a dream, Ann Faraday (1973) suggests that you offer yourself hypotheses about the meanings of images and situations in dreams until you find one that triggers the same sense of being right that you have when you suddenly remember something that has been "on the tip of your tongue." Remember, a dream is a personal message you give yourself while asleep because your waking mind is not ready or willing to accept it. But the message is as much a part of your mental processes as any thought or memory. So when the interpretation of a dream is correct, you may experience a sudden flash of insight — sometimes called the "aha reaction" — as if you had discovered something familiar.

When you are making your hypotheses about the meaning of a dream, first consider the possibility that the images and situations in the dream are

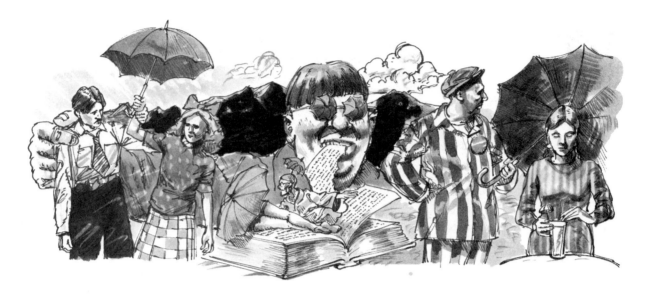

literal representations of reality. If you dream about a mouse, it may be because you saw a mouse in the kitchen that day, or perhaps seeing some movements out of the corner of your eye *suggested* to you that a mouse was around. The dream is reminding you to attend to that even though you are too busy and would prefer not to deal with it.

If the literal interpretation does not give you the sense of being right, then focus on the feeling you had while dreaming the dream, not only on the dream's content. Although you may have dreamed of dancing an incredibly brilliant solo on a stage to the wild applause of an audience, your actual feeling during the dream may have been stark terror. The dream, therefore, is probably about fear and not pride or accomplishment. Perhaps it was the last dance of the show, or the name of the theater is "Testor's." In either case, the dream might be telling you to study for your final exam. Using theater symbolism in this instance is a totally individual matter, arising perhaps because of an earlier conversation about dancing. The same message might have been communicated in images relating to fixing a car. Perhaps there are some strong interconnected feelings about the final exam and dancing. Only the dreamer can truly know.

Some of Calvin Hall's (1966) reminders for people wishing to use dreams to further their health and well-being are:

1. The dream is a creation of your own mind. Even if you dream that the information or images are coming from an outside source, it is still your mind that is producing the dream.

2. You are responsible for everything that appears in your dream. No matter how strange or frightening, the dream is the product of your thoughts and feelings and, as such, represents a part of yourself.

3. All individuals have more than one perception of themselves and of reality; thus, dreams can provide you with insight into alternative ways of handling problems and fears.

4. You should usually rely on a series of dreams rather than on a single dream or episode for your interpretation.

Dreams provide a way for anyone to learn more about the inner self. Dreams can be used to deal with fears and to find ways to resolve emotional distress that cannot be dealt with by thinking about the problem. By suggesting to yourself just before falling asleep each night that you will remember your dreams, you can greatly increase dream recall. Even better is to decide to wake up during the night and immediately write down the dream and what you think it means. It is possible to train your mind to imagine that it is awake in the dream. You can use dreams and positive suggestions while dreaming to increase mind-body harmony and to reduce emotional distress. Best of all, dreams are far more entertaining and instructive than most television shows or movies.

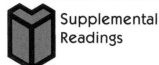

Supplemental Readings

Aggras, Stewart, M.D. *Panic— Facing Fears, Phobias, and Anxiety.* New York: W. H. Freeman and Co., 1985. An excellent, understandable book about the causes and cures for fears and phobias. Emphasizes nondrug approaches to treatment.

Benson, H., and **Proctor, W.** *Beyond the Relaxation Response.* New York: Times Books, 1984. Provides an update on how to use the relaxation response to reduce physical and emotional distress.

Faraday, Ann. *Dream Power.* New York: Berkeley Medallion, 1973. A complete guide to recording and using dreams for better mental health.

Friedrich, O. *Going Crazy.* New York: Avon Books, 1976. The author explores all aspects of the history and ideas of madness. A skeptical inquiry.

Hazelton, Lesley. *The Right to Feel Bad: Coming to Terms with Normal Depression.* New York: Doubleday, 1984. The author argues that depression is a normal reaction to certain experiences and need not be treated like a disease. Also provides ways to help cope with depression.

Summary

Everyone experiences emotional distress at one time or another. These occasions, which generally are brief for most people, result from the inability to fulfill one or more basic human needs. Negative emotions tell you that something is wrong with the way you are conducting your life, and they offer the opportunity to gain more understanding about yourself as you try to overcome them. Viewed in this way, the distressing periods in your life become opportunities for positive personal development.

People employ any number of coping strategies to help them deal with their emotional distress. They can also seek the aid of a psychotherapist or other helping professional to help clarify the problem and arrive at a workable solution.

Several kinds of emotional distress, including depression, organic brain disease, and schizophrenia, may have genetic, biochemical, or nutritional causes.

Sleep and dreams are a normal part of everyone's life, and they play an important part in maintaining mental health. Sleep is characterized by four non-REM stages, which alternate with REM sleep, during which people dream. Many people use their dreams to help them deal with emotionally distressing situations in their lives.

FOR YOUR HEALTH

Keeping a Journal

Our emotions tell us how well we are fulfilling our life needs and how well we are achieving our life goals, but sometimes it is difficult to understand why we feel a certain way at a certain time. One way to clarify thoughts and feelings is to record them in a journal or notebook, which is something like a diary except that thoughts and feelings are recorded instead of specific events. Practice keeping a journal of your thoughts and feelings for a two-week period. Set aside a particular time of each day, perhaps just before you go to sleep, to check in with your feelings by writing how you feel at that moment or how you felt that day and explaining why those feelings may have occurred.

(Continued on next page.)

FOR YOUR HEALTH

Saying No

Many people have a hard time saying no to the requests and demands made by others and an equally hard time saying yes to themselves for something they want. To be generous with time and energy is thought to be a virtue; to accommodate your own wishes selfish. There are times, however, when saying no to others and yes to yourself is highly appropriate. Your emotions tell you those times, too. The time to say no is when saying yes makes you feel angry and resentful. The time to say yes to yourself is when it increases your inner feelings of love and peace.

Think about some recent times when you said yes to others when you really wanted to say no. Write them down like this: I would have liked to have said no when _____ asked me to _____.

Prepare yourself to say no to the same or other requests the next time they occur. Imagine yourself saying no to another, and also imagine yourself firmly and politely dealing with the other person's response.

Learning to say no may take practice, so don't get discouraged if at first you find it difficult.

Keeping a Sleep and Dream Record

Each morning for one week, assess your sleep behavior with the aid of a chart like the one here; also record the details of your dreams in your journal or notebook. Hints for dream recording:

1. Keep a pen or a pencil and a pad of paper near your bed.
2. Remind yourself before going to sleep that you want to remember your dreams.
3. Write down your dreams immediately upon awakening.

Sleep Assessment Chart

	Monday	Tuesday	Wednesday	Thursday	Friday
Time to bed					
Time fell asleep (estimated upon waking)					
Feelings before falling asleep					
Trouble falling asleep? (yes/no)					
Take sleeping aid? (milk/pills)					
Number of times awake in the night					
Time woke up					
Time arose					
Feelings upon awakening					
Dreams? (yes/no)					
Total sleep time					

CHAPTER TWELVE

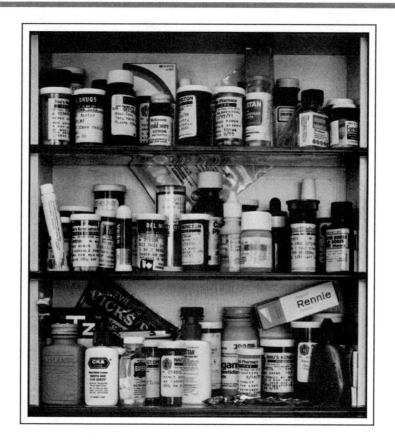

How to be well without drugs.

Drugs and Medicines

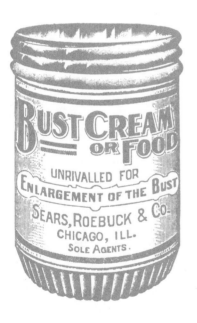

People have been ingesting substances that alter thoughts, feelings, and behavior for thousands of years—ever since somebody first noticed that eating a particular plant changed the way he or she felt or behaved. That eating a particular mushroom or chewing the leaves of a certain plant could bring about pleasant feelings, relieve pain, produce strange visions, or increase physical vigor was probably an accidental discovery made while trying a new kind of food. Throughout the centuries since that discovery, potions, herbals, elixers, and extracts have been used to change consciousness, to produce sleep, to heal the physcially sick and wounded, to drive out evil spirits, and even to restore family and tribal harmony. Today drugs and medications continue to be used for many of these same purposes.

Advances in modern chemistry in the nineteenth century and the rise of new technologies produced a revolution in human drug taking. In 1803 a substance was crystallized from opium poppies that was called morphine, after Morpheus, the Greek god of dreams, because of its numbing effects on the brain. Since that time thousands of biologically active substances have been prepared, no longer from the "eye of newt and toe of frog, wool of bat and tongue of dog," but isolated in pure form from plants, fungi, bacteria, and animals and synthesized by chemists from atoms and molecules. While many prescribed drugs are of enormous value in relieving human pain and suffering, in curing disease, and in facilitating healing, indiscriminate use and overuse of drugs—especially tranquilizers—has become a major health problem in our society. This chapter discusses primarily legal drugs—those that are purchased over the counter or by a doctor's prescription. Chapter 13 discusses what are popularly referred to as **recreational** drugs—those that are taken primarily for pleasure or for reasons that have nothing to do with curing sickness or increasing health.

> A desire to take medicine is perhaps the great
> feature which distinguishes man from other
> animals.
>
> **William Osler**

What Are Drugs?

A **drug** is a single chemical substance that constitutes the active ingredient in a medicine. A particular medicine may contain two or more drugs (aspirin and codeine, for example) because the combined effect is greater than that of either drug alone, which is called **synergism.** (Other drug-drug and drug-food interactions are discussed in a later section.) In the scientific sense, no distinction is made between a drug and a medicine — both are substances used to prevent illness, to cure disease, or to aid the healing process in some other way.

There are three principal ways that drugs are used in medical treatment. One is curative, in the sense that antibiotics can destroy pathogenic microorganisms or that certain drugs destroy cancer cells. In one case we are "cured" of the infection; in the other we are "cured" of cancer. Another way drugs are used is to suppress symptoms. For example, morphine or codeine can suppress pain, and cortisone can suppress inflammation from allergies or arthritis. Third, drugs are used as preventive measures, such as vaccines that protect against viral infections or oral contraceptives that prevent pregnancy.

The **dose** of a drug is the amount that is administered, whether in the form of a tablet, a liquid, or an injection. Once a drug enters the body, the effects and consequences of its chemical activities can vary widely from person to person and from one administration to the next. The correct dose is the amount that will accomplish the desired therapeutic effect with a minimum of other (undesirable) side effects. The effective therapeutic dose is modified by the presence of other drugs or chemicals in the body and by the person's experience with and expectations about the drug. It is important to know the effective therapeutic range for a drug, since too small a dose may provide no relief whereas too large a dose can be dangerous or lethal.

How Do Drugs Act?

The number of chemicals that can act as drugs is large, and so diverse are their chemical structures that it is impossible to classify drugs into single chemical categories. Therefore, drugs are usually classified according to the particular physiological system on which they exert a primary effect (central nervous system, gastrointestinal system, and so on) or by the principal physiological effect they produce (lower blood pressure, relieve pain, stop coughing). For instance, all substances that increase urine production, regardless of their chemical structure, are called diuretics; those that inhibit pain, analgesics; those that relieve anxiety, tranquilizers, and so on.

Nor is there any single biochemical mechanism by which drugs alter physiology. Many drugs have been shown to interact directly with molecules inside cells or with receptor sites on the surface of cells (see Figure 12-1). Once the drug molecules bind to or are absorbed into particular cells and tissues, they can inhibit or activate enzyme functions, stimulate or retard the release and synthesis of hormones and neurotransmitters, and change the flow of chemicals into and out of tissues. Frequently, the chemical structures of drugs mimic (closely resemble) the structures of natural body components, such as enzymes, hormones, neurotransmitters, and vitamins. For example, in Chapter 3 we pointed out that the brain produces molecules called endorphins that block pain by binding to certain pain-receptor sites in brain cells. The drugs morphine and heroin bind to the same cellular receptors as the endorphins, thereby also blocking pain. Another drug, naloxone, inhibits the binding of both morphine and endorphin to receptors and is referred to as an "antagonist" of those substances. Recently, brain cell receptor sites for the tranquilizing drug Valium and for the hallucinogenic drug LSD have also been identified.

The discovery of receptor sites on cells allows scientists to understand the mechanisms of drug action and also allows them to develop new drugs that can produce specific and desirable changes in physiology. For example, it would be of great benefit to have pain-relieving drugs as effective as morphine but that would not cause physical dependence. Solomon Snyder (1980), of the Johns Hopkins Medical School, believes that the rapid advances being made in understanding receptor sites for drugs may soon lead to the development of nonaddicting drugs for pain relief.

Many antibiotics recognize receptors that are specific to bacteria but that are not present in human cells. In this way antibiotics inhibit the growth of disease-causing bacteria in our bodies without interfering with the normal growth and functioning of our own cells. Most drugs used in the treatment of cancer are **antimetabolites.** That is, they adversely affect biochemical reactions that are vital to the growth of cancer cells as well as to the growth of normal cells. The aim of such treatment (chemotherapy) is to destroy the cancer cells completely while allowing the normal, healthy cells to recover once the drug treatment is stopped.

Another type of drug mechanism can be seen with magnesium hydroxide, the active component of milk of magnesia. This drug acts outside the cells, in the body's spaces and fluids. It is poorly absorbed into tissues and while present in the gastrointestinal tract it tends to draw water out of the body, producing a laxative effect.

The Effectiveness of Drugs

The effectiveness of a drug depends on many factors, some of which can be controlled and some not. The amount of the drug taken is something that can be controlled; however, once the drug enters the body, its effect will depend on how rapidly it is absorbed into the tissues, how much reaches the target organs or binds to the appropriate cellular receptors, and how rapidly the drug is broken down and eliminated from the body.

Figure 12-1
Binding of drugs to cellular receptor sites. The molecular structures of many drugs are similar to molecules normally produced in the body. The drugs compete for binding sites on cells and alter the physiological functioning of organs and tissues.

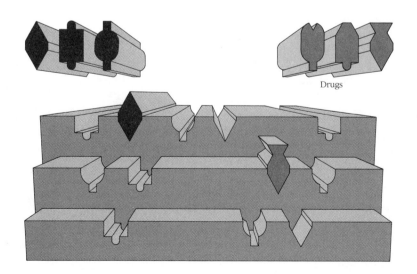

Drugs

Drugs are taken into the body by mouth, by inhalation, by injection into the muscles or skin (from which they diffuse into the surrounding tissues and into the blood), or by injection directly into the bloodstream (intravenous injection). Most drugs remain in the body for a relatively short period of time, often only a few hours, which is why most drugs are prescribed to be taken every few hours.

Inhalatory anesthetics are eliminated from the body with every breath. Other drugs are filtered out by the kidneys and are excreted in the urine. The liver, and to a lesser degree, the lungs, possesses special enzymes that break down drugs so that they become inactive and are excreted. Drug molecules are generally too small to be recognized by phagocytes and other cells of the immune system (see Chapter 9), so drugs usually do not evoke an immune response. An important exception is the allergic response to penicillin, which is discussed in a later section of this chapter.

Interaction of Drugs

The effectiveness of a drug in the body can be markedly altered by interaction with other substances, particularly with alcohol and with certain foods (see Table 12-1). For example, antibiotics such as erythromycin and penicillin are destroyed by excess stomach acid. When taking these drugs, a person is usually instructed to avoid acid foods, such as citrus fruits and juices, vinegar, tomatoes, and cola drinks. The action of tetracycline antibiotics is inhibited by calcium-rich foods, such as milk, cheese, and ice cream. Because both are acidic, the frequent use of aspirin with orange juice can damage the stomach lining and even cause ulcers.

Alcohol interacts with many drugs that affect the central nervous system, such as tranquilizers and sedatives, and should *never* be used while taking such medications. Whenever your physician prescribes a drug ask him or her whether there are any foods that you should avoid or other precautions you should observe while taking the prescribed drug. When in doubt about any drug, ask a physician or pharmacist.

Dangerous Complications of Drug Use

Even though a drug may be intended to have a single therapeutic effect, such a goal is seldom achieved because the chemical reactions in the body are very complex. Drugs may have side effects, may cause allergic reactions, or may be harmful to developing embryos.

Drug Side Effects

Unintended drug actions are called **side effects.** From a biological point of view, they are completely normal reactions. From the patients' point of view, however, the side effects of a drug are undesirable and often dangerous. For example, oral contracep-

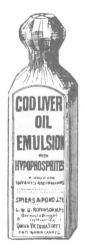

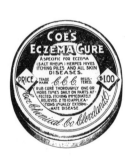

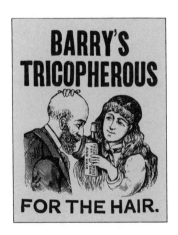

Table 12-1
Drug and Food Interactions That Should Be Avoided

If you take	Avoid	Because
Erythromycin- or penicillin-type antibiotics	Acidic foods: pickles, tomatoes, vinegar, colas	These antibiotics are destroyed by stomach acids
Tetracycline-type antibiotics	Calcium-rich foods: milk, cheese, yogurt, pizza, almonds	Calcium blocks the action of tetracycline
Antihypertensives (to lower blood pressure)	Natural licorice (artificial is OK)	A chemical in natural licorice causes salt and water retention
Anticoagulants (to thin blood)	Vitamin K: green leafy vegetables, beef liver, vegetable oils	Vitamin K promotes blood clotting
Antidepressants (monoamine oxidase inhibitors)	Tyramine-rich foods: colas, chocolate, cheese, coffee, wine, avocados	Tyramine elevates blood pressure
Diuretics	Monosodium glutamate (MSG)	MSG and diuretics both increase water elimination
Thyroid drugs	Cabbage, brussels sprouts, soybeans, cauliflower	Chemicals in these vegetables depress thyroid hormone production

tives are synthetic hormones designed to inhibit ovulation by affecting the activity of the hypothalamus in the brain. But they are so similar to natural hormones that they also affect other hormone-sensitive organs, such as the breasts and vagina, to produce occasionable undesirable side effects. Side effects from the most commonly used tranquilizer, Valium, are numerous and can be quite disturbing (see Box 12-1).

Virtually all drugs produce some undesirable and unpleasant reactions in some people. What one hopes is that the beneficial effects of the drug will far outweigh the undesirable side effects. For many people, however, this is not the case—which is why it is always wise to inquire about the benefits and risks of any drug and not simply to accept another person's assurances (even if that person is a physician). For example, many physicians may prescribe a tranquilizer if a patient seems anxious or stressed, even though it would be much more beneficial to

eliminate the cause of the anxiety or stress. Drugs are often prescribed for hypertension or ulcers when the cause of such symptoms is actually stress that can probably be reduced by other means (see Chapter 10).

Side effects are not a drug's only potential dangers. A drug may also be harmful if it is taken in large doses or if the taker has some medical condition that will be aggravated by that drug. Such conditions are called **contraindications.** The necessity of controlling dosage and the need to screen for possible contraindications are two reasons most potent drugs are available by prescription only.

Physicians should, of course, be knowledgeable about the side effects of drugs and what constitutes safe dosages. Yet it is estimated that about *one-third* of hospital stays are needlessly extended because of doctor-induced illness, called **iatrogenic illness,** caused principally by improper medication (Steel et al., 1981).

BOX 12-1

VALIUM'S UNINTENDED EFFECTS

DEAR DR. MENDEL-SOHN: What do you think of a man (my husband) who has been taking Valium for the past three years? He gets dizzy spells and fuzzy vision, and he is crabby, cranky, and even violent at times. Every time he gets upset, he pops a Valium. He has irregular heartbeats and sometimes can't catch his breath.

Every time he sees the doctor, he's told he's all right and is handed a prescription for Valium. I thought a person who takes Valium over a long period of time should gradually stop.

Can Valium cause impotence? He has sex only once every two months. All he wants to do is sleep.—M.B.

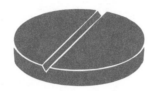

It's been a long time since I've done a column on that old favorite of doctors, Valium.

You say your husband gets dizzy spells? Ataxia (inability to coordinate muscles and to preserve one's equilibrium) and vertigo (dizziness, giddiness) are listed as possible adverse reactions to Valium.

You say that your husband has fuzzy vision? Diplopia (double vision and blurred vision) are also listed as adverse reactions.

You say your husband is crabby, cranky, and violent at times? Anxiety, hyperexcited states and rage also are listed as adverse reactions from this "calming" drug.

While irregular heartbeats are not listed as a side effect, drop in blood pressure (hypotension) is listed. As far as your husband's impotence is concerned, one of the clearly listed adverse reactions is change in libido.

You say your husband only wants to sleep? The first side effects mentioned in the prescribing information are drowsiness and fatigue.

From "Ask the Doctor" by Robert Mendelsohn, M.D., *San Francisco Chronicle,* August 9, 1978.

Drug Hypersensitivity

Some people exhibit an allergic reaction or response to certain drugs. This condition is known as **drug hypersensitivity.** Usually mild reactions, such as a rash, indigestion, or a stuffy nose, may occur on initial exposure. A second exposure to the drug often produces a more severe reaction. Perhaps the best-known example of drug hypersensitivity is the allergic reaction some people have to pencillin.

Such persons produce antibodies specifically directed against penicillin after they have been exposed to the drug. These antibodies are different from the antibodies that are produced in response to infectious bacteria and viruses. Months, even years, later another exposure to penicillin can restimulate antibody production and produce a severe reaction in a sensitive person.

As much as 5 percent of the population exhibits a penicillin allergy. Often the allergy shows up as a rash or inflammation in some part of the body. However, some people have a more severe reaction known as **anaphylaxis,** which can lead to death within hours or even minutes. For this reason repeated use of penicillin to treat bacterial infections may be unwise for some allergic persons, and use of other antibiotics may be safer. A physician will usually inquire if a person has any allergies before prescribing an antibiotic.

Legal Drug Abuse

People take prescription and over-the-counter (OTC) drugs for many reasons that are unrelated to any illness, injury, or therapy. In 1983 the American Medical Association concluded that "The abuse of prescription drugs results in more injuries and deaths to Americans than all illegal drugs combined. . . . Prescription drugs are involved in almost 60 percent of all drug-related deaths." The most abused prescription drugs are the stimulants (amphetamines, anorexiants) and the depressants (opioids, barbiturates, benzodiazepines). OTC drugs that are frequently overused and abused are sleep and cold remedies, analgesics taken for aches and pains, and cough remedies.

People over 65 years of age are the largest consumers of both prescription and OTC drugs, which explains why TV drug ads usually show older persons as sufferers. Older persons often take numerous drugs for a variety of complaints, and these drugs may interact in unforeseen ways to cause additional problems. It is not uncommon to find older people who daily take ten or more different medications that may have been prescribed by different physicians at different times. Older people are physiologically less able to tolerate drugs than younger people and often suffer more serious side effects. Quite often elimination of all drug use for a brief period will cause many symptoms to disappear, which is a clear indication that the combination of drugs is causing problems. Patients need to ask for and use fewer drugs; physicians need to become less eager and willing to prescribe unnecessary drugs.

Teratogenic Drugs

Drugs and other substances that cause defects in developing embryos are called **teratogens.** In the 1960s several thousand babies were born all over the world with an uncommon congenital birth defect characterized by deformation of the arms or legs.

Table 12-2
Drugs That Have Been Proved to Be Teratogenic

Alcohol	Streptomycin
Anticonvulsant drugs	Tetracyclines
Chemotherapeutic drugs	Thalidomide
Folic acid antagonists	Thiourea drugs
Lithium	Trimethadione
Sex steroids	Warfarin

A study subsequently revealed that during early pregnancy all the mothers of the affected children had taken a tranquilizer called thalidomide, which caused the abnormal limb development (see Figure 12-2). The thalidomide incident is a tragic reminder that any drug, no matter how safe it might seem in an adult, may have disastrous effects on the development of a fetus. Many drugs are known or suspected to be teratogenic, including such common substances as antibiotics and alcohol (see Table 12-2). To further complicate matters, drugs that are teratogenic in one animal species may not be in another. Aspirin, for example, is definitely teratogenic in rats but its effect on developing human embryos is still uncertain. Because it is difficult to determine what substances are teratogenic in humans and to what degree, pregnant women are advised to forgo the use of all drugs, including nicotine, alcohol, and caffeine, especially during the first few months.

Figure 12-2
Pregnant women who took the tranquilizer thalidomide frequently gave birth to children whose arms did not develop normally. These individuals are normal in all other respects, including intelligence and the capacity to have normal children when they grow up. (Photo by United Press International.)

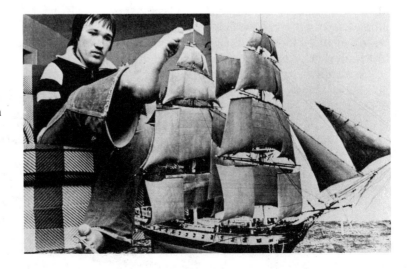

The Overmedicating of Americans

Americans consume an enormous quantity of drugs. Persons in our society have a total of about 1.5 billion drug prescriptions filled a year, which amounts to an average of five prescriptions for every man, woman, and child in the country (Wertheimer, 1983). The total annual cost of prescription drugs is about $16 billion, and another $8 billion is spent on over-the-counter (OTC) medications and remedies (see Table 12-3). In 1982, the annual per capita expenditure for drugs in the United States was almost $100, which is two and a half times the amount that was spent twelve years ago.

In 1980 the U.S. Department of Health and Human Services carried out an extensive survey of drug utilization in office-based medical practices, covering which drugs a doctor recommends for a patient, how often, and for what reason. The survey found that in 1980 Americans made a total of 575,745,000 visits to doctors' offices and that about 60 percent of the time one or more drugs were recommended. It may come as a surprise that in 1981 the top-selling prescription drugs were for stomach ulcers and for high blood pressure—chronic conditions for which nondrug therapies are also quite effective if people are willing to modify their lifestyles.

The use of drugs in our society has become so commonplace and accepted that many people automatically turn to drugs to solve their mental, physical, and emotional problems. So positive and trusting are people's attitudes toward drugs that many fail to appreciate the dangers and health hazards of ingesting drugs. As pointed out by Milton Silverman and Philip R. Lee (1974): "Much of the blame must be placed on the multibillion-dollar-a-year prescription drug industry and its incredibly ef-

Table 12-3
Retail Sales of Prescription and OTC Drugs in 1982

Drugs	Sales (millions of dollars)
Prescription drugs	$16,154
Over the counter pain relievers including aspirin and nonaspirin products	2,451
Digestive aids such as antacids, laxatives, and antidiarrheals	1,996
Cough and cold remedies	1,326
Vitamin supplements	1,031
First aid remedies	839
Diet aids	381
Foot care remedies	278

Data from Statistical Abstracts of the U.S., 1984.

fective promotional campaigns. But reprehensible as some of its huckstering has been, the industry cannot be made the only whipping boy. Others—physicians and patients in particular—must share in the responsibility."

It is in the area of drug use that holistic views of health differ most significantly from those of conventional medicine. When people have symptoms, even for minor complaints such as headache, backache, fatigue, upset stomach, colds, and allergies, most believe and expect that taking drugs is the only solution to their problem. This belief is encouraged by drug companies and physicians, but in the final analysis, it is people who demand, purchase, and use the drugs. Thus, you can ignore or resist advertising that is contrary to your health goals. You can reduce or eliminate the amount and kinds of drugs you take, especially for minor complaints. Learning how drugs affect your body and mind and how they can be harmful is the first step to wise drug usage. The next step is to discover possible nondrug solutions to your particular health problems.

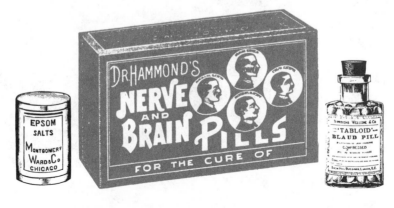

The Effects of Drug Advertising on Health

Drug companies spend approximately $2 billion each year promoting their products both to the general public and to physicians. During the winter months, the TV screen and the pages of popular magazines are loaded with inducements to buy products for coughs and colds. In the summer it's ads for creams and lotions for sunburn and tanning. Ads for pain relievers and upset stomach remedies are ubiquitous and incessant (see Figure 12-3).

Because the lion's share of drug sales comes from prescription medications, it is no wonder that the heaviest drug company advertising is directed toward physicians, the only persons in the United States who can legally dispense these drugs. Drug companies spend thousands of dollars per year per physician (allopathic and osteopathic) trying to persuade him or her to prescribe particular drugs that they manufacture. Drug companies send sales representatives to doctors' offices to inform them of the company's products and to leave free samples. Drug companies sponsor seminars and courses to update physicians on the diagnosis and treatment of particular diseases (for which the company usually manufactures a drug). And drug companies deluge physicians with pharmaceutical "junk" mail. One doctor found that the drug company junk mail he had saved weighed nearly 503 pounds at the end of the year.

Drug company advertising is a major source of revenue for professional medical journals. In 1984, the *Journal of the American Medical Association* was accused of publishing an article favorable to a particular drug (Procardia) to appease Pfizer Laboratories, one of the journal's major advertisers. Indeed, publication of results that are unflattering to a drug company's product can lead to withdrawal of advertising and loss of revenue for a journal.

Although drug company advertising undoubtedly inflates drug costs, a worse consequence is that it may influence a doctor's clinical judgment. Many doctors haven't the time or the inclination to investigate and evaluate the benefits and safety of a new drug, so they utilize drug company courses and advertising literature as the sole basis for making a decision on whether to prescribe the drug.

In 1984 a new pain reliever, **ibuprofen,** was introduced into the OTC drug market. Because aspirin and acetaminophen command over 90 percent

ASPIRIN		
Anacin	8%	
Excedrin	7	
Bayer	7	
Bufferin	6	
Other	18	

ACETAMINOPHEN		
Tylenol	35%	
Anacin	5	
Panadol	2	
Datril	1	
Other	3	

IBUPROFEN		
Advil	6%	
Nuprin	3	

Figure 12-3
OTC pain relievers' share of $1.7 billion market in 1985.

of the $1.7 billion market, manufacturers of the new drug have been heavily promoting it in medical journals. The purpose of these ads is to get physicians to recommend or prescribe the new drug. One advertisement shows that after four hours Nuprin relieves headaches about 8 percent more effectively than acetaminophen (see Figure 12-4). From a holistic health perspective, however, the more significant result is that 40 percent of headache sufferers get the same relief with no drug whatsoever. These people were given a placebo pill (see Chapter 2) that contained no active ingredient. Remember the power of the placebo next time you think you need a pill for minor relief.

The Pharmaceutical Manufacturers Association regularly runs full-page ads in popular magazines to convince the public of the necessity, effectiveness, and safety of drugs. A recent ad opened with this headline: "I'LL HAVE TO TAKE THESE FOR THE REST OF MY LIFE. THANK GOD." Below the headline was a picture of a concerned man holding a bottle of pills. What was this man's problem? High blood pressure, a condition that is often caused by stress (see Chapter 16). Relaxation techniques have been shown to reduce stress and to relieve high blood pressure. Yet the pharmaceutical industry

> ## Too often the wrong drug is ordered for the wrong patient, at the wrong times and in the wrong amounts, and with no consideration of costs. Too often a drug is prescribed when no drug at all is needed.
>
> **Milton Silverman**
> **Philip R. Lee**

recommends to the public that people take drugs for this condition for the *rest of their lives*. No mention is made of other methods for reducing stress or of the serious side effects of these drugs.

An ad in a medical journal shows a photograph of a sad-looking elderly man sitting alone on a park bench. The ad suggests to the physician that the company's antidepressant drug is an appropriate treatment for elderly patients who are depressed because they are alone much of the time. Of greater benefit might be to get the persons involved in meaningful activities and social interactions.

Another medical journal ad shows a man sitting at the console of a complicated electronic device with hundreds of buttons and switches. The man's sleeves are rolled up to indicate he's ready for action, and he's wearing earphones to indicate he is at work. The ad promotes a tranquilizer that promises relief from job anxiety—from the pressure that accompanies this man's responsibility as an electronics expert. If the stress of a job is causing illness, then it is the stress that must be dealt with. Still another drug company ad for a tranquilizer recommends that the physician prescribe this drug for patients who aren't hungry, who feel guilty, who can't calm down, or who can't sleep. None of these conditions necessarily has anything to do with disease, yet drugs are recommended as the appropriate treatment.

It is easy to become angry over the abuses of drug advertising; it is harder to do something about it. We believe that as people become more informed and aware of the undesirable consequences of taking drugs, and of how frequently drugs do little to promote wellness, they will elect to cope with the symptoms of stress and anxiety in ways that do not involve drugs.

When confronted with a person who is in distress but who is not physically sick, most physicians feel obligated to offer some remedy, even if a medically legitimate one does not exist. People *expect* the

Figure 12-4
A study of the effectiveness of ibuprofen (Nuprin) versus acetaminophen in relieving headaches. Note that 40 percent of headache sufferers get relief with no drug at all.

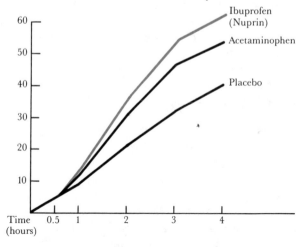

Percent of individuals free of headache pain

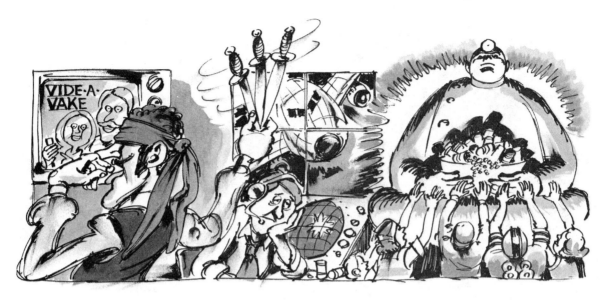

doctor to prescribe something. The answer to this dilemma has been neatly provided by pharmaceutical companies that manufacture and advertise mood-altering drugs for just this situation. If a person is anxious, the drug ads tell the physician to prescribe a tranquilizer. If depression is a problem, give an antidepressant. If the person cannot sleep, prescribe a barbiturate or hypnotic.

The giving and receiving of a drug prescription certifies that a therapeutic interchange has taken place. And, indeed, the tranquilizer or sleeping pill may help temporarily. Sometimes people become so depressed or upset over a life situation that they cannot muster the clear thinking and action necessary to deal with the problem. In such instances, a drug-induced night's sleep or lift from the fog of depression may help achieve a psychological state from which appropriate action can be taken. Unfortunately, too many people and their doctors mistakenly assume that taking the drug in itself will solve the problem, whereas it may instead be preventing proper help and treatment.

Drugs and medications are highly useful substances. But as with so many products of modern technology, benefits also bring problems and risks. We have vaccines to help prevent such dread diseases as polio, antibiotics to help cure infections, and a variety of medications that help people deal with serious illnesses. The availability of so many medications has fostered the belief that drugs can help solve just about any health problem. As recipients of medical care, most people expect some form of medication to signify that their illness is being properly treated. And doctors prescribe medications that may be unnecesary in order to signify to their patients and to themselves that they are giving treatment and care.

To their credit, many physicians recognize this problem and do not like it. They would prefer to deal only with physically ill people—the people whose problems they were trained to treat. But many patients resist the suggestion that they do not have a legitimate medical problem and insist that they receive some form of treatment, usually the prescribing of a tranquilizer or other drug. In our view this is the most serious form of drug abuse, not the illegal use of drugs that receives most of the attention on television and in the press. Being healthy means, among other things, being responsible for the drugs you use. You do not have to resort to "chemical coping" with emotional problems. You can resist being programmed into "pill popping" by a drug company advertising. You can refuse to accept a drug for a condition that results from anxiety, stress, or emotional problems. Saying no to the taking of a drug may be the most healthful action you can take.

When to Take Drugs

Almost everyone takes drugs of one kind or another at one time or another. People take drugs to relieve headaches, heartburn, tension, cramps, fatigue, and anxiety. Drugs are used to get to sleep and to stay

> One of the
> first duties of a physician
> is to educate the masses
> not to take medicine.
> **William Osler**

awake. They are used for everything from skin problems to emotional problems. Many people who don't consider themselves as being dependent on drugs still need several cups of coffee a day to wake up or to keep themselves going.

Drugs can play a vital role in the treatment and prevention of disease. Used with caution, drugs can also provide relief from occasional minor complaints. And used in moderation, certain drugs may occasionally enhance enjoyment of social interactions or increase pleasurable sensations.

But the fact remains that as a society we are overmedicated and overly dependent on drugs. The healthiest approach to living is to be as free of drugs as possible. Wellness is not achieved by taking drugs. No drug should ever be taken casually, whether prescribed, obtained over the counter, or offered in a social setting. It is everyone's responsibility to treat his or her body with respect. Each person can learn when drugs are necessary to maintain or restore health and when the benefits of drug taking outweigh the risks.

 Supplemental Readings

Davis, Lisa. "Custom-Designing Drug Doses to Fit the Genes." *Science News,* July 19, 1986. A short review of the dangers of drugs and how scientists are trying to devise ways to administer the correct dose to each individual.

Hughes, Richard, and **Brewin, Robert.** *The Tranquilizing of America.* New York: Harcourt Brace Jovanovich, 1979, Documents the needless use of pills and the ways in which drug use is encouraged by physicians and pharmaceutical companies.

Morgan, J. P., and **Kagan, D. V., eds.** *Society and Medication: Conflicting Signals for Prescribers and Patients.* Lexington, Mass.: D. C. Heath, 1983. A series of essays on various aspects of the use, action, prescription, and regulation of drugs.

Silverman, Milton, and **Lee, Philip R.** *Pills, Profits and Politics.* Berkeley: University of California Press, 1975. Even though this book was written several years ago, it still provides a useful insight into how drugs are produced, promoted, and priced, and why Americans swallow almost anything.

Weiss, K. J., and **Greenfield, D. P.** "Prescription Drug Abuse." *Psychiatric Clinics of North America,* September 1986. An authoritative medical discussion of the abuse of legal drugs.

Wolfe, S. M., and **Coley, C. M.** *Pills That Don't Work.* Washington, D.C.: Health Research Group, 1981. A consumer's guide to over 600 drugs considered to be ineffective. Can be obtained from Health Research Group, 2000 P Street NW, Washington, D.C. 20036.

Summary

Drugs are chemical substances that can be of great benefit in maintaining health and in treating disease. Medically, drugs are prescribed to cure disease, to suppress or modify distressing symptoms, and to prevent illness or undesired conditions. While drugs are prescribed to modify a particular physiological or psychological condition, all drugs have side effects that may be uncomfortable or harmful. Many drugs mimic natural body substances and interact with cellular receptor sites, thereby altering physiology.

As a society we are addicted to drug use. Far too many drugs are used by people to cope with symptoms and conditions that could be dealt with more effectively by other means. Drug companies encourage the excessive use of drugs for economic reasons. Doctors prescribe drugs excessively because patients expect to receive a drug to alleviate their complaint.

Each person should weigh the risks and benefits before taking any drug. Reducing the kinds and amounts of drugs that are taken should be an important health goal. Such drugs include not only prescription drugs, over-the-counter medications, and illegal drugs but such commonly ingested substances as caffeine, nicotine, and alcohol. Neither wellness nor happiness can be achieved through the use of drugs.

FOR YOUR HEALTH

The Drugs You Take

Make a list of all the drugs that you ingest regularly. Be sure to include birth control pills and such things as coffee, tea, and cola drinks (which contain caffeine), alcohol, nicotine, and aspirin. Try eliminating just one of the nonessential drugs that you ingest most frequently for one week and make notes on how you feel.

Be a Knowledgeable Consumer

If you are taking a prescribed drug, consult the library or your pharmacist or physician to find out any side effects and contraindications of the drug. Evaluate the risks of taking the drug against its thera-peutic benefits. Discuss with your physician ways to deal with your medical needs without the use of drugs.

Drug Advertising and You

Obtain copies of medical journals, such as the *New England Journal of Medicine* or the *Journal of the American Medical Association,* as well as journals directed to pharmacists, such as *American Druggist.* These journals can be found in libraries or may be obtained from doctors and pharmacists. Study the ads to see how drugs are "pushed" by the pharmaceutical industry.

CHAPTER THIRTEEN

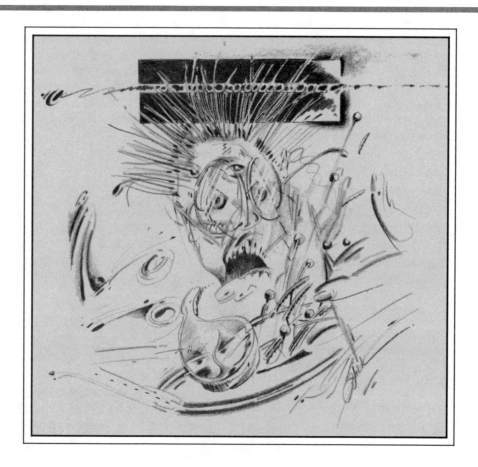

Many drugs used for recreational
purposes are easily abused.

Psychoactive Drugs: Uses and Abuses

Drugs become useful or dangerous depending on how we view them and how we use them.

Andrew Weil, M.D.

People use drugs not only for legitimate health reasons — relief of pain and disease symptoms — but also for reasons that have nothing to do with illness. Some drugs are taken for "fun" or to increase pleasurable sensations. Drugs that produce pleasurable changes invariably contain psychoactive substances and are often referred to as **recreational drugs.** Most people associate psychoactive recreational drugs with illegal substances such as marijuana, LSD, and cocaine, but recreational drugs also include legal substances such as alcohol, tobacco, and caffeine, as well as many legal prescription drugs, such as amphetamines and tranquilizers.

More than one-fourth of illegal drugs sold in the United States and virtually all illegal drugs are **psychoactive**; that is, they alter thoughts, feelings, perceptions, and moods. Millions of Americans use both legal and illegal psychoactive drugs to cope with mental and emotional problems as well as to alter moods and behaviors. Psychoactive drugs include **tranquilizers** that function to calm people; **stimulants** that increase energy and physical activity; **narcotics** that block central nervous system activity, thereby preventing pain and inducing sleep; **sedatives** that slow down the nervous sytem and induce sleep; **analgesics** that block pain; and **hallucinogens** that alter moods and perceptions. A partial list of the many psychoactive substances people use — legally and illegally — to change thoughts, feelings, and behaviors is given in Table 13-1, along with a summary of the drugs' effects.

The legality or illegality of a drug has nothing to do with its proven pharmacological action or even with personal and social dangers associated with its use. The use of tobacco, for example, is both legal and encouraged, yet it is a major cause of disease and death (see Chapter 15). The use of alcohol is also legal and encouraged and a major contributor to disease and death (see Chapter 14). Tranquilizers such as Valium and Librium, which are among the most widely used prescription drugs, are as physically addicting as narcotics. Some prescription drugs, sedatives, and pain relievers also cause physical dependence (see Table 13-1).

The legal status of drugs changes along with changes in social customs and beliefs. For example, alcohol was an illegal drug in the 1920s and 1930s, whereas marijuana use was legal; during the early years of this century, opium, morphine, and cocaine were openly advertised and sold in the form of tonics

Table 13-1

Classifications of Drugs That Affect the Central Nervous System (Psychoactive Drugs)

Drug classification	Common and trade names	Medical uses	Effects of average dose	Physical dependence	Tolerance develops
Narcotics	Codeine Demerol Heroin Methadone Morphine Opium Percodan	Analgesic (pain relief)	Blocks or eases pain; may cause drowsiness and euphoria; some users experience nausea or itching sensations	Marked	Yes
Analgesics	Darvon Talwin	Pain relief	May produce anxiety and hallucinations	Marked	Yes
Sedatives	Amytal Nembutal Phenobarbital Seconal Doriden Quaalude	Sedation, tension relief	Relaxation, sleep; decreases alertness and muscle coordination	Marked	Yes
Minor tranquilizers	Dalmane Equanil/Miltown Librium Valium	Anxiety relief, muscle tension	Mild sedation; increased sense of well being; may cause drowsiness and dizziness	Marked	No
Major tranquilizers (phenothiazines)	Mellaril Thorazine Prolixin	Control psychosis	Heavy sedation, anxiety relief; may cause confusion, muscle rigidity, convulsions	None	No
Alcohol	Beer Wine Liquor	None	Relaxation; loss of inhibition; mood swings; decreased alertness and coordination	Marked	Yes
Inhalants	Amyl nitrite Butyl nitrite Nitrous oxide	Muscle relaxant, anesthetic	Relaxation, euphoria; causes dizziness, headache, drowsiness	None	?
Stimulants	Benzedrine Biphetamine Desoxyn Dexedrine Methedrine Preludin Ritalin	Weight control, narcolepsy; fatigue and hyperactivity in children	Increased alertness and mood elevation; less fatigue and increased concentration; may cause insomnia, anxiety, headache, chills, and rise in blood pressure; organic brain damage after prolonged use	Mild to none	Yes
Cocaine	Cocaine hydrochloride	Local anesthetic, pain relief	Effects similar to stimulants	None	No
Cannabis	Marijuana Hashish	Relief of glaucoma, asthma, nausea accompanying chemotherapy	Relaxation, euphoria, altered perception; may cause confusion, panic, hallucinations	None	No
Hallucinogens	LSD PCP Mescaline Peyote Psilocybin	None	Altered perceptions, visual and sensory distortion; mood swings	None	Yes
Nicotine	(In tobacco)	None	Altered heart rate; tremors; excitation	Yes	Yes

> The use of drugs in our country is very great, and many of the legal ones, such as tobacco, alcohol, coffee, and tranquilizers, cause more social and medical trouble than some of the illegal ones.
>
> Andrew Weil, M.D.

and cough syrups. Coca-Cola, concocted by a Georgia pharmacist in 1886, was sold as both a remedy and an enjoyable drink. "Coke" contained cocaine until 1906, when the cocaine was replaced by caffeine.

Thomas Szasz (1974), a psychiatrist at the State University of New York, argues that our society's views of drug use and abuse are largely based on religious beliefs and on ideas of "good and evil" rather than on the pharmacological facts. In his view,

> . . . the important differences between heroin and alcohol, or marijuana and tobacco—as far as "drug abuse" is concerned—are not chemical but ceremonial. In other words, heroin and marijuana are approached and avoided not because they are more "addictive" or more "dangerous" than alcohol and tobacco but because they are more "holy" or "unholy"—as the case may be.

Szasz contends that our confusion regarding drug abuse is associated with our confusion regarding religion. He defines religion as "any act or idea that gives men and women a sense of what their life is about or for—that, in other words, gives their existence meaning and purpose."

People's motives for taking drugs vary enormously and include curiosity, thrill seeking, relaxation, increased sense of well-being, peer acceptance, and religious experiences. Many people use drugs to escape from the reality of their lives or to achieve happiness and provide meaning to their existence.

In this chapter we discuss the recreational drugs that are widely used (and frequently abused) in American society in the 1980s, without undue emphasis on their legality or illegality. Surveys conducted in 1981 indicate that at least 50 million Americans have some experience with smoking marijuana and 10 million Americans have used cocaine at least once. An estimate of the extent of recreational drug use among college students is shown in Table 13-2. While alcohol and cigarettes lead the way, marijuana and cocaine are not far behind. Obviously, nothing we can say here is going to change the widespread use of recreational drugs in the United States or solve the problems associated with illegal drug use. As with all other aspects of health, we believe that each individual should have access to as much correct information as possible so that he or she can make an informed decision about whether to use recreational drugs.

Table 13-2
National Drug Use Among High School Seniors, 1982

Drug	Percent ever used
Alcohol	93
Cigarettes	70
Marijuana	59
Stimulants	28
Tranquilizers	14
Cocaine	16
Sedatives	15
Hallucinogens	15
PCP	13
Inhalants	18
Heroin and other opiates	12

> In spite of one's personal views concerning the effectiveness or legitimacy of any drug law, society has a tradition of attempting to control drugs and drug-related behavior and, no doubt, will continue to do so in the future.
>
> **Stanley Einstein**

Psychoactive Drugs Change Consciousness

Why do people seek out and use substances that are not needed for any health reasons? The answer seems to be that people enjoy changing their state of consciousness and are eager to ingest substances that promote mental and emotional changes, particularly if the changes seem to be pleasurable. Some drugs are able to produce ecstatic feelings in certain individuals, and psychoactive drugs have been used in religious ceremonies for thousands of years.

Consciousness can be broadly defined as the state of being aware of one's internal mental processes—that is, one's thoughts, feelings, moods, and so on. Each one of us has a "normal" state of consciousness, although many people would have difficulty describing what they mean by "normal." However, every person knows when his or her state of consciousness deviates from normal—for example, during drunkenness, moods of extreme anger or sorrow, or periods of depression or apathy. High fever during illness can change a person's consciousness even to the point of having hallucinations or feeling dissociated from reality.

Numerous activities that we do not generally regard as consciousness-altering do, in fact, produce changes that are comparable in many respects to the changes produced by psychoactive drugs. Long-distance runners may experience a change of consciousness that is described as "high"; dancing can produce psychic "highs" and even ecstatic states of consciousness, which is the goal of whirling dervishes who practice particular forms of Sufi dancing. Food fasts can produce profound changes in consciousness, which is why prolonged fasts are often part of religious training. Many "thrill" activities, such as riding on roller coasters or shooting the rapids on river rafts, change consciousness and presumably are enjoyed partly for that reason. Put into this perspective, ingesting psychoactive drugs is only one of many ways people use to change consciousness.

Drug Abuse

The human body is capable of tolerating and eliminating small quantities of virtually any substance or drug with no permanent harmful effects. However, if large doses are ingested or if a drug is used frequently even though in small quantities, harmful effects on the person's physical or mental health may begin to appear. Generally, any use of a drug to a point where one's health is adversely affected or one's ability to function in society is impaired can be defined as **drug abuse.**

Drug abuse is not so much a problem of the kind or amount of a drug taken but rather of whether the drug is used to cope with life's problems. If a drug is used to mask anxiety or undesirable behaviors, it is being misused or abused. If a drug is used continually to combat the effects of stress, it is being abused. If pleasure is experienced only when the drug is taken, the drug is being abused. Serban (1984) has analyzed the difficulties of eradicating drug abuse:

> Drug abuse is more a disease of
> society than of the individual. The
> task before us is to cure society.
>
> **Michael Smith, M.D.**

Due to the complexity of the problems involved in drug abuse, encompassing psychological, sociological, not to mention the biological aspect of it, the prevention is not necessarily successful, as proven by research, by the simple presentation to the public of the unfavorable consequences of drug use. This approach is not a deterrent for the use of drugs in a hedonistically oriented society. It requires, as well, a change in the attitude of people, a reorientation of life toward work, and toward facing and coping with the inherent adversities of life.

Drug Tolerance and Dependence

The dangers of using a particular drug are often associated with the drug's ability to cause addiction, or **physical dependence** as it is usually referred to nowadays. Many legal drugs, including barbiturates, tranquilizers, analgesics, opiates, alcohol, and tobacco, are addicting and cause physical dependence (see Table 13-1). Among the illegal drugs, only heroin causes severe physical dependence, which means that complex physiological changes result from using the drug, so that **withdrawal symptoms** will occur if the addict abstains from using it. The withdrawal from a physically addicting drug invariably causes moderate to severe physical and mental symptoms.

Besides physical dependence, drugs can create a psychological dependence, called habituation, and a second kind of physiological condition referred to as tolerance. **Habituation** is the repeated use of a drug because the user finds that each use increases pleasurable feelings or reduces feelings of anxiety, fear, or stress. Habituation becomes injurious when the person becomes so consumed by the need for the drugged state of consciousness that all of his or her energies are directed to compulsive drug-seeking behavior. Physically addicting drugs such as heroin and alcohol invariably produce habituation as well, so that the person is trapped into using all of his or her energies and resources for obtaining the drug. As a consequence of this compulsive drug-seeking behavior, relationships, jobs, and families can be destroyed. Many of the widely used recreational drugs, including marijuana, cocaine, LSD, and PCP, do *not* create physical dependence (addiction), but people do become habituated to their use. There are no physical symptoms of withdrawal from stopping use of these drugs, but people may experience uncomfortable psychological symptoms because of the habituation.

Drug tolerance is an adaptation of the body to a drug such that ever larger doses are needed to gain the same effect. Because not all regions of the body become tolerant to the same degree, these higher doses may cause harmful side effects to some parts of the body. For example, a heroin or barbiturate user can become tolerant to the psychological effects of the drug but the brain's respiratory center, which controls breathing, does not. If the dose of heroin, barbiturate, or other depressant be-

> The myth that cocaine is the champagne of drugs is simply stupid. Cocaine is, in fact, an entrapping agent that promises happiness and, in the end, offers nothing but disaster.
>
> Sidney Cohen, M.D.

comes high enough, the brain's respiratory center ceases to function and the person stops breathing.

With these general comments on drug use and abuse as background, we devote the rest of the chapter to brief discussions of the most commonly used recreational drugs: cocaine, marijuana, psychedelics, amphetamines, caffeine, inhalants, PCP, and opiates.

Cocaine

Cocaine is a stimulant obtained from the leaves of the coca shrub, *Erythroxylum coca*, a plant indigenous to the Peruvian Andes. For thousands of years, inhabitants of Peru, Bolivia, and Columbia have been chewing coca leaves to obtain the stimulant effects. After the conquest of the Incan Empire in the sixteenth century, use of coca leaves was introduced to Europe and later to North America. In the late nineteenth century, Angelo Mariani, a Corsican, received a medal from the Pope for manufacturing an extract of coca leaves that "freed the body of fatigue, lifted the spirits, and induced a sense of well-being." In the United States in the 1880s, pharmacist J. C. Pemberton mixed extracts of coca leaves and kola nuts to produce Coca-Cola, claimed at the time to be not only refreshing but also "exhilarating, invigorating, and a cure for all nervous afflictions." Today, of course, Coke no longer contains cocaine, although cocaine-free extracts of coca leaves are still used for flavoring. Sigmund Freud extolled the use of cocaine as a mood elevator, a possible antidote to depression, and a treatment for morphine addiction. However, witnessing a friend's severe and terrifying psychotic reaction to cocaine use tempered Freud's enthusiasm for the drug.

In the doses common to recreational use today, cocaine induces euphoria, a sense of power and clarity of thought, and increased physical vigor. These effects usually occur within 15 minutes after the drug is taken, either by sniffing ("snorting") a cocaine-containing powder, by injection, or by smoking. A typical cocaine high lasts 30 minutes to an hour, after which the user usually experiences a letdown and a craving for another dose of the drug.

Cocaine increases heart rate and blood pressure. Overdose may induce seizures, heart stoppage, and cessation of breathing. Continued use of the drug can result in loss of appetite, weight loss, malnutrition, sleep disturbance, and altered thought and mood patterns. Frequent cocaine sniffing can inflame the nasal passages and possibly cause permanent damage to the nasal septum.

In a strict sense cocaine does not induce tolerance, physical dependence, or withdrawal. However,

Cocaine ("free base").

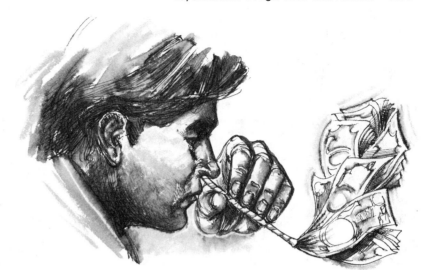

- Blurred vision
- Panic attacks
- Crushing headaches
- Debilitating nausea
- Paranoia
- Convulsions
- Depression
- Hallucinations
- Respiratory arrest
- Cardiac arrest
- Death

Symptoms of cocaine use.

the potential for psychological dependence is great, and some people develop such a strong craving for the drug that their lives and fortunes are consumed by their cocaine habit.

In today's society, cocaine use is associated with a lifestyle of high status, wealth, glamour, and excitement. In 1980, cocaine sales in the United States were estimated to have a value of over $30 billion, making the cocaine business one of the biggest industries in the country. From the mid-1970s to the mid-1980s cocaine use increased enormously. In the United States in 1982 about 22 million people admitted to having tried cocaine and about 4 million were current users. In 1985 the cocaine hotline (800-COCAINE) received nearly a thousand calls a day requesting help. The use of cocaine has reached the state of a national public health emergency.

One of the factors that has contributed to the problem has been the introduction of "free base" forms of cocaine known as "crack" that can be smoked or added to tobacco and inhaled along with the smoke. The cocaine that is generally snorted through the nose consists of cocaine hydrochloride and is sold in the form of a powder. Crack is sold in small quantities costing $10 to $20, making it available to a great number of people, especially

Cannabinol.

young persons who previously could not afford to buy cocaine. People who use crack either by inhalation or injection become psychologically addicted and dependent on it very quickly. In animal experiments, monkeys that are fed cocaine will choose it over available food and water until they die. Awareness of the dangerous symptoms of cocaine use should deter any sensible person who values his or her health from trying or experimenting with cocaine in any form.

Marijuana

Marijuana and **hashish** are products of the plant *Cannabis sativa* and other *Cannabis* species that grow in temperate climates all over the world. *Cannabis* has been cultivated for thousands of years, principally as a source of hemp fiber used in rope. A number of ancient cultures, including those of China, India, Japan, Greece, and Assyria, used marijuana for its psychoactive properties. In the United States today, marijuana is the most widely used illegal recreational drug, with an estimated one-third of all persons between 18 and 25 years of age using it.

The principal psychoactive ingredient in marijuana and hashish is a chemical compound called delta-9-tetrahydrocannabinol, or THC. Ingestion of THC usually occurs either by inhaling the smoke from marijuana cigarettes or pipes or by taking pills or eating substances that contain THC (such as cookies or brownies). Once inside the body, THC is absorbed rapidly in the tissues. In most in-

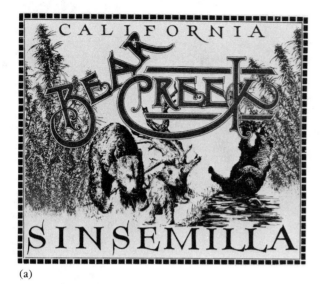

(a)

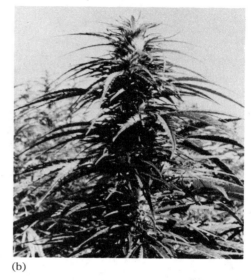

(b)

Figure 13-1

Sinsemilla marijuana cultivation in California. (a) A label used by a marijuana grower. (b) A field of mature female marijuana plants.

dividuals, low doses of THC produce a high characterized by euphoria, a sense of relaxation, and occasionally altered perception of space and time. Speech may be impaired and short-term memory is affected (Nicholi, 1983c). Because perception, motor coordination, and reaction time are also impaired, driving a car or operating other machines while intoxicated with THC is considered unsafe.

Sometimes marijuana use, especially among first-time or naive drug users, may evoke such psychological reactions as confusion, anxiety, panic, hallucinations, and paranoia. Marijuana may also worsen a prior mental health problem or negative mood states. Long-term use does not cause permanent changes in brain function or impaired cognitive abilities. Some of the possible health dangers of chronic, long-term marijuana use include the risk of developing bronchitis caused by marijuana smoke, increasing heart rate and blood pressure, and possibly a slight depression of immune system functions. Contrary to what was once popular belief, marijuana does not turn users into crazed murderers and rapists (see Box 13-1).

In an exhaustive study, *Marijuana and Health*, conducted by the National Academy of Sciences, a panel of experts concluded that "the verdict of the experts is—that there is no verdict . . . Marijuana cannot be exonerated as harmless, but neither can

it be convicted of being as dangerous as some have claimed" (Relman, 1982b). The study did state with some conviction that there was no evidence supporting the belief that marijuana use inevitably leads to the use of any other drug.

Marijuana sold in the illegal drug market used to consist of a mixture of leaves, stems, and seeds. In the past few years, however, sophisticated marijuana growers in California, Hawaii, and elsewhere have begun producing **sinsemilla** (literally, "without seeds") marijuana that consists exclusively of mature dried flowers of female plants (see Figure 13-1). Sinsemilla marijuana is usually about ten times more potent than marijuana mixtures containing leaves and seeds. Persons who smoke a "joint" of this high-potency marijuana may hallucinate or experience a severe anxiety attack. Frequently, just one or two puffs (hits) of a potent marijuana cigarette are sufficient to produce a high; if one is not certain of a drug's potency, it is wise to take one or two hits and wait 15 to 20 minutes to see what the effects are.

In some studies marijuana has been shown to be effective in treating glaucoma (by reducing ocular fluid pressure) and in relieving the symptoms of nausea and vomiting that frequently accompany cancer chemotherapy. The federal government cultivates a limited amount of marijuana to supply phy-

---

BOX 13-1

MARIJUANA MADNESS

Much of the paranoia and misinformation over marijuana use that has persisted over the years can be traced to the fervent antidrug attitudes of Harry J. Anslinger, who was chief of the U.S. Bureau of Narcotics in the 1930s. It was largely at Anslinger's urging that Congress passed the Marijuana Tax Act in 1937, which provided stiff penalties for using and selling marijuana. Prior to that date, marijuana was completely legal in the United States and, in fact, was often prescribed by doctors for a variety of ailments.

Anslinger lectured and wrote widely on the evils of marijuana. He staunchly believed (even contrary to the evidence available at the time) that marijuana was a narcotic (like opium or heroin) and was a "killer drug." Here is an excerpt from an article entitled "Marijuana—Assassin of Youth" he wrote for *The American Magazine* in 1937:

Not long ago the body of a young girl lay crushed on the sidewalk after a plunge from a Chicago apartment window. Everyone called it suicide, but actually it was murder. The killer was a narcotic known to America as marijuana, and to history as hashish. Used in the form of cigarettes, it is comparatively new to the United States and as dangerous as a coiled rattlesnake.

How many murders, suicides, robberies, and maniacal deeds it causes each year, especially among the young,

can only be conjectured. In numerous communities it thrives almost unmolested, largely because of official ignorance of its effects.

Marijuana is the unknown quantity among narcotics. No one knows, when he smokes it, whether he will become a philosopher, a joyous reveler, a mad insensate, or a murderer.

The young girl's story is typical. She had heard the whisper which has gone the rounds of American youth about a new thrill, a cigarette with a "real kick" which gave wonderful reactions and no harmful aftereffects. With some friends she experimented at an evening smoking party.

The results were weird. Some of the party went into paroxysms of laughter; others of mediocre musical ability became almost expert; the piano dinned constantly. Still others found themselves discussing weighty problems with remarkable clarity. The girl danced without fatigue through a night of inexplicable exhilaration.

Other parties followed. Finally there came a gathering at a time when the girl was behind in her studies and greatly worried. Suddenly, as she was smoking, she thought of a solution to her school problems. Without hesitancy she walked to a window and leaped to her death. Thus madly can marijuana "solve" one's difficulties. It gives few

warnings of what it intends to do to the human brain.

Last year a young marijuana addict was hanged in Baltimore for criminal assault on a ten-year-old girl. In Chicago, two marijuana-smoking boys murdered a policeman. In Florida, police found a youth staggering about in a human slaughterhouse. With an ax he had killed his father, mother, two brothers, and a sister. He had no recollection of having committed this multiple crime. Ordinarily, a sane, rather quiet young man, he had become crazed from smoking marijuana. In at least two dozen comparatively recent cases of murder or degenerate sex attacks, marijuana proved to be a contributing cause.

These lurid portrayals have not been supported by any study carried out then or since, but Anslinger's views influenced a generation of American citizens and law enforcement officials. Other antimarijuana laws have been passed by most states in addition to the federal law. None of the laws, however, has been successful in curbing the growing, selling, or use of marijuana in the United States. Today, most persons have a better understanding of the actual consequences of smoking marijuana and the dangers of its use. A jazz musician Mezz Mezzrow said a few years ago, "I know one very bad thing that marijuana can do to you—it can put you in jail."

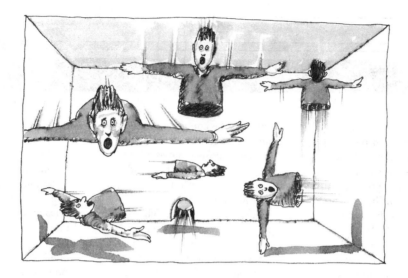

sicians who prescribe it for patients and for medical research. However, the widespread illegal cultivation of marijuana is intended solely for sale to those who use it as a recreational drug. A survey by drug enforcement officials in California estimated that the 1981 marijuana crop in that state had a value of between $5 billion and $6 billion; nationwide estimates of marijuana sales are in excess of $50 billion, which equals the amount of money Americans spend each year on alcohol and tobacco combined.

By many health criteria, marijuana is a safer substance than either alcohol or tobacco in terms of morbidity and mortality. (Keep in mind that no drug is entirely harmless.) That is why many people believe that the time has come to legalize or decriminalize marijuana use. If 50 million Americans have indeed broken the law, it is argued, it may be time to consider the possibility that something is wrong with the law. Despite the fact that marijuana is a relatively safe substance in a pharmacological sense does not mean that it is without danger to individuals who use it or to society as a whole. People can become dependent on marijuana use just as they become dependent on many other substances. Marijuana affects brain and motor functions and decreases alertness and intellectual abilities. Its use can adversely affect the performance of students and workers and can be a threat to public safety. For example, marijuana use by pilots, bus drivers, ship officers, physicians, and others clearly is a threat to persons who depend on their skills and judgment.

Tests for illegal drugs such as marijuana and cocaine are extremely sensitive and have become rela-

tively inexpensive ($15 to $50). Cocaine can be detected in urine samples up to 48 hours after ingestion; marijuana usually can be detected up to a week after use and in heavy, chronic users traces may persist for a month or more after use has stopped.

Psychedelic Drugs

Drugs whose primary effects are to produce changes in perceptions and thoughts and that may evoke dreamlike and mystical experiences are called **hallucinogens,** or **psychedelic drugs**. The most potent psychoactive drug known is the hallucinogen D-lysergic acid diethylamide, commonly called LSD. As little as a few millionths of a gram of pure LSD can produce hallucinations; 50–100 micrograms is an average dose that produces an "acid trip" lasting several hours. The psychedelic effects of LSD were discovered accidently by a Swiss chemist, Albert Hofmann, who subsequently described the experience:

> Last Friday, April 16, 1943, I was forced to stop my work in the laboratory in the middle of the afternoon and to go home, as I was seized by a peculiar restlessness associated with a sensation of mild dizziness. Having reached home, I lay down and sank in a kind of drunkenness which was not unpleasant and which was characterized by extreme activity of imagination. As I lay in a dazed condition with my eyes closed (I experienced daylight as disagreeably bright) there surged upon me an interrupted stream

Table 13-3
Substances Considered to Be Hallucinogenic or Psychedelic

Substance	Common name
D-lysergic acid diethylamide	LSD
Trimethoxyphenylethylamine	Mescaline (peyote)
2,5-Dimethoxy-4-methyl-amphetamine	STP
Dimethyltryptamine	DMT
Diethyltryptamine	DET
Tetrahydrocannabinol	Marijuana (*Cannabis*)
Phencyclidine	PCP
Psilocybin	Mushrooms
Atropine	
Bufotenin	
Datura	
Harmine	
Ibogain	
Kava	
Khat	
Morning glory seeds	
Nutmeg	

of fantastic images of extraordinary plasticity and vividness and accompanied by an intense, kaleidoscope-like play of colors. This condition gradually passed off after about two hours.

The hallucinogens comprise a wide variety of chemical substances derived from as many as 100 different kinds of plants as well as from chemical synthesis in the laboratory (see Table 13-3). Despite their variety, these substances possess the common quality of being able to alter perception, thought, mood, sensation, and experience. The similarity of their effects to psychotic hallucinatory experience is one reason they are called hallucinogens, but in many respects the psychedelic drug experience is not the same as a psychotic hallucination. Psychotic hallucinations are generally auditory and frightening, and the hallucinator believes them to be real. Drug-induced hallucinations tend to be visual, they are usually enjoyable or fascinating, and the individual is aware that the experience is exceptional or unusual and is not part of his or her normal state of consciousness.

Regardless of the specific substance, hallucinogens are most often ingested orally, either by eating the plant itself or by ingesting powder containing the active chemical. Normally, a hallucinogenic drug begins to take effect in 45 to 60 minutes, with the first effects being physical: sweating, nausea, increased body temperature, and pupil dilation. These symptoms eventually subside, and the psychological effects become manifest within an hour or two after ingestion. Depending on the particular substance and the amount ingested, the "trip" will last anywhere from 1 to 24 hours.

A common feature of the hallucinogenic experience is that the drugs suspend the normal psy-

LSD.

Psilocybin.

Mescaline.

> A study of 279 marijuana smokers shows people who smoke three to five joints daily suffer lung symptoms comparable to smoking 20 tobacco cigarettes a day.
>
> **Donald Pashkin, M.D.**
> **UCLA School of Medicine**

chic mechanisms that integrate the self with the environment. The distortion of self-environment interactions makes the user extremely open to conditions in the surroundings. For this reason, experience in any particular drug episode is highly influenced, for better or worse, by the environmental setting in which the trip takes place and by the "psychic set"— the expectations and attitudes—of the user.

Some of the more common effects induced by hallucinogenic drugs include:

1. *Changes in mood.* Hallucinogenic drugs can induce mood changes ranging from euphoria and giddiness to terror and deep despair. In the worst case, a person can experience a complete loss of emotional control, becoming frightened, anxious, and paranoid. At the other extreme, some users occasionally experience a state of complete joy, blessedness, and inner peace.

2. *Changes in sensation.* While a person is "tripping," colors may seem brighter, sounds richer and louder, and tastes more intense and pleasurable. There may be a sensation of the merging of the senses (synesthesia), such that sounds are experienced as colors or vice versa.

3. *Changes in perception.* The hallucinogenic experience may involve time distortion: seconds may seem like an eternity. Vivid colors and shapes may be seen with the eyes closed. Things that normally go unnoticed, such as pores in concrete, may seem fascinating. Small objects may seem unusually large or plain objects strikingly beautiful.

The tripper may visualize intricate geometric forms and patterns.

4. *Changes in relations.* The hallucinogenic drug experience often brings a sense of depersonalization—the user feels simultaneously outside and within. The user's ego boundaries are suspended, so there is a sense of merging with others or with objects in the environment. Occasionally there is a sense of complete merging—a oneness with the universe. There may be a sense of profound understanding, and many diverse aspects of life suddenly become clear and meaningful.

Hallucinogenic drugs produce tolerance to the psychedelic effect but do not create physical dependence or produce symptoms of withdrawal, even after long-term use. However, as with most psychoactive drugs, there is a danger of psychological dependence. There is no evidence that hallucinogens have permanent harmful effects on health, and they do not cause genetic damage or birth defects in humans, contrary to what is often stated (Grinspoon and Bakalar, 1979).

Many psychedelic drugs have chemical structures quite similar to those of normal brain neurotransmitters (see Chapter 3, Figure 3-4). Serotonin, one of several different brain neurotransmitters, is synthesized from tryptophan, an amino acid obtained from proteins in food. Such hallucinogenic drugs as LSD and DMT have chemical structures derived from the basic ring structure of trytophan or serotonin. Because of this chemical similarity, hallucinogens are able to bind to neurotransmitter

I see the true importance of LSD in the possibility of providing material aid to meditation aimed at the mystical experience of a deeper, comprehensive reality.

Albert Hofmann

receptor sites on brain cells or to alter the pattern of binding of neurotransmitters that are normally synthesized in the body. Even slight changes in brain chemistry can result in profound changes in brain activity and thought patterns.

Hallucinogenic drugs are powerful mediators of brain function and can dramatically alter perceptions and thoughts. They can precipitate psychotic reactions and behaviors in persons who are mentally unstable or who fear the effects of the drug. Because they are illegal, hallucinogenic drugs can only be obtained from unreliable sources. Most hallucinogenic drugs sold as LSD or mescaline, for example, actually contain other psychoactive drugs, and the buyer has no way of knowing what is being ingested.

Amphetamines

Amphetamines are manufactured chemicals that act as stimulants of the central nervous system. The most commonly used amphetamines are dexedrine ("dexies," "footballs," "orange"), benzedrine ("bennies," "peaches"), and methedrine ("meth," "speed"). Another psychoactive amphetamine that is manufactured and sold illegally is called MDA (methylenedioxyamphetamine), which produces a hallucinogenic state lasting several hours. This drug is not safe and has been shown to cause destruction of brain cells as well as less severe symptoms (Ricaurte et al., 1985). Amphetamines are usually taken orally but they can also be injected ("mainlined"). The effects of an oral dose usually last several hours.

Although amphetamines are sometimes prescribed to suppress appetite or to counteract fatigue, they are by and large useless as therapeutic agents. Overweight and fatigue are not illnesses that require drug intervention. Both conditions are better managed by improved diet and exercise and, in the case of fatigue, by less work, better time management, and more sleep. Another dubious use of amphetamines is to counteract the effects of overuse of drugs that depress the central nervous system.

The principal uses of amphetamines are recreational. These drugs produce feelings of euphoria, increased energy, greater self-confidence, an increased ability to concentrate, increased motor and speech activity, and improved physical performance. Besides being used by those wishing to experience the amphetamine high, these drugs are frequently abused by people who fight sleep, such as truck drivers, students who cram for exams all night, and nightclub entertainers. Athletes often use amphetamines to improve physical performance and self-confidence.

Excessive use of amphetamines can produce headaches, irritability, dizziness, insomnia, panic, confusion, and delirium. After extensive amphetamine use, the user often experiences a rebound

Metamphetamine.

"crash," during which he or she usually sleeps for long periods, is very tired, and is depressed.

Prolonged use of amphetamines can lead to tolerance, especially for the euphoric effects and for appetite suppression. Amphetamines do not cause physical dependence, but they can create a psychological dependence and a particular pattern of use called the "yo-yo." The yo-yo is a cycle of drug abuse in which a person uses amphetamines for the stimulatory effect and then uses a nervous system depressant to calm down enough to sleep, only to be followed with more amphetamines in order to get going the next day. Chronic use can cause an amphetamine psychosis, which consists of auditory and visual hallucinations, delusions, and mood swings.

Caffeine

Caffeine is a natural substance found in a variety of plants. Nearly all Americans regularly ingest caffeine in one form or another: coffee, tea, chocolate, and soft drinks (see Table 13-4). These beverages and foods are such an integral part of American eating habits that it cannot be argued that they are consumed solely for the pharmacological effects of the caffeine. Nevertheless, these products do have psychoactive properties and in addition to caffeine contain theophylline (principally in tea) and theobromine (principally in cocoa).

The effects of caffeine are familiar to most people. They include a lessening of drowsiness and fatigue (especially when performing tedious or boring tasks), more rapid and clearer flow of thought, and increased capacity for sustained performance (for example, typists work faster with fewer errors). In higher doses, caffeine produces nervousness, restlessness, tremors, and insomnia. In very high doses (10 grams, or 60 cups of coffee) it can produce convulsions and can be lethal.

In the past, caffeine was prescribed for a variety of complaints, but it is rarely used therapeutically nowadays. However, it is still compounded into over a thousand over-the-counter drugs (see Table

Table 13-4
Caffeine Content of Beverages, Foods, and Drugs

Item	Milligrams caffeine (average)	Item	Milligrams caffeine (average)
Coffee (5 oz. cup)		Dark chocolate, semisweet (1 oz.)	20
Brewed, drip method	115	Baker's chocolate (1oz.)	26
Brewed, percolator	80	Chocolate-flavored syrup (1 oz.)	4
Instant	65	Soft drinks	
Decaffeinated, brewed	3	Mountain Dew	54.0
Tea (5 oz. cup)		Mello Yello	52.8
Brewed, major U.S. brands	40	TAB	46.8
Brewed, imported brands	60	Coca-Cola	45.6
Instant	30	Diet Coke	45.6
Cocoa beverage (5 oz. cup)	4	Shasta Cola	44.4
Chocolate milk beverage (8 oz.)	5	Dr. Pepper	39.6
Milk chocolate (1 oz.)	6	Pepsi-Cola	38.4
		RC Cola	36.0
Weight-control aids		Cold/allergy remedies	
Dex-A-Diet II	200	Coryban-D capsules	30
Dexatrim, Dexatrim Extra Strength	200	Triaminicin tablets	30
Dietac capsules	200	Dristan decongestant tablets and	
Alertness tablets		Dristan A-F decongestant tablets	16.2
Nodoz	100	Prescription drugs	
Vivarin	200	Cafergot (for migraine headache)	100
Analgesic/pain relief		Fiorinal (for tension headache)	40
Anacin, Maximum Strength Anacin	32	Soma Compound (pain relief, muscle	
Excedrin	65	relaxant)	32
Diuretics		Darvon Compound (pain relief)	32.4
Aqua-Ban	100		
Maximum Strength Aqua-Ban Plus	200		

SOURCE: *FDA Consumer*, March 1984.

> One out of six TV commercials tells you
> and me and our youngsters that if you're
> not feeling well there is a substance that
> will make you feel better, be it something for
> a headache, something to give you energy,
> something to lose weight.
>
> **John C. Lawn**
> **Drug Enforcement Administration**

13-4). For example, many "energizers" and "stay-awake" products are pure caffeine. Analgesics, cough medicines, and cold remedies contain caffeine to counteract the drowsiness produced by the other ingredients in those medications. Caffeine is also put into weight control and menstrual pain products because it is a potent diuretic (it increases urine output and water loss).

A mild psychological dependence can result from the chronic use of caffeine, and tolerance to the stimulant effect can gradually develop. Mild withdrawal symptoms (headache, irritability, restlessness, and lethargy) may occur in consumers who are habituated.

Central Nervous System (CNS) Depressants

Central nervous system depressants comprise a vast number of drugs that have the common effect of reducing a person's level of arousal, awareness of the environment, and level of motor activity, and increasing drowsiness and sedation. The CNS depressants include alcohol (discussed in Chapter 14), drugs that affect sleep (discussed in Chapter 12), **sedatives, tranquilizers,** and **hypnotics** (see Table 13-5). A number of other drugs, such as opiates, antihistamines, and some medications used in the treatment of high blood pressure or heart disease, may also depress the activity of the central nervous system.

The CNS depressants have effects similar to those of alcohol. In low doses, they may produce a mild state of euphoria, reduce inhibitions, or induce a feeling of relaxation and lessened tension. In high doses they may impair mood, speech, and motor coordination.

CNS depressants are dangerous. All carry the potential for physical and psychological dependency, tolerance, unpleasant withdrawal symptoms, and toxicity from continual use or overuse. Acute overdoses may produce coma, respiratory or cardiovascular collapse, and even death. Aggravating the potential for toxic and possible lethal overdose is the synergistic actions of CNS drugs. That is, when taken together, two or more different CNS depressants can produce a much stronger effect than either drug would produce if taken alone. The most commonly seen synergistic effect occurs when people drink alcohol while taking depressant drugs, such as barbiturates.

CNS depressants are the largest class of medically prescribed drugs—more prescriptions are written for tranquilizers than for any other class of drugs. Although many depressants are medically useful in the treatment of seizure disorders and insomnia, preparation for anesthesia, and alleviation of acute anxiety that may accompany certain severe mental or emotional problems, the extent of their use far exceeds appropriate therapeutic indications. Millions of prescriptions for depressant drugs are handed out for complaints that are more effectively and safely handled by counseling or changes in lifestyle. CNS depressants are among the most abused of drugs, but because they are not illegal, their abuse receives little attention from the media or from government regulatory agencies.

Inhalants

Inhalants include a wide variety of chemical substances that vaporize readily and that, when inhaled, produce various kinds of intoxicating effects similar to the effects of alcohol. Like alcohol, inhalants are depressants of the central nervous system. Generally, their intended effect is to produce a sense of euphoria, a loss of inhibition, and a sense of excitement. Some of the unintended effects include dizziness, amnesia, inability to concentrate, confusion, postural imbalance, impaired judgment, hallucinations, and acute psychosis (Nicholi, 1983b).

The inhalants that are commonly used for recreational purposes include:

1. Commercial chemicals such as model airplane glue, nail polish remover, paint thinner, and gasoline, and substances such as acetone, toluene, naphtha, hexane, and cyclohexane.
2. Aerosols—the substances that are found in aerosol spray products.
3. Anesthetics such as amyl nitrate, nitrous oxide ("laughing gas"), diethyl ether, and chloroform.

Because they are vaporous, these substances get into the body quite rapidly. The fumes are usually inhaled from plastic bags. The intoxicant effects are often felt within minutes, and the high lasts less than an hour. Regular users tend to be preteens and teenagers of low socioeconomic status whose home lives are unstable and often violent. They use inhalants because they do not have the money to buy other drugs. Some adults use amyl nitrate ("poppers") during sexual relations, believing that the drug enhances the sexual experience. Some medical personnel are frequent users of nitrous oxide because it is so available to them.

The inhalant chemicals do not produce tolerance or withdrawal, nor do they induce physical dependence. However, they are quite dangerous. In addition to any harm that may ensue because of uncontrolled behavior (such as driving while intoxicated), these chemicals damage the kidneys, liver, and lungs and can upset the normal rhythmic beating of the heart. Some users have suffocated while inhaling the fumes from the plastic bags, and the potential for explosion is ever present.

Phencyclidine (PCP)

Phencyclidine, also known as PCP, angel dust, hog, crystal, killer weed, and a variety of other names, was developed originally for medical use as an anesthetic. But because of the drug's many adverse effects, it was taken off the market and became an illegal recreational drug. In the 1960s, phencyclidine was called the *PeaCePill*—a serious misnomer when one considers what the drug does to the user.

The effects of PCP are quite variable. Depending on the dose and the route of administration, PCP can be a stimulant, a depressant, or a hal-

Table 13-5
Central Nervous System (CNS) Depressant Drugs

Minor Tranquilizers (Benzodiazepines)	*Nonbenzodiazepine–Nonbarbiturates*
Chlordiazepoxide (Libritabs, Librium)	Hydroxizine (Atarax, Orgatrax, Vistaril)
Chlorazepate (Tranxene)	Meprobamate (Equanil, Meprospan,
Diazepam (Valcaps, Valium, Valrelease)	Miltown)
Flurazepam (Dalmane)	
Halazepam (Paxipam)	*Hypnotics*
Prazepam (Centrax)	Chloral hydrate
Lorazepam (Ativan)	Ethchlorvynol (Placidyl)
Oxazepam (Serax)	Ethinamate (Valmid)
Temazepam (Restoril)	Glutethimide (Doriden)
Barbiturate Sedatives	Methaqualone (Mequin, Parest,
Butabarbital (Butisol)	Quaalude)
Phenobarbital	Methyprylon (Noludar)
Mephobarbital (Mebaral)	Paraldehyde (Paral)
Amobarbital (Amytal, "blues")	Diphenhydramine (Sominex Formula 2)
Pentobarbital (Nembutal, "yellow	Doxylamine (Unisom)
jackets")	Pyrilamine (Nervine, Nytol, Sleep-Eze,
Secobarbital (Seconal, "reds")	Sominex)

> ## PCP may induce an acute psychosis in some individuals . . . Treatment of PCP-precipitated psychosis should be considered a psychiatric emergency, and the patient should be hospitalized immediately.
> **Armand M. Nicholi, Jr., M.D.**

lucinogen. Some of the intended effects are heightened sensitivity to external stimuli, mood elevation, relaxation, and a sense of omnipotence. Some of the unintended and frequent effects are paranoia, confusion, restlessness, disorientation, feelings of depersonalization, and violent or bizarre behavior. In high doses the drug can cause coma, interruption of breathing, and psychosis. Many admissions to psychiatric emergency rooms are for PCP intoxication. The drug impairs perception and muscular control, and users are prone to accidents such as falling from heights, drowning, walking in front of moving vehicles, and collisions while driving under the influence of the drug. PCP does not induce

tolerance or physical dependence, but because it is eliminated slowly from the body, chronic users may experience the drug's effects for an extended period.

The effects of PCP are unpredictable and frequently unpleasant, if not actually horrible and life-threatening. PCP produces more unwanted and dangerous symptoms of drug intoxication than any other psychoactive substance (see Table 13-6). Persons who sell illegal recreational drugs often surreptitiously mix PCP with marijuana or cocaine or sell PCP while claiming it to be LSD, DMT, or some other drug. Because PCP is relatively easy to manufacture, it is one of the more readily available and dangerous of the illegal recreational drugs.

Table 13-6
Common Signs and Symptoms of Drug Intoxication

Signs and symptoms	PCP	Stimu-lants	Hallucin-ogens	Sedative-hypnotics	Nar-cotics
Aggressive and violent behavior	X	X			
Ataxia	X			X	
Coma	X			X	X
Confusion	X		X		
Convulsions	X	X			
Drowsiness	X			X	X
Hallucinations	X		X		
Hyperreflexia	X	X			
Nystagmus	X			X	
Hypertension	X	X			
Paranoia	X	X	X		
Psychosis	X	X	X		
Respiratory depression				X	X
Slurred speech	X			X	

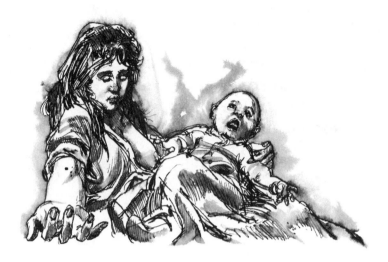

Opiates

The **opiates** are a group of chemically similar drugs that depresss the central nervous system (see Figure 13-2). These substances do cause physical dependence, habituation, tolerance and produce serious withdrawal symptoms. The opiates are derived from the opium poppy, *Papaver somniferum,* extracts of which have been used for thousands of years in a variety of cultures to produce euphoria, to relieve pain, and to treat various diseases.

Opium is a complex mixture of plant alkaloids; its principal psychoactive substances are morphine and, to a much lesser degree, codeine. Heroin is derived from morphine. Morphine and other opiates block nerve transmission in the central nervous system, thereby suppressing mental and physiological functions. Opiates bind to the nervous system cell receptors and mimic the actions of the body's natural pain-relieving substances, endorphins, and enkephalins (see Chapter 3). Morphine and codeine are used medically for pain relief, while heroin is used primarily as an illegal recreational drug.

The sensations produced by injecting heroin into the circulatory system are markedly different from those of morphine and codeine, even though the opiate drugs have similar structures. As one heroin user described the sensation: "It's so good, don't even try it once" (Smith and Gay, 1972). Regular use of opiates can produce many unwanted effects in addition to the psychological high. Among the adverse reactions are constipation, loss of appetite, depression, loss of interest in sex, constriction of the pupil of the eye, disruption of the menstrual cycle, and drowsiness. Very large doses or prolonged use can be lethal because of respiratory failure.

Street heroin may contain as little as 1 to 3 percent heroin; the rest is sugar, cornstarch, cleansing agents, strychnine, or almost any white powder. Heroin is converted to morphine in the body, and the morphine is eventually excreted in urine, saliva, sweat, and the breast milk of lactating women. Because morphine crosses the placenta, a developing fetus can become addicted even before birth and will experience withdrawal symptoms after it is born.

Figure 13-2
Chemical structures of opiate drugs. Morphine and codeine occur naturally in opium extracts of poppies. Heroin is synthesized by chemically modifying morphine. Opiates bind to receptor sites on brain cells (different from hallucinogen receptor sites) and change consciousness.

Morphine

Heroin

Codeine

> War is but a spectacular expression
> of our daily conduct.
> **Krishnamurti**

In 1983 researchers at Stanford University School of Medicine observed that people who used a "synthetic heroin" acquired a Parkinson-like disease that involved destruction of the brain and nerve cells leading to irreversible neurological damage. The substance in the synthetic heroin that was responsible for these serious symptoms was identified as MPTP (1-methyl-4-phenyl-1,2,3,6-tetrahydropyridine). For scientists the discovery of the neurotoxic effects of MPTP provided a powerful tool for investigating the chemistry of brain diseases and brain functions. However, for the unfortunate users of MPTP the consequences are irreversible brain damage and destroyed lives.

Recreational Drugs Are Not Always Fun

No one knows why people use drugs. Peer pressure seems to be a strong motivating force. The fact is that drugs have been used by people in all cultures since recorded history and probably much earlier. The following imaginary interview probably contains all the relevant information on why people use drugs:

> Question: Why do you use drugs?
> Answer: Why not?
> Question: What would convince you to stop?
> Answer: Show me something better.

All drugs are dangerous, and illegal recreational drugs are especially so, since one cannot be sure of either the drug or the dose. While it may be true that marijuana is less dangerous than either alcohol or cigarette smoking, that still does not make it absolutely safe. Some persons may benefit psychologically or feel spiritually uplifted by hallucinogenic drugs; others may "freak out" or suffer a mental breakdown. It is impossible to reliably predict the experience any individual will have with a particular drug.

Recreational drugs are not essential to health and well-being. Yet most people, especially young people, will experiment with one or more illegal drugs. For those who are determined to experiment, we offer the following cautions:

1. All illegal drugs are dangerous because of the uncertainty of the drug and the dose. Never use an illegal drug that has not already been taken by someone you know and trust.
2. Never forget that use of illegal drugs can lead to arrest, a criminal record, jail, costly legal defense, and unnecessary stress.
3. Never take an illegal drug to solve personal problems or to try to alleviate anxiety or depression. All psychoactive drugs enhance negative feeling states and can produce severe anxiety attacks or psychotic behaviors.

The fact that as we get older we are less inclined to experiment with drugs, particularly illegal recreational drugs, means that we have found other ways to make our lives satisfying and interesting. The earlier in life we discover how to be healthy and happy without drugs, the more satisfied with ourselves we will become. One sign of maturity is being able to say no to the use of drugs.

> Words are the most potent drug that
> mankind uses.
>
> **Rudyard Kipling**

 ## Supplemental Readings

Abel, E. L. *Marijuana: The First Twelve Thousand Years.* New York: Plenum Press, 1980. An excellent book on the history and uses of marijuana. Of especial value is the summary, which debunks a lot of marijuana folklore.

Jacobs, B. L., ed. *Hallucinogens: Neurochemical, Behavioral,* and *Clinical Perspectives.* New York: Raven Press, 1984. A detailed discussion of all aspects of hallucinogenic drugs.

Jacobs, B. L. "How Hallucinogenic Drugs Work." *American Scientist,* July/August 1987. Explains the mechanisms by which these drugs affect brain functions.

Lieber, J., "Coping with Cocaine." *Atlantic Monthly,* January 1986. A lucid and factual discussion of the problem of cocaine use in the United States.

Marijuana and Health. Washington, D.C.: National Academy Press, 1982. A balanced and comprehensive review of the effects of smoking marijuana. A summary of the report's findings appeared in *Science,* 215 (1982), 1488.

Murray, T. H.; Gaylin, W.; and Macklin, R., eds. *Feeling Good and Doing Better.* Clifton, N.J.: Humana Press, 1984. An excellent collection of essays covering the medical, social, and psychological aspects of the use and abuse of mood-altering drugs.

Nicholi, H. M., Jr. "The College Student and Marijuana: Research Findings Concerning Adverse Biological and Psychological Effects." *Journal of American College Health,* October 1983. An article that emphasizes the adverse consequences of smoking marijuana.

Summary

All recreational drugs contain psychoactive substances that affect moods, perceptions, and thoughts. Humans have always sought out ways to change states of consciousness, first by eating or smoking natural plant and fungal materials, and more recently by ingesting purified and manufactured chemicals. No one really understands why people seek out and use psychoactive drugs. For some, these drugs increase pleasurable sensations and feelings; for others, they mask negative and depressed mood states. In many cultures the use of psychoactive drugs is an integral part of religious practices or increases the intensity of mystical and spiritual experiences.

Marijuana is the most commonly used recreational drug in the United States and has been smoked and eaten by people all over the world for thousands of years. The use of cocaine, which is purified from coca leaves grown in South America, has increased dramatically in this country in recent years. Neither marijuana nor cocaine causes physical dependence (addiction) or tolerance (need for increased doses), but both substances create psychological habituation. Some people's lives are disrupted or destroyed because all of their energy and resources are devoted to obtaining the recreational drug they crave.

The hallucinogenic drugs, such as LSD and mescaline, are among the most potent psychoactive drugs known. The hallucinogens change patterns of nerve transmissions in the brain by temporarily modifying neurotransmitter activity in the nervous system. Perceptions, moods, thoughts, and feelings are drastically altered from what is normally experienced. Many other substances, such as inhalants, phencyclidine (PCP), and opiates are also used as recreational drugs and produce both physical and mental effects that are dangerous to well-being. All recreational drugs that are commonly used (except for alcohol and tobacco and, to a lesser degree, amphetamines and caffeine) are illegal, and using or selling these drugs is a crime. Rightly or wrongly, society has always regulated the use of drugs in the past and will probably continue to do so in the future.

FOR YOUR HEALTH

Drug Attitudes and Behaviors

Make a list of the behaviors or attitudes of people that you know who use recreational drugs. Compare your list with those of other students. Are there any common behaviors and attitudes that are associated with recreational drug use? Do you have any of those attitudes or behaviors?

Drug Habits

List all chemicals or substances that you use that change your state of consciousness—drinking beer, drinking caffeine-containing drinks, using chewing tobacco, smoking marijuana, and so on. Try to give up one or more of these substances for a period of time, and keep a record of how you feel and any changes you notice in your health or behavior.

CHAPTER FOURTEEN

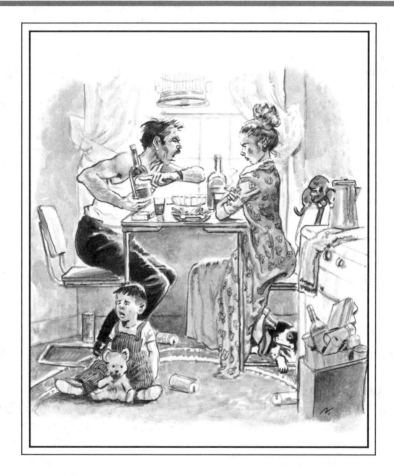

Learn to drink in moderation
if you drink.

Alcohol Use and Abuse

Alcohol abuse is one of the most significant health-related drug problems in the United States and in many other countries. Although the use of heroin, marijuana, cocaine, and other illegal drugs receives much more attention from governments and the news media, these drugs affect far fewer people and cause far fewer health problems than alcohol. In 1986, over 100,000 deaths were alcohol related, and alcohol abuse was responsible for approximately $120 billion in health and social costs. Excessive alcohol use is associated with thousands of divorces, perhaps as many as 50 percent of the incidents of family violence, and millions of hours of school and job absenteeism. Alcohol abuse is also linked to a long list of diseases and disorders (see Figure 14-1).

Alcohol use has long been a part of social events such as parties, dinners, weddings, ballgames, and picnics. The liquor industry encourages alcohol use by spending over $1 billion per year advertising its products in newspapers and magazines and on radio and television. Whereas no direct link between advertising alcohol-containing products and alcohol abuse has been established, public health authorities and organizations such as the American Medical Association are concerned that advertising that associates drinking with athletic prowess, material wealth, social prestige, relaxation, and sex without also cautioning of the dangers of alcohol consumption encourages irresponsible drinking behavior. Breweries and distributors are especially active on college campuses, spending approximately $2 million per year on advertising in campus newspapers and promoting their products by sponsoring "pub nights" and drinking contests, giving away items with product logos, and underwriting some of the costs of college athletic events.

Alcohol's positive public image makes many people skeptical that they can benefit from learning about alcohol use and abuse. Most people who drink believe that they can "hold their liquor" and that alcoholic beverages, especially beer, are no more harmful to health than soft drinks. It is not our intention to argue that some consumption of alcohol is unhealthy. As with so many other aspects of health, for most people responsibility and moderation are more desirable than fanatical adherence to a single course of action. Everyone can benefit from knowing more about the effects of alcohol on the brain and body.

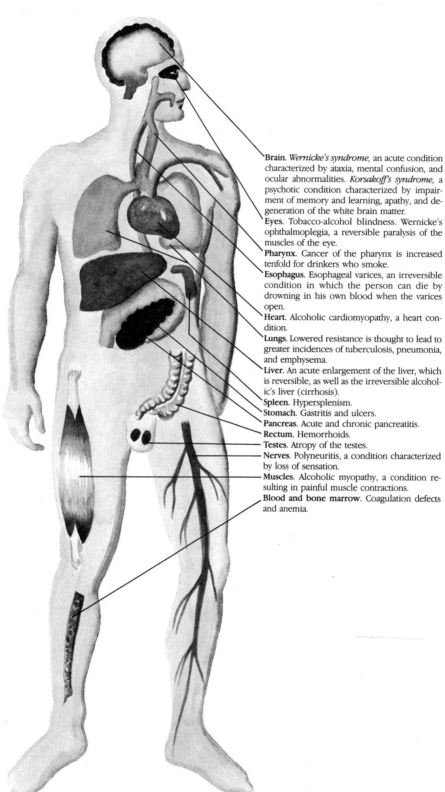

Brain. *Wernicke's syndrome,* an acute condition characterized by ataxia, mental confusion, and ocular abnormalities. *Korsakoff's syndrome,* a psychotic condition characterized by impairment of memory and learning, apathy, and degeneration of the white brain matter.

Eyes. Tobacco-alcohol blindness. Wernicke's ophthalmoplegia, a reversible paralysis of the muscles of the eye.

Pharynx. Cancer of the pharynx is increased tenfold for drinkers who smoke.

Esophagus. Esophageal varices, an irreversible condition in which the person can die by drowning in his own blood when the varices open.

Heart. Alcoholic cardiomyopathy, a heart condition.

Lungs. Lowered resistance is thought to lead to greater incidences of tuberculosis, pneumonia, and emphysema.

Liver. An acute enlargement of the liver, which is reversible, as well as the irreversible alcoholic's liver (cirrhosis).

Spleen. Hypersplenism.

Stomach. Gastritis and ulcers.

Pancreas. Acute and chronic pancreatitis.

Rectum. Hemorrhoids.

Testes. Atropy of the testes.

Nerves. Polyneuritis, a condition characterized by loss of sensation.

Muscles. Alcoholic myopathy, a condition resulting in painful muscle contractions.

Blood and bone marrow. Coagulation defects and anemia.

Figure 14-1

Diseases and disorders associated with alcohol abuse.

> What alcoholics have in
> common is drinking and damage.
> **Elvin M. Jellinek**

History of Alcohol Use

It is likely that humans have been drinking alcohol since someone accidently noticed the psychological effects of drinking fermented liquids. Anthropological evidence indicates that Stone Age people drank the fermented juice of berries. Perhaps this first fruit wine was produced when some berry juice was left too long in a covered earthen jar and yeasts in the mixture converted the sugar in the juice to alcohol by **fermentation.** The first recorded use of alcohol dates from the Mesopotamian agrarian cultures of around 5000 B.C.

Through the ages, the drinking of fermented grains (beer); fermented berries, grapes, and fruits (wine); and the distilled products of natural fermentations (brandies and "hard" liquors) has become commonplace in almost every human society. Alcohol is used in some religious ceremonies, is given as medicine, is used to ratify contracts, agreements, and treaties, and is offered to display hospitality. Alcohol consumption has been an integral part of American life since the landing of the Mayflower at Plymouth Rock. Yet over the years many people have regarded drinking as a social evil and drunkenness as a sin. The United States government tried to legislate alcohol use out of American lives in 1919 by the Volstead Act, a Constitutional amendment that prohibited the sale and consumption of alcoholic beverages. This attempt to control alcohol consumption failed, however, and in 1933 prohibition was ended by another amendment to the Constitution.

Today, alcoholic beverages come in many varieties. Not only are there the old stand-bys of beer, wine, and the traditional hard liquors, but beverage manufacturers also market a variety of pre-mixed cocktails, often sweetened with sugar and containing various flavors to make the drink more palatable.

Alcohol and the Body

The alcohol in beverages is a chemical called **ethyl alcohol.** There are many other kinds of alcohol, such as methyl alcohol (wood alcohol) and isopropyl alcohol (rubbing alcohol). Most alcohols are poisonous if ingested in small amounts. In large amounts even ethyl alcohol is toxic, but the body has ways to detoxify and eliminate some of it.

The amount of ethyl alcohol in a commercial alcoholic product is listed on the product label. The amount of alcohol in beer and wine is given as the percentage of the total volume. Beer, for example, is generally about 4 percent alcohol, although some beers may contain more and some less (so-called light beers have nearly the same alcohol content as regular beers); wine is about 12 percent alcohol. The amount of alcohol in distilled liquors (scotch, vodka, bourbon, tequila, rum, and so on) is given in terms of **proof,** a number that represents twice the percentage of alcohol in the product. Thus, an 80 proof whiskey is 40 percent alcohol; a 100 proof vodka is 50 percent alcohol.

Most standard portions of alcoholic drinks contain about ½ ounce of ethyl alcohol. For example,

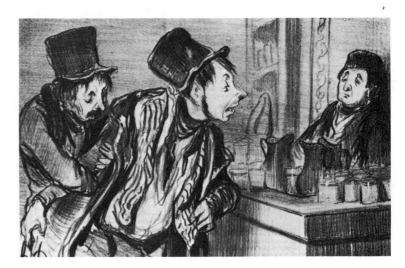

A cartoon by the French artist Honore Daumier, a keen observer of drunkenness. The leader of the two drinkers is saying, "Everything is paid for? We didn't do anybody any harm did we? . . . Goodbye then . . . " (Courtesy World Health Organization.)

a 12-ounce can of beer that is 4 percent alcohol contains .48 ounces of alcohol. The same amount of alcohol is contained in a 4 ounce glass of wine. And the alcohol content of a cocktail mixed with one shot (1 ounce) of a 100 proof bourbon is 0.5 ounce. So a can of beer, a glass of wine, and a highball contain approximately the same amount of alcohol.

After alcohol is ingested, it is readily absorbed into the body through the gastrointestinal tract. About 20 percent of ingested alcohol is absorbed by the stomach and the rest by the small intestine. Once inside the body the alcohol is carried through the bloodstream to all the body's tissues and organs. Although not strictly a food (it contains no protein, vitamins, or minerals), alcohol does contain calories — in fact, almost twice as many calories per gram as sugar.

Several factors affect the rate at which alcohol is absorbed into the body tissues. For example, food in the stomach — especially fatty foods or proteins — slows the absorption of alcohol. Nonalcoholic substances in beer and wine and cocktails can also slow absorption of alcohol. The presence of carbon dioxide in beverages such as champagne, sparkling wines, beer, and carbonated mixed drinks increases the rate of alcohol absorption. That is why people feel intoxicated more quickly when drinking champagne or beer, especially on an empty stomach. The higher the alcohol content in a drink, the faster it is absorbed.

The concentration of alcohol in the blood is called the **blood alcohol content** (BAC). A simple way to estimate BAC is to assume that ingesting one standard drink per hour (one beer, one glass of wine, one mixed drink), which contains approximately ½ ounce of ethyl alcohol, gives a BAC of .02 in a 150 pound male. Thus, the BAC of an average-sized man who drinks five beers during the first hour at a party will be .10; this is the level of alcohol in the blood that violates the drinking-and-driving laws of most states. This shorthand method of approximating BAC changes with body size, body composition, and gender. All other things being equal, the BAC of a large person is less than that of a smaller person because the alcohol is diluted more in the large person's tissues. According to Jones and Jones (1976), women tend to have a higher BAC from the same number of drinks as men because they generally weigh less than men, have proportionately more body fat (which does not absorb alcohol as readily as muscle and other tissues), and have sex hormones that tend to increase alcohol absorption and decrease its elimination.

Alcohol is eliminated from the body in two ways. About 10 percent is excreted unchanged through sweat, urine, or breath (hence the use of breath analyzers to test for drinking). Alcohol that is not excreted is broken down primarily by the liver, ultimately winding up as carbon dioxide and water. The liver detoxifies alcohol at a rate of about ½ ounce per hour, and there is no way to speed up the process. Sobering-up remedies, such as drinking a lot of coffee, taking a cold shower, or engaging in vigorous exercise, do not accelerate the rate at which the liver removes alcohol from the body.

Alcohol and Behavior

Pharmacologically, alcohol acts as a central nervous system depressant, which means that it slows certain functions in some parts of the brain. In moderate amounts, alcohol may affect the parts of the brain that control judgment and inhibitions, which is why many people have a drink or two at a party—drinking may help them "loosen up," to become less shy and able to interact more freely with others. They may talk or laugh more than usual. Unfortunately, the effects of alcohol are unpredictable, and some people become boisterous, argumentative, irritable, or depressed.

The effects of alcohol on sexual desires and performance vary from person to person and with the BAC. Pinhas (1980) points out that in some individuals small amounts of alcohol may dispel uncomfortable feelings about sex and therefore may facilitate sexual arousal. Higher amounts of alcohol, however (.10 BAC), may produce problems getting and maintaining an erection or ejaculating in males and a reduction in vaginal lubrication and difficulty reaching orgasm in females. Even at moderate BACs, some individuals are too intoxicated to effectively give and receive sexual pleasure.

The behavioral effects of alcohol depend on the BAC, as shown in Table 14-1. At a BAC of .05, the "loosening-up" effects of alcohol become manifest. At a BAC of .10, the depressant effects of the drug become pronounced, the person may become sleepy, and motor coordination is affected. Speech may become slurred and postural instability may become noticeable. Alcohol's effects on motor skills, judgment, and reaction times make driving after drinking extremely dangerous (see Box 14-1). Approximately *half* of all highway fatalities each year involve people who have been drinking and are intoxicated. Highway accidents are among the ten leading causes of death in the United States.

Physical and psychological tolerance to the effects of alcohol can be acquired through regular use. The nervous system can adapt over time to the effects of alcohol so that higher amounts are required to produce the same physiological and psychological effects (see Chapter 13 for a discussion of drug tolerance). Some people learn to modify their behaviors so that they appear sober even though their BAC is quite high. This phenomenon is called **learned behavioral tolerance.** In general, the more experience a person has with certain behaviors, the less likely alcohol will be to impair those behaviors, although not all behaviors are affected by alcohol to the same degree.

Studies indicate that some people may experience the sensation of being intoxicated without actually ingesting alcohol. This placebo effect (see Chapter 2) can occur in individuals who are familiar with the state of being "high" or drunk from previous experiences. On the other hand, some people who drink can decide they do not want to feel drunk even after several drinks and, in fact, feel and act sober. Most people who drink alcohol know that the psychological and behavioral effects of alcohol are strongly influenced by their mental and emotional states.

Table 14-1
Behavioral Effects of Alcohol

Number of drinks	Ounces of alcohol	BAC (g/100 ml)	Approximate time for removal	Effects
1 beer, glass of wine, or mixed drink	½	0.02	1 hour	Feeling relaxed or "loosened up"
2½ beers, glasses of wine, or mixed drinks	1¼	0.05	2½ hours	Feeling "high"; decrease in inhibitions; increase in confidence; judgment impaired
5 beers, glasses of wine, or mixed drinks	2½	0.10	5 hours	Memory impaired; muscular coordination reduced; slurred speech; euphoric or sad feelings
10 beers, glasses of wine, or mixed drinks	5	0.20	10 hours	Slowed reflexes; erratic changes in feelings
15 beers, glasses of wine, or mixed drinks	7½	0.30	15–16 hours	Stuporous, complete loss of coordination; little sensation
20 beers, glasses of wine, or mixed drinks	10	0.40	20 hours	May become comatose; breathing may cease
25–30 beers, glasses of wine, or mixed drinks	15–20	0.50	26 hours	Fatal amount for most people

---

BOX 14-1

DRIVING UNDER THE INFLUENCE OF ALCOHOL (DUI)

Early in the morning last summer, I was arrested for driving under the influence of alcohol.

It's not easy to recall what actually happened—I see it through a fog, as if I was watching someone else.

The actual arrest is the blurriest. I was running for those few moments on pure adrenaline and fear. For awhile I don't even think I was breathing.

It's hard to explain the exact emotions.

It's hard to explain what it feels like to want more than anything to be sober.

It's hard to explain losing complete control of your life for even a short time.

It is hard to explain the feeling of handcuffs.

It's hard to explain what it feels like to sit in a holding cell and bite your lip in the hopes of not going to sleep.

One thing for sure is that when those flashing lights appeared in my rearview mirror, all the rationalizations that got me into that car vanished. "It's just around the corner," "I need to get a friend home," or "No one is on the road at this hour"—none of them mean a thing—zero.

At the jail, it took what seemed like days to be finger printed and photographed and to fill out the required forms. Each step was just a little more humiliating than the last.

I am still overwhelmed at how a single, incredibly poor judgment could affect so many parts of my life.

The ramifications will be with me in various ways for the next three years—which is as far ahead as I have ever cared to plan.

These shock waves include probation for three years, an exorbitant increase in the cost of my car insurance, restricted driver's license for 90 days (which was agreed upon in lieu of two days in jail) and a $600 fine, to name a few.

Many of the ramifications cannot be quantified. There was the call home, a couple of days of generally feeling lousy and the unshakable sense that I had proven myself a fool.

Through all of it, however, I have some things to be thankful for.

On the top of that very short list is the fact that I didn't kill anyone.

Having struggled to come to terms with the arrest, it is impossible to imagine . . . for that there is no atonement.

Also on that list is the discovery of some very supportive people in my life, all of whom said not that what happened was OK, but that I was going to be OK. I turned to my parents and friends for help, and no one turned away—I am thankful.

Whether this column will keep anyone from driving drunk is doubtful. If I had read this column before my arrest, I would have thought of a 100 reasons why it would never have applied to me—but I would have been wrong.

Ethan Watters, editor, *The Aggie.*
University of California, Davis.
(Reprinted by permission.)

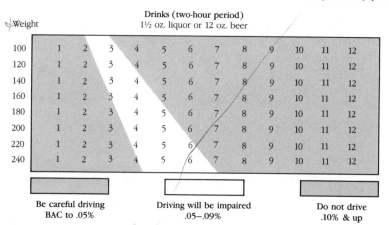

Effects of drinking on driving.

Table 14-2
Alcohol and Drugs That Don't Mix
Alcohol should not be consumed when taking drugs such as those listed below.

Drug	Dangerous interaction
Acetaminophen (Tylenol, Anacin-3)	Heavy use plus alcohol can cause liver damage.
Aspirin (Anacin, Excedrin)	Heavy use plus alcohol can cause bleeding of stomach wall.
Antihistamines (Chlor-Trimeton, Benadryl)	Drowsiness and loss of coordination increased by alcohol.
Tranquilizers, sedatives (Valium, Dalmane, Miltown)	Alcohol increases their effects.
Painkillers (codeine, Percodan, morphine)	Alcohol increases sedation and reduces ability to concentrate.
Barbiturates (Amytal, Seconal, phenobarbital)	Potentially FATAL. Don't ever use with alcohol.

Other Effects of Alcohol

Alcohol can impair the functioning of other body organs in addition to the brain. Alcohol can irritate the organs of the gastrointestinal (GI) tract—the esophagus, stomach, intestine, pancreas, and liver—causing upset or irritability, nausea, vomiting, or diarrhea. Alcohol can also dilate arteries and cause bloodshot eyes. Dilation of arteries in the arms, legs, and skin can cause a drop in blood pressure and loss of body heat. This is why people occasionally feel flushed and their faces redden when they drink. Giving people alcohol to warm them up can actually produce the opposite physiological effect.

Alcohol should not be ingested simultaneously with other CNS depressant drugs such as tranquilizers and sedatives. In many instances, the depressant effects of alcohol and the other drug interact so that the combined effect of the two drugs is greater than the simple additive effects. What may seem like reasonable amounts of alcohol, when taken with another drug, can dangerously suppress brain function and respiration (see Table 14-2).

The Hangover

An occasional consequence of drinking alcohol is a **hangover,** which may involve stomach upset, headache, fatigue, weakness, shakiness, irritability, and sometimes vomiting after a drinking episode. The frequency and severity of hangovers vary. The particular factors in alcohol that cause a hangover are unknown, but several causes have been suggested:

1. When alcohol is present in the body, normal liver function may slow in order to break down the alcohol. This may reduce the amount of sugar the liver releases into the blood, resulting in temporary hypoglycemia and its resultant fatigue, irritability, and headache.

2. Alcohol may inhibit REM sleep, resulting in fatigue, irritability, and trouble concentrating.

3. **Congeners,** which are other chemical substances in an alcoholic beverage, or the breakdown products produced in the liver may cause a hangover.

4. Acetaldehyde, a toxic intermediate produced when the liver breaks down alcohol, may be responsible for hangover symptoms.

The best way to deal with a hangover is to sleep, to drink juice to replace the lost body fluid and blood sugar (alcohol increases urine output), and perhaps to take an analgesic for headache. Ingesting more alcohol will only prolong the hangover symptoms.

> The evolution to stable moderate drinking appears to be a rare outcome among alcoholics treated at medical or psychiatric facilities.
>
> *New England Journal of Medicine*

Fetal Alcohol Syndrome

Alcohol can harm the health of anyone, man or woman, young or old. Even the unborn fetus can be damaged by alcohol. Over the last ten years evidence has accumulated showing that numerous kinds of birth defects and mental retardation may result from ingestion of alcohol by pregnant women — a condition known as **fetal alcohol syndrome.** Fetal alcohol syndrome is estimated to be the third leading cause of birth defects and mental retardation among newborns. Since the harmful effects on fetal development are believed to occur during the first few weeks or months of prenatal development, a time during which much of the nervous system is being formed, it is important that women refrain from drinking if they are trying to

become pregnant or if they suspect that they are pregnant. Studies have also shown that the level of alcohol in the fetus's blood may be ten times greater than the BAC of the mother. This explains why even a couple of drinks during pregnancy can endanger normal fetal development.

Alcohol Abuse and Alcoholism

Alcohol abuse is the principal drug abuse problem in the United States. Approximately 12 million Americans of different ages, religions, races, educational backgrounds, and socioeconomic status have problems with alcohol. Over 3 million American teenagers (ages 14–17) have a drinking problem.

Figure 14-2
Fetal alcohol syndrome. (Photo courtesy Kenneth Lyons Jones, M.D.)

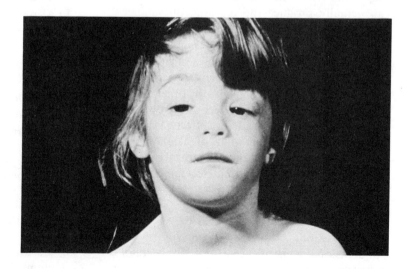

More than a third of all suicides involve alcohol. Approximately 6 million adults have personal and health problems with alcohol that are severe enough to warrant the label "alcoholic" and to suffer **alcoholism**. These people are unable to control their

Figure 14-3
Percentage and types of drinkers among adults age 18 and older, 1981. (Data from National Institute of Alcohol Abuse and Alcoholism.)

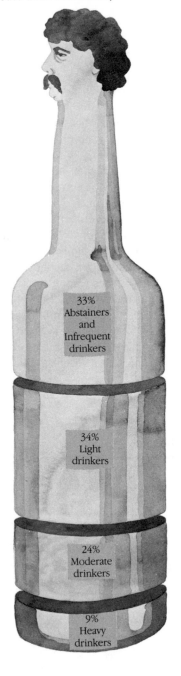

33%
Abstainers
and
Infrequent
drinkers

34%
Light
drinkers

24%
Moderate
drinkers

9%
Heavy
drinkers

drinking and some are physically dependent on alcohol and may experience withdrawal symptoms, including **delirium tremens** (DT's), when deprived of alcohol. Delirium tremens is characterized by hallucinations and uncontrollable shaking.

Problem drinking can cause numerous problems in a person's life. Job and school performance can be impaired, family relationships and friendships can be destroyed, and drunk driving may cause legal problems. Because alcohol supplies calories, constant drinkers are rarely hungry, and they may suffer from vitamin deficiency syndromes, which result in loss of muscular coordination and mental confusion. After years of heavy drinking, a person may suffer serious liver, stomach, heart, and neurological damage.

The cause or causes of problem drinking and alcoholism are unknown although hypotheses abound. Before the advent of modern psychology and medicine, alcohol abuse was thought to be a manifestation of immorality and irreligiousness. Some people still hold that view, but most professionals (and problem drinkers) interpret alcohol abuse as a behavioral disorder or a medical disease. For example, some people with low self esteem or seemingly unmanageable life conflicts may drink in order to feel better about themselves or to try to cope with life. Instead they may add a drinking problem to their other problems.

There is some evidence that, at least for some people, alcoholism may have a biological basis, either because people metabolize alcohol differently or because their brains respond differently to alcohol. Some experts resist considering alcohol abuse a disease because doing so may remove the sense of personal responsibility for problem drinking. Others argue that calling alcohol abuse a disease fosters successful treatment because it removes the stigma and lessens guilt associated with such behavior and offers a supervised and presumably scientifically based plan for treatment.

The Development of Alcoholism

Alcoholism usually develops from a prealcoholic stage of needing to drink to relieve tensions and anxieties. The prealcoholic phase may last for years, during which tolerance to alcohol gradually develops. Progression to a state of alcoholism is characterized by three phases (Jellinek, 1960):

> Treating the alcoholic is like the
> recipe for rabbit stew: first you must
> catch the rabbit.
>
> **Cecil Carle**

1. *The warning phase.* In this first stage of alcoholism, problem drinkers have an increased tolerance to alcohol and a preoccupation with drinking. For example, when they are invited to a party they may ask what alcoholic beverages will be served rather than who is going to be there. In this stage problem drinkers may sneak drinks often and may deny that they are drinking too much. Blackouts may also occur. Blackouts are not periods of unconsciousness. Others observe the drinker as behaving normally, but he or she has no recall of events that happened while drinking. Some of the signs of the warning phase of alcoholism are presented in Table 14-3.

2. *The crucial phase.* This phase of alcoholism is characterized by the problem drinker's loss of control over how much he or she drinks. The person may not drink every day, but he or she cannot control the amount of alcohol consumed once drinking has begun. In this stage, the problem drinker may rationalize his or her drinking behavior and actually believe that there are good reasons for heavy drinking. An alcoholic may still carry out his or her responsibilities (housework, job, doing well in school) for some period of time and may employ a series of strategies to keep the family from rejecting him or her. These may include promising to stop drinking. Often the alcoholic's extrava-

Table 14-3
Warning Signs of Problem Drinking or Alcoholism

1. Gulping drinks.
2. Drinking to modify uncomfortable feelings.
3. Personality or behavioral changes after drinking.
4. Getting drunk frequently.
5. Experiencing "blackouts"—not being able to remember what happened while drinking.
6. Frequent accidents or illness as a result of drinking.
7. Priming—preparing yourself with alcohol before a social gathering at which alcohol is going to be served.
8. Not wanting to talk about the negative consequences of drinking (avoidance).
9. Preoccupation with alcohol.
10. Focusing social situations around alcohol.
11. Sneaking drinks or clandestine drinking.

**Alcoholism is the most common social disease
picked up in a bar.**

gant measures to prove he or she doesn't
have a drinking problem appear successful,
and eventually the person begins drinking
heavily again. Perhaps at this point the
problem with alcohol is blamed on the kind
of drinks that the person prefers or on the
usual place of drinking; so the problem
drinker changes to a different form of alcoholic beverage or to a different place in
which to drink.

3. *The chronic phase.* In this phase, the alcoholic is usually totally dependent on the
   drug, and drinking behavior has consumed
   all aspects of life. Friends and family have

resigned themselves to the problem and may
be angry and ignore the alcoholic. At this
stage of alcoholism the person may be unable to work or attend school. In this phase
the health consequences of alcohol abuse
may intensify and the person may need
medical attention and even hospitalization.
If physical addiction to alcohol has occurred, continual drinking is needed to prevent withdrawal symptoms. Drinking may go
on for days at a time, which is called a
bender. The great majority of alcoholics do
not wind up on "skid row" but instead
struggle with their problem within their families and communities.

(Pierre Brebiette, "The Triumph of
Bacchus," 1630, courtesy The Christian
Brothers Collection, San Francisco.)

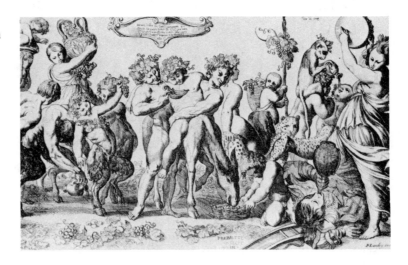

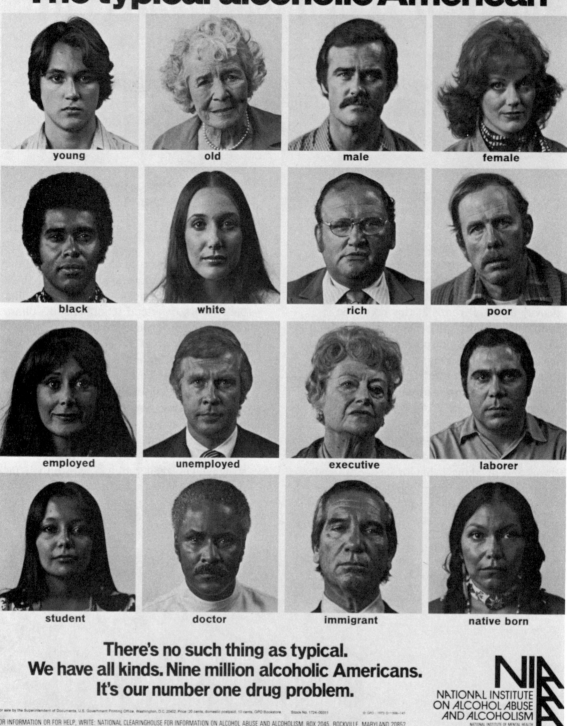

Figure 14-4
This poster demonstrates that there is no such thing as a typical alcoholic. (Courtesy National Institute on Alcohol Abuse and Alcoholism.)

If alcohol is a major public health problem—you could not find this out from watching television.

Lawrence Wallack
Professor, University of California

Alcoholism and the Family

Alcoholism can severely disrupt marriage and family relationships. One family member's drinking problem can stress all the other family members, causing them mental and emotional suffering and sometimes financial hardship. Alcoholism is costly to many persons, not just the alcoholic.

Close relatives of a problem drinker can experience a variety of emotions, ranging from joy and relief when the problem drinker stops drinking for a time to feelings of failure and depression when the problem drinker begins actively drinking again. In between the highs and lows, family members can feel rage, shame, guilt, pity, and constant anxiety. They may try to cope with the situation in different ways.

Some may try to assume responsibility for the problem; others may be blamed for it (scapegoats). Some may withdraw in silence, while others try to maintain their sense of humor. These behaviors are all defense mechanisms against the family's psychological pain.

Like the problem drinker, family members may deny the problem, try to rationalize it, isolate themselves from friends and relatives, and in some cases actually feel responsible for the other's drinking problem. This enabling or protection process keeps the alcoholic from feeling responsible for his or her drinking—which is part of the paradox experienced by families of alcoholics. In their attempts to protect, family members may unwittingly be contributing to the drinking problem and may even protect

Figure 14-5
The largest meeting of Alcoholics Anonymous ever held. About 25,000 AA members, families, and friends from thirty-three countries gathered at the Superdome in New Orleans in 1980 for the organization's forty-fifth anniversary convention. AA's first meeting was held in Akron, Ohio, in 1935, with two people in attendance. They were AA's co-founders, a New York stockbrocker named Bill W. and an Akron physician named Dr. Bob. (Photo courtesy Alcoholics Anonymous.)

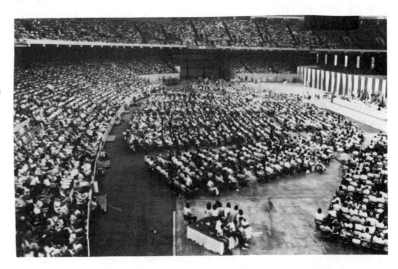

> It ain't what we don't know that gives us trouble.
> It's what we know that ain't so
> that gives us trouble.
> **Will Rogers**

the alcoholic from some of the serious social consequences of drinking too much (such as making excuses for absenteeism from work or school).

Family members of alcoholics may attend Alanon, an organization that helps spouses, families, and friends of alcoholics. Alateen is a similar organization that helps children of alcoholics. Alanon and Alateen help family members understand how alcoholism has affected their lives and help them to explore the family relationships that contribute to the alcoholic problem. Family therapy (with or without the problem drinker's participation) may help a family find ways to cope with the problem and regain a harmonious family life.

Seeking Help

The situation of problem drinkers and alcoholics is serious but not necessarily hopeless. Recovery is possible if the person is strongly motivated to stop drinking. Moreover, as in other aspects of health, "an ounce of prevention is worth a pound of cure." To help you determine whether you have a potential drinking problem, a simple questionnaire is provided at the end of this chapter.

Sometimes the motivation to stop drinking comes in the form of a threat—a drinking-related legal problem, severe disruption of family life, loss of job, or a serious drinking-related illness. The motivation to stop drinking can also come from the person's own resolve to stop his or her self-destructive behavior and to stop feeling helpless, hopeless, and confused.

Alcoholics Anonymous (AA), the worldwide nonprofit self-help organization, has assisted many people to get on the road to wellness and enjoyment of life again. AA bases its program on total sobriety, anonymity, and a step-by-step program of recovery. The environment at AA meetings is relaxing, caring, and open. Members share their experiences, strengths, and hopes with each other, with the goal of helping new and old members identify and learn more about their own problems with alcohol. Practical tips on how to remain sober are shared, and telephone numbers are exchanged so that a member can contact another member if stressful situations arise that previously led to drinking.

Alcoholics Anonymous emphasizes that sobriety is a state of mind, which means that recovering from a drinking problem involves changing values, attitudes, and lifestyles. The AA program helps problem drinkers honestly examine their feelings, recognize their limitations, and accept responsibility for past wrongs. For problem drinkers, remaining sober is an ongoing process, which involves finding new ways to satisfy emotional, spiritual, and environmental needs. Of course, AA may not be the answer for everyone who has a drinking problem. Individual and group psychotherapy with a therapist skilled in helping problem drinkers can also be successful.

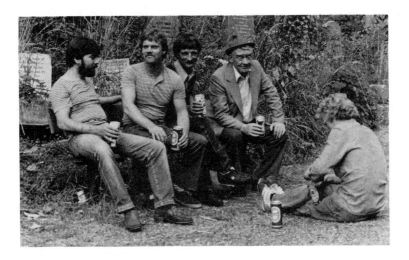

Responsible Drinking

Each person has the option of drinking or abstaining from alcohol. Each of you has responsibility for determining the occasions for drinking and the amounts of alcohol that you consume. If you are one of the millions of people who already enjoy drinking, here are some guidelines to remember:

1. Make sure that alcohol use improves your social interactions and does not harm or destroy them.
2. Drink slowly and avoid mixing alcohol with other drugs.
3. Be sure that using alcohol enhances your general sense of well-being and does not make either you or other persons feel disgusted with your actions.
4. If you plan to drink, decide beforehand that you will not drive and designate someone who will not drink to be the driver.

In addition to being responsible for your own drinking habits, you can also help other people to drink responsibly. Respect the wishes of the person who chooses to abstain from drinking and don't "push" drinks on people at parties. If you are giving a party, be sure to provide alternatives to alcohol. You may also offer places to sleep for those who have been drinking and should not drive home. Remember to eat when you drink and to provide food at parties that you give.

There is no evidence to indicate that abstaining from alcohol use is necessary to health. On the other hand, there is a great deal of evidence showing that excessive alcohol use can destroy personal health and family relationships, can cause traffic deaths and suicides, and can produce birth defects in newborns. We believe that you can significantly improve your health and happiness by developing responsible drinking habits while you are young and maintaining moderate drinking habits throughout life.

Supplemental Readings

Alcoholics Anonymous. *Twelve Steps and Twelve Traditions.* New York: Alcoholics Anonymous World Services, Inc., 1978. Explains the Alcoholics Anonymous way to stop drinking.

Mendelson, Jack H., and **Mello, Nancy K.** *Alcohol: Use and Abuse in America.* Boston: Little, Brown, 1985. A comprehensive treatise on all aspects of alcohol abuse in the United States including its history, sociology, biology, and current methods of understanding and treatment.

Olson, Steve. *Alcohol in America: Taking Action to Prevent Abuse.* Washington, D.C.: National Academy Press, 1985. This book was commissioned by the National Academy of Sciences to make available to the public its 1984 report on preventing alcohol abuse in the United States.

The Whole College Catalogue About Drinking. Washington, D.C.: National Institute on Alcohol Abuse and Alcoholism, 1976. All about drinking problems and their solutions.

Summary

Alcohol abuse is the major drug problem in the United States. Consumption of alcohol is responsible for almost half of all highway fatalities and for numerous social, family, and health problems.

Alcoholic beverages contain ethyl alcohol, which is produced by the action of yeast on sugar (fermentation) in the juices of grains, berries, and fruits. Beer and wine are direct products of fermentation; "hard" liquor, such as whiskey, vodka, rum, and brandy, is made from distilled fermented liquids. Most standard portions of any alcoholic beverage contain ½ ounce of ethyl alcohol.

Alcohol enters the bloodstream within minutes after ingestion. The physical and behavioral effects of alcohol depend on the blood alcohol content (BAC). A BAC of 0.02 produces a "loosening up" effect. A BAC of .10 seriously impairs motor coordination and judgment; in most states it is illegal to drive with a BAC of .10.

Frequent and constant use of alcohol can lead to physical dependence and tolerance to the drug (alcoholism). Alcoholism develops in stages, starting with not being able to control drinking and advancing to complete physical dependence. Alcoholics may encounter severe health problems and their personal lives, and family relationships and friendships may be disrupted.

Organizations such as Alcoholics Anonymous and individual or group psychotherapy can help people recover from problem drinking and alcoholism. Alcohol abuse can be prevented by taking responsibility for one's drinking behavior.

FOR YOUR HEALTH

This questionnaire is designed to help you determine whether you have a problem with alcohol. Answer each question yes or no and record you choice in the right-hand column.

	YES	NO
1. Do you feel you are a normal drinker?	___	___
2. Have you ever awakened the morning after drinking the night before and found that you could not remember a part of the evening before?	___	___

(Continued on next page.)

FOR YOUR HEALTH

	YES	NO
3. Does your wife, husband, a parent, or other near relative ever worry or complain about your drinking?	___	___
4. Can you stop drinking without a struggle after one or two drinks?	___	___
5. Do you ever feel bad about your drinking?	___	___
6. Do friends or relatives think you are a normal drinker?	___	___
7. Do you ever try to limit your drinking to certain times of the day or to certain places?	___	___
8. Are you always able to stop drinking when you want to?	___	___
9. Have you ever attended a meeting of Alcoholics Anonymous?	___	___
10. Have you gotten into fights when drinking?	___	___
11. Has drinking ever created problems between you and your wife, husband, boyfriend, girlfriend, a parent, or other near relative?	___	___
12. Has your wife, husband, boyfriend, girlfriend, a parent, or other near relative ever gone to anyone for help about your drinking?	___	___
13. Have you ever lost friends because of drinking?	___	___
14. Have you ever gotten into trouble at work because of drinking?	___	___
15. Have you ever lost a job because of drinking?	___	___
16. Have you ever neglected your obligations, your family, or your work for two or more days in a row because you were drinking?	___	___
17. Do you drink before noon fairly often?	___	___
18. Have you ever been told you have liver trouble? Cirrhosis?	___	___
19. After heavy drinking have you ever had delirium tremens (DT's) or severe shaking?	___	___
20. After heavy drinking have you ever heard voices or seen things that weren't really there?	___	___
21. Have you ever gone to anyone for help about your drinking?	___	___
22. Have you ever been in a hospital because of drinking?	___	___
23. Have you ever been a patient in a psychiatric hospital or in a psychiatric ward of a general hospital?	___	___
24. Have you ever been in a hospital to be "dried out" (detoxified) because of drinking?	___	___
25. Have you ever been in jail, even for a few hours, because of drunk behavior?	___	___

Scoring: Item keying for alcoholic responses are 1. N; 2. Y; 3. Y; 4. N; 5. Y; 6. N; 7. Y; 8. N; 9–25, Y.

To score, add one point for each alcoholic response. The total score is the number of alcoholic responses.

No. of Alcoholic Responses	Interpretation
0–2	No problem with alcohol
3–5	Early warning signs that drinking is becoming problematic
6 or more	Problem drinker/alcoholic

CHAPTER FIFTEEN

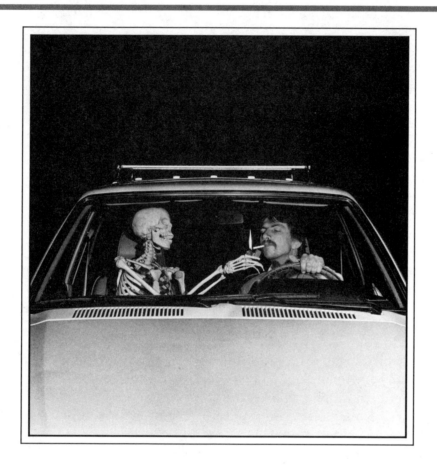

A good thing to give up—
or never start.

Smoking

Cigarette smoking is the single most preventable cause of death.

The U.S. Surgeon General's Report on Health Promotion and Disease Prevention, 1979

In recent years antismoking efforts in this country have increased markedly but America still has a long way to go to become a "smokeless society by the year 2000," a goal of C. Everett Koop, the U.S. Surgeon General. Many towns, cities, and states have enacted legislation prohibiting smoking in public places and have mandated no-smoking areas in restaurants and working areas. Some companies have designated no-smoking areas and have used various incentives to encourage their employees to stop smoking. American society as a whole seems to be moving toward less acceptance of tobacco use and smoking; however, as of 1986 about 50 million Americans still smoked cigarettes.

The health costs of smoking are staggering. Each year about 350,000 Americans die as a direct result of smoking. Almost one-third of all cancer deaths—about 125,000 each year—are caused by smoking. Alan Dershowitz (1986), a professor of law at Harvard University, defends the right of tobacco companies to advertise and sell cigarettes so long as they are legal. But he also says:

> Cigarettes kill, maim, and sicken. Anyone who doubts the truth should have his (and increasingly her) head (and probably lungs) examined. There really is no longer any room for rational debate about the dangers of smoking, both to those who inhale and to those upon whom they exhale.

It is estimated that cigarette smoking costs our society about $26 billion per year in lost manpower and $13 billion in direct medical costs (U.S. Surgeon General, 1984). Yet tobacco companies continue to deny that smoking is harmful and continue to advertise vigorously. In 1984 cigarette companies spent $2.1 billion on advertising; cigarette companies rank first in newspaper advertising and second in magazine advertising (Davis, 1987). Few newspapers or magazines can afford to turn down cigarette ads. The irrationality of tobacco advertising is pointed out by Kenneth E. Walker (1987) of the University of Michigan School of Public Health.

> Ironically, the object of the nation's most expensive marketing campaign is also the only legal product that is hazardous when used as intended. It is the leading cause of premature death, a product so pervasive and lethal that is causes more

> Ninety percent of the 149,000 people
> who will have lung cancer in the U.S.
> in 1986 will die of their disease.
>
> **National Cancer Institute**

deaths than the combined total caused by all illicit drugs and alcohol, all accidents, and all homicides and suicides.

More and more people realize that the time has come to ban cigarettes and smoking despite personal motivations or economic hardship (tobacco-growing regions of the country will suffer). The consequences to health justify the statement by Richard Peto (1985), a renowned epidemiologist: "The reason one wants to prevent smoking is not just because it is dangerous — lots of things are dangerous — but because it is *so* dangerous." In this chapter we discuss the facts about smoking and its health hazards. We will also attempt to alert you to the dangers of smokeless tobacco and to the blandishments of tobacco advertising.

Tobacco

The use of tobacco in our culture probably originated with the introduction of tobacco smoking in sixteenth-century Europe by Spanish sailors returning from voyages to the New World. Apparently the sailors had learned about smoking from American Indians who used tobacco in much the same way it is used today. In fact, the word "tobacco" is an Indian word signifying the pipe used to smoke the minced or rolled leaf of the tobacco plant.

The smoking habit spread quickly in Europe, fueled by tobacco imports from Spain's New World colonies. By the nineteenth century, changing social customs had caused smoking to be largely replaced by tobacco chewing — and by the even more popular habit of sniffing it in the form of snuff. It wasn't until the 1880s, when the cigarette-making machine was invented in the United States, that cigarette smoking became an increasingly popular habit among the people of the world. Today about 3 trillion cigarettes are smoked worldwide each year and in the United States, the number of cigarettes smoked annually is about 600 billion.

Tobacco used for smoking, chewing, or snuff is a processed product of the leaves of the plant *Nicotiana tabacum*. This plant is indigenous to the Western Hemisphere, where it grows best in semitropical climates. Since its discovery by European explorers, it has come to be cultivated in many regions of the world. In the United States tobacco is grown primarily in thirteen states, and the tobacco industry is vital to their economies.

The preparation of tobacco for consumption involves harvesting the tobacco leaves and curing them by any one of several drying methods. The cured tobacco leaves are shredded, and various strains of leaves are blended to give whatever mixture is commercially desirable. Often flavorings and colorings are added to enhance the tobacco mixture's desirability, as well as chemicals that facilitate even burning. Finally, the mixture is used to manufacture cigarettes, pipe tobacco, and chewing tobacco or is wrapped in specially cured tobacco leaves to make cigars.

The most familiar chemical constituent of tobacco is **nicotine,** but when tobacco is burned, approximately 4000 other chemical substances are released and carried in the smoke — including acetone, acrolein, carbon monoxide, methanol, ammonia, nitrous dioxide, hydrogen sulfide, traces of various mineral elements, traces of radioactive elements, acids, insecticides, and other substances (see Table 15-1). Besides these chemical compounds, tobacco smoke also contains countless microscopic particles that contribute to the yellowish brown residue of tobacco smoke known as **tar**.

Most of the physiological effects of tobacco smoking are attributable to the pharmacological effects of nicotine. The most prominent effects include increased heart rate, increased release of adrenalin, and a direct stimulatory effect on the brain. These effects combine to produce the "rush" cigarette smokers experience when they light up. Nicotine is also responsible for the nausea and vomiting experienced by most beginning smokers. Habituation to nicotine is probably responsible for the perpetuation of many a smoker's habit, either by causing a psychological dependence—a wish to experience the immediate psychological effects of the drug—or by causing actual physiological dependence (addiction).

The harmful effects of cigarette smoking probably come from nicotine and carbon monoxide, which are thought to contribute to the development of heart and blood vessel disease (Kaufman, 1983), and from a host of other chemicals that contribute to the development of cancer and diseases of the respiratory tract. Among these chemicals are benzo(a)pyrene, aza-arenes, N-nitrosamines, the

radioactive isotope of the element polonium (^{210}Po), and the radioactive isotope radon with its decay products, known as "radon daughters." Polonium-210 is a product of the breakdown of radioactive lead-210 (^{210}Pb), a natural constituent of soil. Radioactive particles in the soil become deposited on sticky tobacco leaf hairs and eventually become part of tobacco smoke. Radon and radon daughters are present in soil and building materials and from these sources condense on airborne particles in tobacco smoke that is inhaled.

Smokeless Tobaccos

An alternative to smoking cigarettes that has gained popularity in recent years is the use of smokeless tobaccos such as snuff and chewing tobacco. This form of tobacco is used by placing a pinch of snuff or plug of chewing tobacco in the mouth. The tobacco mixes with saliva and the nicotine and other chemicals are absorbed into the bloodsteam. Dr. Gregory N. Connolly (1986) and other researchers have concluded that smokeless tobacco causes oral-pharyngeal cancer and is associated with cancers of other organs as well. Despite what tobacco companies say, smokeless tobaccos are not safe.

In 1986 Congress passed a law banning TV advertising of smokeless tobaccos (cigarette advertising was previously banned on TV). Congress also required companies to put warning labels on pack-

Table 15-1
A Partial List of Chemical Substances in Cigarettes

Aromatic hydrocarbons	Radioisotopes	Phenols	Insecticides
Benzo[*a*]pyrene	Polonium-210	Phenol	Arsenic
Dibenz[*a,h*]anthracene	Radium-226	*o*-Cresol	DDT
Dibenzo[*a,l*]pyrene	Radon-222	*m* + *p*-Cresol	TDE
Dibenzo[*a,i*]pyrene	Potassium-40	Dimethyl phenols	Endrin
Chrysene	**Aldehydes and ketones**	**Acids**	**Fungicides**
Methylbenzo[*a*]pyrene	Formaldehyde	Formic acid	Dithiocarbamates
Methylchrysene	Acrolein	Acetic acid	**Vapor phase components**
N-Nitrosamines	Crotonaldehyde	Propionic acid	Hydrogen cyanide
Diethylnitrosamine	**Esters and alcohols**	Lauric acid	
Methyl-*n*-butylnitrosamine	Solanesol		
Nitrosopiperidine	Phytosterol		
Nitrosopyrrolidine	Phytol		
Other nitrosamines	Oleic alcohol		
	Long-chain unsaturated alcohols		

Adapted from E. Wynder and D. Hoffman, *Tobacco and Tobacco Smoke* (New York: Academic Press, 1967).

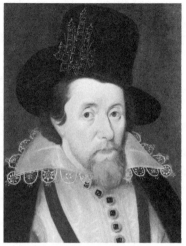 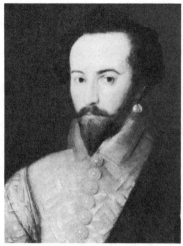

Figure 15-1

"A custom loathsome to the eye, hateful to the nose, harmful to the braine, dangerous to the lungs, and in the blacke, stinking fume thereof, nearest resembling the horrible Stigian smoke of the pit that is bottomlesse." So concluded James I of England in his *Counterblaste to Tobacco,* published in 1604. Sir Walter Raleigh had promoted and popularized the habit of smoking in the court of Queen Elizabeth of England in the late sixteenth century. But James I, who became king when Elizabeth died in 1603, was strongly opposed to the habit. He eventually had Raleigh beheaded for political reasons, but perhaps Raleigh had also smoked too much in the king's presence. (Courtesy National Portrait Gallery, London.)

ages. Despite these efforts, the use of smokeless tobaccos has increased markedly in recent years due to advertising and people's belief that chewing tobacco is less dangerous than smoking it.

Sales of snuff rose from 23 to 37 million pounds between 1978 and 1984. During the same period sales of chewing tobacco increased from 80 to 87 million pounds. Unfortunately the increase has occurred largely among teenage boys. Surveys show that from 8 to 36 percent of high school males use smokeless tobacco; one study showed that more than 10 percent of eight- and nine-year-olds were using it.

Besides causing various kinds of cancer, smokeless tobaccos cause other less serious diseases of the mouth, such as the occurrence of hard white patches (**leukoplakia**) and inflammatory lesions of the gum (**gingivitis**). Some users show a marked increase in blood pressure, which is a major factor in heart disease (see Chapter 16). There is good evidence that smokeless tobacco products produce dependence on and possibly addiction to nicotine. Smokeless tobacco ads have been all too succesful in getting a young, suggestible group to use these dangerous products.

Smoking and Illness

Almost from the very beginning of tobacco's use in Europe and colonial America, people have been concerned about the possible harmful effects of smoking (see Figure 15-1). Several articles in the medical literature of the eighteenth and nineteenth centuries claimed that tobacco smoking is a cause of cancer of the lip, tongue, and lung. Twentieth-century research into the health consequences of cigarette smoking has provided widely accepted evidence that among smokers as a group the incidence of certain diseases is greater—sometimes very much greater—than among people who do not smoke. Smoking is cited as a factor in the development of coronary artery disease, lung cancer, bronchitis, emphysema, cancer of the larynx, lip, and oral cavity, cancer of the bladder and stomach, duodenal ulcer, and allergies (Surgeon General, 1979b).

An enormous amount of data demonstrates that the death rate from causes such as cancer, heart disease, and respiratory diseases is higher among cigarette smokers than among nonsmokers (see Figure 15-2). The data also show that the death rate

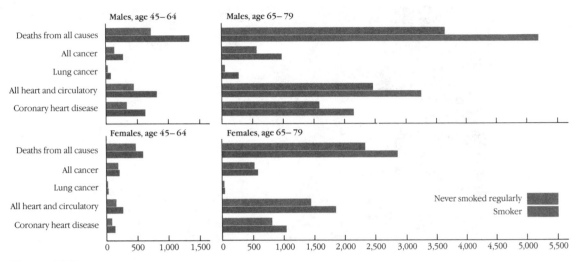

Figure 15-2
Death rates per 100,000 population of smokers versus nonsmokers.
(Data from National Cancer Institute Monograph No. 19.)

for smokers is greater than for nonsmokers whatever the listed cause of death. The death rate from lung cancer for adult male smokers is 8 to 10 times that for nonsmokers. For heart disease, the death rate for smokers is almost twice that for those who do not smoke. Although the data vary somewhat for adult women, a similar pattern is nevertheless observable.

Other studies indicate that babies born to mothers who smoke have lower birth weights than babies born to nonsmoking mothers and that smokers' babies show a higher risk of dying early in infancy. There is also evidence that pregnant women who smoke are more likely to have spontaneous abortions than those who do not. A father who smokes a pack a day risks having his baby's weight reduced by over 4 ounces at birth.

One feature that emerges from all these studies is the risk of developing smoking-related diseases and other complications depends in part on the nature as well as the extent of exposure to tobacco smoke. For example, pipe and cigar smokers show an incidence of death and disease for the smoking-related illnessess somewhere between that for cigarette smokers and nonsmokers—presumably because pipe and cigar smokers inhale less smoke than cigarette smokers. Light smokers (4 to 10 cigarettes per day) are at less risk than heavy smokers (more than 25 cigarettes per day). The mortality rates for heart disease and cancer for those who stop smoking for 15 years are about the same for nonsmokers.

Cessation of smoking also improves breathing and reduces the chance of premature death from noncancerous respiratory disease.

Smokers' apparent concern for their health has produced a tremendous demand for low-tar/low-nicotine cigarettes. Approximately 60 percent of all the cigarettes now sold in North America are of the "low-yield" variety. Whereas the use of low-tar/low-nicotine cigarettes may reduce somewhat the risk of developing lung cancer, smoking these kinds of cigarettes apparently does not lessen the risk of developing heart disease (Rickert, 1983). One principal reason for this is that smokers of low-yield cigarettes change their smoking behavior: They increase the depth of inhalation, increase the frequency of puffing, increase the time that smoke is held in the lungs, and increase the number of cigarettes consumed. Consequently, smokers of low-nicotine cigarettes do not consume less nicotine than smokers of brands with a higher nicotine yield (Benowitz et al., 1983), and they also increase their consumption of other constituents of tobacco smoke, including carcinogens and tar.

Lung Cancer

Lung cancer has long been the most common form of cancer among men and, in recent years, among women also. In 1986 approximately 125,000 persons died of lung cancer in the United States. The num-

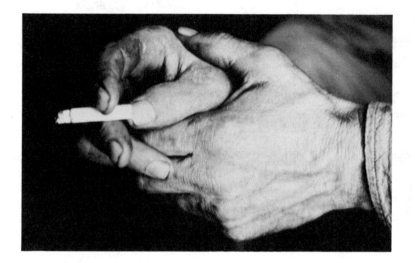

ber of men dying of lung cancer has increased steadily since 1940 (see Figure 15-3). While the rate of increase among men is beginning to decline (fewer men are smoking cigarettes), the increase in lung cancer among women is still rising (more women are smoking cigarettes). In 1984, for the first time in U.S. history, lung cancer surpassed breast cancer as the leading cancer-related cause of death in women.

As shown in Figure 15-4, the increase in lung cancer deaths is the principal reason that the overall death rate from cancer continues to increase. If lung cancer death rates are excluded from the statistics, the actual death rate from cancer has been falling steadily for many years, principally because of preventive efforts and improved diagnosis and treatment of cancers not associated with cigarette smoking. This situation is ironic as well as tragic, for lung cancer is one of the most preventable of all diseases. People simply need to stop smoking cigarettes.

It should be noted that not all lung cancer deaths are attributable to cigarette smoking. The data suggest that about 80 percent of lung cancer deaths are related to smoking; the other 20 percent may be due to any number of environmental factors, including air pollution (some studies indicate that twice as many city dwellers die of lung cancer than do people who live in rural areas) and airborne substances encountered in work environments such as particles of chromate, iron, or asbestos.

A full biological explanation of how smoking causes lung cancer (and contributes to cancer in other body sites) is not yet available. A number of known **carcinogens**—cancer-causing chemicals—are found in tobacco smoke, and it is thought that they are at least partly responsible for the onset of the cellular changes leading to the disease. For example, some evidence suggests that lung cancer may

Figure 15-3
Lung cancer rates per 100,000 population in the United States. (Data from U.S. National Center for Health Statistics and U.S. Bureau of the Census.)

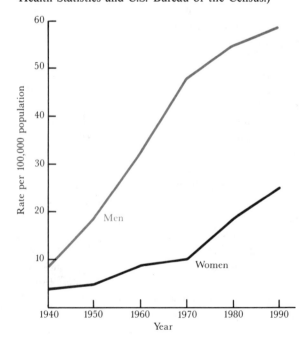

> Of the 12,000 lung cancer deaths in 1985 among nonsmokers, over 2400 were caused by environmental tobacco smoke.
>
> **James Robins**
> **Harvard School of Public Health**

be caused by deposition of radioactive particles such as polonium-210, radon, or radon daughters in lung tissues (Martell, 1983). These radioactive elements, which are known to be present in tobacco smoke, become trapped in the lungs and accumulate over the years. The long-term exposure to the radioactivity at specific sites in the lungs may eventually trigger the conversion of normal cells into cancer cells (see Chapter 17). Transfer of the radioactive particles or of cancer cells to other parts of the body could also account for the increased risk smokers have of developing cancers in other organs as well.

Bronchitis and Emphysema

Bronchitis and emphysema are respiratory diseases that are sometimes classified along with asthma as **chronic obstructive pulmonary diseases (COPD)**. Each of these maladies is associated with difficulty in breathing caused by obstruction of some part of the respiratory system. Often persons suffer from more than one of these conditions at the same time.

Bronchitis is an inflammatory condition of the upper part of the respiratory tract, principally the trachea or the larger bronchial airways. It is characterized by an excessive production of mucus by cells that line the airways, which is the cause of the major symptoms of bronchitis—a continual cough (smoker's cough) and the production of large amounts of sputum. Some affected people also experience shortness of breath, particularly during exertion.

Unquestionably, smoking is a factor in the development of chronic bronchitis, although air pollution and the breathing of hazardous chemicals and particles encountered in certain occupations are also suspected of contributing to it. Apparently the excessive production of mucus by the glands of the bronchi is a reaction to the irritation caused by cigarette smoke and other air pollutants.

Fortunately, the pathology that produces the symptoms of bronchitis can be almost completely reversed by giving up smoking, reducing one's exposure to polluted air, or both. It is not uncommon, however, for people to "live with" their persistent

Figure 15-4
Death rates per 100,000 population from all cancers, lung cancer, and all cancers other than lung cancer 1950–1978. (From "Health Consequences of Smoking Cancer." U.S. Department of Health and Human Services, 1982.)

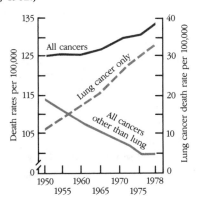

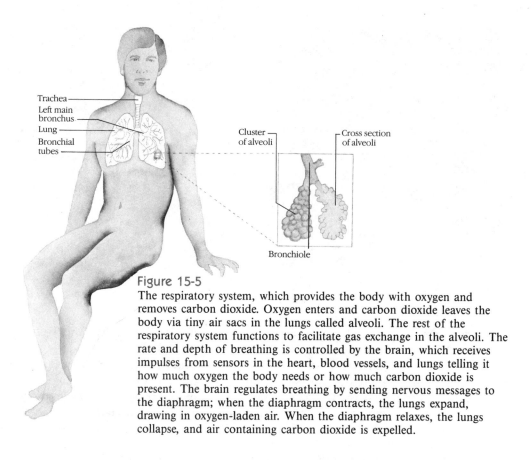

Trachea
Left main bronchus
Lung
Bronchial tubes

Cluster of alveoli
Cross section of alveoli

Bronchiole

Figure 15-5
The respiratory system, which provides the body with oxygen and removes carbon dioxide. Oxygen enters and carbon dioxide leaves the body via tiny air sacs in the lungs called alveoli. The rest of the respiratory system functions to facilitate gas exchange in the alveoli. The rate and depth of breathing is controlled by the brain, which receives impulses from sensors in the heart, blood vessels, and lungs telling it how much oxygen the body needs or how much carbon dioxide is present. The brain regulates breathing by sending nervous messages to the diaphragm; when the diaphragm contracts, the lungs expand, drawing in oxygen-laden air. When the diaphragm relaxes, the lungs collapse, and air containing carbon dioxide is expelled.

cough for many years and not be concerned with the message their body is giving them. If the disease is left to run its course, the person increases his or her vulnerability to developing other respiratory illnesses, and the airways may become irreversibly blocked.

Emphysema is the result of the destruction of the tiny air sacs deep in the lungs called **alveoli** (see Figure 15-5). Each lung contains millions of alveoli. It is across their thin membranes that the function of breathing is accomplished—the exchange of the respiratory gases, oxygen and carbon dioxide.

Upon inhaling, about 500 ml of air (which is 20 percent oxygen) flows through the nose and mouth into the trachea and bronchial tubes to the lungs, where it fills the approximately 300 million alveoli. Oxygen diffuses through the membranes of the alveoli into tiny blood vessels in the lung tissue. Having entered the bloodstream, it is carried by red blood cells throughout the body, where it is used to provide energy for cellular activities. One of the by-products of cellular energy production is carbon

dioxide, which is carried by the blood to the lungs, where it diffuses into the alveoli and is eliminated from the body upon exhalation.

When the alveoli become destroyed in emphysema, they lose their shape and become distended with trapped air, which ultimately results in the impairment of gas exchange. Emphysema involves a slow, irreversible process of alveoli destruction; thus, as the disease progresses, affected people have greater and greater trouble breathing.

As with lung cancer, the exact mechanism by which tobacco smoking or air pollution contributes to emphysema is still under investigation. One hypothesis suggests that body cells in the lung normally engaged in the destruction of material foreign to the body (macrophage and leukocyte cells produced by the immune system, discussed in Chapter 9) release large amounts of destructive enzymes in response to the presence of respiratory pollutants, and these enzymes inadvertently destroy lung tissue, thereby causing emphysema. Normally, a protein in the blood called alpha-one-antitrypsin, or AAT, in-

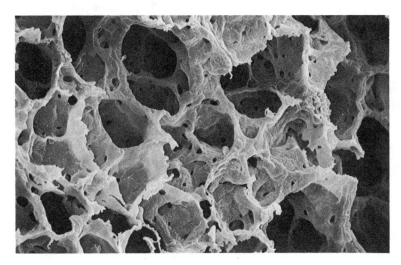

Figure 15-6
Photomicrograph of alveoli in a normal lung. (Photo courtesy Lawrence Berkeley Laboratories.)

hibits the destructive enzymes. Some studies have shown that people with emphysema have low levels of AAT, either because of genetic factors that may increase their susceptibility to emphysema or because of some as yet unknown correlation between respiratory pollution and the impaired production of AAT.

Tobacco Smoke's Effects on Nonsmokers

Many people are surprised to learn that nonsmokers who are exposed to tobacco smoke run some health risk as well. People who work or live in environments that are heavily laden with tobacco smoke inhale the same smoke-borne substances as do smokers. In fact, about two-thirds of the smoke from a burning cigarette enters the environment, and anyone who has been in a roomful of smokers can attest that such an environment is considerably more polluted than the worst smoggy day in a big city. A nonsmoker in a smoke-filled room can inhale in one hour the equivalent of a cigarette's worth of nicotine, carbon monoxide, and other substances. Many people are allergic to tobacco smoke, and such an environment can bring about eye irritation, headache, cough, nasal congestion, and asthma. Nonsmokers forced to inhale tobacco smoke for long periods of time, such as those who work in enclosed work environments routinely filled with tobacco smoke, can suffer impairment of lung func-

tion equivalent to smokers who inhale 10 cigarettes a day (White and Froeb, 1980). A study of the risks of passive smoking among Japanese adults found that the wives of men who smoked had a one-third higher cancer mortality rate as compared to wives of nonsmoking men (Hirayama, 1981).

Passive cigarette smoking can also affect children. Studies have shown that the children of parents who smoke are more prone to bronchitis, episodes of pneumonia, chronic cough, more missed school days, and more hospital admissions (Weiss, 1983). Substances in tobacco smoke have been found in the urine of infants whose parents smoke (Greenberg et al., 1984). Maternal cigarette smoking has been shown to hinder the development of the lungs of children and to impair respiratory function, which may predispose these children to respiratory illnesses later in life (Tager et al., 1983).

Following an exhaustive review of all the evidence for and against the effects of passive smoke on health, the 1986 Surgeon General's report concluded that involuntary smoking *is* a cause of disease and that "it is certain" that some nonsmokers' lung cancers are caused by exposure to tobacco smoke. Despite numerous studies demonstrating the harmful effects of passive smoke, the Tobacco Institute steadfastly maintains that "proof of harm to nonsmokers from passive smoking remains as wispy as cigarette smoke itself" (Stapf, 1987). We believe that a smoke-free environment will benefit both nonsmokers and the millions who desire to quit smoking.

> The ongoing epidemic of smoking has taught us that prevention as a strategy is particularly hard to sell as long as treatment and cure are bandied about as alternatives, so we must be very sure not to dilute the message with false or distant hopes.
>
> June E. Osborn, M.D.

Why People Smoke

Most people begin to smoke in their teenage years, emulating parents or celebrities who smoke. Teenagers also smoke to attain acceptance in their peer group. About half of the people who experiment with smoking continue the habit into adulthood. There must be some very compelling reasons that people continue to smoke despite the unpleasant taste, the initial adverse physiological reactions to smoke and nicotine, and the knowledge—now widespread—that tobacco smoke can cause serious, even life-threatening, illness.

The reasons people give for smoking are many and varied. According to the American Cancer Society, however, the motivations of smokers can be grouped into six general categories:

1. *Stimulation*—some people experience a psychological lift from smoking. They say that smoking helps them to wake up in the morning and organize their energies. They often report that smoking increases their intellectual capacities.
2. *Handling*—some people enjoy the mere handling of cigarettes and smoking paraphernalia, such as lighters.
3. *Pleasurable relaxation*—some smokers say they smoke simply because they like it. Smoking brings them true pleasure and is often practiced to enhance other pleasurable sensations, such as the taste of a good meal.
4. *Reducing negative feelings* (crutch)—approximately one-third of smokers say they smoke because it helps them deal with stress, anger, fear, anxiety, or pressure.
5. *Craving*—some people crave cigarettes and have no other explanation for their habit other than they have frequent needs to smoke, irrespective of the pleasurable or tension-relieving effects that smoking might bring.
6. *Habit*—some smokers light up only because of habit. They no longer receive much physical or psychological gratification from smoking; they often smoke without being aware of whether or not they really want the cigarette.

The American Cancer Society has developed a self-administered test to help smokers determine their strongest motives for smoking (see Box 15-1).

The question that still eludes a definitive answer is: What distinguishes people who smoke from those who do not? The list of suggested answers includes a biological susceptibility to dependence on nicotine, a variety of personality and sociological traits, and a need for an effective way to deal with stress. There may be as many reasons as there are smokers. Whatever the case, people smoke because they want to. Many biological, psychological, and sociological explanations of smoking behavior have been offered by various researchers, but in the final analysis, smoking—like any other habitual, non-life-supporting behavior—is a matter of choice.

BOX 15-1

WHY DO YOU SMOKE?

Here are some statements made by people to describe what they get out of smoking cigarettes. How often do you feel this way when smoking? Circle one number for each statement.

Important: Answer every question.

	Always	Frequently	Occasionally	Seldom	Never
A. I smoke cigarettes in order to keep myself from slowing down.	5	4	3	2	1
B. Handling a cigarette is part of the enjoyment of smoking it.	5	4	3	2	1
C. Smoking cigarettes is pleasant and relaxing.	5	4	3	2	1
D. I light up a cigarette when I feel angry about something.	5	4	3	2	1
E. When I have run out of cigarettes I find it almost unbearable until I can get them.	5	4	3	2	1
F. I smoke cigarettes automatically without even being aware of it.	5	4	3	2	1
G. I smoke cigarettes to stimulate me, to perk myself up.	5	4	3	2	1
H. Part of the enjoyment of smoking a cigarette comes from the steps I take to light up.	5	4	3	2	1
I. I find cigarettes pleasurable.	5	4	3	2	1
J. When I feel uncomfortable or upset about something, I light up a cigarette.	5	4	3	2	1
K. I am very much aware of the fact when I am not smoking a cigarette.	5	4	3	2	1
L. I light up a cigarette without realizing I still have one burning in the ashtray.	5	4	3	2	1
M. I smoke cigarettes to give me a "lift."	5	4	3	2	1
N. When I smoke a cigarette, part of the enjoyment is watching the smoke as I exhale it.	5	4	3	2	1
O. I want a cigarette most when I am comfortable and relaxed.	5	4	3	2	1
P. When I feel "blue" or want to take my mind off cares and worries, I smoke cigarettes.	5	4	3	2	1
Q. I get a real gnawing hunger for a cigarette when I haven't smoked for a while.	5	4	3	2	1
R. I've found a cigarette in my mouth and didn't remember putting it there.	5	4	3	2	1

(Continued on next page.)

BOX 15-1 (Continued)

How to Score

1. Enter the numbers you have circled in the spaces below, putting the number you have circled to Question A over line A, to Question B over line B, etc.

2. Add the three scores on each line to get your totals. For example, the sum of your scores over lines A, G, and M gives you your score on *Stimulation,* lines B, H, and N give the score on *Handling,* and so on.

Totals

_____ A	+	_____ G	+ _____ M =	_____ Stimulation
_____ B	+	_____ H	+ _____ N =	_____ Handling
_____ C	+	_____ I	+ _____ O =	_____ Pleasurable relaxation
_____ D	+	_____ J	+ _____ P =	_____ Crutch: tension reduction
_____ E	+	_____ K	+ _____ Q =	_____ Craving: psychological addiction
_____ F	+	_____ L	+ _____ R =	_____ Habit

Scores of 11 or above indicate that this factor is an important source of satisfaction for the smoker. Scores of 7 or less are low and probably indicate that this factor does not apply to you. Scores in between are marginal.

Smoker's Self-testing Kit developed by Daniel Horn, Ph.D. Originally published by National Clearinghouse for Smoking and Health, Department of Health, Education, and Welfare.

Quitting

There's an old joke among smokers: "It's easy to quit. I've done it over fifty times!"

Each year millions of smokers try to kick their habit. The major problem they face, as the little joke recognizes, is that stopping for awhile is not nearly as difficult as permanently eliminating the habit. Each year, however, thousands of people successfully quit smoking. They do so for a variety of reasons: to reduce the risk of early death from heart or lung disease, to enjoy once again the unpolluted taste of food, to please nonsmoking loved ones, to eliminate the ever-present ashes and smell of cigarette smoke from the house, and to fulfill a simple commitment to get healthy. Frequently a positive change in other aspects of one's lifestyle leads to an unplanned cessation of smoking. For example, many people who take up meditation, t'ai chi ch'uan, jogging, or other physical activity automatically stop smoking. They simply lose the desire to smoke cigarettes.

In recent years many psychologists and human behavior specialists have been involved in a search for a "quitter's magic bullet"—a single therapeutic approach that will help people stop smoking, not only during the several weeks of the treatment, or the six months to a year after the treatment has stopped, but for the rest of their lives.

There are now a dozen or more different therapeutic strategies to help people stop smoking. Often these strategies are applied in special smoking clinics, where smokers are exposed to health information, encouragement, moral support, social pressure, and suggestions about how to resist the temptation to light up.

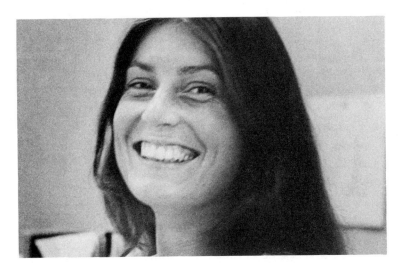

Figure 15-7
Confession of an ex-smoker: "Quitting was my New Year's resolution. I tore up my pack of cigarettes and threw them in the fireplace and haven't smoked a cigarette since. I'd been smoking a pack to a pack and a half for about 5 years. Both my parents smoked; everybody I knew smoked. I got hooked when I was 13. I had tried to quit several times before this one, but not bad enough. I really wanted to quit this time because I was really sick of smoking, and I had a cough that kept getting worse and worse. As soon as I quit, my cough went away. I would never smoke cigarettes again."

A chemically based therapy makes use of the idea that people smoke because they are addicted to the effects of nicotine. Thus, the therapy provides smokers with nicotine or a nicotine-like drug that satisfies their dependence on nicotine while eliminating the tar and other harmful chemicals in tobacco smoke from their system.

Still other therapies are based on the idea that smoking is a response to personal stress—and so stress-reduction techniques such as meditation and biofeedback are employed to give the smoker another, healthier way to deal with stress.

Some basic tips for smokers who want to quit are presented in Box 15-2. Whatever the specific technique, most people involved in helping smokers quit agree that the major factor in stopping smoking is the personal resolve of the smoker to do so (Schwartz, 1978). There is no quitter's magic bullet. No single therapeutic technique in itself stops the smoking habit. This does not mean that smokers have to exercise will power or employ unusual behaviors like putting money in a piggy bank each time they resist the urge to smoke. Such artificial practices rarely stop smoking permanently. Successful elimination of the smoking habit can be accomplished by becoming aware of one's personal motives for smoking. It is possible to reprogram the mind to eliminate the thoughts and behaviors that lead to smoking. A person can then integrate positive and rewarding activities, thoughts, and feelings in place of those that lead to smoking. In so doing, people stop smoking because they feel good without having to smoke, and in fact, feel better by not smoking at all.

The War of Words Between the Pros and the Antis

There exists a long-standing war of words between antismoking groups (most notably the American Cancer Society and The American Heart Association) and the tobacco industry (tobacco growers and other businesses involved in the production and sale of smoking products). At stake are the loyalties of millions of smokers and prospective smokers. The health groups try to persuade these people not to smoke; the tobacco industry encourages them to smoke more and more. Legal experts such as Alan Dershowitz (1986) reluctantly concluded that, "in the end, the cigarette industry's right to free speech may well cost lives. The First Amendment requires us all to tolerate views we find offensive as the price of being able to present views we deem essential."

The medical war of words takes place in relative obscurity compared with the propagandizing carried on in the form of advertising. Each year the tobacco industry spends hundreds of millions of dollars to promote its products and to recruit smokers. Perusal of many major magazines and newspapers reveals that cigarette advertising relies heavily on imagery that portrays smoking as healthful and enjoyable and smokers as attractive, sexy,

> In the operating room, the surgeon sees, all too often, the triumph of the cigarette maker's art. My operating room could aptly be called "Marlboro Country" indeed.
>
> **William Cahan, M.D.**

slim, and of high social status (see Box 15-3). Most magazines depend heavily on the financial rewards of cigarette advertising. When cigarette advertising was banned from radio and television in 1970, tobacco companies actually increased their advertising budgets and began spending hundreds of millions of dollars on newspaper and magazine ads. They also developed costly promotional campaigns (such as the Virginia Slims Tennis Tournament) that attempt to associate smoking cigarettes with health, fun, and fitness. Tobacco companies began to support health research, exotic travel excursions, rock concerts, and major athletic events to promote the virtues of smoking. To combat this promotional blitz by the tobacco industry, antismoking groups put forth hundreds of messages each year about the health consequences of smoking, using not only the printed media but also radio and television.

In other parts of the world, particularly the developing countries of Africa and Asia, cigarette advertising is having an enormous impact. In Africa, for example, per capita cigarette consumption in the 1970s increased 33 percent. Many Third World governments do not warn their citizens of the health risks of smoking, and some are in economic partnership with tobacco companies. If this trend continues, the World Health Organization fears that "smoking disease will appear in developing countries before communicable disease and malnutrition have been controlled, and the gap between the rich and poor countries will thus be further widened."

People would benefit if the land and resources used for the cultivation of tobacco were used to grow food crops, and if the desire to eradicate worldwide hunger were as important to governments and corporations as the promotion of tobacco use.

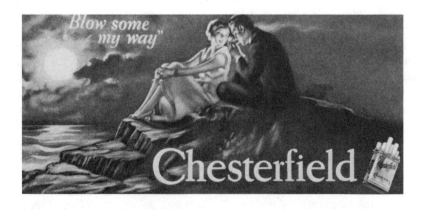

The federal government plays a predictably paradoxical role in the war of words. It supports both sides. Through the Department of Agriculture, the government provides price supports and other financial aids to tobacco growers and other members of the tobacco industry. Through the Public Health Service the government supports antismoking educational programs and finances research into the health effects of smoking. Given the pluralistic nature of our governmental system, one could hardly expect anything else, which points up once again that it would be foolish to depend entirely on the federal government—or on any other organization—to be the guardian of your personal health.

BOX 15-2

TIPS FOR SMOKERS WHO WANT TO QUIT

When Thinking About Quitting . . .

1. List all the reasons you want to stop smoking.
2. Keep a diary of the times of the day and the circumstances of your smoking behavior. Be particularly mindful of your feelings that lead you to light up.
3. Tell your family and friends you are going to quit and ask for their support.
4. Switch to a brand of cigarettes you dislike. Try not to smoke two packs of the same brand in a row.

Cut Down the Number of Cigarettes You Smoke

1. Smoke only half of each cigarette.
2. Don't smoke when you first experience a craving. Wait several minutes. During this time change your activity or talk to someone.
3. Do not buy cigarettes by the carton. Wait until one pack is empty before buying another.
4. Make cigarettes difficult to get. Don't carry them with you.

5. Don't smoke automatically. Smoke only when you really *want* to.
6. Reward yourself in some way other than smoking.
7. Reach for a glass of juice instead of a cigarette for a pick-me-up.

Immediately After Quitting

1. Whenever you feel uncomfortable sensations from having stopped smoking, remind yourself that they are signs of your body's return to health and that they will soon pass.
2. If you miss the sensation of having a cigarette in your hand, play with something else—a pencil, a paper clip, a marble.
3. Instead of smoking after meals, get up from the table and brush your teeth or go for a walk.
4. Temporarily avoid situations you strongly associate with the pleasurable acts of smoking.

5. Develop a clean, fresh nonsmoking environment around yourself—at work and at home.
6. Until you are confident of your ability to stay off cigarettes, limit your socializing to healthful, outdoor activities or to situations in which smoking is prohibited.
7. Look at cigarette ads more critically. Remind yourself that cigarette companies are making money at the expense of your health and well-being.

Find New Habits

1. Change your habits to make smoking difficult and unnecessary.
2. Keep a clean-tasting mouth.
3. Substitute relaxation and deep breathing for stressful situations.
4. Absorb yourself in activities that are meaningful to you.
5. Never allow yourself to think that "one won't hurt"—it will!

Based on *Calling It Quits,* U.S. Department of Health, Education, and Welfare Publication No. (NIH) 79–1824.

BOX 15-3

WOMEN AND CIGARETTE ADVERTISING

For over 50 years tobacco companies have tried to entice women to smoke cigarettes by emphasizing sexiness, slimness, elegance, and fun in advertisements. (The Lucky Strike ad is from 1931; the other ad is from the 1980s.) The success of such ads over the years in getting women to smoke is borne out by the current number of lung cancer deaths among women who smoke. Currently about 23 million American women smoke cigarettes. Between 1935 and 1983 the percentage of women who smoked increased from 18 percent of all women to 30 percent. (During the same interval the percentage of men who smoked actually decreased from 52 to 35 percent.)

The female group that increased its smoking most dramatically in 1986 was white women in their twenties. In 1983 tobacco companies spent $329 million on advertising cigarette brands designed exclusively for women.

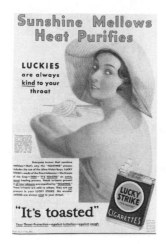

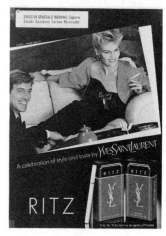

As one observer put it: "The cigarette industry has mastered the art of sending the subliminal message to the susceptible consumer."

In 1985 about 40,000 women died from cigarette-caused lung cancer. Lung cancer has surpassed breast cancer as the leading cause of cancer deaths among women. Smoking also increases women's chances for heart disease and cervical cancer. And if that's not

enough, the beauty editor of *Harper's* magazine points out that "smokers' skin wrinkles up to 10 years sooner than that of nonsmokers." Not believing cigarette ads and not smoking are the individual's responsibility. As long as tobacco is legal companies have a right to advertise. You also have the right to not smoke, which is one of the single most important health decisions you can make.

Supplemental Readings

Blum, Alan, ed. *The Cigarette Underworld—A Front Line Report on the War Against Your Lungs.* New York: Lyle Stuart, 1985. An exposé of the tobacco industry.

Ferguson, T. "The Best Bet Yet for Worried Smokers." *Prevention,* June 1987. Describes how to kick the smoking habit by using nicotine gum.

Fielding, Jonathan E. "Smoking: Health Effects and Control." *The New England Journal of Medicine,* 313 (1985), 491–498 and 555–562. Two excellent articles that discuss the medical and social consequences of smoking.

Inglehart, J. K. "Smoking and Public Policy" and "The Campaign Against Smoking Gains Momentum." *The New England Journal of Medicine,* February 23, 1984, and April 17, 1986. A discussion of the politics and policies involved in antismoking campaigns and legislation.

Surgeon General of the United States. *Report on Smoking and Health.* Washington, D.C.: U.S. Government Printing Office, 1984. The complete up-to-date report on the many health risks associated with smoking.

U.S. Congress, Office of Technology Assessment. "Passive Smoking in the Workplace." Washington, D.C.: U.S. Government Printing Office, 1986. An analysis of the health effects of passive smoke on workers who are nonsmokers.

Summary

No public health message is disseminated as widely as that which appears on every package of cigarettes and in every cigarette advertisement: "Warning: The Surgeon General Has Determined That Cigarette Smoking Is Dangerous to Your Health." Yet in spite of the overwhelming evidence that cigarette smoking is associated with higher death rates from cancer, heart disease, and respiratory diseases, approximately 50 million Americans smoke.

Smoking is an acquired habit; it is not a life-sustaining activity. Therefore, the primary motivation for all smokers is the desire to smoke. For some, that desire comes from the stimulation they receive from smoking; for others, smoking is a means to increase pleasure or to decrease stress.

The fact that smoking is a matter of personal choice means that people *can* stop smoking if they choose to. An abundance of stop-smoking programs is available to assist the motivated quitter. The success of any attempt to quit smoking relies on the smoker's resolve to quit and on replacing the unhealthy smoking habit with personally rewarding behaviors.

One of the reasons that people continue to smoke is that the tobacco industry spends millions of dollars each year for advertising and other promotional activities that encourage people to smoke. The federal government is also partly to blame. While the Public Health Service campaigns against smoking, the Department of Agriculture provides tobacco growers with price supports for their crop.

The war of words will probably continue for a long time. But you need not be confused by the real issue: smoking is a serious risk to your health. Anyone who smokes, and anyone who is thinking of trying it, should keep in mind the dangers and not bemoan the fact that there is no cure for heart disease, emphysema, or lung cancer.

FOR YOUR HEALTH

Smokers: Here's Your Chance to Quit

If you smoke, determine your strongest motivations for doing so by taking the self-assessment test in Box 15-1. Once you have determined your motives for smoking, make a list of nonsmoking, healthful activities you can substitute for smoking behavior. If you decide to quit smoking cigarettes, you can try this four-week program designed to help smokers stop smoking.

First week: List the positive reasons you want to quit smoking, and read the list daily. Wrap your cigarette pack with paper and rubber bands. Each time you smoke, write down the time of day, what you are doing, how you are feeling, and how important that cigarette is to you on a scale from 1 to 5. Then rewrap the pack.

Second week: Keep reading your list of reasons, and add to it if possible. Don't carry matches, and keep your cigarettes some distance away. Each day, try to smoke fewer cigarettes, eliminating those that, at the time, seem the least or most important (whichever works best).

Third week: Continue with the second week's instructions. Don't buy a new pack until you finish the one you're smoking and never buy a carton. Change brands twice during the week, each time choosing a brand lower in tar and nicotine. Try to stop smoking for 48 hours sometime during the week.

Fourth week: Quit smoking entirely. Increase your physical activity. Avoid situations you most closely associate with smoking. Find a substitute for cigarettes. Do deep breathing exercises whenever you get the urge to smoke.

CHAPTER SIXTEEN

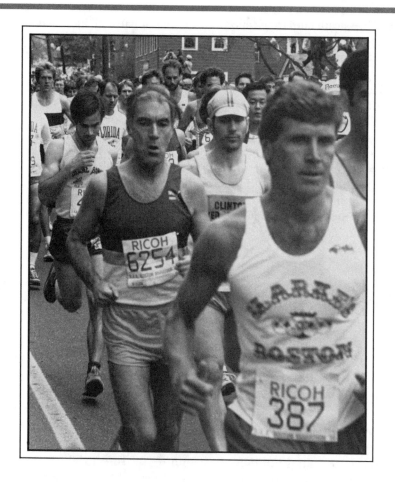

How to take care of your heart as a
means to promote wellness.

The Heart: Preventing Cardiovascular Disease

Have a heart that never hardens
A temper that never tires
A touch that never hurts.

Charles Dickens

The human heart has long been accorded special attention by poets, lovers, and sentimentalists. Everyday language still reflects the venerable notion that the heart is the repository of love, feelings, and emotions. When love relationships collapse, people express anguish by reference to a "broken heart," by becoming "heartsick," or by complaining of the "heartlessness" of the loved one. People are described by the character of their hearts—cruel hearts, kind hearts, hard hearts, cold hearts, warm hearts, or even hearts of stone or of gold. When referring to the distressing experiences of life, people speak of heartaches, whereas intense happiness prompts them to say that the heart leaps for joy.

Of course, few people today believe that love and emotions reside in the human heart. Most know that the scientific evidence points to the brain as the center of feelings and emotions. The heart's true function is to pump blood. Indeed, it is an extraordinarily effective device for maintaining the circulation of blood (about a gallon in the adult body) through approximately 60,000 miles of blood vessels.

The poets and sentimentalists didn't have it all wrong, however. There *is* a very important connection between one's heart and feelings and emotions. Under stress, the brain may send signals to the heart that cause it to beat erratically—even cause a **heart attack** (a condition in which the heart stops beating and pumping blood). A recent study showed that rabbits that were touched, played with, and talked to a number of times during the day had much healthier **aortas** (the main artery that carries blood from the heart to the rest of the body) than a control group of rabbits that were fed the same but were otherwise ignored (Nerem, Levesque, and Cornhill, 1980). As we will explain in this chapter, emotions, stress, and thoughts can—and do—affect the health and functions of the human heart.

The heart you were born with is going to have to serve you throughout life. Because healthy heart function is critical to the enjoyment of an active, fulfilling life, everyone can benefit from knowing how to help keep the heart free of disease and how to keep it functioning efficiently.

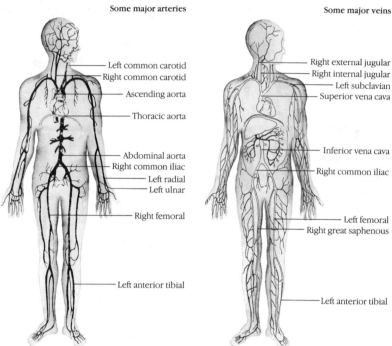

Some major arteries

- Left common carotid
- Right common carotid
- Ascending aorta
- Thoracic aorta
- Abdominal aorta
- Right common iliac
- Left radial
- Left ulnar
- Right femoral
- Left anterior tibial

Some major veins

- Right external jugular
- Right internal jugular
- Left subclavian
- Superior vena cava
- Inferior vena cava
- Right common iliac
- Left femoral
- Right great saphenous
- Left anterior tibial

Figure 16-1
The circulatory system. The arteries (*above*) supply oxygen and nutrients to all the body's cells, and the veins (*opposite*) carry away carbon dioxide and dissolved waste products.

The Heart and Blood Vessels

The circulatory system of the human body consists of the heart (the pump) and the various vessels that transport the blood: **arteries** for carrying oxygenated blood to organs and tissues, **veins** for returning blood to the heart after oxygen and nutrients have been exchanged for waste products and carbon dioxide in the cells (see Figure 16-1), and **capillaries**—tiny blood vessels that branch out from arteries and veins and supply blood to all the tissues and individual cells of the body. The blood vessels can be injured or they can become obstructed by disease processes that ultimately may lead to a heart attack (resulting from damage to the **coronary arteries,** which supply blood and oxygen to the heart itself) or a **stroke** (resulting from damage to arteries in the brain). The organ that pumps the blood and keeps it circulating continuously through the arteries and veins is, of course, the heart.

The heart isn't shaped quite like the version on Valentine cards. It looks more like the drawing in Figure 16-2. The heart is a highly specialized muscle about the size of your fist that is designed to pump blood continuously and to respond to the

body's needs. The muscular wall of the heart is called the **myocardium.** There are four separate chambers in the heart: the upper right and left **atria** (also called **auricles**), which receive blood returning from the body via the veins; and the lower right and left **ventricles,** which pump blood out of the heart into the lungs and body. Blood flow is maintained in one direction by one-way valves that separate the atria from the ventricles. If these heart valves are not formed correctly during embryonic development, or if they become defective as a result of disease (such as rheumatic fever), heart action and blood circulation may be impaired.

The pattern of blood flowing through the chambers of the heart is diagrammed in Figure 16-3. Blood depleted of oxygen enters the right atrium after returning from various parts of the body. The blood flows from the right atrium into the right ventricle and from there it is pumped to the lungs. In the lungs carbon dioxide is exchanged for oxygen and the blood, now bright red, returns to the left atrium through the pulmonary vein. The blood flows into the left ventricle and finally is pumped to all parts of the body through the heart's main artery, the aorta.

This remarkable pump circulates over a gallon of blood a minute through the blood vessels by contracting and relaxing about 60 to 75 times, the heart rate being determined by the body's needs. During an average human life span of 70 years, the heart will pump between 30 to 40 million gallons of blood. It will beat nearly a billion times.

The arteries and veins through which the blood flows are hollow tubes that are normally soft, elastic, and pliable. These blood vessels can stretch and expand to allow more blood to flow, or they can constrict to impede the flow of blood. By means of the sympathetic and parasympathetic nervous systems (see Chapter 3), the brain can influence the rate of the heartbeat as well as blood flow and blood pressure in veins and arteries.

A healthy heart beats rhythmically at a pace that is initiated by the heart itself. In the right atrium a region called the **sinoatrial node** (pacemaker) generates a periodic electrical impulse that causes the heart muscle to contract and pump blood from the ventricles. The pace of the heartbeat, however, is influenced by nerves originating in the brain, which explains how emotions, excitement, or stress can suddenly change the rhythm of the heartbeat.

The heartbeat can also be initiated by nerve impulses that originate in areas of the heart other than the sinoatrial node. If these additional signals interfere with the normal pacemaker signal, the heart may beat irregularly or contract prematurely. Multiple signals may also cause different areas of the

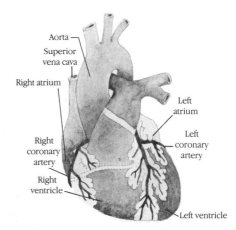

Figure 16-2
The heart has four chambers that pump blood. Oxygenated blood leaves the heart to the body through the aorta and is returned through the superior vena cava.

heart muscle to beat independently of one another, causing **fibrillation** (irregular heartbeat), which sometimes precedes a heart attack. However, it should be noted that many people experience irregular heartbeats without suffering a heart attack. Nowadays persistent, irregular heartbeats can be controlled with drugs. In some instances, electrical pacemakers are permanently installed in a person's chest to provide a steadying electrical stimulus.

Figure 16-3
Circulation of the blood to and from the separate chambers of the heart.

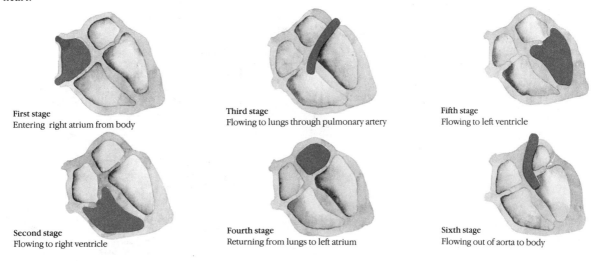

First stage
Entering right atrium from body

Second stage
Flowing to right ventricle

Third stage
Flowing to lungs through pulmonary artery

Fourth stage
Returning from lungs to left atrium

Fifth stage
Flowing to left ventricle

Sixth stage
Flowing out of aorta to body

> Don't worry about your heart:
> it will last you all your life.
>
> **Evan Esar**

Heart Valves and Blood Vessels

To maintain uniform blood flow in one direction through veins and arteries, the cardiovascular system has been equipped with valves that are located not only in the chambers of the heart but in blood vessels as well (see Figure 16-4). The most important valves are the four located in the heart, as shown in Figure 16-5. With every heartbeat, these valves open and close to allow the pumping action to be maximally effective.

In a small number of persons, one or more of these valves is defective at birth because of developmental abnormalities. With modern techniques for open-heart surgery, defective heart valves often can be repaired or even replaced with artificial valves, if necessary, so that a person can live a normal life (see Figure 16-6).

A more frequent way that heart valves become damaged is by certain forms of streptococcal infection during childhood, which occasionally produce an illness called **rheumatic fever**. If streptococcal infections reoccur frequently, rheumatic heart disease may eventually develop—even years later. It seems that in certain susceptible individuals, the immune system overreacts to the presence of certain kinds of streptococcal bacteria, and the result is inflammation of body joints and also heart tissue, especially the mitral and aortic valves. Scar tissue forms on these valves and may eventually prevent them from opening and closing correctly. By listening to the sounds the heart valves make as they open and close, a physician can determine whether they are defective. The incidence of rheumatic heart disease has decreased in the United States in recent years, but children with strep throat should still

Figure 16-4
William Harvey, a seventeenth-century physician, was the first to describe the circulation of the blood. In one of Harvey's experiments, shown in this drawing, he used a tourniquet to stop flow in order to identify the veins and the position of the valves in the veins. (Courtesy World Health Organization.)

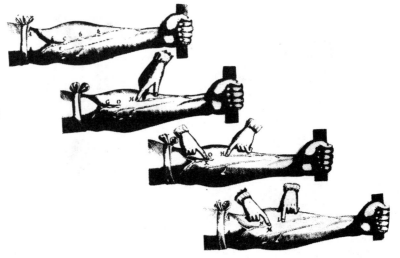

> The only effective way to deal with coronary disease is to prevent it. In essence, we are dealing with a failure of the health system every time somebody comes in with a heart attack.
>
> **Eugene Passamani, M.D.**

receive prompt medical attention because the streptococcus infection is a threat to their hearts.

Another common form of valve defect occurs in the veins and results in a blood circulation disorder commonly known as **varicose veins.** These unsightly bluish, bulging veins usually occur in the legs, where blood returning to the heart has to flow against the pull of gravity. One-way valves in the leg veins normally prevent blood from draining backward in the legs. If valves in the leg veins become weakened, blood tends to accumulate in the leg, distending the veins and producing the visible varicosities. However, faulty blood flow in veins should not be confused with the more serious diseases of the arteries collectively called **arteriosclerosis,** or hardening of the arteries. It is arterial diseases that may eventually lead to heart failure or stroke.

Atherosclerosis and Heart Disease

Arteriosclerosis includes all kinds of arterial diseases, but the one that is of primary concern is the disease known as **atherosclerosis.** This disease begins with damage to cells of the arterial inner walls and the formation of a fatty fibrous deposit called an **atherosclerotic lesion,** or **plaque.** The plaque gradually increases in size until the amount of blood flowing through the artery is greatly reduced or even completely blocked. The formation of atherosclerotic plaque inside an artery is depicted in Figure 16-7.

The reason that obstruction of any artery is so serious is that the arteries carry oxygenated blood

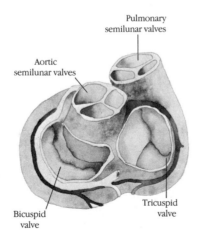

◄Figure 16-5
The heart's valves keep the blood flowing in one direction into and out of the chambers of the heart.

Figure 16-6 ▼
An artificial valve used to replace a defective aortic valve in a human heart. (Photo courtesy World Health Organization.)

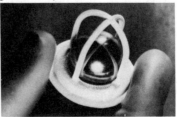

to all parts of the body. Cells require a continuous supply of oxygen to remain alive. If nerve cells in the brain are oxygen-starved for even a few minutes, they die and cannot regenerate. Interrupted blood supply to the brain causes a stroke. The muscle cells of the heart itself are heavy consumers of oxygen. Oxygen is supplied to the heart by the coronary arteries, which are the first to branch from the aorta (see Figure 16-8). Despite its small size, the heart uses about 20 percent of the total blood circulated to supply its own muscle cells with oxygen, since, unlike other muscles in the body, the heart muscles work unceasingly—even while a person is asleep.

If the coronary arteries become partially blocked by atherosclerotic lesions, the heart does not get sufficient oxygen, which may cause severe chest pain called **angina pectoris.** If a coronary artery should become partly or completely blocked, the person may suffer a heart attack, or **myocardial infarction**—a term that refers to the death of regions of heart muscle that have been deprived of oxygen.

The heart is a remarkably resilient organ. Even after a heart attack, heart functions can often recover if the damaged area is not too extensive. With time, minor arteries within the heart can augment its blood supply. Although stroke and myocardial infarction are recorded as the cause of death in more than 1 million deaths in the United States each year, the underlying cause is invariably arterial disease—atherosclerosis—that interrupts the essential flow of blood to the heart or brain.

Recently, medical researchers have discovered that angina pectoris and even heart attacks may be caused by coronary artery spasms (Marx, 1980). Because the heart and arteries contain muscle tissue, they can spasm (cramp) just like a muscle in an arm or a leg. These spasms can restrict the blood flow to the heart. If the coronary arteries are already partially blocked by atherosclerotic plaque, the spasms may complete the blockage. Since even young persons can suffer heart attacks, it is possible that coronary artery spasms are the cause in some instances. Although there is no scientific evidence linking spasms with mental stress and tension, we do know that the brain regulates heartbeat as well as the constriction and dilation of blood vessels. Recall the case of Anna described in Chapter 3 (see Box 3-1), who suffered symptoms of stroke without any evidence of arteries being permanently blocked or damaged. Each year in the United States approxi-

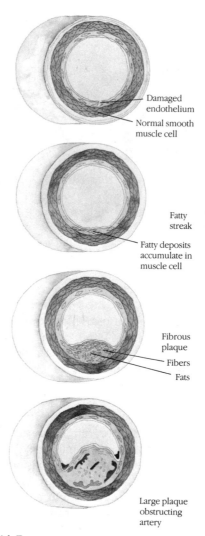

Figure 16-7
Development of an atherosclerotic lesion (plaque) inside an artery. Such lesions can eventually block blood flow, causing a heart attack or stroke. Many factors are suspected to cause the formation of arterial plaque, but none have been proven.

mately 1.5 million persons are admitted to hospital coronary care units because of suspected heart attacks. Tests eventually rule out a heart attack in at least 50 percent of those individuals who have chest pains, shortness of breath, or some other symptom of heart attack. These unnecessary hospital admissions constitute a considerable financial burden to patients and a drain on the resources of the medical care system (Pozen et al., 1984).

Persons whose coronary arteries are blocked by atherosclerotic lesions are often advised to undergo an operation known as **coronary bypass surgery.**

> The greatest single curse in medicine is the curse of unnecessary operations, and there would be fewer of them, if the doctor got the same salary whether he operated or not.
>
> **Richard Cabot, M.D.**
> **Harvard Medical School**
> **1938**

In this operation the diseased portions of the arteries are surgically removed and a portion of vein, usually taken from the person's leg, is grafted onto the coronary arteries to replace the diseased segments. A $24 million study recently completed by the government's National Heart, Lung, and Blood Institute showed that, for patients with mild coronary artery blockage, there was no advantage to having coronary bypass surgery over the use of medication to treat symptoms; that is, patients' five-year survival rate was unchanged. As a result of its study, the Institute also concluded that as many as 25,000 bypass operations a year are performed unnecessarily. As might be expected, this conclusion has met with considerable criticism and opposition from the medical profession (Kolata, 1983). There is great controversy (see Box 16-1) regarding the usefulness of this heart operation. The controversy provides an opportunity to compare the value of a holistic medical approach to the prevention and treatment of heart disease with that of conventional medicine and surgery.

A new technique for opening blocked coronary arteries that does not require open-heart surgery has recently been developed. Called **angioplasty,** it utilizes a balloon that is threaded to the site of the blockage in the artery and then inflated. The balloon squashes the atherosclerotic plaque and opens the artery. A newer refinement of angioplasty employs a miniature laser located inside the ballon-tipped catheter. The laser beam is used to heat and dissolve the clot in the artery. Also, there is a new clot-dissolving enzyme, **tissue plasminogen activator** (t-PA), that can be released directly into the blocked artery through a catheter.

What Causes Atherosclerosis?

Virtually the only uncontested fact about the cause of atherosclerosis and coronary artery disease is that nobody really knows what causes it. As one prominent heart researcher, R. A. Stallones (1983), poetically put it: "In the best of all possible worlds, we could now look back over this trail of research findings . . . and pluck the flower of truth from the nettle of confusion. However, (in the case of heart disease), truth is not readily apparent." After decades of research, scientists investigating the causes

Figure 16-8
The coronary arteries supply blood to the heart itself. Obstruction of blood flow in any part of these arteries can damage the heart and cause a heart attack.

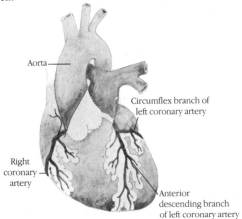

Aorta

Circumflex branch of left coronary artery

Right coronary artery

Anterior descending branch of left coronary artery

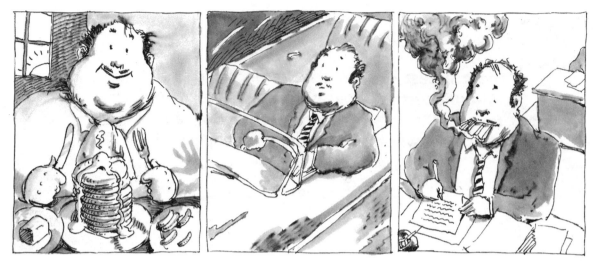

Figure 16-9
Among lifestyle factors that contribute to the risk of cardiovascular disease are excessive cholesterol in the blood, high blood pressure, smoking, stress, and a high-fat diet. Although there is no proof that any one or combination of these risk factors actually causes cardiovascular disease, it is recommended that people reduce these risk factors in their lives.

of cardiovascular disease can only point to certain associated risk factors. The factors shown in Figure 16-9 are associated with an increased risk of developing artery and heart disease, but there is no compelling evidence demonstrating that these factors actually cause atherosclerosis and heart attacks.

Consider these observations. Atherosclerosis is largely a disease of technologically developed countries. Many human populations show a low incidence of cardiovascular disease, especially preliterate societies such as tribes in New Guinea, !Kung tribes in the Kalahari Desert, and Eskimos in Canada and Greenland. Most mammals other than humans do not develop atherosclerosis with increased age. Animals in the wild are usually free of the disease — but some animals in captivity do develop atherosclerosis. These observations all suggest that cardiovascular disease is not inevitable and that the particular style of American living (overeating, lack of exercise, smoking, stress, and so forth) is the real cause for the high incidence of atherosclerosis in this country. This lifestyle would include nutritional, psychological, and environmental risk factors as well as those already mentioned. The key question still remains: what causes or starts atherosclerotic plaques?

Environment

Research studies by Earl P. Benditt (1977) at the University of Washington School of Medicine have led to the idea that chemicals in the environment, in air, food, and water, can permanently alter cells in the linings of the arteries. Most ingested chemicals ultimately circulate through the blood supply. Benditt hypothesizes that mutagenic chemicals damage the DNA in arterial cells causing them to grow abnormally. This abnormal growth subsequently leads to development of the atherosclerotic plaque. The strongest evidence in support of this hypothesis is the finding that all the cells in plaque frequently appear to be identical and to have arisen from a single genetically altered cell. If Benditt's ideas are correct, chemicals that are known to cause cancer (see Chapter 17) may also be responsible for atherosclerotic lesions. His hypothesis is consistent with the observation that smoking tobacco, which is known to contain cancer-causing chemicals, increases a person's risk of developing cardiovascular disease as well as cancer. His hypothesis also accounts for findings, mentioned previously, that isolated human communities that have not been

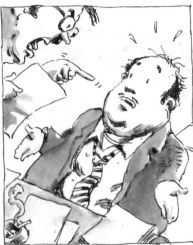
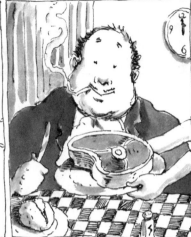
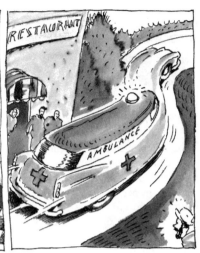

exposed to large amounts of modern chemicals and industrialized lifestyles have a low incidence of cardiovascular disease.

That environmental factors contribute significantly to heart disease is borne out by epidemiological studies of human populations that move from one environment to another. Japanese men living in Hawaii have half the incidence of fatal and nonfatal heart disease as white U.S. citizens living on the mainland but twice the incidence of Japanese men living in Japan. That is, the rate of heart disease of Japanese men in Hawaii is almost exactly halfway between the low rates in Japan and the high rates in the United States and can only be due to environmental differences (Yano, Reed, and McGee, 1984). Other epidemiological studies have not shown any association between the different diets that people eat and development of heart disease; however, no specific environmental chemicals have been investigated in these studies. (It is virtually impossible to determine different degrees of chemical exposures among people.)

Nutrition and Diet

In regard to heart disease, almost everyone in our society has heard of the dangers of excess cholesterol in the blood and of eating saturated animal fats. Elevated levels of cholesterol in the blood are associated with increased risk of heart attack, and the risk is compounded if a person has high cholesterol and also is a smoker (see Figure 16-10).

Research on different human populations that consume different diets has shown a strong association between serum (blood) cholesterol levels and heart disease. (Cholesterol levels in adult Americans vary between 150 and 260 mg/dl; the average is about 210 mg/dl.) However, the same population studies show either no association or negative associations between diet and serum cholesterol or between diet and heart disease. Since food habits and other cultural customs are so intertwined that they cannot be separated, it is impossible to sort out the contribution of particular diets to the development of heart disease (Stallones, 1983).

Thus, all one can conclude for certain is that elevated levels of cholesterol in the blood (beginning around 200 mg/dl) increase the risk of coronary heart disease and heart attack. It is not proved that diet, particularly the kind and amount of fat in the diet, leads to elevated blood cholesterol levels. It is likely that people differ with regard to how their cholesterol levels change in response to dietary fat consumption. That is part of the reason why it is difficult, even impossible, to establish dietary guidelines appropriate for everyone (Grundy, 1986).

Cholesterol is an essential component of cells and is synthesized in the body as well as being obtained in food. Cholesterol circulates in the blood in the form of large particles called **high-density lipoprotein** (HDL) and **low-density lipoprotein** (LDL). The cholesterol that gets deposited in atherosclerotic plaques is derived mainly from LDL particles, which are thought to be the primary contributors to heart disease.

BOX 16-1

CORONARY BYPASS SURGERY

Coronary bypass surgery is one of the most frequently recommended surgical procedures in the United States. In 1977, about 70,000 bypass operations were performed. In 1979, the number had grown to 110,000 at an average cost of $15,000 each. By 1986, the number had swelled to 250,000 and the total cost to the nation was estimated to be $2.5 to $5 billion. Clearly, coronary bypass surgery is big business. Despite the popularity of this operation, it has never been proved that most patients' heart functions really improve after surgery, although most patients report "feeling better." A ten-year government study (CASS), recently completed, showed no improvement in survival in patients suffering from mild heart disease after bypass surgery over conventional medical treatment. However, in another study (European Coronary Surgery Study), it was concluded that the operation did prolong life in patients who had three blocked coronary arteries and in some patients with only two blocked arteries.

The bypass operation involves splicing one or more sections of a vein (usually taken from the saphenous vein in the person's leg) from the aorta to one of several of the coronary arteries, thus creating new pathways for blood flow to the heart (see Figure A). Blockage of the coronary arteries by atherosclerotic lesions can be

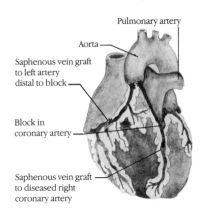

Figure A.

detected by **angiography**—injection of a dye into the blood so that the coronary arteries can be visualized by x-rays. If blockage of one or more coronary arteries is detected, coronary bypass surgery is usually recommended.

Most heart surgeons point out that coronary bypass surgery does provide relief from **angina,** the chest pain that results when insufficient oxygen reaches heart cells. Indeed, it is widely accepted that about 90 percent of bypass patients experience angina relief after surgery. While bypass surgery (as well as medications) relieves angina, other factors can also explain the chest-pain relief. For example, patients undergoing surgery are forced to rest during hospitalization and recuperation, and many change their lifestyles

after surgery. And it is likely that the placebo effect (Chapter 2) plays an important role in pain relief.

In the 1950s, angina pain from partially blocked coronary arteries was relieved by an operation in which a chest artery was tied off in the hope that more blood would be supplied to the patient's heart. About 40 percent of the patients felt better following this operation. To see whether the relief of angina pain was a placebo effect or really resulted from the surgery, a number of mock operations were done in which anesthesia was given, the person's chest was cut open, but nothing was done to the artery. The patients receiving the mock operations experienced just as much relief as those whose artery was actually tied off, so the operation was abandoned (Frank, 1975).

Despite mounting criticism of coronary bypass surgery, many physicians still recommend it to patients over milder forms of treatment. Recently, Dr. Thomas A. Preston, chief of cardiology at Pacific Medical Center in Seattle, summed up his opposition to coronary bypass surgery: "The operation does not cure patients, it is scandalously overused, and its high cost drains resources from other areas of need. Fully half of the bypass operations performed in the United States are unnecessary."

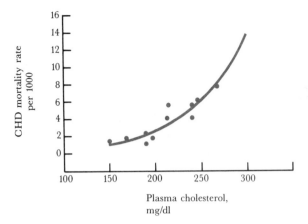

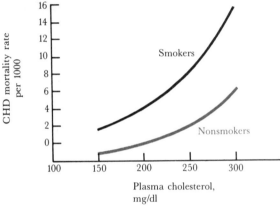

Figure 16-10

The graph on the left shows that rate of death from heart attack increases with cholesterol level, particularly above 200 mg/dl. The graph on the right shows the same data but separates out smokers from nonsmokers. Note the markedly increased risk that smokers have of dying from a heart attack at every level of cholesterol. (Data are from the Multiple Risk Factor Intervention Trial (MRFIT).)

Each LDL particle contains over a thousand molecules of cholesterol along with a large protein called apoprotein B-100 (APO-B). It is the job of the APO-B protein, which is synthesized in the liver, to deliver the cholesterol to body cells. It does this by binding to specific receptor sites on cells (LDL receptors) and releasing the cholesterol, which is used to synthesize and repair cell membranes.

It is in this process that potential problems may arise (Brown and Goldstein, 1984). If the number of LDL receptors on cells is normal, then the LDL particles and cholesterol are removed promptly from the blood and utilized efficiently by cells. However, if the number of LDL receptors is abnormally low in people, the LDL particles accumulate in the blood. Now these fatty particles may begin to attach to the walls of arteries and form atherosclerotic plaques that eventually may result in a blocked artery. If the blockage occurs in a coronary artery, a heart attack ensues; if the blockage occurs in a blood vessel in the brain, a stroke results. What controls the level of LDL cell receptors is probably a combination of the particular genes a person has inherited plus unidentified environmental factors.

George V. Mann (1977) of the Vanderbilt University School of Medicine, a severe critic of the hypothesis linking cholesterol to formation of atherosclerotic lesions, points out that the well-known Framingham, Massachusetts heart study failed to show any correlation between people's dietary habits and their blood-serum cholesterol levels. He also emphasizes that both diet therapy and drugs that reduce cholesterol blood levels in patients with atherosclerosis produce no improvment in their coronary artery disease.

Mark D. Altschule (1974) of the Harvard Medical School is also unconvinced by assertions that dietary cholesterol causes atherosclerosis. He speculates that it may not be dietary cholesterol that is harmful but the extent to which food is commercially processed that creates potentially harmful substances.

In May 1980 the Food and Nutrition Board of the National Academy of Sciences issued a report concluding that there is no need for the average healthy American to cut down on dietary cholesterol. This conclusion sparked considerable controversy, and the panel was accused of conflict of interest because some of the panel's members had financial ties to food industries.

Scientists have identified numerous risk factors that are associated with increased risk of heart disease. Recently, however, a factor has been identified that appears to *reduce* the risk of heart disease. This factor is high fish consumption. Greenland eskimos, Japanese fishermen, and other maritime populations that eat large quantities of fish have a low incidence of heart attacks and mortality from heart disease. A current hypothesis is that particular polyunsaturated fatty acids in fish (see Figure 16-11) that people eat affords some protection against atherosclerosis and heart attacks. While it probably is

> About 63.4 million Americans (one out of four persons) suffer from one or more forms of cardiovascular disease, including 57.7 million with high blood pressure.
>
> **American Heart Association**

beneficial to include more fish in your diet, it is not recommended that people take fish oil supplements, as these supplements may create other health problems.

The precise relationship between diet in general and cholesterol in particular to atherosclerosis and heart disease is unsettled. It remains true that animals fed diets high in saturated fats, cholesterol, and sugar develop atherosclerosis. But it is possible that disease develops not because of the dietary excesses but because of dietary deficiencies. In addition to possible vitamin B_6 deficiency, deficiencies of chromium and manganese may also result in atherosclerosis. Both elements are required for metabolism of carbohydrates and fats, and mineral deficiencies can lead to blood vessel damage.

Finally, mention should be made of a study showing that blood cholesterol levels could be reduced by meditation (Cooper and Aygen, 1979). Stress may not only adversely affect blood vessels but may also elevate cholesterol levels in the blood.

From the viewpoint of maintaining the health of the heart and arteries, the nutritional message seems clear. Eat reasonable amounts of a variety of natural, uncooked foods. Minimize consumption of processed foods as much as possible because they are probably lacking in essential trace nutrients and, in addition, may contain toxic substances that are added to the food or formed during processing. It may take years for nutritional deficiencies to be manifested, but it's also true that cardiovascular disease progresses for many years before symptoms are noticed.

High Blood Pressure

It is estimated that one out of every six adult Americans has **hypertension,** or high blood pressure—that is, blood pressure above what is regarded as normal. Each time the heart contracts, blood is pumped through the arteries, exerting a pressure on the ar-

Figure 16-11
This molecule is called an omega-3, omega-6 polyunsaturated fatty acid. It is unsaturated because it is not completely hydrogenated. The carbon at the left is designated omega-1; the unsaturated carbons occur at the omega-3 and omega-6 carbons. Fish contain mostly omega-3 monounsaturated fatty acids; meat contains mostly omega-6 monounsaturated fatty acids.

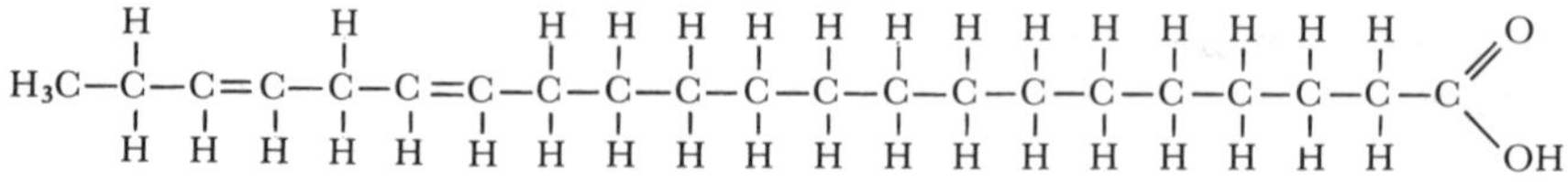

Figure 16-12

Blood pressure is measured by listening for certain changes in the sound of blood flowing through the brachial artery in the arm as the pressure in the pneumatic cuff, which has been raised sufficiently to cut off arterial blood flow, is gradually reduced. When the pressure in the cuff equals the maximum pressure in the artery, the artery opens and the sound of the blood rushing through the artery is amplified by the stethoscope. This is the systolic pressure. As the cuff pressure is reduced further, the sound suddenly becomes faint. This is the diastolic pressure—the relaxation of the heart between contractions.

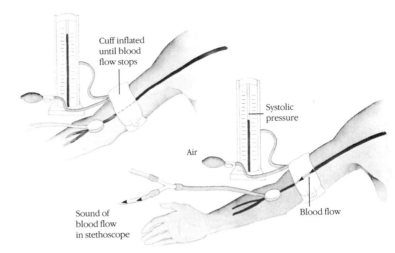

terial wall that can be measured as shown in Figure 16-12. Actually, two pressures are measured, both of which are important diagnostically. The maximum pressure in the arteries occurs when the heart contracts (**systole**), pumping blood from the heart to the lungs and the body. Between contractions, the pressure falls to a lower value (**diastole**) as blood flows from one chamber to another. In a young adult, normal systolic pressures range between 110 and 140, and diastolic pressures range between 70 and 90. Mild hypertension is arbitrarily defined as a diastolic pressure of 90–104; about 15 percent of men and 13 percent of women fall in this range. Diastolic pressure is significant because higher diastolic pressures are associated with increased risk of death (see Figure 16-13).

Long-term studies show that chronic high blood pressure increases the chances for heart disease, stroke, atherosclerosis, and kidney disease. (In some cases kidney disease causes high blood pressure.) All blood vessels are elastic tubes, and increasing the pressure can cause a rupture, especially if the vessel is damaged or weakened. In the case of the arteries it may be that high blood pressure actually helps to begin an atherosclerotic lesion and probably contributes to plaque formation once the arterial wall has been damaged.

High blood pressure has serious consequences. Life insurance company statistics show that life expectancy for a 35-year-old American male is reduced by 16 years if he has a blood pressure of 150/100 as compared to a normal pressure of 120/80. In the

Figure 16-13

Relationship of high diastolic blood pressure and risk of death.

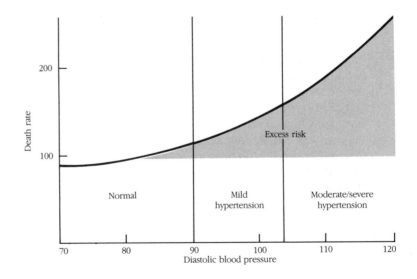

Table 16-1
Side Effects of Antihypertensive Drugs

Drug	Side effect
Diuretics	Low blood potassium levels (except for potassium-sparing diuretics)
	Excess uric acid and sugar in blood (thiazide diuretics)
	Breast enlargement
Sympatholytics (beta-adrenergic blockers)	Edema (water retention)
	Depression
	Diarrhea
	Fever (methyldopa)
	Impotence
	Lethargy
Vasodilators (hydralazine)	Palpitation
	Edema
	Rapid heartbeat
	Drug-induced lupus erythematosus

U.S. population, blood pressure increases with age, yet among the South American Yanomano Indians blood pressure decreases significantly as they get older. High blood pressure is not an inevitable biological consequence of aging and most certainly is related to living habits, although occasionally it can be caused by diseases in other body organs. The idea that lifestyle may cause hypertension and heart disease is not new. C.P. Donnison (1938), working on a tribal reservation in Kenya in the 1930s, measured blood pressure in all patients admitted to his hospital. Among 1800 African patients of all ages there was not a single case of high blood pressure. He concluded that it is primarily cultural patterns and lifestyles that cause high blood pressure.

Joseph Eyer (1979) also views hypertension as a disease of modern society:

> Medical science divides hypertension into two broad varieties: types of elevated pressure for which specific cause can be found, and all the rest, termed essential hypertension, for which causation has not yet been fully worked out. Among the populations of present-day developed countries, essential hypertension comprises about 90 percent of all hypertension.

A variety of factors have been proposed as causing hypertension—salt, heredity, smoking, coffee, alcohol, stress—but none of these hypothetical risk factors is substantiated by any evidence except for stress, which is discussed in the next section (Castelli, 1982). Salt consumption as a cause in hypertension has been the subject of controversy for years. Recent findings indicate that low-sodium (salt) diets are of little or no value in preventing or reducing hypertension in the general population. Reduced salt consumption (2 grams a day or less) may benefit a small subgroup of hypertensives, but even that fact is questionable. Michael Alderman of Cornell University Medical School says bluntly: "There is no correlation between sodium consumption and blood pressure levels. . . . I think it is incumbent on those who want to change our diets to provide evidence that we should do so" (Kolata, 1982).

Most Americans who have high blood pressure have no medically detectable disease that causes the increase in blood pressure. Today the accepted treatment for high blood pressure is drug therapy, and many drugs are effective in lowering blood pressure. Yet every one of these drugs has side effects that are dangerous (see Table 16-1).

Elmer and Alyce Green (1980) of the Menninger Foundation have shown that four out of five persons with severe hypertension can restore and maintain normal blood pressure without drugs through biofeedback and psychophysiologic training. In fact, more than a dozen studies over the past ten years have shown that any one of a variety of different relaxation techniques is effective in lowering blood pressure in hypertensive patients (Agras, 1983). Given this fact, it is unfortunate that more people

Table 16-2
Prevalence of Hypertensive Heart Disease Among White and Black American Adults by Age and Sex, 1960–1962

Age	Men		Women	
	White	Black	White	Black
18–24	0.2	1.9	—	1.6
25–34	1.1	5.2	0.7	4.7
35–44	4.0	15.2	2.7	14.0
45–54	7.7	24.4	6.8	31.5
55–64	11.7	33.1	19.5	46.4
65–74	16.3	50.2	37.5	66.4
75–79	24.0	32.3	37.1	69.5
Total 18–79 years	6.5	19.1	9.8	22.2

Data from U.S. Department of Health, Education, and Welfare, *Blood Pressure of Adults by Race and Area, United States, 1960–1962* (National Health Examination Survey, National Center for Health Statistics, Series 11, Number 5, 1964).

with hypertension are not advised to try a relaxation technique to lower their blood pressure before being advised to take drugs for the rest of their lives to control blood pressure.

That high blood pressure is caused by the lifestyles of modern industrialized societies probably cannot be proven with absolute certainty. Yet the data shown in Table 16-2 would certainly support the view that stress and/or other social factors can cause hypertension. Black males in the United States between the ages of 18 and 34 are afflicted with hypertension at a rate five to ten times higher than that found in white males. Black women are even more seriously afflicted with high blood pressure. How is this enormous difference in the incidence of hypertension between black and white populations to be explained? Some investigators look for genetic, nutritional, or environmental differences between black and white populations. Others believe the answer lies in the day-to-day frustrations blacks encounter in educational, social, and employment opportunities.

Tiny receptors in the walls of the arteries respond to any change in blood pressure. If the blood pressure goes up these receptors usually send signals to the nerves to relax the arteries and to slow down the heartbeat, thereby returning blood pressure to normal. But this normal regulatory mechanism can be counteracted by signals originating in the brain. Arteries can be constricted and blood pressure raised by thoughts and feelings. Fear, tension,

anger, apprehension, anxiety—all activate the sympathetic nervous system, which transmits signals that constrict the arteries. When arteries are constricted, blood pressure goes up and can remain high as long as the stressful situations persist. If one's daily life is overly stressful or full of apprehension, anger, or frustration, arteries may stay constricted and blood pressure will rise, as will the risk for developing serious heart disease.

Stress

A few years ago two doctors, Meyer Friedman and Ray Rosenman (1974), created a medical furor by suggesting that almost all heart disease is of behavioral origin. They claimed that in the absence of a human behavior pattern they called **type A behavior,** all the other risk factors we have discussed in relation to heart disease would not by themselves cause heart and artery disease. These other factors—lack of exercise, smoking, cholesterol, obesity—would contribute to development of heart disease, but the main factor is stress resulting from the way a person lives and acts. Type A behavior is

a particular complex of personality traits including excessive competitive drive, aggressiveness, impatience, and a harrying sense of time urgency. Individuals displaying this pattern seem to be engaged in a chronic, ceaseless, and often fruitless struggle—with

> It is the type A man's ceaseless striving, his everlasting *struggle* with time, that we believe so very frequently leads to his early demise from coronary heart disease.
>
> Meyer Friedman and Ray H. Rosenman

themselves, with others, with circumstances, with time, sometimes with life itself. They also frequently exhibit a free-floating but well-rationalized form of hostility, and almost always a deep-seated insecurity.

Some examples of common type A behaviors are:

Becoming irritated and impatient while waiting in lines.

Constantly feeling pressed for time.

Insisting that everything always be done on time.

Not letting other persons finish what they are saying.

Always trying to show others how to do things correctly.

Playing games to win every time.

Not allowing time for relaxation and doing nothing.

Many people in our society are familiar with the term "type A person" and have some idea of what it means in terms of people's behaviors. Friedman and Rosenman originally defined the term *type A* on the basis of clinical observations with patients—that is, patients with heart disease seemed to behave differently in a number of ways when compared to patients with other kinds of diseases. Since the original definition of type A behaviors, a number of psychological tests have been developed that are now used to characterize a person as type A or type B. In a number of studies using these tests, it was found that the frequency of heart attacks and deaths was positively correlated with type A individuals but not with type B persons. As a result of these studies, it was argued that type A persons are more likely to die of a heart attack than type B persons are.

However, the association between type A behavior and heart attack has not been easy to document and is far from being proved. At least five large research investigations including the MRFIT study involving 12,700 men at high risk for coronary heart disease (CHD) failed to find an association between type A behavior and heart disease. On the other hand, an equal number of different studies did find an association between type A behavior and heart disease. No one has been able to resolve the different findings in the various studies or why the results were in conflict. What all of the studies do demonstrate is the difficulty of measuring particular human behaviors and proving that such behaviors cause disease.

One idea that has been suggested is that type A behavior itself does not cause heart disease but that hostility does. In terms of people's personalities it may be that ambition and impatience are not risk factors but constant annoyance and hostility are. Until the issue is resolved most researchers agree that changing type A behavior is useful. As one former type A patient concluded: "I am doing more business, with less stress, and I am a more loving, understanding person. The fact is my life has improved 100 percent" (Fischman, 1987).

Stress may be a major risk factor in human heart disease, but the connection between the two

> Since our hearts can speak a language that no one hears or sees and therefore cannot understand, we can get sick at heart.
>
> **James J. Lynch**
> *The Language of the Heart*

has been difficult to prove. An individual is neither type A nor type B all of the time, which is part of the problem of classifying people. People's reactions to other people and to the environment change continually. For example, we may exhibit type A behaviors on a day that we have to take an exam and type B behaviors on all other days. Or we may exhibit type A behavior when we are with a person we dislike and type B behavior with others. Scoring as type A or type B on a psychological test has little or no predictive value as to whether or not you will die from a heart attack. Stress in particular situations is not easily measured by a psychological test. Individually, each one of us knows what stress "feels" like, but so far no one really knows how to measure it.

We live in a society that encourages and rewards competitive drive and ambition. Material wealth and status are cherished goals. Most of us strive to be at the top of our class, business, profession, or bowling league. In some respects, setting goals and striving for success is to be admired, but each of us must decide what price we are willing to pay. Is what we earn and achieve worth risking health and possibly life for?

The Artificial Heart

On December 2, 1982, the first completely artificial heart was implanted into the chest of Dr. Barney Clark at the University of Utah Medical Center.

Some medical researchers heralded this event as opening up a glorious new era in cardiovascular medicine; others regarded it as an untimely experiment at best and questioned the ethics of the entire procedure (Woolley, 1984). Although Clark did give informed consent to the procedure, the subsequent medical treatments and interventions were seldom under his control. He never fully recovered from the implantation and died some four months later. It is estimated that $200,000 was spent to prolong his life by a few months. It is not obvious that Barney Clark would have chosen those few months if he had known how the quality of his life would deteriorate.

Artificial heart research has been going on in this country since the early 1960s, mostly with dogs and other animals. The ultimate goal of the animal research was to develop an artificial human heart, and to this end the federal government has invested about $200 million (Strauss, 1984). The motives behind the artificial heart program have been largely political and economic, not medical or humanitarian (this criticism also applies to much cancer reseach). In 1969, and again in 1981, Dr. Denton Cooley of the Texas Heart Institute implanted early versions of the artificial heart in terminally ill patients, without success. The entire U.S. artificial heart program was examined by a panel of experts in 1972. They recommended continuing with the research but also were concerned with the ethical and economic issues raised by artificial hearts. The concerns and issues surrounding artificial heart implantation have not been resolved, nor are they likely to be in the near future.

BOX 16-2

A CARDIAC RISK ASSESSMENT

Listed below are eight categories that pertain to the health of your heart. Select the number in each category that applies to you. If you don't know your blood cholesterol level, assume that it is less than 200 mg, which is the case for most college students of normal weight. You can estimate your risk by comparing your score with the risk table shown at the end of the test.

1. Age	10 to 20 1	21 to 30 2	31 to 40 3	41 to 50 4	51 to 60 6	61 to 70 and over 8
2. Heredity	No known history of heart disease 1	1 relative with cardiovascular disease over 60 2	2 relatives with cardio-vascular disease over 60 3	1 relative with cardiovascular disease under 60 4	2 relatives with cardio-vascular disease under 60 6	3 relatives with cardio-vascular disease under 60 8
3. Weight	More than 5 lbs. below standard weight 0	Standard weight 1	5–20 lbs over-weight 2	21–35 lbs overweight 3	36–50 lbs overweight 5	51–65 lbs overweight 7
4. Tobacco smoking	Nonuser 0	Cigar and/or pipe 1	10 cigarettes or less a day 2	20 cigarettes a day 3	30 cigarettes a day 5	40 cigarettes a day or more 8
5. Exercise	Intensive occupational and recre-ational exer-tion 1	Moderate occupational and recre-ational exer-tion 2	Sedentary work and intense recre-ational ex-ertion 3	Sedentary occupational and moderate recreational exertion 5	Sedentary work and light recre-ational exer-tion 6	Complete lack of all exercise 8
6. Cholesterol or percent fat in diet	Cholesterol below 180 mg. Diet contains no animal or solid fats 1	Cholesterol 181–205 mg. Diet contains 10% animal or solid fats 2	Cholesterol 206–230 mg. Diet contains 20% animal or solid fats 3	Cholesterol 231–255 mg. Diet contains 30% animal or solid fats 4	Cholesterol 256–280 mg. Diet contains 40% animal or solid fats 5	Cholesterol 281–330 mg. Diet contains 50% animal or solid fats 7
7. Blood pressure	100 upper reading 1	120 upper reading 2	140 upper reading 3	160 upper reading 4	180 upper reading 6	200 or over upper reading 8
8. Sex	Female 1	Female over 45 2	Male 3	Bald male 4	Bald, short male 6	Bald, short, stocky male 7

Your total score _____

Degree of risk

6 to 11 = Very low risk   26 to 32 = High risk
12 to 17 = Low risk   33 to 42 = Dangerous risk
18 to 25 = Average risk   42 to 60 = Extremely dangerous risk

Adapted from a test designed by John L. Boyer.

> As a result of the artificial heart, our society must again confront such issues as defining death, considering health care as a right, and deciding who is to receive a scarce form of therapy.
>
> **Michael J. Strauss, M.D.**

Keeping the Heart and Blood Vessels Healthy

Mortality from heart disease and strokes has been declining in the United States, and no one really knows why. Since 1964 the rate of deaths from heart attacks and strokes has dropped over 30 percent for people between the ages of 35 and 75, and somewhat less for people over 75 (Walker, 1983). Improved medical care cannot account for this dramatic decline over the past two decades, although it may have contributed slightly. What has changed significantly are people's lifestyles, particularly changes in their diets. Since the mid-1960s Americans have been smoking less and have reduced their consumption of butter, milk and cream, eggs, and animal meats and fats. However, association between these dietary changes and lower mortality does not prove that the changes in diet actually produced the decline in heart attacks and strokes. And, of course, the industries that manufacture these foods are quick to point out that association does not prove guilt. Whatever the reason for the decline in the rate of heart attacks, it does seem prudent to maintain a lifestyle that serves to minimize the risk of heart disease.

Nearly everyone is born with a healthy heart and blood vessels. An impressive body of evidence strongly suggests that one's lifestyle profoundly determines whether these organs and tissues remain healthy or whether they become diseased. The health of the heart and blood vessels truly does depend on how you live — what you eat and drink and whether you smoke or exercise. Arterial disease can begin at a young age — years before anyone is aware of any problem. By deciding while you are young to reduce the risk factors that have been shown to be associated with atherosclerosis and heart disease, you *can* preserve the health of your cardiovascular system.

John L. Boyer of San Diego State University has developed a short test for measuring cardiac risk. The test is presented in Box 16-2. We recommend that you take it to determine for yourself how your lifestyle is contributing to your risk of heart disease later in life. Although the test does not include an estimate of stress, which might be a serious omission, you can compare your own behaviors with those associated with Type A personalities as described by Friedman and Rosenman.

We close this discussion by returning to the idea of love. Does love affect the human heart? In examining the medical consequences of loneliness on the heart, author James J. Lynch (1977) observed:

> Even though the effects of human love on the heart are still largely ignored by most scientists, times are changing. The larger question of the effects of human emotions on the development of cardiac disease is now being seriously considered by many scientists. Growing numbers of physicians now recognize that the health of the human heart depends not only on such factors as genetics, diet, and exercise, but also to a large extent on the social and emotional health of the individual.

Thus, it may well be that the emotions poetically associated with the heart really do affect its health.

Supplemental Readings

American Medical Association. *Heart Care.* New York: Random House, 1984. A practical guide to heart disease and treatments.

DeYoung, H. G. "State of the Heart." *High Technology,* May 1984. An up-to-date article on heart disease and new techniques for its diagnosis and treatment.

Fischman, J. "Type A on Trial." *Psychology Today,* February 1987. Discusses the controversy over type A behavior and heart disease.

Grady, D. "Can Heart Disease Be Reversed?" *Discover,* March 1987. Describes a new program of nutrition and relaxation to reduce the risk of heart attack.

Lands, W. E. M. *Fish and Human Health.* New York: Academic Press, 1986. Everything you want to know about this subject—and probably more.

Lynch, J. J. *The Language of the Heart: The Body's Response to Human Dialogue.* New York: Basic Books, 1985. What we say and hear affects blood pressure and the functioning of the heart. Lynch shows how feelings and speech affect the heart.

Summary

The heart is a pump that maintains blood circulation in the arteries and veins. The arteries carry oxygen and nutrients to all body cells, and the veins carry carbon dioxide and waste products back to the lungs to exchange for fresh oxygen. Valves in the heart and blood vessels keep blood circulating in one direction.

Cardiovascular disease is the leading cause of death in the United States. It accounts for more than half of all deaths. There are many risk factors that are associated with the development of arterial disease that eventually can result in a heart attack or stroke. High blood pressure, cigarette smoking, excessive cholesterol in the blood, lack of exercise, overweight, stress, and type A personality all may contribute to the development of cardiovascular disease. Although all these risk factors are significant, poor nutrition, stress, and smoking stand out as major factors in the occurrence of hypertension, heart attack, and stroke.

Heart and vascular disease are preventable. There are human societies in which people rarely suffer from heart disease, even as they get older. The lifestyle of modern civilization seems to be the chief cause of deaths from cardiovascular disease. Coronary bypass operations and antihypertensive drugs are of debatable value. Prevention is the key to the continued health of the heart and vascular system. Every person can examine his or her lifestyle and try to reduce or eliminate those factors that contribute to the risk of developing heart disease.

FOR YOUR HEALTH

Slowing Your Pulse

Learn to take your pulse by pressing two fingers on the inside of the wrist of your opposite hand. Every artery expands and contracts with each heartbeat, so measuring the pulse is the same as counting heartbeats. Move your fingers around and press slightly until you find an artery and can feel your pulse (heartbeat). Count the number of beats for 30 seconds or a minute. Now practice slow, regular deep breathing for 5 minutes. Inhale slowly to a count of 6 or 8, hold for a count of 2, and exhale slowly for the same count of 6 or 8. (The count should be comfortable but as slow as you can make it.) After breathing in this way for a short time, take your pulse again. Most persons will notice a significant decrease in the rate of their heartbeat. You can use this exercise to calm yourself and slow down the pumping of your heart whenever you become anxious or overexcited. After a while you can use the breathing exercise to calm yourself without even taking your pulse.

Changing Your Habits

Make a list of any habits you have that might contribute to heart disease. Resolve to change at least one of these habits for a given period of time. Then try to make the healthy new habit a permanent part of your lifestyle.

CHAPTER SEVENTEEN

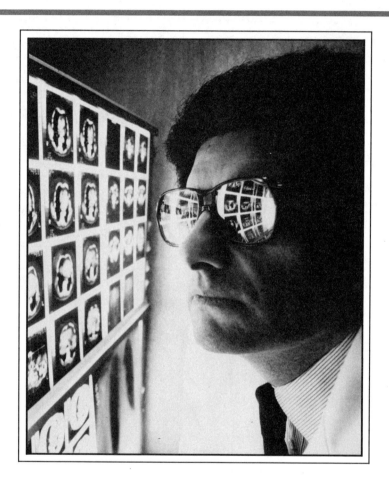

Understanding cancer can reduce the
risk and fear of getting this disease, as
well as help with preventing its
occurrence.

Cancer: Causes and Prevention

By now it is abundantly clear that the incidence of the common human cancers is determined by various controllable, external factors. This is surely the single most important fact to come out of all cancer research; for, it means that cancer is a preventable disease.

John Cairns

One person in four in the United States is likely to develop some form of cancer during his or her lifetime, and one person in five is likely to die from it. This is the bleak picture presented by the most recent statistical data (see Figure 17-1). Cancer is the second most frequent cause of death in the United States, accounting for more than 400,000 deaths annually. Only heart disease kills more people each year. While deaths from most other major diseases, including heart disease, have decreased in recent years, the incidence of cancer in the United States has increased primarily due to the increase in lung cancer.

Death from cancer seems to many people to be more frightening and odious than death from any other disease. Almost everyone has some fear of contracting cancer. For reasons that cannot be explained adequately, being told that one has serious heart disease or dangerously high blood pressure does not evoke the same fear and stigma as being told that one has cancer. In an editorial in the *New England Journal of Medicine,* F. J. Ingelfinger (1975) describes this consuming popular fear as "cancerophobia":

> American cancerophobia, in brief, is a disease as serious to society as cancer is to the individual—and morally devastating. For this state of affairs many are to blame—not only high-pressure advertisers who foment and exploit our cancerophobia, but also the well-meaning but yet baneful practices of other groups: activist consumer organizations, politicians, and even the American Cancer Society, which points directly accusatory fingers at you if you do not give money to "cure cancer." Among the guilty are the media. Because of our society's disease, any news about cancer, no matter how trivial, is ipso facto sensational.

There is some suggestive evidence (discussed at the end of this chapter) that fear of cancer, by creating stress and anxiety that lowers immune system response, may even contribute to the development or progression of the disease. No one should be resigned to the idea that cancer is inevitable or that a diagnosis of cancer assuredly means suffering, pain, and death. As with many other diseases there is a great deal that each person can do to reduce the risk of getting cancer. Everyone's goal should

> In biblical times, the symbolic disease was leprosy. Later, it was plague, then tuberculosis and syphilis. All of these diseases, long before the discovery of bacteria and protozoa, carried a fatal taint, an aura of accursedness that required some holy intervention to cure. Meanwhile, victims were shunned, segregated, often exiled. We may be somewhat *more* temperate today, but cancer is still thought of, by some, as a dirty, deadly disease, and its victims may be set apart.
>
> Avery D. Weisman, M.D.

be the *prevention* of cancer—adoption of a lifestyle that minimizes the risk of developing cancer—and also understanding the early warning signs of cancer, because many cancers *are* curable by surgery and drugs if they are detected early enough. Approximately one-third of *all* cancers are caused by cigarette smoking and other forms of tobacco use. It is estimated that 80 percent of all cancers could be prevented by changes in diet, smoking, and other unhealthy behaviors.

Many risk factors contribute to cancer formation—radiation, mutagenic chemicals in the environment, genetic predisposition, nutritional factors, immunological deficiencies—possibly even stress and negative mental states. In order to adequately evaluate the environmental and psychological risks associated with developing the various diseases labeled as "cancer," you need to understand something about the biology and causes of cancer. Then you can intelligently decide how to reduce the risk of cancer as well as to understand how to cope with the disease if it should arise.

What Is Cancer?

The term "cancer" comes from the Latin word meaning "crab." The characterization of this disease as crablike was used by the Greek physician Hippocrates because it seemed to creep in all directions through the body, eventually cutting off life with its pincers.

Cancer is the unregulated multiplication of cells in the body. This definition applies to every form of cancer—of which there are several hundred—regardless of the specific medical description.

Each one of the body's cells must be able to regulate its growth and functions, which, in turn, regulate the size and functions of tissues and organs. If a normal cell somehow loses its ability to regulate its growth and reproduction, it may form a **tumor.** A tumor is a mass of abnormal cells (generally more than a billion before it becomes detectable) that most likely has arisen as the consequence of a genetic alteration of a single normal cell. The growth and reproduction of the cell become unregulated as a consequence of the mutation and of other factors (Nowell, 1976). Another term used to describe unregulated cell growth is **neoplasm** (literally "new growth"), which also refers to a mass of cells whose growth and reproduction are no longer regulated. The words neoplasm, tumor, and cancer are often used interchangeably.

If the cells of the tumor remain localized at the site of origin and multiply relatively slowly, the tumor is said to be **benign.** Benign tumors (cysts, moles, warts, and polyps) do not spread to other parts of the body, can usually be removed surgically, and generally are not a threat to life. Once removed, benign tumors seldom regrow.

Malignant neoplasms, or **malignant tumors,** are composed of cells that usually multiply much more rapidly than normal cells and have a number of other properties that distinguish them from normal cells. Neoplastic cells have altered cell surfaces as well as other tissue differences that enable a pathologist (a physician who specializes in the nature and causes of diseases) to determine whether

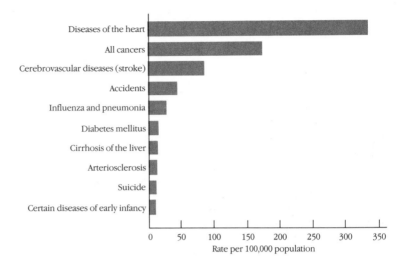

Figure 17-1
Major causes of death in the U.S. (Data from National Center for Health Statistics, U.S. Public Health Service, 1981.)

the cells are normal or malignant. The abnormal cells of a malignant tumor also commonly revert to a more embryonic, undifferentiated state and they may have abnormal chromosomes. Whatever the specific changes, it is the unregulated cell multiplication that is the characteristic and destructive feature of all cancer cells.

Cancers are classified medically according to the organ or kind of tissue in which the tumor originates. The four major categories of cancer— **carcinomas, sarcomas, leukemias,** and **lymphomas**—are described in Figure 17-2. Within these major classifications there are hundreds of subgroups.

Figure 17-2 also give the relative frequencies of the major kinds of cancer. Most cancers are carcinomas, which arise from cellular changes in skin and membrane tissues surrounding vital organs. In fact, about *half* of all human cancers in the United States originate in one of three organs: the lung, the breast, or the large intestine. Considerable research effort is directed toward finding the factors that contribute to development of cancer in these organs.

The cells of some malignant tumors also may undergo **metastasis,** a process in which cells detach from the original tumor, enter the bloodstream, and are carried to other organs of the body. The life-destroying property of malignant tumors derives

Figure 17-2
Major classifications and frequency of kinds of cancer.

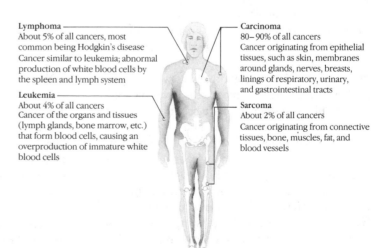

Lymphoma
About 5% of all cancers, most common being Hodgkin's disease Cancer similar to leukemia; abnormal production of white blood cells by the spleen and lymph system

Leukemia
About 4% of all cancers Cancer of the organs and tissues (lymph glands, bone marrow, etc.) that form blood cells, causing an overproduction of immature white blood cells

Carcinoma
80–90% of all cancers Cancer originating from epithelial tissues, such as skin, membranes around glands, nerves, breasts, linings of respiratory, urinary, and gastrointestinal tracts

Sarcoma
About 2% of all cancers Cancer originating from connective tissues, bone, muscles, fat, and blood vessels

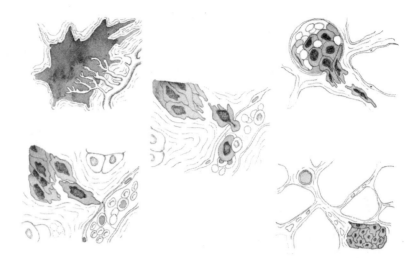

Figure 17-3
The stages of metastasis: (a) tumor cells invade surrounding tissue, (b) they squeeze into a capillary and enter the bloodstream, (c) then they are carried to the lungs and other body organs, (d) they may become arrested in a capillary of the lung, where (e) they may form new tumors.

from the ability of cancer cells to migrate (metastasize) to vital body organs and form new tumors. Most cancer patients are killed not by the primary tumor but by its metastasis. The main stages in metastasis, which is a complex biological process, are shown in Figure 17-3.

Cancer does not develop abruptly but rather results from several cellular changes that accumulate over many years, often over several decades. The progression of tumor development is defined by four relatively distinct stages. In stage I, cancer cells can be distinguished from normal cells under the microscope. The cancerous cells are still localized in the body, and surgical removal of the abnormal mass of cells often results in a complete cure. By stage II the cancer cells have begun to metastasize (move from their original site) and are also found in nearby lymph nodes. This is why lymph nodes are sometimes removed along with a breast in advanced stages of breast cancer. In Stage III, the cancer cells have proliferated through many lymph nodes and may have invaded nearby organs as well. Stage IV is often a final stage of cancer; cells have now spread into the blood system and have become established at many sites throughout the body.

What is it about unregulated cell multiplication and metastasis that eventually leads to death? Benign tumors usually do not kill people, because the cells remain localized, and unless the tumor mechanically interferes with some essential body function—for example, by pressing against some vital nerves—it can grow to enormous size without being lethal. Single tumors weighing many pounds have been surgically removed from patients who have then fully recovered from the operation.

However, malignant tumors whose cells metastasize can result in death. In addition to diverting essential nutrients from normal cells, the growth of tumors in vital organs such as the lungs, heart, liver, or brain can interfere with the functioning of those organs so that serious illness and possibly death ensues. The extent to which malignant tumors metastasize and the rate of growth of malignant tumor cells are extremely variable and depend on many factors, including the kind of therapy the patient receives, the person's nutritional state, emotional and mental attitudes, and hormonal and immunological responsiveness. These are some of the reasons why it is so difficult to predict the eventual course of cancer for a particular person. It is worth remembering that statistics do not apply to the individual—only to populations of individuals.

The Causes of Cancer

The causes of cancer—or perhaps it is better to speak of the risk factors associated with the development of cancer—are numerous and complex. It is difficult, if not impossible, to point to a single cause for even one kind of cancer. For each person, the development of cancer probably derives from many cellular events accumulated over time, which culminate in one or a few cells becoming transformed so that they commence to grow and multiply in an unregulated, abnormal way.

Table 17-1
Lifestyle Causes of Cancer

Cause	Estimated percentage	Types of cancer	Approximate number of daily deaths
Nutrition and diet	45 percent of cancer deaths are mainly due to nutritional problems including: 1. Excess calories. 2. Excess intake of fats of all kinds. 3. Obesity — 40 lbs or more overweight. 4. Nutritional deficiencies, especially of fiber and vitamin A.	Most cancers of the colon, rectum, stomach, breast, and many cancers of the ovaries	450
Cigarettes and alcohol	35 percent of cancer deaths are mainly due to smoking high-tar cigarettes and drinking excessive amounts of hard liquor.	Cancers of the lungs, mouth, larynx, esophagus, liver and some cancers of the urinary bladder	350
Occupation	5 percent of cancer deaths are due to past occupational exposures to substances now known to cause cancer.	Cancers of the bladder, lung, stomach, blood, liver, bones, and skin	50
Radiation	3 percent are mainly due to ionizing radiation, including "background" and medical radiation.	Leukemia and various others	30
Other	The rest of cancer deaths are due to a variety of causes, including genetic and chronic diseases, drugs, chemotherapy, and so forth.	Various	120

Data from J. A. Cimino and H. B. Demopoulos, "Determinants of Cancer Relative to Prevention in the War on Cancer," in H. B. Demopoulos and M. A. Mehlman (eds.), *Cancer and the Environment* (Park Forest South, Ill.: Pathotox Publishers, 1980).

Scientific studies indicate that most cancers are caused by the ways in which people live (see Table 17-1). Three classes of environmental agents have been shown to produce cancer in animals and humans. **Ionizing radiation, tumor viruses,** and certain chemicals all appear to cause cancer, presumably by a common mechanism. The most reasonable hypothesis at present says that all of these agents can mutate or change the genetic information (DNA) in any cell of the body (see Figure 17-4). It is also thought that expression of these genetic changes can be helped by substances called **tumor promoters.** That is, a cell with the genetic potential for becoming cancerous can be pushed further in that direction by small amounts of certain chemicals. Thus, genetic changes as well as cellular changes are required for unregulated cell growth to occur. Other factors in the body, such as the lack of certain nutrients, abnormal hormone levels, and reduced activity of the immune system may also contribute to the process of cell transformation and cancer formation.

We know that ionizing radiation, numerous chemicals, and certain viruses can cause cancer to develop, because exposure of experimental animals to these agents produces tumors in many of them, especially if the doses are large. Moreover, epidemiological studies of human populations have shown that exposure to environmental agents such as cigarette smoke, coal tars, asbestos, x-rays, atomic fallout, and other forms of radiation is associated with more frequent development of cancer.

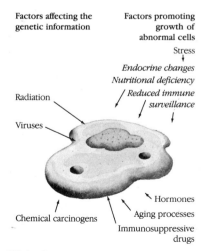

Factors affecting the genetic information

Factors promoting growth of abnormal cells

Stress
Endocrine changes
Nutritional deficiency
Reduced immune surveillance

Radiation

Viruses

Hormones

Chemical carcinogens

Aging processes

Immunosuppressive drugs

Figure 17-4
Factors involved in the formation of a cancer cell.

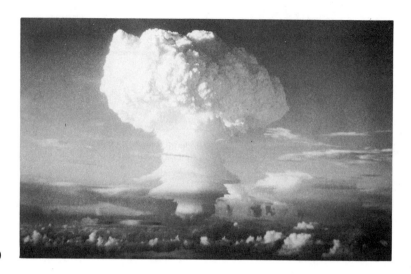

Figure 17-5
A nuclear bomb test. The mushroom is 10 miles high and 100 miles wide. (Courtesy U.S. Department of Energy.)

Evidence supporting the assertions by the U.S. National Cancer Institute and the World Health Organization that most human cancers are caused by environmental factors is presented in the following sections. John Higginson (1983), founding director of WHO's International Agency for Research on Cancer, has concluded that 80–90 percent of all human cancers are environmentally caused and, in principal, are preventable. It is his view that "epidemiologic analysis of cancer patterns in advanced and underdeveloped countries indicates that, for the most part, they are associated with behavioral, cultural and dietary factors." People need to realize that cancer *is* a preventable disease and they need to become more aware of the factors that contribute to its development.

Radiation

The significantly higher-than-normal incidence of leukemia and other forms of cancer among survivors of the Hiroshima and Nagasaki atomic bomb blasts leaves no doubt that atomic radiation is a potent **carcinogen**—that is, an agent that can cause cancer. More recently in our own country, it has been demonstrated that leukemia deaths among children born in southern Utah (who were exposed to fallout from above-ground atomic bomb tests in Nevada) were two to three times greater than those among children born in the years before and after the atomic tests (Lyon et al., 1979) (see Figure 17-5). In a landmark legal decision a federal court ruled in 1984 that the U.S. government was negligent in

conducting the atomic bomb tests in Nevada in the 1950s that released radioactive material into the atmosphere. The court ruled that the families who were exposed to the radioactivity, and whose members died as a result of the exposure are entitled to compensation.

Some types of radiation—for example, visible light and infrared radiation, commonly called "radiant heat"—are not carcinogens. But there are types of radiation with energy levels high enough to knock electrons out of atoms. Such radiation is called **ionizing radiation** because an atom (or molecule) lacking one or more electrons is called an **ion**. Alpha, beta, and gamma radiation, as well as x-rays, are types of ionizing radiation. All are emitted by radioactive substances (x-rays are actually a form of gamma radiation). And all radiation—x-rays are the most familiar example—can be produced by man-made devices.

The amount of radiation absorbed by a tissue is expressed in terms of energy per weight of tissue. A common unit of radiation is the **rad** (**r**adiation **a**bsorbed **d**ose), defined as 100 ergs of energy per gram of tissue. Because radiation can come from a variety of sources, including x-rays, ultraviolet light, and radioactive elements, another unit of radiation called the **rem** (**r**oentgen **e**quivalent **m**an) is often used. For most purposes the rem and the rad are equivalent.

While almost all scientists agree that exposure to large amounts of ionizing radiation can increase the occurrence of cancer, there has been considerable disagreement about whether exposure to low levels of atomic or x-ray irradiation increases the

It is, I believe, just as practicable to contemplate starting a 10–20 year project to achieve the prevention of most forms of cancer as it was in 1963 to start a 10 year project to land a man on the moon; each could be done with existing technology.

John Cairns

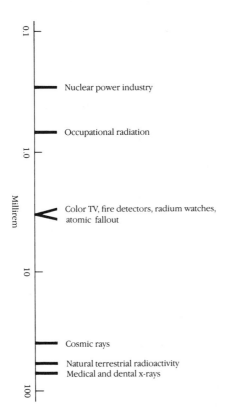

Figure 17-6
Estimates of whole-body radiation to an average American each year (based on U.S. government BEIR Report, 1972). About 40 percent of all radiation exposure comes from medical and dental x-rays. The values given are an estimated average. For some people—x-ray and dental technicians or workers in the nuclear industry, for example—radiation exposures will be higher; for other people, exposures will be less than average.

probability of cancer. Recent studies, however, support the contention of many scientists that even low doses of ionizing radiation are dangerous. In England, dockyard workers exposed to low-level radiation from the nuclear reactors of nuclear-powered ships over a 10 year period were shown to have increased chromosomal damage. And a statistical study in the United States concluded that frequent medical x-rays may make a person ten times more susceptible to getting leukemia (Evans et al., 1979; Bross, Ball, and Falen, 1979; Kohn and Fry, 1984). It is estimated that several million American children who grew up in the 1940s and 1950s received large doses of x-rays to shrink tonsils and to treat other neck and chest ailments. At that time x-ray treatment of these organs was considered standard medical procedure, although it is now realized that this group of individuals has a greatly increased risk of developing thyroid and salivary gland tumors. In a study of 15,000 children who were treated with radiation for various cancers, the rate of secondary tumor development was ten times greater than expected. For this group the benefits of the radiation treatment clearly outweighed the risks of subsequent tumor formation; however, the study does demonstrate the hazard of radiation exposure and the subsequent risk of cancer.

The radiation we are exposed to comes from many sources in the environment (see Figure 17-6). Radioactivity from ores and other material in the environment and the atomic particles in cosmic rays are sources of natural radiation. Man-made radiation is generated by nuclear power plants, atomic tests, radioisotopes used in laboratories, medical and

> It is the general scientific consensus,
> clearly indicated not in words but in the efforts
> that are being expended, that cancer is
> a solvable problem.
> **Michael Shimkin, M.D.**

dental x-rays, and even color television sets. Because it is believed that any amount of radiation, however small, has the potential for causing chromosomal damage and genetic changes in cells, it seems sensible to minimize one's exposure to all sources of radiation as much as possible. For example, if you are healthy, periodic chest x-rays may be unwarranted. Routine dental x-rays with every checkup definitely pose a cumulative risk. Neither does it make sense to build your house on top of debris from a uranium mine. (Unfortunately, more than a few people have done just this.)

Viruses and Oncogenes

In 1911 Peyton Rous, a scientist working at the Rockefeller Institute in New York, showed that tumors could be induced in chickens by injecting them with a particular virus. This **oncogenic** (cancer-causing) virus subsequently was named after its discoverer and is called the Rous sarcoma virus. Since then, numerous oncogenic viruses have been identified that produce specific kinds of cancer when injected into susceptible animals. For example, mouse mammary tumor virus (MMTV) causes mammary cancer in female mice, and feline leukemia (FTV) causes leukemia in cats. As a general rule, tumor viruses are specific both for the species of animal they can infect and for the kind of cancer they initiate.

Enormous expenditures of money and research effort have been devoted to determining whether at least some human cancers are caused by viruses. Now, the finding of a virus in cancer cells does not

prove that cancer is actually caused by the virus any more than your presence in a car that is involved in a crash means that you caused the accident. To date, no oncogenic virus has been shown conclusively to cause cancer in humans, although in a few instances the presence of a particular virus is associated with increased risk of developing a particular kind of cancer. Epstein-Barr virus (EBV) is the only virus in humans that shows a strong association with a particular cancer, **Burkitt's lymphoma,** which occurs primarily in the regions of Africa and usually in children. A curious and unexplained fact about EBV is that almost all children in the United States and other countries have been infected with EBV yet hardly any cases of lymphoma develop. Outside of Africa EBV appears to cause mononucleosis, a mild infectious disease that occurs frequently among college students. What this information about EBV tells us is that a virus that is potentially oncogenic causes cancer only under specific environmental conditions. Under other conditions it may cause a mild disease or, in the majority of people, no disease at all.

Strictly speaking, tumor viruses are environmental agents, but few cancers are thought to be caused just by viral infections. Cancer is not a contagious disease nor is it passed from person to person. The **oncogene hypothesis** says viral genetic information (DNA) is normally present in the chromosomes of animals, including humans (the viral genes are inherited along with all the other genes). This viral genetic information remains unexpressed and harmless unless it becomes activated by exposure to an environmental agent such as ionizing radi-

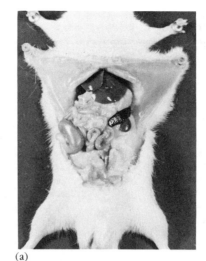 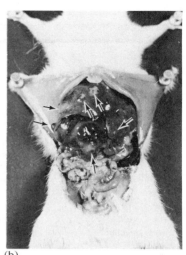

(a)   (b)

Figure 17-7
(a) Abdominal organs of a normal rat and (b) abdominal organs of a rat that was administered dimethylnitrosamine, a carcinogen identified in a variety of foods, including fish, cheese, cured ham, and fried bacon. In (b), liver tumor masses (arrows) are plainly visible. (Courtesy Joseph Arcos, Environmental Protection Agency, Washington, D.C.)

ation or carcinogenic chemicals. Viruses may then proliferate and alter the properties of cells. Eventually, the unregulated multiplication of the virus-transformed cells may produce a possibly malignant tumor.

The current scientific excitement over oncogenes in tumor viruses (cancer-causing genes carried in the RNA or DNA molecules of viruses) derives from the hope that by understanding oncogenes we will begin to understand the biological mechanisms that convert a normal cell into a cancer cell. Without such basic understanding, cancer prevention is largely guesswork and cancer treatment is not as safe and effective as it might be. So far, scientists have shown that viral oncogenes are derived from closely related genes that are normally present in all cells. At least some of the cellular oncogenes appear to perform essential functions in cells, and it may be that these cells become cancerous only after the cell's oncogenes are altered by radiation or carcinogenic chemicals. It is the view of J. M. Bishop (1982), a prominent cancer researcher at the University of California, San Francisco, that

normal cells may bear the seeds of their own destruction in the form of cancer genes. The activities of these genes may represent the final common pathway by which many carcinogens act. Cancer genes may be not unwanted guests but essential constituents of the cell's genetic apparatus, betraying the cell only when their structure or control is disturbed by carcinogens.

Despite all of the research that has been carried out over the past quarter century on oncogenic viruses and cancer, there still is no proof or compelling evidence that viruses cause any of the commonly occuring human cancers such as lung, breast, stomach, or colon cancer. In fact, to date none of the predictions of the virus theories of human cancer causation have been confirmed by experiments. It may be that viruses are simply associated with tumors and do not actually cause them unless other properties of the cell have already been altered by other factors such as genetic aberrations.

The reason that so much effort in cancer research has focused on viruses and cancer-causing genes (oncogenes) is that if specific cellular genes or viruses actually cause cancer, then it may be possible to design and develop effective therapies. For example, it might be possible to find drugs that block cancer-causing genes or their products, or it might be possible to develop vaccines against tumor viruses. However, because it is not even clear that viruses or oncogenes actually cause cancer, no one anticipates that cures for cancer caused by viruses or for AIDS (see Chapter 18) will be forthcoming in the foreseeable future.

Chemical Carcinogens

A **chemical carcinogen** is a substance that can interact with cells' genetic material to produce cancer. Suspected chemical carcinogens are usually tested in experimental animals such as rats, mice, and guinea pigs under scientifically controlled conditions (see Figure 17-7). Many substances to which you are

Table 17-2
Substances Proven to Be Carcinogenic

Chemical	Site of cancer	Chemical	Site of Cancer
Aromatic amines	Bladder	Alkylating agents	Bladder
Arsenic	Skin and bronchus		Hematopoietic tissue
Asbestos	Bronchus, pleura, and peritoneum	Anabolic steroids	Liver
		Arsenic	Skin
Benzene	Marrow	Chlornaphazine	Bladder
Beryllium	Prostate	Diethylstilbestrol	Vagina
Bis(chloromethyl) ether	Bronchus	Immunosuppressive drugs	Lymphoid tissue
Bis(chloroethyl)sulfide	Respiratory tract	Phenacetin (acetophenetidin)	Kidney
Cadmium	Prostate	Chloramphenicol, melphalan	Marrow
Chrome ores	Bronchus	Aflatoxins	Liver
Coke ovens	Bronchus	Tobacco smoke	Bronchus, mouth, pharynx, larynx, esophagus, bladder
Nickel ores	Bronchus and nasal sinuses		
Soots, tars, and oils	Skin and lungs	Oral contraceptives	Liver
Wood dust	Nasal sinuses	Betel nut and lime	Mouth
Vinyl chloride	Liver	Nitrates, nitrites, and nitrosamines	Stomach, liver, bladder, kidney
Wood and leather dust	Respiratory tract		

exposed in your daily living can increase the likelihood that some cells in the body will become genetically altered, thereby acquiring the potential for becoming cancerous. The list of carcinogenic substances is unfortunately quite long. It includes cigarette smoke, hair dyes, food additives, artificial sweeteners, pesticides, anesthetics, asbestos, fire-retardant chemicals in clothing, benzene, nitrosamines, vinyl chloride, soot, and aflatoxins. In fact, so many substances are proving to be carcinogenic that people are confused about what is safe to eat, drink, or wear—or even when and where it is safe to breathe. Table 17-2 lists substances present in people's diets, in prescribed drugs, and in certain occupations that have been proven to cause human cancers. Exposure to these substances should be avoided. Many other substances are suspected carcinogens but have not been adequately tested to be included in this list.

Scientific experts often disagree among themselves about what is safe and what is likely to cause cancer and other diseases. In the face of conflicting statements, some people tend to disregard all warnings. Others become overly concerned about everything they eat or drink. A healthy viewpoint lies somewhere in between these two extremes.

Environmental substances that can cause cancer have increased drastically in the last 20 years but the situation is not yet hopeless. As Bruce Ames (1978), professor of biochemistry at the University of California, Berkeley, and originator of the most widely used test for identifying carcinogens, puts it:

Since the late 1950s we have been exposed to a flood of chemicals—from flame retardants in our children's pajamas to pesticides accumulating in our body fat—that were not tested for carcinogenicity or mutagenicity before their use. A few of these chemicals are now being tested in animals, but for most of them the human population is serving as the test animal. We are exposed to a very large number of chemicals that are mutagens and carcinogens, many of them quite useful to society, and it is clearly impractical to ban them all, yet foolish to ignore their potential danger. We must have some way of setting priorities for regulation of these chemicals, and this requires an assessment of human risk.

Ames (1979) took an important first step in the risk assessment of chemicals by developing "tester" bacteria that can measure the mutagenic potential of most chemicals. The importance of the Ames test and others since developed is that they make it possible to rapidly test many chemicals for their carcinogenic potential (in a few days as compared to months or years in animals) and cheaply (a few hundred dollars as compared to tens or hundreds of thousands of dollars for animal tests). Ames and his collaborators have shown that there is a high correlation between carcinogenicity (causing cancer in animals) and mutagenicity (causing mutations in cellular DNA). Over 90 percent of chemicals known

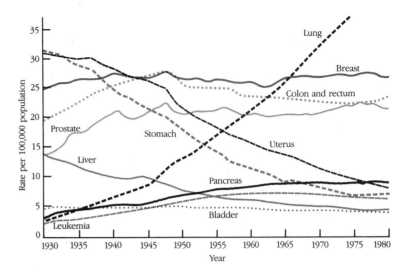

Figure 17-8
Cancer death rates by site over the past 50 years. Rates for breast and uterus are calculated for female populations and prostate for male populations. (Data from the National Center for Health Statistics and Bureau of the Census; courtesy American Cancer Society.)

to be carcinogenic are also mutagenic, so chemical companies can now save considerable time and money by early testing of a new chemical to determine its carcinogenic hazard.

It is estimated that at least 63,000 chemicals are in common use in this country. Of the 7000 that have been tested to some extent in animal experiments, over half have been reported to be carcinogenic. Each year approximately 1000 new chemicals are introduced into the environment in one form or another (Maugh, 1978).

Despite the mutagenic tests performed on bacteria and the carcinogenic tests on animals, can we be sure these substances cause cancer in people? To answer this we have to turn to epidemiological studies. Figure 17-8 shows how the death rates from specific cancers have changed over the past 50 years. While the rates for most cancers have remained constant or have declined somewhat, lung cancer has increased dramatically since 1940. All of the available scientific evidence points to cigarette smoking as being responsible for most cases of lung cancer. Men began to smoke heavily during the 1940s and women more recently. Since lung cancer generally takes 20 years or more to develop in an individual, we are now witnessing an epidemic of lung cancers caused by many years of smoking.

Cigarette smoking and lung cancer are inextricably linked (see Chapter 15). But as the tobacco companies argue, this does not constitute absolute proof that smoking causes cancer since not every person who smokes will develop lung cancer. Some may die

of other causes before lung cancer develops. Others may be biologically more resistant to developing cancer, but that still does not mean that smoking is safe. Epidemiological studies also link other environmental substances with specific cancers. Cancer of the large intestine varies in frequency around the world and generally seems to correlate positively with meat consumption (see Figure 17-9). This is not to say that meat is carcinogenic per se, but excessive meat consumption or the production of substances in meat while cooking may act as cancer promoters when other precancerous changes have already occurred in body cells. Moreover, in the United States antibiotics, hormones, and other chemicals are often added to animal feed to fatten cattle before slaughtering.

Among the most convincing epidemiological studies are those that analyze changes in cancer incidence among genetically similar groups of individuals living in different environments. For example, cancer of the stomach is quite frequent in Japan and relatively infrequent in the United States. The converse is true for colon cancer: it is common in the United States but rare in Japan. When the incidence of these two kinds of cancer is measured among Japanese living in Japan and among Japanese who have moved to Hawaii and adopted American lifestyles, the effect of environmental factors becomes more evident. As Figure 17-10 shows, Japanese who moved to Hawaii have considerably less stomach cancer than those who stayed home. These studies show that the incidence of certain

Figure 17-9
Geography of cancer suggests a probable cause of the disease. The incidence of cancer of the large intestine among women in twenty-three countries is closely related to per capita meat consumption in those countries. The data are adjusted to eliminate differences in age distribution in the populations. An alternative explanation attributes cancer of the large intestine to a low consumption of cereals. The two hypotheses are hard to distinguish from each other because high meat consumption and low cereal consumption tend to go together. (Data from J. Cairns, "The Cancer Problem," copyright © 1975 by Scientific American, Inc. All rights reserved.)

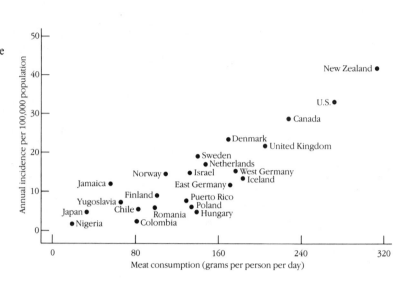

cancers can be increased or decreased by environmental factors. Taken all together, epidemiological studies make a convincing case that environmental factors contribute to the formation of 70–90 percent of all cancers.

If one examines occupational carcinogenesis (occurrence of specific cancers among workers in particular industries) the evidence becomes overwhelming. More than 200 years ago, an English physician, Percivall Pott, reported a high rate of scrotal cancer among London chimney sweeps. Today coke-oven workers in the U.S. steelmaking industry inhale the same sooty substances that eighteenth-century London chimney sweeps did, and these workers die of lung cancer at a rate ten times higher than that of other steel workers. For more than 25 years, asbestos dust has been known to cause a particular kind of lung cancer, and of the million or so current and former asbestos workers who still survive, about 300,000 will eventually die of cancer (Wagoner, 1976). If one examines the incidence of a number of kinds of cancers across the United States, another disturbing correlation emerges. The greatest numbers of certain cancers cluster in highly industrialized areas of the country, thus supporting the view that these cancers are of environmental and occupational origin (see Box 17-1).

We have delved at length into the environmental basis for cancer because as individuals we can elect where to live, the conditions we choose to work

Figure 17-10
Incidence of stomach and colon cancer among Japanese men and women. Stomach cancers decrease for Japanese who move to Hawaii but now colon cancer is more frequent, showing that the environment affects the frequency of these types of cancer. (Data from Hawaii State Department of Health, The Cancer Center, 1976.)

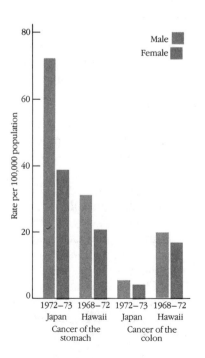

BOX 17-1

CARCINOGENS ON THE JOB: THE MOST HAZARDOUS INDUSTRIES

What industry exposes its workers to the greatest cancer risks? It is not, as many would guess, the chemical industry. Neither is it uranium mining. According to a study prepared for the National Institute for Occupational Safety and Health (NIOSH), the most hazardous industry is the manufacture of industrial and scientific instruments (Hickey and Kearney, 1977).

The study ranked the fabricated metal products industry as second most hazardous and placed the electrical equipment industry third. The chemical industry didn't even have the dubious distinction of being placed among the top ten industries in terms of worker exposure to carcinogens—although it was lower down on the list, in twelfth place.

According to the study, the most hazardous industries and some of the carcinogens used in them are:

1. Industrial and scientific instruments (asbestos, lead, solder).
2. Fabricated metal products (lead, nickel, asbestos, certain solvents).
3. Electrical equipment and supplies (lead, asbestos, mercury, chlorohydrocarbons, certain solvents).
4. Machinery (except electrical: cutting, quenching, and lubricating oils).
5. Transportation equipment (ingredients of plastics, including formaldehyde and phenol).
6. Petroleum and petroleum products (benzene, napthalene).
7. Leather products (chrome salts and organic compounds used in the tanning of hides).
8. Pipeline transportation (petroleum derivatives, metals used in welding).

The rankings in the study are based on (1) the relative toxicity of the carcinogens involved and (2) the extent of workers' exposure to them. Relatively small amounts of carcinogens are used in the industry ranked most hazardous: industrial and scientific instruments. But these substances are used in devices that have handmade components, so workers' exposure levels to them are high. Earlier studies of carcinogens in the workplace had been based on amounts produced but not on workers' exposure to them. This is why the chemical industry had been ranked much higher on older "hazardous" lists. It produces relatively huge amounts of carcinogens, but relatively few workers are involved in their production. Thus total worker exposure to these carcinogens is low compared with worker exposure in several other industries.

What of the carcinogens themselves— which are the most hazardous? The study assessed the toxicity, amount of worker exposure, and annual production of the various carcinogens. It concluded that the ten most hazardous ones are, in order, asbestos, formaldehyde, benzene, lead, kerosene, nickel, chromium, "volatiles" in coal tar, carbon tetrachloride, and sulfuric acid.

The study was commissioned as part of NIOSH's long-range plan for reducing exposure to carcinogens on the job. Carcinogenic dusts were found by researchers to be the biggest problem in many of the industries studied. The researchers recommended that a major effort be made to seal off the dust-producing processes from the workers. They also proposed that more workers use masks and other apparatus to protect themselves from carcinogens in their workplaces.

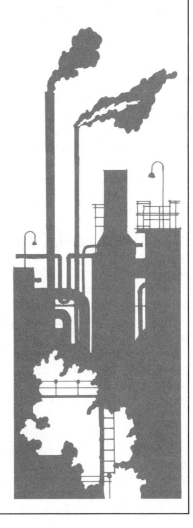

under, what to eat, and whether to dye our hair or to spray our gardens with pesticides. We do have choices as individuals and we can also exhort the government regulatory agencies to ban the use of proven, widely used carcinogenic substances. Most of the environmental decisions in our country are made for political and economic reasons. The responsible individuals in industry and government must continually weigh the risks versus the benefits for each substance and product. What would be the consequences of banning the use of asbestos in brake linings, pipe fittings, and home insulation? How will food production be affected if pesticide use is sharply curtailed? What are the health hazards from spoilage of meat if use of the traditional preservatives, sodium nitrate and sodium nitrite, is prohibited? The answers to such questions are not simple. Joseph C. Arcos (1978) of the Environmental Protection Agency expresses the dilemma thusly: "Viewed against the complexity of the problem, the steady increase of cancers in the industrialized countries is seen as a consequence as well as an indictment of our technological lifestyles."

As individuals you can choose a lifestyle that minimizes your exposure to environmental carcinogens. You can educate yourself to the hazards of any chemical substances you use frequently—cosmetics, insect spray and garden pesticides, artificial food additives, cleaning solutions and solvents, and so forth. The solution to cancer—as it is for other major diseases—is prevention.

Nutrition and Cancer

Because cancer rates differ appreciably among populations that have different diets, considerable scientific and public attention has become focused on food as a contributing factor in the development of certain cancers. It is also becoming apparent that certain diets and food may actually protect against cancer formation. Vitamin E, vitamin C, beta-carotene, fiber, and other substances have all been identified as possible anticarcinogens (see Table 17-3).

Even with the strong epidemiological evidence supporting the view that certain cancers are caused by particular diets, there still is no unambiguous way to identify the specific foods or substances in the diet that may cause cancer. Despite this scientific uncertainty, the Committee on Diet, Nutrition and

Cancer of the National Research Council recommended certain dietary guidelines in 1982. The committee felt that, despite the lack of conclusive scientific data, certain dietary practices were prudent and might help reduce the future incidence of cancer. These recommended cancer-reducing nutritional guidelines are summarized in Table 17-4.

Preventing Cancer

Cancer prevention depends primarily on reducing your exposure to environmental agents that can mutate the cells' genetic information or cause other deleterious cellular changes. This includes minimizing your exposure to radioactivity and medical x-rays except when necessary and reducing, as much as possible, ingestion of carcinogenic substances in air, food, and water. Your work and living environments should be as free as possible from known carcinogenic substances.

Such precautions are only common sense. Yet many people are still unable to apply common sense in their personal health habits. This is apparent from a comparison of cancer mortality statistics over the years. In 1962 in the U.S. the age-adjusted cancer mortality rate was 170.2 deaths per 100,000 persons; in 1982 the rate had actually increased to 185.1 deaths per 100,000. Presumably the increase is due to the lack of improved treatments for most cancers

Table 17-3
Foods That Act as Cancer Inhibitors in Animal Studies
Note that most of the inhibitors are in vegetables.

Inhibitor	Food source
Vitamin A	Milk, butter, liver
Vitamin C	Citrus fruits, leafy vegetables, tomatoes
Vitamin E	Vegetable oils, nuts, asparagus
Beta-carotene	Carrots, sweet potatoes, leafy vegetables
Aromatic isothiocynanates	Cruciferous vegetables, (brussels sprouts, cabbage, cauliflower, broccoli)
Coumarins, lactones	Citrus fruits, vegetables
Flavinoids	Fruits, vegetables, grains
Indoles	Cruciferous vegetables
Phenolic acids	Coffee, tea, soybeans, potatoes, oats
Selenium	Grains, mushrooms, clams
Fiber	Whole grains, fruits, vegetables

> Man-made toxic chemicals are a significant source
> of death and disease in the United States today.
> We estimate that occupational exposure to
> carcinogens is a factor in more than 20 percent of
> all cancers.
>
> **Gus Speth**
> **Chairman, U.S. Council on Environmental Quality**

and to the dramatic increase in cigarette smoking during those years. It seems paradoxical that as a society we can be angered by carcinogenic pollutants in our environment and lobby for more government regulation and yet continue to smoke more than 600 billion cigarettes a year.

In addition to chemical carcinogens and radiation, poor nutrition, drugs, and stress may initiate or promote the cellular changes that result in cancer. The immune system protects the body from aberrant cells and tissues as well as from infectious organisms (see Chapter 9). The idea that the immune

Table 17-4
Nutritional Guidelines That May Help to Prevent Cancer*

1. Eat moderately. Maintain body weight within acceptable limits for height and age.
2. Reduce consumption of animal products, especially fats. No more than one-third of dietary energy should be supplied by fats.
3. Increase consumption of *fresh* vegetables, fruits, and whole-grain cereals.
4. Make sure diet contains adequate amounts of vitamin A, vitamin C, and vitamin E.
5. Avoid frequent consumption of smoked, pickled, and barbecued meats. The scorched skin and fat of barbecued meat contain potent carcinogens.

*It should be noted that experts disagree, sometimes vehemently, over the interactions of diet, carcinogens, anticarcinogens, and cancer. For example, see the exchange of letters in *Science,* May 18, 1984.

system can normally detect and destroy cancer cells as they arise in the body—known as the **immune surveillance hypothesis**—was proposed by the Nobel prize-winning immunologist F. M. Burnet (1976). While the precise mechanism is not understood, it is thought that particular cells of the immune system are able to distinguish normal cells from cancer cells and to destroy the abnormal cells.

As long as you are healthy and your immune system is functioning optimally, abnormal cells will probably be eliminated from the body as they arise. However, if your immune response is depressed, the cancer cells may proliferate and become too numerous for the immune system to be able to handle. People with immunological deficiency diseases, for example, are much more prone to developing cancer. Even people without any immunological disease can depress their immune responsiveness by poor nutrition, stressful lifestyles, and emotional problems. Therefore, all of the factors we have discussed that contribute to health may also help to prevent cancer from developing. One of the goals of holistic medicine as well as of conventional medicine is prevention of cancer, but the primary responsibility for prevention rests with each one of us.

Detecting Cancer

Since medicine has not been particularly effective up until now in preventing cancer, an enormous effort is being made to detect and treat it. But this approach has not been very effective either, as evi-

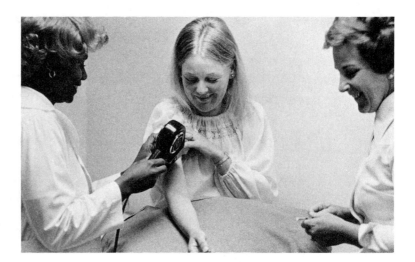

Figure 17-11
One of the major approaches to cancer treatment today is immunotherapy. Here a woman is being given an injection to help her immune system deal with cancer cells. (Courtesy Mount Zion Hospital and Medical Center, San Francisco.)

denced by the high cancer death rates. For years the American Cancer Society has attempted to educate the American public to cancer's early warning signals. These symptoms include any change in a mole or wart, the appearance of a lump in a breast or elsewhere, unusual bleeding, and persistant respiratory or digestive disturbances. Only a physician using a variety of diagnostic tests can determine whether a symptom is the result of a serious disease. The holistic approach to health emphasizes being "in touch" with your body (see Chapter 3). If your intuition tells you something "feels" wrong, heed the message and arrange for a medical checkup. The earlier a tumor is detected, the greater the chances for successful treatment.

The **Pap smear** is a simple test for cervical cancer in women. If a woman has had several negative Pap smears over a period of years, she has a low risk of developing cervical cancer. However, if a pap smear discloses any abnormal cells, more frequent checkups are advised. A woman can also examine her breasts regularly by feeling for any areas of thickening or for lumps (see Appendix B). It is also recommended that men feel their testicles periodically for any unusual lumps. While it is counterproductive to be constantly preoccupied with the dangers of developing cancer, a periodic checkup can ease one's mind.

Some promising new techniques for early detection and for identifying persons especially susceptible to cancer have been reported. One test measures the blood levels of a protein called **fibrinopeptide A** (FP-A). Persons suspected of

having cancer that may be undiagnosable by other techniques often show high levels of FP-A in their blood. Another test measures the blood level of specific immunological T-cells, which are thought to play a role in immune surveillance. Persons with inactive T-cells in their blood or with depressed levels of T-cells often develop cancer within a short while. Recently a promising new test for detecting malignant tumors by nuclear magnetic resonance (NMR) was reported (Fossel et al., 1986). It involves analyzing the NMR spectrum of blood samples. In preliminary tests patients with malignant cancers could be distinguished from other kinds of patients, and it is hoped that eventually this test might be used to detect cancers in the earliest stages of development, when treatments are most effective.

Treating Cancer

The three medical treatments for cancer, once it develops, are surgery, radiation therapy, and chemotherapy. Whenever possible, surgery is used to remove the mass of tumor cells while trying to minimize damage to surrounding healthy tissue. Removal of all cancerous tissue that is accessible to surgery has been an unquestioned medical practice throughout this century. However, in a careful critique of breast cancer treatments, researchers Klim McPherson and Maurice S. Fox (1977) point out that

the intuitive notion that the maximum purging of possibly offensive tissue is the most

> It seems far more sensible to prevent cancer than to try to cure it, particularly since present treatments are unusually traumatic, sometimes life-threatening, and can cure on the average only about one victim in four.
>
> **David M. Prescott**
> **Abraham S. Flexer, M.D.**

effective approach to the treatment of breast cancer, and of cancer in general, continues to dominate medical procedures. While it is possible that this notion is correct, there is little, if any, evidence to support it.

This point is of particular concern when one considers that over 120,000 American women are diagnosed as having breast cancer each year. Until quite recently, the recommended medical treatment for this disease was radical mastectomy—surgical removal of the breast or breasts along with considerable underlying tissue. Less radical surgery for breast cancer has been shown to be just as effective as rad-

Figure 17-12
Mammography exam. The breast on the left is normal; the one on the right shows a dark spot indicative of a tumor. The dark lines are veins and arteries.

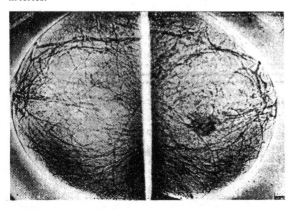

ical mastectomy, particularly if the tumor is detected while it is quite small. Any woman diagnosed with breast cancer would be well advised to obtain several opinions before making a final decision on the best surgical procedure and follow-up therapy. A panel of NIH physicians concluded recently that chemotherapy following breast cancer surgery may be of some benefit to premenopausal women in terms of length of survival but appears to be of no benefit to postmenopausal women. Several diagnostic techniques such as mammography, ultrasound, and thermography are used to detect the presence of breast tumors. The most reliable of the tests is mammography, which involves taking an x-ray picture of the breast (see Figure 17-12).

If there is evidence that tumor cells have metastasized (spread to other organs), then radiation therapy and/or chemotherapy may be necessary. These treatments destroy and damage normal cells as well as cancer cells. However, cancer cells are destroyed more readily than normal cells, which apparently can repair cellular damage and regenerate healthy tissue.

Cancer has also been treated by directly stimulating the patient's immune system with vaccines derived from bacteria such as the bacillus Calmette-Guerin (BCG) strain. Some dramatic cures by immunologic therapy have been reported, but there have also been some cases in which the growth of the tumor was enhanced by the vaccine.

Vitamin C has received considerable notoriety in the treatment of cancer and other diseases. Linus Pauling, a scientist of international fame, having

> Whether or not dynamic hope is a factor in cancer survival, it must never be denied to the cancer patient. . . . Even if there is no firm evidence that dynamic hope can prolong life beyond its expected duration, it is almost certain that absence of hope can shorten life, apart from vitiating its quality.
>
> **Basil A. Stoll, M.D.**

received two Nobel prizes (one for chemistry and another for peace), and Ewan Cameron administered 10 grams — 70 to 100 times the adult RDA — of vitamin C daily to 100 patients with untreatable (terminal) cancer. These persons survived from three to twenty times longer than patients who did not receive vitamin C (Cameron and Pauling, 1976). Pauling, Cameron, and others believe that high doses of vitamin C might be effective in preventing cancer and other stress-related lifestyle diseases, as well as being a useful adjunct in the treatment of cancer. However, the results of their studies have not been confirmed by controlled clinical trials with cancer patients, and vitamin C is not regarded as a useful agent in the treatment of cancer (Moertel et al., 1985).

A number of more exotic drugs have been used experimentally in the treatment of terminally ill cancer patients. These drugs include various kinds of interferon (see Chapter 9), **interleukin-2,** and **tumor necrosis factor** (TNF). Despite some sensational reports in the press, none of these agents so far have proved effective in treating the more common forms of cancer. These experimental drugs cannot be used on any but the most seriously ill persons since they are extremely toxic in the amounts that must be administered. A few cancer patients have died from high doses of interferon and others have experienced serious complications.

Cancer victims often become desperate and depressed, and they sometimes lose hope. In this state of mind some cancer patients turn to unconventional medicines, illegal drugs, and many other forms of nonmedical assistance.

One substance that has aroused both public enthusiasm and much controversy is **laetrile,** which is extracted from almond and apricot pits. The active ingredient in laetrile is actually a compound called **amygdalin,** which also happens to contain cyanide. Laetrile is not an innocuous substance, and several deaths have been attributed to cyanide poisoning resulting from excess laetrile ingestion. Numerous human and animal cancer experiments have been performed with laetrile, all yielding negative results, which is why the medical profession condemns its use in treating cancer. The results of a comprehensive clinical trial involving treatment of cancer patients with laetrile were published in 1982 (Moertel et al., 1982). No substantial benefit to the patients was observed.

The effects of cancer treatment vary from person to person. Anyone whose medical condition is diagnosed as cancer should insist on a full discussion and understanding of the problem, including an appraisal of the risks and benefits of any recommended therapy. It goes without saying that your authors believe strongly in a holistic approach to cancer treatment. So does Neil Fiore, a young psychologist who survived a cancer that had metastasized. He describes, in Box 17-2, his views of a holistic medical approach based on his own successful battle with testicular cancer.

BOX 17-2

A HOLISTIC APPROACH FOR THE PATIENT WITH CANCER

Neil Fiore, a psychologist, discovered a small lump in his scrotum, which was diagnosed as testicular cancer. Using a combination of medical and holistic approaches, his cancer was cured. The following passages are excerpts from his longer article that outlines his holistic philosophy for cancer treatment.

Fighting cancer must come to mean more than excising a tumor and focusing the latest weapons on the metastases. It must include a recognition, by both the medical professionals and the patient, that the patient's mind and body are powerful factors in this fight . . .

A holistic approach to the patient with cancer uses a team of experts, including the patients, as experts on their own feelings and the reaction of their bodies, and as the ones ultimately responsible for their lives . . .

Instead of keeping patients compliant and sedated, therapists should be encouraging exuberance, independence and individual responsibility. Vivacity and direct communication of complaints and fears can be healthy signs that the patient is fighting and wants to get better. To avoid the danger of increasing the sense of patient helplessness, one must ensure that active patient behavior is neither punished nor suppressed. Whenever possible, it must be demonstrated to patients that they can be effective in communicating and in influencing their environment . . .

It is my belief that patients with cancer, like those with heart disease, must change their behavior and lifestyles to achieve complete health. I am suggesting that in all likelihood most such patients come from a lifestyle that has been extremely stressful or one in which their mechanisms for coping with stress have been inadequate and inefficient. Often, however, patients would rather have the doctor cut out or deaden the pain resulting from a stressful life than to change old habits. Patients thereby remove the annoying messenger from their bodies that tells them to slow down and avoid excesses.

Patients with cancer are in a situation that makes it likely that they will be highly suggestible. This circumstance is also true of patients coming out of an anesthetic or those who are in shock. All the conditions necessary for a hypnotic trance are present: the patient needs and expects help; the patient sees the doctor as an authority; the patient is often confused and shocked by the diagnosis and the medical procedures; and the patient is placed in a passive role from the time he or she talks to the nurse or receptionist. Physicians, by their attitudes and words, can lead patients to imagine and expect a hopeless situation with much pain. Examples of this approach are, "You will have a lot of pain but we have the drugs to help you," or "Chemotherapy is highly toxic and you will lose your hair and become nauseated." By the same token, aware physicians can use the patient's suggestible state to calm and to increase the chances for a positive outcome.

They can say, "You will be receiving some very powerful medicine capable of killing rapidly producing cells. Cancer is the most rapidly producing cell, but there are other rapidly producing cells such as hair. And since the medication cannot tell the difference between hair and cancer cells, you may lose some hair temporarily. Fortunately, your normal healthy cells can recover from the medication and reproduce themselves, but the weak, poorly formed cancer cells cannot."

The patient's mental image of his or her disease and body can, through the workings of ideomotor responses, influence the direction of the body, toward health or disease. I therefore see it as a healthy sign when patients refuse to accept fully that they have "cancer." Rather than assume that these patients are "in denial," I believe that physicians need to explore with patients what their concepts of cancer are and how they see the healthy parts of themselves fighting or containing the disease . . .

The positive statement uses the word "medication" instead of "drugs" to emphasize the helpful nature of chemotherapy, and uses "powerful" instead of "toxic" to emphasize the point that this is a strong ally to the body. The loss of hair and other side effects are presented as possible, and not certain, to avoid self-fulfilling prophecies. Most importantly, the statement allows patients to conceptualize the side effects as a sign that their powerful ally is working at killing rapidly producing cells. Without this kind of intervention, patients often concluded that the side effects are proof that they are dying—if not from cancer, from its treatment.

---

* Reprinted with permission from *New England Journal of Medicine,* February 8, 1979, pp. 284–289.

> Too many cancer patients have their last days or weeks or months made wretched by intensive treatment with drugs, or radiation, or both when there is no reasonable prospect of a cure, and when they should have been allowed to die in dignity and peace.
>
> **Donald Gould**
> *Black and White Medicine Show*

Coping with Cancer: The Crucial Role of the Mind

The diagnosis of cancer raises a host of problems for the patient as well as for his or her family and friends. Everyone involved has to cope with new problems — the therapy itself, fears of death, loss of a loved one, loss of income, change in living habits — and above all the uncertainty as to the outcome, which may last for months or years. Avery D. Weisman (1979), professor of psychiatry at the Harvard Medical School, observes:

> Cancer, like war, is too serious to be left to the physician. A cancer patient is more than a vessel for a neoplastic process. Jobs are lost, never regained. Families are split, or drawn closer together. Close relationships disintegrate; friendships falter. Conflicts may be aggravated. Values can be sullied. Goals are given up for the pursuit of a cure that may never come. Even new diseases arise as a result of treatment.

These are but a few of the reasons why coping with cancer is different, say, from coping with pneumonia or heart disease. The coping strategies discussed in Chapter 11 for dealing with emotional distress apply to cancer patients as well. Perhaps the whole issue of cancer therapies and of coping with the disease can be put into a useful perspective by examining the effects of the mind on cancer development and treatment.

In 1897, W. S. Halstead, a surgeon at Johns Hopkins Medical School, reported on the mysterious disappearance of some breast cancers in women. Today the spontaneous regression of tumors and remission of cancer in some patients is becoming accepted medical fact. What is the scientific basis for the disappearance of untreated tumors? Although there is no definitive answer to this question, most doctors and psychologists would agree that the mind plays a critical role in the healing process.

Meditation techniques and image visualization (discussed in Chapters 2 and 3) can help the person with cancer and assist the physician in making treatments more effective. A number of studies have shown that mental states affect the outcome of cancer therapy and may facilitate cures (Magarey, 1983). By using mental relaxation techniques, a person can muster powerful defenses against the development of cancer cells as well as assist in their destruction by modulating the immune system. Stress and emotional upset can depress the body's normal immune system responses (Riley, 1981). There is scientific evidence that hostile feelings, resentment, deeply felt personal loss, and feelings of hopelessness all might be important factors contributing to cancer formation and to a general lowering of disease resistance.

As explained in Chapters 2 and 3, belief, suggestions, placebo effects, and faith can all affect physiology and health. The course of cancer growth is unpredictable. In persons with diagnostically iden-

> If psychological stress factors, acting upon the immune system, can induce cancer, then there is the further possibility that this negative process can be reversed and immunity stabilized or enhanced through stress-reduction practices.
>
> **Kenneth Pelletier**
> *Mind as Healer, Mind as Slayer*

tical cancers that go untreated the tumors may disappear completely, may regress and reappear over a period of many years, or may grow rapidly and lead to death within months.

A dramatic illustration of the power of belief in altering the course of even terminal cancer is the case of a Mr. Wright, a cancer patient of the 1950s. At that time the drug krebiozen (subsequently shown to be ineffective) was believed by some people to be a wonder drug that could cure cancer. Wright, who had terminal lymphosarcoma, was given a life expectancy of two weeks by his doctor. Wright, however, had enormous faith in this new wonder drug. After a single injection, his doctor noted, "the tumor masses had melted like snowballs on a hot stove, and in only these few days, they were half their original size" (Klopfer, 1957).

Mr. Wright was symptom-free for two months until newspapers began reporting that krebiozen was a worthless drug in treating cancer. Wright relapsed. With nothing to lose, his doctors assured him that a fresh, double-strength injection of krebiozen would cure him. Actually, however, they gave him an injection of water—and he was again symptom-free, this time for two months. The American Medical Association (AMA) then announced that "nationwide tests show krebiozen to be a worthless drug in treatment of cancer." Wright again relapsed and died after two days in the hospital.

O. Carl Simonton has pioneered the use of mental imagery along with conventional medical therapy in treating patients with cancer. He encourages the use of meditation, biofeedback, hypnosis, and especially image visualization in his cancer patients. His view of the healing process in cancer is that

when we look at spontaneous remission or at unexpectedly good responses and try to figure out what happens in common, we find the same spontaneous occurrence of visualizing oneself being well. You analyze these people, you sit down with them and you find out what their thoughts are during that period of time, from the time they were given their diagnosis to the time that they were over their disease with no medical treatment. I have not found any patient that did not go through a similar visualizing process. It might be a spiritual process, God healing them, up and down the whole spectrum. But the important thing was what they pictured and the way they saw things. They were very positive, regardless of the source, and their picture was very positive. (Simonton and Simonton, 1975)

The human mind has the power to keep a person healthy as well as the power to heal the body. Dealing with cancer requires courage. It takes conviction. One mustn't give up. The person must believe that a cure is possible. Some positive mental images that the Simontons recommend to cancer patients are listed in Table 17-5.

Most cancers are preventable diseases. Cancer is predominantly a "disease of civilization"—that is, of our contemporary Western lifestyles. As an individual responsible for your own health, you can take measures that will reduce the chance that you will develop cancer during your lifetime (see Table

Table 17-5
Some Positive Mental Images for Dealing with Cancer

1. The cancer cells are weak and confused.
2. The treatment is strong and powerful.
3. The healthy cells can repair any slight damage the treatment might do.
4. The army of white blood cells is vast and destroys the cancer cells.
5. The white blood cells are aggressive and quick to find the cancer cells and destroy them.
6. The dead cancer cells are flushed from the body normally and naturally.
7. I am healthy and free of cancer.
8. I still have many goals in life and reasons to live.

Table 17-6
Measures That Should Help Prevent Cancer

STOP	Smoking or chewing tobacco.
AVOID	Excessive exposure to sunlight (use sunscreen lotions).
AVOID	Exposure to proven carcinogens in your diet, at home, and in work environments.
AVOID	Excess consumption of alcohol; pickled, smoked, and charred foods; and animal fats.
AVOID	Unnecessary exposure to ionizing radiation.
INCREASE	Consumption of fresh fruits and vegetables rich in vitamin A, vitamin C, and vitamin E.
REDUCE	Overeating and psychosocial stress.

17-6). Making these relatively simple changes early in your life can help you maintain a high resistance to disease—including cancer.

Supplemental Readings

American Cancer Society. "Facts and Figures." A yearly update on cancer statistics and recent developments in detection and treatment.

Barbacid, M. "Mutagens, Oncogenes and Cancer." *Trends in Genetics,* July 1986. Explains how the activation of certain genes (oncogenes) may be the cause of some cancers.

Cairns, John. "The Treatment of Diseases and the War Against Cancer." *Scientific American,* November 1985. One of the best articles describing cancer and the reasons it is a preventable disease.

Fiore, Neil A. *The Road Back to Health: Coping with the Emotional Side of Cancer.* New York: Bantam Books, 1985. Based on his own experience with cancer, Fiore recounts

what you need to know to wage the best battle.

Gallo, R. C. "The First Human Retrovirus." *Scientific American,* December 1986. Describes how leukemia and AIDS are caused by special kinds of viruses.

Levy, S. M. *Behavior and Cancer: Life-style and Psychosocial Factors in the Initiation and Progression of Cancer.* San Francisco: Jossey-Bass, 1985. Presents the evidence that supports the idea that how we live may contribute to the development of cancer.

Prescott, D. M., and **Flexer, A. S.** *Cancer—The Misguided Cell.* 3rd ed. New York: Charles Scribner's Sons, 1986. An excellent introductory book that discusses the biology of cancer as well as its treatment and prevention.

Simone, C. B. *Cancer and Nutrition.* New York: McGraw-Hill, 1983.

A good introduction to the dietary risk factors in cancer.

Simonton, S. M., and **Shook, R. L.** *The Healing Family: The Simonton Approach for Families Facing Illness.* New York: Bantam Books, 1986. An integrated, holistic approach to coping with cancer and other catastrophic illnesses.

"Viruses." *Time,* November 3, 1986. Explains how viruses are involved in cancer and AIDS.

Weisman, Avery D. *Coping with Cancer.* New York: McGraw-Hill, 1979. A psychiatrist's sensitive and practical guide for coping with cancer.

Willett, W. C., and **MacMahon, B.** "Diet and Cancer—An Overview." *New England Journal of Medicine,* March 8, 1984, and March 15, 1984. A detailed analysis of the "diet and cancer" controversy.

Summary

Cancer is a group of diseases all of which share the common property of unregulated and abnormal cell multiplication. Ionizing radiation, radioactivity, and carcinogenic chemicals can alter the genetic information in a cell to initiate the cancer process. Other substances can promote the growth of cancer cells. Physiological factors, including immunological deficiencies, hormone imbalances, poor nutrition, and psychological factors can affect cancer development.

The treatments for cancer include surgery, radiation, and chemotherapy all of which attempt to remove or destroy the cancer cells. All treatments for cancer are rather drastic procedures and their efficacy can be helped by a patient's attitudes as well as by support from medical personnel, family, and friends.

Most cancers are believed to be environmentally caused and consequently cancer is a preventable disease. To significantly reduce the incidence of cancer in our society, however, will require significant changes in personal lifestyles and social values.

Prevention of cancer should be an important health goal for every person. To prevent cancer you should reduce your exposure to carcinogenic substances, maintain good nutrition and health habits, and have a positive mental outlook on life.

FOR YOUR HEALTH

Reduce Environmental Cancer Risks

Make a list of environmental agents and substances that you think have been exposed to recently that are known to be carcinogenic. Some common examples are x-rays, cigarette smoke, asbestos dust, and household pesticides. In what ways can you reduce your exposure to these and other carcinogenic substances?

Self-Exams for Health

Women: Establish a routine for periodically doing the breast self-exam (see Appendix B).

Men: Become aware of the signs of testicular cancer and periodically check yourself for them.

Help Someone You Care About

If you have a relative or a friend who smokes cigarettes or whose occupation or lifestyle increases his or her cancer risk, embark on a plan to encourage that person to reduce his or her cancer risk.

Are You at Risk?

Try to find out how many of your close relatives have had cancer or have died of it. This may help you to learn whether you are at risk for a particular type of cancer and may also encourage you to adopt a lifestlye that can help prevent cancer.

CHAPTER EIGHTEEN

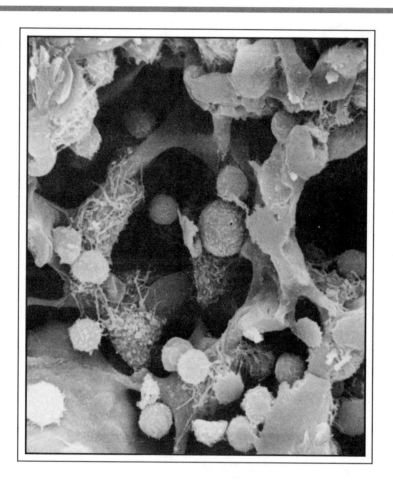

Prevention through education
and responsible behavior is the
way to stop AIDS.

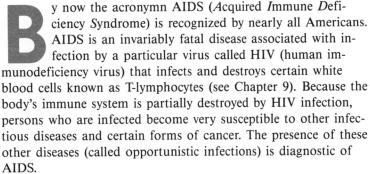

AIDS: The New Epidemic

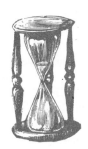

By now the acronymn AIDS (*A*cquired *I*mmune *D*eficiency *S*yndrome) is recognized by nearly all Americans. AIDS is an invariably fatal disease associated with infection by a particular virus called HIV (human immunodeficiency virus) that infects and destroys certain white blood cells known as T-lymphocytes (see Chapter 9). Because the body's immune system is partially destroyed by HIV infection, persons who are infected become very susceptible to other infectious diseases and certain forms of cancer. The presence of these other diseases (called opportunistic infections) is diagnostic of AIDS.

The most common and serious infection of AIDS victims causes a special kind of pneumonia; however, other infections such as oral candidiasis (thrush) and herpes zoster (shingles) are also quite common. Not everyone who becomes infected with HIV will necessarily come down with AIDS; some people have a less severe form of disease known as ARC (*A*IDS *R*elated *C*omplex). Still other people who are infected by HIV, for reasons that are unclear, have no symptoms of disease whatsoever, or the symptoms may appear many years after the infection. However, people who test positive for HIV antibodies and are asymptomatic carriers of the virus usually can infect others either during sexual intercourse or by sharing blood.

AIDS is classified by medical epidemiologists as an epidemic, that is, a disease that spreads rapidly in a population and causes sickness among many individuals. Strictly speaking, AIDS is classified as a pandemic disease because it occurs worldwide, but we will refer to it as an epidemic in this chapter. AIDS cases have been reported in over one hundred countries. Worldwide it is estimated that 5–10 million people are infected with the AIDS virus. About three-fourths of all AIDS cases reported in the United States have occurred in homosexual or bisexual men. As a consequence, AIDS has become known as "the gay disease." However, women, heterosexual men, and children are as likely to be infected by the AIDS virus as are homosexual men. It is important to realize that viruses do not discriminate as to whom they infect.

The AIDS epidemic is potentially the most serious infectious disease to emerge in this century. The epidemic is still in its infancy in the United States, and many thousands—possibly many millions—of people may contract the virus and either AIDS or

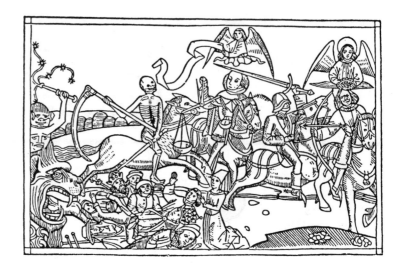

The Four Apocalyptic Horsemen.
From the Cologne Bible, printed by
Bartholomäus von Uncle, 1479.
(*Picture Book of Devils, Demons and
Witchcraft,* E. and J. Lehner; Dover
Publications, 1971.)

ARC. It is estimated that by 1991 there may be as many as 250,000 AIDS patients in this country and that there may be 50,000 deaths from AIDS in that year alone. Some people may become infected and yet be fortunate enough to have no serious symptoms of disease. Nevertheless, it is certain that the lives of millions of Americans, particularly young, sexually active persons, are going to be affected by the AIDS epidemic. As we have emphasized throughout *Health and Wellness,* the only reliable path to personal health is through *prevention of disease* and through *self-responsibility* for one's nutrition, sexual habits, and life-style. The *only sure way* to safeguard yourself from AIDS is to avoid becoming infected. As was pointed out in the *Harvard Medical School Health Letter* (November 1985), "Once HTLV-III* infection is established, it is probably permanent. The conservative assumption—for purposes of preventing the disease—is that infection is lifelong and that individuals who are carrying HTLV-III are potentially infectious to others." This chapter presents the information and guidelines you need to help control the AIDS epidemic and to protect yourself from infection during your lifetime.

What Is AIDS?

AIDS is now known to be caused by a special class of viruses called **retroviruses,** which are so named

because they are able to integrate their genetic information back into the chromosomes of cells (hence the term *retro*). The specific retrovirus that almost always is associated with AIDS was first called HTLV-III, which stands for *h*uman *T*-cell *l*ymphotropic *v*irus type III. Other researchers have called it LAV (*l*ymphadenopathy *a*ssociated *v*irus) or ARV (*A*IDS *r*elated *v*irus). To avoid confusion scientists have now agreed to call the virus HIV or AIDS virus. These are the terms we will use in this chapter.

Infection by the AIDS virus is a necessary but not always sufficient condition to cause AIDS. Some infected persons may have no symptoms of sickness and yet have antibodies to the virus in their blood. This means that the person is either presently infected by the virus or has a persistent infection that cannot be completely eliminated. Other infected persons may have only mild symptoms (ARC) or all of the symptoms characteristic of AIDS. There is no way to predict how serious the disease will become in any HIV-infected individual.

Preliminary studies of populations in Africa indicate that as many as 10 percent of people in eastern Africa carry antibodies to HIV in their blood but most of them are not sick and do not have AIDS. Because of the prevalence of the AIDS virus in Africa, it has been suggested that the virus originated in Africa and spread to other areas of the world as people moved from country to country. This suggestion has caused consternation among African nations and among black Americans, as it may rekindle racial prejudices in this country and elsewhere. At present, any suggestion as to the origin of the AIDS virus is purely speculative. Viruses

---

* HTLV-III is another name for HIV.

> Law may require all of us to be vaccinated against some diseases, especially when we are threatened by an epidemic, but in general, it has no way of controlling habits, even those inevitably leading to disease.
>
> **Earl Warren (1962)**
> **Former Chief Justice, U.S. Supreme Court**

that appear to be related to human AIDS virus have been detected in African green monkeys as well as in domesticated sheep. The AIDS virus has been detected in patients in Alaska, northern Scandinavia, and Japan. Because the origin of the human virus is uncertain, victims of AIDS who are already burdened by the disease itself do not deserve additional suffering deriving from racial, national, or sexual prejudices.

Remember that we still do not understand a great deal about viral infections in general and about the AIDS virus in particular. Nevertheless, it is

known that a person infected by HIV can be free of symptoms for years and then suddenly become sick. The longest documented disease-free period following HIV infection was discovered in a young child who was infected shortly after birth as a result of a blood transfusion. The child was well until age 5½ when he became sick and was diagnosed as having AIDS. This long latency means that some persons may remain well for many years after becoming infected and may not even be aware of their infected condition until symptoms appear. It is quite likely that during the asymptomatic period infected persons appear healthy but still can transmit the virus by sexual intercourse or from blood. This means that the AIDS virus can be spread by healthy persons—a matter of considerable concern. The shortest documented period from the time of diagnosis of HIV infection to development of symptoms is about two months; this case also occurred in an individual who received virus-contaminated blood in a transfusion.

About 5 percent of AIDS cases in the United States have resulted from blood transfusions in which the blood contained HIV viruses. Presently all blood that is donated to blood banks is tested for the presence of antibodies to the AIDS virus. Blood supplies are now as safe as medical science can make them. However, because antibodies to the AIDS virus take several days or weeks to develop in an infected individual, it is still remotely possible that a person might become infected by HIV and donate blood before antibodies to the virus develop. Current estimates of the risk of HIV infection from a blood transfusion in hospitals in this country are about 1 per 100,000 transfusions.

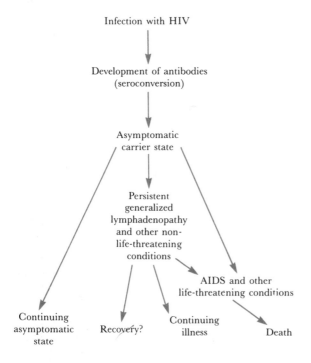

Prevention is the best approach to
any public health problem.
James Lieber
Atlantic Monthly

Symptoms and Diagnosis of AIDS

Many of the early symptoms of AIDS are also signs of other diseases or health problems that have nothing to do with AIDS. For example, some early signs resemble those of mononucleosis, a serious but nonfatal virus infection that is unrelated to AIDS. Particular symptoms that should receive prompt medical attention are persistent fever, skin rash, sore throat, painful or swollen lymph nodes, and mental or neurological abnormalities. Other vague symptoms that require medical attention and diagnosis are prolonged loss of appetite or continued weight loss over a period of months that is not deliberate, and recurrent, profuse sweating while sleeping.

A diagnosis of AIDS is contingent on finding that a person has been infected with HIV. This is done by sampling a person's blood and testing for the presence of antibodies to the virus. Several tests have been developed and some are more sensitive than others. The simpler and less expensive tests for antibodies to the virus do give some false positives; that is, they indicate an HIV infection when, in fact, the person has not been infected by the virus and does not have AIDS. Therefore, healthy individuals who test positive should not panic (easy to say, hard to do), and should insist on a second and more sensitive test known as a Western Blot. Soon even more sensitive and accurate tests to detect the presence of the virus itself should be available.

Because the virus infects special white blood cells (so-called helper T-cells) that are essential to the functioning of the immune system, a person with AIDS has a severe immune system deficiency and is especially susceptible to infections, particularly ones called **opportunistic infections.** A lung infection commonly observed in AIDS patients is caused by a protozoan (*Pneumocystis carinii*) that almost never causes sickness in individuals whose immune systems are healthy. Other common infections in AIDS patients are due to fungi; these infections may appear as white spots on the tongue or in the mouth or elsewhere in the body and are generally caused by a yeast (*Candida albicans*). AIDS patients also frequently contract an otherwise rare form of cancer known as **Kaposi's sarcoma.** An early indication of this cancer is numerous colored spots on the skin. Both opportunistic infections and Kaposi's sarcoma in AIDS patients ultimately lead to death despite all treatments and care. Because the virus also infects the brain and nerve cells, AIDS patients often exhibit neurological disorders.

The AIDS Virus

To understand how infection by any retrovirus can cause disease, you must first understand what biological and molecular changes occur in virus-infected cells. This knowledge also helps you to understand why there is no cure for AIDS and why cures cannot be anticipated in the foreseeable future. Development of a vaccine that would be able to protect against HIV infection is still problematical and, in any case, is still many years in the future

Although AIDS may never touch you personally,
the societal impact certainly will.
C. Everett Koop
U.S. Surgeon General

(some scientists guess from 10 to 20 years). A vaccine may be able to protect the next generation but cannot help the millions of people who already are, or who will become infected by the AIDS virus. Vaccination against viruses or bacteria only protects individuals who are uninfected; vaccination *cannot* help or protect anyone who already has been infected (see Chapter 9).

Retroviruses can infect many different kinds of cells, but infection of specific T-cells of the immune system by HIV (see Figure 18-1) can destroy the body's principal defense against pathogenic microorganisms. Once T-cells have become infected, the small RNA molecule of the retrovirus is copied into a corresponding DNA molecule, which is permanently integrated into the chromosome of T-cells located in the bone marrow. Subsequently, the millions of viruses or viral RNA copies produced by

the infected cells destroy all T-cells in the body, so the body then becomes susceptible to opportunistic infections by microorganisms. More insidiously, the HIV virus can infect other kinds of cells, particularly nerve cells, and eventually will spread to the brain. This is especially worrisome because infected persons who do not become sick or manifest symptoms of AIDS or ARC may eventually show neurological signs of brain deterioration. It is simply not known, nor can predictions be made about the outcome of any retrovirus infection in any individual. Frequently these viruses only produce disease symptoms after many years. That is yet another reason why infection by HIV is so serious—it places an individual at lifelong risk for serious or fatal disease as well as imposing the psychological distress of not knowing when or how the disease may ultimately appear.

Figure 18-1
Cells of the human immune system.

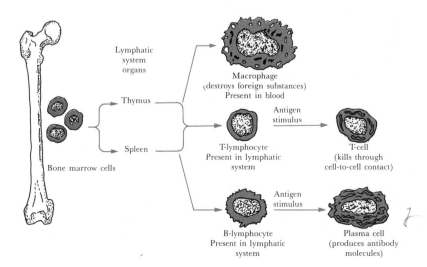

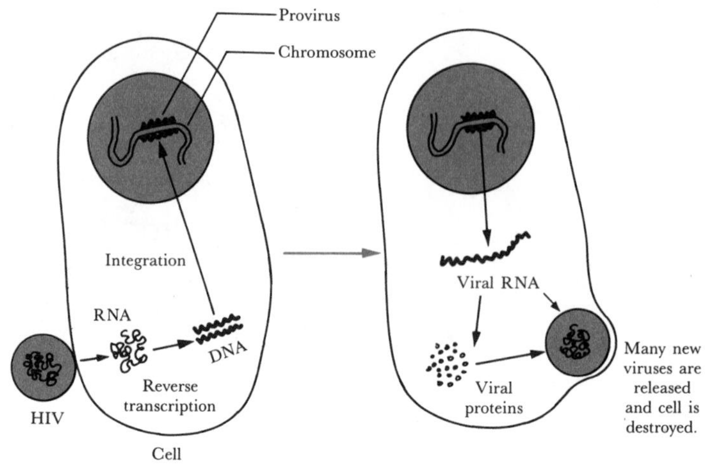

Figure 18-2
Life cycle of the AIDS retrovirus.
Virus RNA enters the cell and is
converted to DNA, which is integrated
into the cell's chromosome, becoming
a provirus.

Once the retrovirus penetrates a T-cell, the RNA is released and the DNA copy is inserted at random into a cell's chromosomes (see Figure 18-2). The integrated form of the retrovirus is called the **provirus**. From its integrated position, the provirus can direct the synthesis of countless new virus particles or RNA molecules. The HIV provirus is particularly adept at destroying T-cells by mechanisms that are still unclear. When all of the T-cells are destroyed, a vital part of a person's immune system also is destroyed. Other retroviruses do not usually destroy T-cells but instead cause them to grow abnormally and become cancer cells, eventually producing leukemia or lymphoma.

Because the genetic information of the virus is integrated into the chromosomes, the viral genes are indistinguishable from the normal genes of the cell (except by sophisticated laboratory techniques). Thus, there is no way to cure or to eliminate the virus from infected cells or from infected persons. At most, physicians can try to slow down or block the production of new viruses with drugs, and thus slow down the spread of the viruses to uninfected cells. It is hoped that some of the numerous experimental drugs that are being tested on AIDS patients, such as azidothymidine (AZT), will prove effective in reducing the spread of the virus in the body. If this could be accomplished, and if sufficient numbers of uninfected T-cells remained, the uninfected T-cells might proliferate and restore some measure of normal function to the immune system.

Nevertheless, the development of effective antiviral drugs is still problematical. To date no drug has ever been effective in curing a viral disease, even common ones such as flu, herpes, or mononucleosis. The diseases caused by retroviruses are thought to be even more resistant to drugs because the viruses become an intimate part of the cell's own chromosomes. Any effective anti-viral drug would, by its very nature, also be toxic to normal cells, particularly if it interfered with the replication of virus DNA. Moreover, a person infected with HIV would have to continue to take the yet-to-be-discovered anti-viral drug for the rest of his or her life because there probably is no way completely to rid the body of the virus. The sad fact is that medical science does not expect to cure AIDS victims. It may be possible in the future to mitigate symptoms and to prolong life, but complete cures are not in the offing.

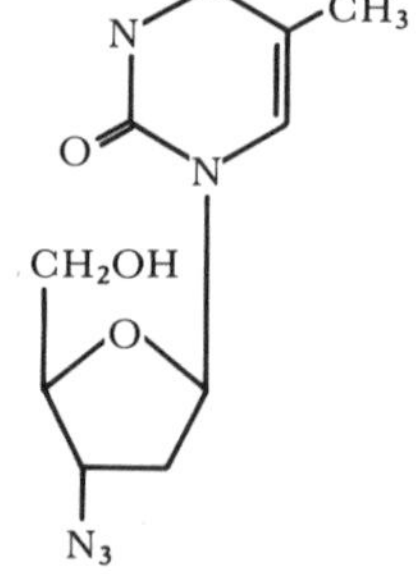

> The recognition that there are
> probably neurological consequences of
> infection by HIV makes a serious problem of
> public health still worse.
>
> **John Maddox**
> *Nature*

Vaccines

The official long-range health policy of the United States government is to try to control the AIDS epidemic by the year 2000. The only realistic hope is to develop a safe, effective vaccine and vaccinate all or most of the population. Development of an effective AIDS vaccine is far from a sure thing. A few vaccines that protect mice or cats against retrovirus infections have been developed, but it is not certain that effective human vaccines can be developed. It is already known that there is not just one unique AIDS virus, because the viruses isolated from AIDS patients are all subtly different in structure. Thus, any human vaccine might have to be effective against many different types of viruses. Like the flu virus, HIV seems to be able to change its genetic information and antigenic properties quite easily and quite often. A vaccine effective against this year's virus might prove to be useless against next year's crop of viruses. Again, it simply is not known what lies ahead and whether the AIDS epidemic can be contained by a yet-to-be-developed vaccine.

Who Is at Risk?

The answer to this question is that everyone who is sexually active with more than one partner is at risk to some degree. However, certain groups of individuals have a potentially high risk and certain sex-

Table 18-1
Distribution of AIDS Cases

Group	Total AIDS cases
Male homosexuals	72%
Intravenous drug users	18%
Haitians	4%
Hemophiliacs	1%
Others	5%

ual habits surely increase one's risk. Table 18-1 shows how the reported cases of AIDS are distributed presently among various high-risk groups.

The AIDS virus is present in body fluids—principally in semen and blood and to a lesser degree in saliva, tears, breast milk, and possibly vaginal fluids. In principal, intimate contact with any body fluid from an infected individual can result in transmission of the virus. Nevertheless, among thousands of AIDS cases that have been investigated, nearly all occur from contact with semen and blood. These fluids appear to be the most effective sources of virus transmission. No AIDS cases are known to have been caused by contact with virus-containing saliva—from biting or kissing, for example—but the possibility of infection in this manner cannot be completely excluded. Public health officials have stressed the fact that the AIDS virus is not transmitted by casual contacts between infected and uninfected persons. Some communities (San Francisco,

> Shaking hands, hugging, social kissing,
> crying, coughing, or sneezing will not transmit
> the AIDS virus.
>
> **C. Everett Koop**
> **U.S. Surgeon General**

for example) have already passed laws preventing discrimination against AIDS victims in housing, jobs, and services. While health laws can be based on scientific evidence, it is difficult to legislate against people's fears and individuals' sexual habits. That is another reason why an understanding of AIDS is so important for individuals and for society.

Transfer of virus-containing semen during either homosexual or heterosexual intercourse can transmit the virus to uninfected sexual partners. AIDS is classified as a sexually transmitted disease (for a discussion of STDs see Chapter 22) and is preventable by avoiding sexual contact with infected persons and to a lesser degree by using condoms and spermicides. In addition to sexual contact, individuals who take drugs, either legal or illegal, by injection and who do not use sterile syringes and needles are at high risk of infection. At least one case of AIDS has been reported in a body-builder who used a shared syringe to inject himself with steroids.

A high proportion of prostitutes are also intravenous drug users and many may be infected with HIV even though they are without symptoms or sickness. Thus, prostitutes represent a significant source of possible AIDS transmission that is still difficult to evaluate. Dr. William A. Haseltine of Harvard Medical School estimates that 50% of prostitutes in Berlin are infected, 30% in New York, 15% in San Francisco, and 5% in Phoenix. Overall, about one-third of prostitutes are intravenous drug users. Thus, the possibility exists that AIDS could be introduced into any population, even a college student population, as a result of individuals having sexual intercourse with infected female or male prostitutes. The subsequent spread of the virus would then depend on how promiscuous newly-infected individuals were, and how early or late their symptoms appeared.

Because the virus is present in blood, infected women who become pregnant can infect the developing fetus. A significant number of children with AIDS has already been diagnosed and many more are expected. These children represent a particularly tragic group of AIDS victims because they will have to cope with the disease as long as they live. So far there is no indication that these children can spread the disease to other children or adults by ordinary contacts, and health authorities have opposed preventing AIDS children from attending school or from other social activities. Again, the recommendations could change if new evidence indicates transmission of the virus is possible by casual contact. Because no absolute certainties exist with respect to preventing transmission of the virus by casual contact, a certain amount of public unease—even some hysteria—exists despite repeated assurances by public health officials.

Safer Sex or No Sex?

By now you must realize that the only solution to the AIDS epidemic in this country and throughout the world is to prevent the spread of the AIDS virus from infected to uninfected individuals. Since the primary mode of transmission of the virus is by sexual intercourse, either homosexual or heterosexual,

> Liberty means responsibility.
> That's why most men dread it.
>
> **George Bernard Shaw**

the focus is primarily on sex education with emphasis on increased responsibility of everyone in her or his sexual interactions. Because the epidemic can only be stopped with people's cooperation, widespread public information programs have been initiated by federal, state, and local health officials. Everyone needs to be familiar with the basic facts about AIDS (see Table 18-2).

The U.S. Public Health Service recommends that educational AIDS material be provided to adolescents and preadolescents. Sex education and the dangers of AIDS need to be taught to children as early as possible. Some states and cities have already begun AIDS education programs in their schools and more will soon follow their lead. It is not easy for most people to discuss sexual diseases openly, and for many persons such discussion is offensive or conflicts with their religious beliefs. However, the threat of the AIDS epidemic is so great that personal convictions must be put aside. Universal sex education is essential.

The surest way to avoid AIDS is to avoid all sex. The next surest way is to have only one sexual partner who also is uninfected. The more sexual partners a person has, the greater the risk of becoming infected. For that reason attitudes in our society inevitably must change and the risks of casual sexual intercourse must be understood by everyone. For those who do not, or will not, refrain from frequent sexual interactions with multiple partners, the use of condoms and spermicides afford considerable protection and are essential. If you are unsure what constitutes safer sex, then you should avoid that behavior or sexual act until you can talk to a counselor or physician about your concerns.

Table 18-2
Basic Facts About AIDS

1. AIDS is a fatal disease that cannot now be cured.
2. AIDS is *not* spread by casual contact.
3. AIDS is spread by sexual intercourse, by contaminated blood, and by contaminated hypodermic needles.
4. An infected woman can give AIDS to her child during pregnancy.
5. A stable, sexually exclusive relationship with another uninfected person is safest.
6. For the sexually active, always using condoms is good protection against AIDS.
7. A person can look and feel healthy and still be able to spread the infection that causes AIDS.

The Effect of AIDS on Society

Society has already begun to react to the AIDS epidemic in a variety of ways, and the inevitable spread of the epidemic in the next decade and beyond will evoke further responses. The AIDS epidemic has the potential to change radically social values and sexual norms in the United States and other countries. Indeed, the AIDS epidemic could shred the fabric

> No tropical storm has the economically
> devastating potential of the new cases of AIDS
> expected in the next few years.
> **June E. Osborn, M.D.**

of this society if the disease spreads to a significant degree in the heterosexual population. Listed below are some of the recent decisions and steps that have already been taken in response to the AIDS epidemic.

1. The United States Defense Department has decided to test all 2.2 million service personnel for the presence of antibodies in their blood that would indicate infection by the virus. All new recruits also will be tested and no infected individuals will be inducted. The first tests of 35,000 recruits showed that 40 persons were infected.

2. Some school districts have sought to ban children with AIDS from public schools; other school districts and towns have made it illegal to ban children with AIDS or to discriminate against persons with AIDS.

3. Some companies have begun to test all food handlers for AIDS and to remove them from food handling jobs if they are infected.

4. Insurance companies have begun to require the AIDS test before issuing life or health insurance.

The United States has a history of protecting the rights of its citizens that dates back to the adopting of the Bill of Rights. People in our society have come to expect that their sexual rights, religious beliefs, and political convictions will be legally safeguarded. However, when a lethal epidemic spreads through a society, the rights of the individual may become secondary to the rights of the society. In time of threat to everyone's health, society's rights may be greater than individual rights. Dr. John A. Knowles (1977), a leading health educator, expressed this view in an article written almost ten years ago:

> The idea of individual responsibility has been submerged to individual rights—rights, or demands, to be guaranteed by government and delivered by public and private institutions. The cost of sloth, gluttony, alcoholic intemperance, reckless driving, sexual frenzy, and smoking is now a national, and not an individual, responsibility. This is justified as individual freedom—but one man's freedom in health is another man's shackle in taxes and insurance premiums. I believe the idea of a "right" to health should be replaced by the idea of an individual moral obligation to preserve one's own health—a public duty if you will.

History provides evidence that even advanced civilizations can be destroyed by disastrous epidemics. The plague of Athens (430–427 B.C.) destroyed as many as ten percent of Athens' 300,000 citizens, including Pericles, and the decline of the Greek civilization can be traced to the plague. Recent evidence suggests that the epidemic in Athens may have been caused by an influenza virus and by

> A great scourge never appears unless
> there is a reason for it.
> Henry Miller
> *The Air-Conditioned Nightmare*

subsequent bacterial infections in weakened persons. Within 30 years of the outset of this epidemic Athens was defeated by Sparta in the Peloponnesian War.

The course of the AIDS epidemic in our society and its consequence on sexual behaviors and health habits cannot be predicted. So far the number of heterosexual AIDS cases in the U.S. is relatively small. It may be several years before we know how many heterosexual men and women are infected in the United States, although recent estimates are between one and two million individuals. Young persons who are just entering their sexually active years need to be especially careful and responsible in their sexual behaviors if they want to avoid HIV infection and the possibility of AIDS. It *is* possible for a dedicated citizenry to wipe out all sexually transmitted diseases. China has been able to accomplish this — a fact little publicized in the west — by intensive educational and medical efforts over the past 30 years. Time will tell whether people in our society can become as dedicated and sexually responsible as the Chinese are with respect to preventable sexually transmitted diseases and especially with regard to AIDS.

Note: A national AIDS informational hot line exists. The number is 1-800-342-AIDS.

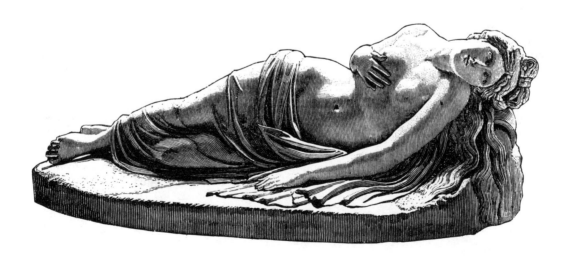

Supplemental Readings

Altman, Dennis. *"AIDS—In the Mind of America."* New York: Anchor Press, 1986. This book discusses the political and social implications of AIDS.

Curran, J. W., et al. "The Epidemiology of AIDS: Current Status and Future Prospects." *Science,* 229 (1985), 1352–1357.

Gallo, Robert C. "The First Human Retrovirus" and "The AIDS Virus." *Scientific American,* December 1986 and January 1987. Two articles that explain how viruses that cause AIDS were discovered and how they function.

Harris, J. E. "The AIDS Epidemic: Looking into the 1990s." *Technology Review,* July 1987. Forecasts the spread and consequences of the AIDS epidemic in the U.S. through 1992.

Koop, C. Everett. "Surgeon General's Report on AIDS." *Journal of the American Medical Association,* November 28, 1986. A factual, honest, and detailed description of what AIDS is and how people can cope with this public health problem. Copies of this report can be obtained free-of-charge from: AIDS, Box 14252, Washington, D.C. 20044.

Langone, J. "AIDS." *Discover,* December 1985. A good general introduction to the AIDS virus and the AIDS epidemic.

Osborne, J. E. "The AIDS Epidemic—An Overview of the Science." *Issues in Science and Technology,* Winter 1986, National Academy of Sciences, pp. 40–55.

Weisburd, S. "Will There Be an AIDS Vaccine?" *Science News,* May 9, 1987, and May 23, 1987. A realistic appraisal of the prospects for an effective AIDS vaccine.

Summary

AIDS, Acquired Immune Deficiency Syndrome, is a lethal disease caused by human immunodeficiency virus (HIV). AIDS is a new disease in human history, and it is spreading rapidly throughout the world. In the United States and other western countries, AIDS has struck hardest among the population of homosexual men, whereas in eastern Africa, the disease has affected primarily adult heterosexual women and men. The message is that anyone can get AIDS.

AIDS is transmitted from person to person via blood and semen. Inside the body HIV particles attack and destroy certain cells of the immune system (called T-lymphocytes or T-cells). Viral infection of T-cells weakens the immune system and renders the infected person susceptible to a variety of infections and cancer. It is these secondary or opportunistic infections that eventually cause death.

Anyone can be infected with the AIDS virus. The major routes of transmission are by blood (through transfusions with HIV-contaminated blood or sharing needles) and semen, and possibly vaginal fluids. Casual social contacts, such as shaking hands or touching objects that other people have touched, are not routes of transmission. Neither can the AIDS virus be transmitted through the air. Some children have AIDS because their mothers were infected with the virus during pregnancy.

At present there is no way to rid the body of HIV and cure AIDS. Nor is an effective vaccine available or likely to be for many years. The only way to stop the spread of AIDS is to take precautions not to become infected. This means that sexually active individuals must become informed about AIDS and they must adopt sexual practices that eliminate the risk of transmission. People exposed to others' blood must do the same.

If the AIDS epidemic is not stopped, we can expect that the risk of the disease and the large number of infected individuals will cause major social changes and possibly even threats to liberties that we now take for granted.

FOR YOUR HEALTH

Assessing the Risk for Getting AIDS

What do you think are your and your friends' risks for getting AIDS at this time in your lives?

	Me	Men friends	Women friends
None	☐	☐	☐
Low	☐	☐	☐
Moderate	☐	☐	☐
High	☐	☐	☐
Very high	☐	☐	☐

Why did you answer this questions the way you did? Compare your responses with your friends'.

What do you think your and your friends' risks will be two years from now? Five years from now? Why?

Taking Precautions

What, if anything, are you and your friends doing to lower your risk for getting AIDS?

	Me	Men friends	Women friends
Discussing AIDS occasionally	☐	☐	☐
Becoming more knowledgeable about AIDS	☐	☐	☐
Using condoms more often	☐	☐	☐
Abstaining from sexual intercourse	☐	☐	☐
Engaging in sex with only one person	☐	☐	☐
Asking new partners about their sexual history	☐	☐	☐

CHAPTER NINETEEN

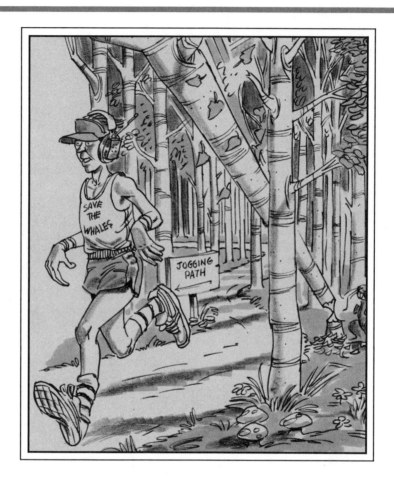

Each person contributes in many ways
to making a healthy environment.

Environmental Hazards to Health

What is this thing called health? Simply a state in which the individual happens transiently to be perfectly adapted to his environment.

H. L. Mencken

The environment includes everything to which we are exposed, both internally and externally. The term **environment** in this chapter refers to all external factors, natural and manmade, that affect health and well-being. In order to survive, all animals, including humans, have certain basic biological needs that must be met, including adequate air, water, food, and shelter. To the extent that individuals are deprived of any of the essential environmental factors, or that the factors are impure or toxic in some manner, health is adversely affected. Anyone who has experienced difficulty breathing or persistent eye irritation from "smoggy," dusty, or pollen-laden air realizes that health is diminished by poor air quality. Anyone who has become sick from inhaling chemical fumes, drinking contaminated water, or eating spoiled food knows how important the quality of air, water, and food is to health.

Optimizing health means keeping the quality of the environment high. Unfortunately, magazine and newspaper headlines tell us almost daily that the environment is becoming increasingly polluted and unhealthy and that people's lives are becoming increasingly affected by this pollution. The effects of environmental pollution are widespread and some damage may be long-lasting or even irreversible. It may be many more years before our society realizes the extent of air, water, and land pollution that has occurred and before we are prepared to pay the price, both in money and lifestyle changes, that will be required to clean up and maintain a healthy environment. For example, the pesticides DDT and 2,4,5-T were introduced into wide use in the mid-1940s, but it wasn't until the 1970s that the health hazards became so apparent that further use of these chemicals was banned in the United States.

Environmental health hazards stem from many diverse causes—which is the reason why solutions to environmental problems are not easily found. Many factors have to be considered in assessing pollution problems and deciding what to do about them.

The United States is making progress in reducing environmental pollution, preserving natural resources, and protecting plant and animal wildlife. But much remains to be done to help restore the environment to a more healthy condition. Despite enactment of environmental protection bills, six of which were modified and renewed in 1984, much of this country's air, water, and land is becoming increasingly polluted. At least 700 toxic industrial chemicals have been identified in underground and surface water supplies, and it is estimated that 30 percent of all groundwater systems used to supply drinking water are contaminated. In checking almost 1000 hazardous waste sites, the Environmental Protection Agency (EPA) found that 90 percent of the sites had caused some contamination and that about 25 percent of them were health hazards.

Table 19-1
Causes of Death in the United States by Rank Order (1984)
Note that nine out of the sixteen most frequent causes of death are due to accidents or are self-inflicted.

Number of deaths	Cause
738,000	Heart disease
328,000	Cancer
209,100	Stroke
55,350	**Motor vehicle accidents**
38,950	Diabetes
24,600	Suicide
21,730	Emphysema
18,860	**Homicide**
7,380	**Drowning**
7,380	**Fire**
3,690	Tuberculosis
2,563	**Poison**
2,255	**Firearm accident**
1,886	Asthma
1,517	**Motor vehicle collisions with trains**
1,025	**Electrocution**
902	Appendicitis
677	Infectious hepatitis
451	Pregnancy, birth, and abortion
410	Syphilis
334	**Excess cold**
205	**Flood**
129	Nonvenomous animal
107	**Lightning**
90	**Tornado**
48	**Venomous bite or sting**
17	Polio
15	Whooping cough
8	Smallpox vaccination
6	**Fireworks**
5	Measles
2	**Botulism**
1	**Poisoning by vitamins**
0	Smallpox

We cannot expect the government—or any organization, for that matter—to solve this country's pollution and health problems. As the character Pogo the possum declared a number of years ago in a comic strip created by Walt Kelly: "We have met the enemy and he is us!" Each of us must assume responsibility for living in a manner that brings the greatest personal health and satisfaction while at the same time causing the least damage to the environment that we share with all living organisms. Environmental hazards and accidents frequently result in death (see Table 19-1).

Our dependence on the automobile and the vast amount of gasoline and oil that we use provide a graphic example of how people's lifestyles contribute to pollution and endanger the health of everyone (see Figure 19-1). The emissions from millions of gasoline engines pollute the air with lead and other chemicals that are harmful to lungs and other body tissues. The giant petrochemical industries that manufacture gasoline, oil, plastics, and chemicals dump uncounted tons of toxic wastes into the environment annually. Highways, parking lots, and junked automobiles destroy millions of acres of fertile land each year. About 50,000 people die and another 2 million are seriously injured in automobile accidents every year in the United States. Still, our lifestyles and physical comforts depend on automobiles, on trucks, and on petroleum products. Therein lies the dilemma: How can each one of us achieve a healthy lifestyle and at the same time live in ways that pollute the environment and that create health hazards for everyone? Solutions to environmental problems will require major changes in the values of our society.

This chapter discusses the various kinds of environmental hazards to health.

Air Pollution

Every person breathes about 35 pounds of air a day—more than 6 tons over the course of a year. Pure, unpolluted air is essential for all body functions and for health. Fresh, clean air consists of about 21 percent oxygen, 78 percent nitrogen, and trace amounts of seven other gases. It is the oxygen in air that is essential to human life. If the oxygen content of air drops below 16 percent, body and brain functions are affected. If breathing stops, even

> I do not think that the measure of a civilization is how tall its buildings of concrete are, but rather how well its people have learned to relate to their environment and fellow man.
>
> **Sun Bear**
> **Chippewa tribe**

for a brief period, the person becomes unconscious and will die within a few minutes unless breathing is restored.

Air pollution reduces the quality of the air we breathe by limiting the availability of oxygen and by forcing us to breathe substances that are harmful to the lungs, blood, and other body tissues. The American Lung Association estimates that one out of five people suffers from chronic obstructive pulmonary disease (COPD) (see Chapter 15), which includes asthma, emphysema, bronchitis, and chronic cough.

In addition to causing breathing problems and serious illness, air pollution can damage vegetation, can diminish the growth of vegetables, grains, and flowers, and can even reduce milk and egg production. It can also corrode metal and erode stone and cause paper, leather, and rubber products to disintegrate.

Everybody has heard of **smog** (see Figure 19-2). The term was first used in England to describe a hazardous combination of smoke and fog (hence, "smog") that is largely responsible for the chronic cough and bronchitis that affected many British citizens. In many U.S. cities smog is not associated with fog but results from the action of sunlight on various airborne chemicals and from particles and gases in the air emitted by automobiles, electricity generating plants, blast furnaces, oil refineries, and from many other sources. The major kinds of "aer-

Figure 19-1
Automobiles contribute to air, water, and land pollution. (Courtesy Environmental Protection Agency.)

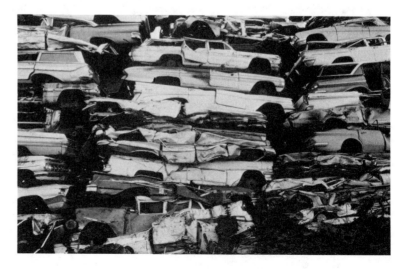

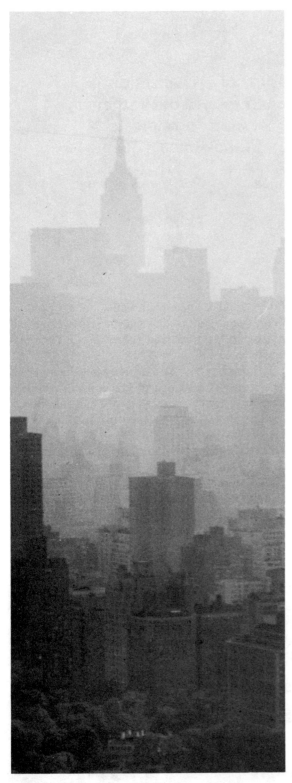

Figure 19-2
New York City smog. (Courtesy Environmental Protection Agency.)

ial garbage" are described in Figure 19-3. The EPA has developed a numerical scale for measuring air pollution called the Pollutant Standards Index (PSI). The hourly concentrations of six constituents of polluted air are measured and the total amounts are expressed as a number whose value ranges from zero to 500. Values below 100 are regarded as safe, whereas values above 100 are increasingly unhealthy. Values above 300 mean that the air is hazardous to the health of people breathing it.

Smoggy, polluted air is not only irritating to the eyes and lungs but also, as we have already indicated, contributes to more serious health problems such as allergies, lung infections, and heart disease. Carbon monoxide, one of the components of smog, interferes with the binding of oxygen to the hemoglobin in red blood cells. If the air contains 80 ppm (parts per million) of carbon monoxide, the body's supply of oxygen is reduced about 15 percent. In heavily congested traffic the levels of carbon monoxide may reach 400 ppm, and people are frequently stuck in traffic jams for hours at a time. It is no surprise that many commuters in large cities arrive home with headaches. Car mechanics and parking lot attendants are often exposed to high levels of carbon monoxide for extended periods of time and may develop health problems as a consequence.

Sulfur oxides are produced when coal or oil containing sulfur is burned. If the air is damp, sulfuric acid, a very corrosive substance, is formed. Damp air laden with sulfur oxides can pit metals and erode stone buildings as well as damage lung tissue. Acid rain is produced in air containing sulfur oxides and can damage crops and forests far from the site of the initial air pollution.

Most scientists and environmentalists who are familiar with the facts concerning the dispute over acid rain agree that forests, lakes, and rivers are damaged by acid rain. Many kinds of fish are finding it more and more difficult to survive and reproduce in water that is becoming increasingly acidic. For example, fish eggs are damaged and fish hatchlings develop abnormally in acid water below pH 5.0. Water that is neutral—that is, neither basic nor acidic—has a pH value of 7.0. Since pH values are based on a logarithmic scale, a pH change from 7.0 to 5.0 means that the acidity has increased 100 times.

Canada began to monitor the acidity of rain in 1976 and the United States began its monitoring two

Carbon Monoxide
A poisonous gas from car exhaust that drives out oxygen in the bloodstream. Large amounts can kill; small amounts can cause dizziness, headaches, and fatigue. Often exists in tunnels, garages, and heavy traffic. Especially dangerous for people with heart disease, asthma, anemia, and so on.

Hydrocarbons
Unburned chemicals in combustion, such as car exhaust, which react in air to produce smog. Hydrocarbons have produced cancer in animals.

Sulfur Oxides
Poisonous gases that come from factories and power plants burning coal or oil-containing sulfur. Forms sulfur dioxide, a poison that irritates the eyes, nose, and throat, damages the lungs, kills plants, rusts metals, and reduces visibility.

Particulates
Solid and liquid matter in air such as smoke, fly ash, dust, and fumes. They may settle to the ground or stay suspended. They soil clothes, dirty window sills, scatter light, and carry poisonous gases to lungs. They come from autos, fuels, smelters, building materials, fertilizers, and so on.

Nitrogen Oxides
A result of burning fuels that convert the nitrogen and oxygen in the air to nitrogen dioxide. Can cause a stinking brown haze that irritates the eyes and nose, shuts out sunlight, and destroys the view.

Photochemical Smog
A mixture of gases and particles oxidized by the sun from products of gasoline and other burning fuels. They irritate the eyes, nose, and throat, make breathing difficult, and damage crops.

Figure 19-3
Components of smog. Almost 200,000 tons of "aerial garbage" are released into the air annually in the United States. (Data from Environmental Protection Agency.)

years later. In 1982 the United States spent almost $20 million on research into the acid rain problem (see Figure 19-4). However, despite the expenditure of vast amounts of time and money, no acceptable federal policy or solution to the acid rain problem is in sight. Ore smelters and related industries spew millions of tons of sulfur dioxide, the principal cause of acid rain, into the U.S. atmosphere each year. Acid rain consists of about 70 percent sulfur dioxide, and the remaining 30 percent is derived from nitrogen oxides. The sulfur and nitrogen oxides released into the atmosphere react with water to produce sulfuric and nitric acids that fall into lakes and rivers thereby raising their acidity. Worldwide about 130 million tons of sulfur dioxide is put into the atmosphere annually, which makes acid rain a global problem.

Solutions to the acid rain problem involve difficult economic and political decisions and require the cooperation of many countries to control emissions. Acid rain can fall thousands of miles from the source of the sulfur dioxide emissions, which explains why it is difficult to pinpoint who is to blame. Meanwhile forests continue to be damaged and many forms of animal life will suffer and die because of the acid rain falling into their aquatic environments.

Nitrogen oxides, which are mostly produced by automobile exhausts, interfere with the oxygen-carrying capacity of the lungs and blood cells. Photochemical smog, containing nitrogen oxide, is formed over large cities such as Los Angeles by the action of sunlight on the various nitrogen compounds in the polluted air. This gives the air a hazy, brownish appearance, limits visibility, and irritates eyes and lungs.

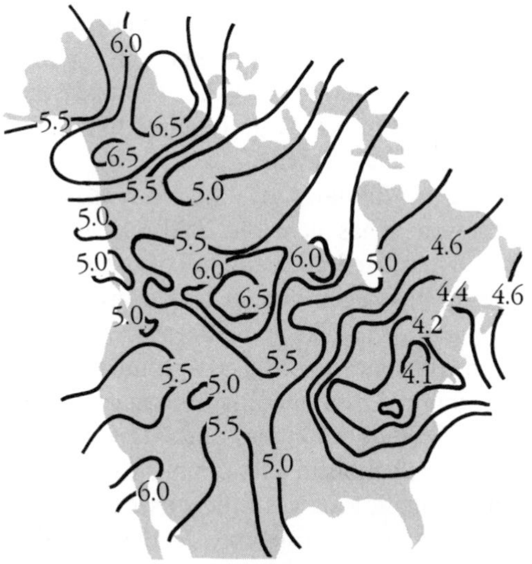

Figure 19-4
Acidity of rain in North America. On the average, rain in the eastern part of the country (pH 4.1–4.6) is five to ten times more acid than the rain falling in other parts of the country (pH 5.0–5.6). Winds tend to blow from west to east and carry industrial emissions in an easterly direction. These data were compiled by various U.S. and Canadian agencies in 1982.

Table 19-2
Symptoms of Carbon Monoxide Poisoning

Percentage of CO in hemoglobin	Symptoms
0–2	No symptoms.
2–5	No symptoms in most people, but sensitive tests reveal slight impairment of arithmetic and other cognitive abilities. Levels of 2–5% are found in light or moderate smokers.
5–10	Slight breathlessness on severe exertion. Levels of 5–10% are found in smokers who inhale one or more packs of cigarettes per day.
10–20	Mild headache, breathlessness on moderate exertion. These levels are sometimes seen in smokers who are exposed to additional CO from other sources.
20–30	Throbbing headache, irritability, impaired judgment, defective memory, rapid fatigue.
30–40	Severe headache, weakness, nausea, dimness of vision, confusion.
40–50	Confusion, hallucinations, ataxia, hyperventilation, and collapse.
50–60	Deep coma with possible convulsions.
Above 60	Usually results in death.

In addition to widespread outdoor pollution, the lungs are further assaulted by indoor pollutants. Cigarette smoking is not only harmful to the person who smokes but "second-hand smoke" often creates indoor air pollution that is more harmful than all but the worst forms of outdoor smog (see Chapter 15). Carbon monoxide levels indoors may be increased by cigarette smoke to levels that are regarded as hazardous to workers in industry and that are prohibited by law. For example, factories are not allowed to exceed carbon monoxide levels of 50 ppm and the Federal Air Quality Standard Act sets the allowable level in air outdoors at 9 ppm. Yet, the air in bars, conference rooms, and other places where many people are smoking may contain levels of carbon monoxide as high as 50 ppm.

Experimental animals that were exposed for several months to 50–100 ppm of carbon monoxide showed heart and brain damage, and it is responsible to assume that people would also suffer some adverse affects from these levels (see Table 19-2). Particulate matter such as dust, soot, lead, and asbestos in polluted air also creates serious public health problems but is of particular concern to workers who are exposed to these substances in large amounts.

The human lungs have a remarkable capacity for extracting vital oxygen from the air and for expelling unwanted gases and contaminants. Tens of millions of **cilia,** tiny hairlike projections in the breathing passageways, sweep out airborne microorganisms and particulate matter before the air ever reaches the lungs. Within the lungs, special macrophage cells (shown in Chapter 9) scavenge the foreign substances that do manage to reach the alveoli, the tiny air sacs that exchange incoming oxygen for the carbon dioxide that has been produced by the body. Years of breathing polluted air and smoking tobacco can weaken and destroy cilia, alveoli, and lung cells.

Air pollution is not confined to the immediate vicinities of factories, oil refineries, or cities. The air supply is, of course, global, and eventually air pollutants are carried to all areas of the planet. This fact is dramatically demonstrated by studies showing the increase in lead content in the Greenland snowpack over the last 100 years. The amount of lead in the snowpack has increased sharply since 1900 due to the lead in the air that is carried and deposited in this isolated area of the world. Most of the airborne lead is presumed to have originated from automotive exhausts. (This is one reason why auto manufacturers are now required to design cars that run on lead-free gas.)

Since pre-Roman times the amount of lead in the atmosphere has increased 2000-fold. It has been suggested that the decline and fall of the Roman empire could have been due, at least in part, to lead poisoning of its leaders and citizens (Nriagu, 1983). It is thought that the physical and mental deterioration exhibited by numerous Roman emperors, including Claudius, Caligula, and Nero, could have been due to alcoholism and chronic lead poisoning. In Roman times, lead was widely used to store food and wines and was also used in plates and wine goblets. In short, Romans ate a daily dose of lead.

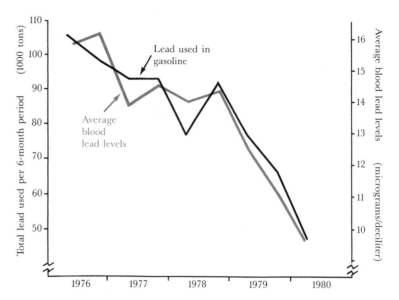

Figure 19-5
Total lead used in gasoline versus the average level of lead in people's blood. The chart shows that blood lead levels have declined at about the same rate as the use of lead in gasoline. The EPA decided in 1985 to phase out the use of lead in all gasoline.

Today, the primary source of lead pollution is lead-contaminated air. There is evidence that the introduction of lead-free gasoline several years ago has reduced blood levels of lead in the general U.S. population to a significant degree (see Figure 19-5). In 1984, after ten years of studies, hearings, and legal maneuvering by lead and gasoline companies, the EPA proposed reducing the amount of lead in gasoline by a factor of ten. The eventual goal would be to eliminate lead in gasoline completely. The EPA decision was based mainly on a cost analysis showing that by 1988 the country would save almost $800 million. The estimated savings would come partly from longer engine life and reduced wear and tear on exhaust systems. More than half of the savings would result from healthier children who would not require treatment for lead poisoning or remedial education because of their diminished capacity to learn.

Water Pollution

After air, water is probably the body's most essential requirement. We can survive without air for only a few minutes and without water perhaps several days. The human body is composed of about 60 percent water, which is essential to every function carried out by the body, including digestion, blood circulation, and excretion.

Agriculture and industry in this country are enormous consumers of water. For example, several hundred gallons of water are necessary to produce a pound of flour; brewing a barrel of beer consumes a thousand gallons; a ton of newspaper takes about a quarter of a million gallons; a ton of steel requires over half a million gallons; and irrigating an acre of orange trees requires almost a million gallons of water a year. Water is as vital to the maintenance of our lifestyle as it is to the body's continued health.

Water is continuously recycled in the environment by evaporation and rain. However, as more and more water becomes polluted from pesticides, chemicals, oil spills, and sewage, less and less water is suitable for human consumption and agricultural use. Of special concern is the chemical contamination of rivers, lakes, and underground water supplies, which provide most of our water needs (see Figure 19-6).

Waterborne diseases such as cholera, typhoid fever, and dysentery have been virtually eliminated in North America through sanitation and water treatment methods. In many communities the water supplied to homes is purified by sedimentation filtration and/or chlorination. The addition of chlorine to water to kill dangerous bacteria, however, may create other health hazards. Interaction of chlorine with other chemicals in the water produces toxic substances such as chloroform and chloramines, which are carcinogens (cancer-causing agents). The widespread use of detergents, herbicides, pesticides, fertilizers, and other chemicals has also contributed to increase water pollution.

Love Canal, formerly a charming waterway in New York near Niagara Falls, was recently declared a federal disaster area. Between 1947 and 1952, the

Hooker Chemical Company disposed of its chemical wastes in the area around Love Canal. Years later, as the chemicals oozed to the surface of the land and into the canal, the incidence of cancer and birth defects among people living in the area was found to be unusually high. No one knows for certain how much it will cost to clean up Love Canal, and some areas near the canal may remain a permanent health hazard. Recent studies have found that small field mice called voles living around the canal have a reduced life expectancy compared to voles living some distance from the canal. The closer to the canal the voles live, the younger they die

(Christian, 1983). Many of the voles that have been trapped, especially those living close to the canal, show evidence of liver damage and also have high tissue levels of the pesticides that were dumped into the canal years ago.

Analysis of drinking water from communities across the United States has shown that much of the water is unsafe and unhealthy (see Box 19-1). In the early 1970s, the Environmental Protection Agency found that the water supplies of many towns and cities were dangerously contaminated with pathogenic organisms and toxic chemicals. (It found 66 organic chemicals in the drinking water of New

---

BOX 19-1

WIDESPREAD CONTAMINATION OF DRINKING WATER EXISTS IN THE UNITED STATES

Over one hundred chemicals potentially hazardous to health have been introduced into drinking water supplies across the country as a result of environmental pollution from various sources. The Environmental Protection Agency (EPA), which is responsible for monitoring our drinking water and for setting standards, has established safe levels for about twenty of the more common pollutants in drinking water (see table).

In addition to these chemicals, other compounds have seeped into underground water supplies in many areas from nearby industrial complexes or toxic waste dumps. Other hazardous substances found in drinking water are benzene, carbon tetrachloride, dioxin, ethylene dibromide (EDB), polychlorinated biphenyls (PCBs), and vinyl chloride. All of these chemicals are carcinogens (see Chapter 17). Children are usually more vulnera-

ble to ingestion of toxic substances than adults because of their smaller size and because they are still growing.

Many kinds of home water purifiers are now on the market,

but many of them are not very efficient at filtering out hazardous substances despite manufacturers' claims. Safe drinking water is going to be increasingly hard to find in the future.

Pollutant	Maximum level (mg/l)	Pollutant	Maximum level (mg/l)
INORGANIC CHEMICALS			
Arsenic	0.05	Lead	0.025
Barium	1.0	Manganese	0.05
Cadmium	0.01	Mecury	0.002
Chromium	0.05	Nitrites and nitrates	10.0
Copper	10.0	Selenium	0.045
Detergents	0.5	Silver	0.05
Fluoride	1.4	Sulfate	250.0
Iron	0.3	Total dissolved solids	500.0

ORGANIC CHEMICALS		RADIOACTIVE SUBSTANCES	
Endrin	0.0002	Radium 226 and 228	5 pCi/l
Lindane	0.004	Gross alpha particle activity	15 pCi/l
Methoxychlor	0.1		
Toxaphene	0.005		
Total trihalomethanes (THM)	0.1*		

*EPA has slated a future goal of 0.01–0.025 mg/l for THM.

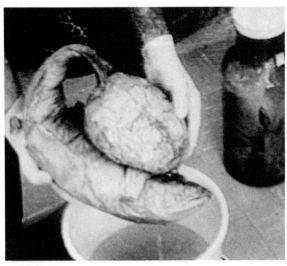

Figure 19-6
A giant tumor on a fish caught in Lake Michigan. Toxic chemicals introduced into rivers, lakes, and underground water pose a major health threat to anyone using contaminated water. (Courtesy Cable Network News.)

Orleans, for example.) As a result of these findings, Congress passed the Safe Drinking Water Act of 1974, which covers 40,000 community water supply systems and another 200,000 private systems. The act requires that these systems meet new federal drinking water safety standards. But it is one thing to pass such a law and another thing to enforce it,

and many community water supplies are still contaminated. Many people today are forced to drink bottled, distilled, or spring water to protect their health.

Land Pollution

Until recently, little public attention was given to the disposal of solid wastes. Each year in the United States we junk about 7 million autos; 75 billion cans, bottles, and jars; and 200 million tons of trash and garbage. The U.S. Public Health Service has labeled over 90 percent of the thousands of authorized hazardous waste disposal sites as posing "unacceptable" health risks. Hazardous wastes consist of materials that are flammable, corrosive, toxic, or chemically reactive, and about 35 million tons of such wastes are produced each year in the United States. In 1979, the EPA documented 400 cases of health and environmental damage due to improper hazardous waste disposal, and this number is thought to represent only a tiny fraction of the actual health problems caused by disposal of toxic substances. The magnitude of the environmental pollution and of health problems posed by disposal of hazardous chemicals is indicated by the data in Table 19-3. Because most of these toxic substances are not readily broken down or inactivated in the environment, the health problems resulting from such wastes may increase in the years ahead.

Table 19-3
Annual Disposal of Some Hazardous Chemicals in the United States, 1977

Substance	Amount (millions of pounds)	Source	Health effects
Mercury	2.6	Sludge from chloralkali plants; electrical equipment, fluorescent lights	Tremors, mental retardation, loss of teeth, kidney damage, neurological damage
Arsenic	110.0	Arsenic trioxide from coal combustion and from metal smelters	Diarrhea, vomiting, paralysis, skin cancers
Cadmium	1.8	Waste from electroplating industry; paint containers, nickel-cadmium batteries	Lung diseases
Cyanide	21.0	Electroplating industry waste	Poisoning, interferes with cellular energy metabolism
Pesticides	230.0	Solid wastes and wastes in solutions	Multiple effects including rashes, respiratory and gastrointestinal symptoms, neurological disorders, hemorrhages

Data from Janice Crossland, "The Wastes Endure," *Archives of Environmental Health*, 19 (1977), 9.

> Surely the protection of life in all its beauty and richness and diversity is the most compelling environmental cause of all, and the most urgent.
>
> **Russell E. Train**
> **Former director of EPA**

Pesticides and Related Chemicals

Soil and water in America have become increasingly polluted by chemicals that have been used to control weeds, insects, and plant diseases. Any substance capable of killing or limiting the growth of living organisms is called a **pesticide.** Chemicals that are specific for certain classes of organisms are called insecticides, rodenticides, fungicides, or herbicides. Pesticides are important to the agricultural industry of this country, which claims it could not produce such an abundant food supply without them, although some experts disagree (Van den Bosch, 1978). Billions of pounds of DDT and other polychlorinated hydrocarbons have been used in the last 20 years to kill insects and other pests that destroy valuable crops. Pesticide use has been beneficial to agriculture, but it has also created serious environmental and health problems, which are not easily resolved. DDT, probably the most widely disseminated pesticide in the world, was banned from use in the United States.

The principal health danger from continued widespread use of pesticides is that most are carcinogens and teratogens (cause damage to developing embryos). Pesticides are found in farmland and forest soils and, because they are washed out of the soil by rain and irrigation, are found in the water of rivers, lakes, and oceans. Their harmful effects on health are enhanced further because they accumulate in animal and human tissues. The chemicals become more and more concentrated in organisms as they move up the food chain. The fish, fowl, and beef that people eat nowadays may have high levels of pesticides in them, which then become part of human body tissues. Several agencies of the federal government monitor pesticide contamination in various foods, and the government then has the difficult task of determining what levels are safe and what levels should be regarded as dangerous to health. It is easy to understand how governmental decisions could provoke heated controversy between consumers concerned with health and producers of food who are concerned with productivity (see Box 19-2).

Recent studies by the National Cancer Institute (NCI) show that farmworkers exposed to the weed killer 2,4-D have a five to ten times higher risk of cancer than farmworkers not exposed to the chemical. After several farmworkers died following exposure to Dinoseb, a widely used, highly toxic herbicide, the EPA issued an emergency ban on its use. About ten million pounds of Captan, a potent fungicide, are used in the United States each year, primarily on fruits such as grapes and apples. Captan is a carcinogen, a mutagen, and a teratogen, but because it is not acutely toxic like Dinoseb, it has been regarded as safe. However, increased public pressure may force EPA to ban the use of Captan also.

The lesson from these and numerous other studies is that no pesticide is safe and most can cause short- or long-term health problems (see Figure 19-7). Evidence is also beginning to show that common pesticides used around the home and garden can cause headaches, allergies, and flu-like symptoms. Everyone needs to be aware that pesticides are

---

BOX 19-2

SOME COMMON PESTICIDES AND PRECAUTIONS FOR THEIR USE

Organophosphates
diazinon
malathion

Organophosphates have a relatively short persistence in the environment. These chemicals can cause acute nervous system poisoning in people. Malathion is less acutely toxic than many other pesticides.

Carbamates
carbaryl (Sevin)
aldicarb (Temik)

These chemicals are similar to the organophosphates in their persistence and toxic effects on the nervous system. The chemical involved in the mass poisonings in Bhopal, India, has been used in manufacturing each of these two pesticides.

Organochlorines
DDT
chlordane
lindane

Compared to the previous groups, these chemicals have relatively long persistence in the environment and low acute toxicity. Each of these three chemicals has been shown to cause cancer in experimental animals. Chlordane is widely used to control termite infestations. Lindane has been used in home pesticide vaporizers and as a drug in treating scabies (mite infestations). DDT is no longer used in the United States but is used in other countries to control insects that spread disease such as malaria.

**Phyenoxyacetic acids
and related compounds**
2,4,5-T
2,4-D
pentachlorophenol

This group of compounds is generally used to kill weeds. Several have been found to be contaminated with dioxins, chemicals that are deadly both on an acute and a long-term basis.

**Pesticides derived
from plants**
pyrethrum
nicotine
rotenone

Exposure to some of the botanical pesticides can cause allergic reactions and other adverse reactions. Pets and people may be affected. These chemicals have fairly long persistence in the environment.

1. *Before you buy* a pesticide product, read the instructions for use and any health and safety warnings. Do not purchase the product if you can't use the pesticide properly (you may not have the right equipment). If you don't understand, or feel completely comfortable with, the health and safety information provided, get more information before you buy the product. Also, consider whether you have adequate storage space for the pesticide. A bigger bottle may be cheaper, but can you store it safely?

2. Use the least toxic pesticide available for your pest control problem. Try to strike a balance between effective pest control and the safety of people, pets, and other nontarget organisms.

3. Minimize skin and respiratory contact with pesticides. Wear protective gloves. When you select gloves, consider both the solvent used in the pesticide formulation and the possibility that the pesticide itself can penetrate skin. A local safety equipment store (check the telephone directory) can be help-

ful. You may want to use a respirator to guard against inhaling pesticide spray or dust.

4. Use pesticides only for the uses for which they are intended. For instance, some wood preservatives are meant for outside use only, so don't use them inside the house!

5. Don't leave seemingly empty pesticide containers where children can get them. Children have been poisoned by drinking from "empty" containers that actually contained leftover pesticide.

> ## Suppose the Russians had poisoned our earth and contaminated our water. We would call that chemical warfare. That is what we are now allowing corporations to do to us.
> **Reverend Jesse Jackson**

dangerous and, if they must be used, all precautions against exposure should be observed.

Dioxin, a chemical present as a contaminant in some herbicides, is an extremely potent carcinogen. It has been detected in samples of human breast milk, which creates a problem for mothers who have to decide whether to nurse their babies or not. The U.S. Forest Service still sprays forests with herbicides to control brush, although there is some evidence suggesting that the health of people living near forests that are sprayed is adversely affected. Some veterans of the Vietnam War believe that their health was impaired by the herbicides (such as Agent Orange) they were exposed to in Vietnam, and some have sued the government for damages. In 1984 the U.S. military agreed to establish a fund of $180 million to be distributed over the next 25 years to Vietnam veterans and their families who were affected by exposure to Agent Orange (Raloff, 1984). Despite this enormous settlement, the official policy of the federal government and chemical companies is that no adverse health effects have been proven except for the occurrence of skin rashes (chloracne) among people who are exposed (Tschirley, 1986).

Because of extensive chemical contamination of their town, about 800 residents of Times Beach, Missouri will never return to their homes (Sun, 1983a,b; Garmon, 1983). These people had to abandon their town because dirt roads and other dusty areas had been sprayed over a period of years with oil that was heavily contaminated with **dioxin** (2-3-8 tetra-chlorodibenzopara dioxin, TCDD). Horses, dogs, cats, birds, and insects died after coming into contact with sprayed areas. Children broke out in rashes and came down with other medical problems. The residents of Times Beach were eventually compen-

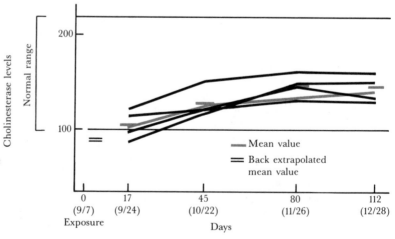

Figure 19-7
Cholinesterase levels in five office workers exposed to pesticides. After their office was sprayed by an exterminator, all five workers became ill within an hour. They were told that they had the flu. Cholinesterase is an enzyme essential for functioning of the brain and nervous system. Their enzyme levels remained abnormal for over a month after pesticide exposure. (Data from Hodgson and Parkinson, 1985.)

> Children stricken with moderate to severe lead
> poisoning who do not receive immediate
> treatment risk permanent brain damage.
>
> **John Graef, M.D.**
> **Boston Children's Hospital**

sated for the loss of their homes, and continuing efforts are being made to decontaminate the area.

Ethylene dibromide (EDB) is a pesticide widely used to fumigate fruit and to control insect infestation in stored grain. For the past 20 years it has been assumed that EDB is safe despite many studies showing it to be a highly toxic chemical and a potent carcinogen in mice and rats. After almost 7 years of deliberation, in 1984 the EPA finally decided to ban further use of EDB (Sun, 1984a).

Polybrominated biphenyls (PBBs) were widely used in the 1970s as fire-retardant chemicals. In 1973 several thousand pounds of PBBs were accidentally added to livestock feed and distributed to about 800 dairy farmers in Michigan. Some months later, when cattle became sick and calves began to die, the accident was discovered. In the meanwhile, people had eaten PBB-contaminated milk and meat and had assimilated the substance into their tissues. Public health scientists are continuing to monitor these people to see whether their health is adversely affected over the long term.

Polychlorinated biphenyls (PCBs) are compounds used in electrical transformers, hydraulic fluids, paints, and many other products. Although the EPA banned the manufacture of PCBs a number of years ago, the chemicals continue to find their way into the environment. It is estimated that there are still 340 million pounds of PCBs in air, water, and soil and another 750 million pounds of various pieces of equipment still in use (Garmon, 1982).

What is certain in the controversy over the use of pesticides is that billions of pounds of chemicals have been diffused into the environment and that these chemicals will continue to pollute the land and water for generations to come. Increased rates of cancer, stillbirth, and birth defects tomorrow may be the terrible harvest of the widespread use of pesticides, herbicides, and toxic chemicals now and in the past.

Heavy Metal Pollution

Many heavy metals are toxic to living organisms when they are present in the body in more than minute amounts. These metals include beryllium, cadmium, nickel, arsenic, manganese, and especially lead and mercury. Because these heavy metals are vital to many manufacturing processes and industries, the amounts entering the environment have increased sharply in recent years. Heavy metals affect health in a variety of ways—all of them detrimental. They inhibit many essential enzyme reactions in body cells. They damage blood cells, producing symptoms of anemia. And they damage cells of the nervous system, causing headaches, loss of coordination, drowsiness, mental retardation, and even death.

Lead

Lead is a cumulative cellular poison and presents the most serious health hazard because of the enormous amounts that are used and because it contaminates air, food, and water. Early symptoms of **plumbism** (lead poisoning) are loss of appetite,

> All messianic leaders should come with a warning label attached to their foreheads, saying: "This leader could be hazardous to our health."
>
> **Frank Herbert**

weakness, and anemia. Because such general symptoms can result from many causes, a diagnosis of plumbism often is not made until more serious symptoms develop (see Table 19-4).

One of the tragedies of lead poisoning is that children are the chief victims. In 1970 the Surgeon General estimated that 400,000 children in the United States had dangerous levels of lead in their blood, and that number may be higher today. More than one-fourth of those children will suffer some brain damage. The number of children suffering lead poisoning is particularly high in city slums (Berwick and Komaroff, 1982).

In addition to airborne lead pollution poisoning, small children become poisoned because of a condition known as **pica,** an appetite for unusual substances or abnormal kinds of food. Many older paints contain lead and are sweet to the taste. As paint flakes off walls in old buildings, children crawling around are apt to eat the paint flakes.

Mothers do not usually notice any unusual symptoms until the lead poisoning has advanced to a stage where brain damage has already occurred. Studies of children with learning disabilities suspected to have been caused by lead poisoning have shown them to have more than five times the amount of lead in their bodies as normal children (Pihl and Parkes, 1977).

In 1975, about 900,000 tons of lead were used in the manufacture of batteries and other metal products. An additional 200,000 tons of lead were used in the production of gasoline as an "antiknock" additive. The lead added to gasoline is the more serious source of pollution because almost all of it ends up in the air we breathe. It is estimated that without man-made lead pollution, the natural body burden of an adult would be about .25 mcg of lead per 100 ml of blood. Today the average adult living in a large city has a blood level *one hundred times* that amount, or 25 mcg of lead per 100 ml of blood. Be-

Table 19-4
The Effect of Lead Accumulation in People

Amount of lead in blood (micrograms/100 ml)	Observable effects
10	Enzyme inhibition, learning disabilities
15–40	Red blood cells affected
40–50	Anemia
50–60	Central nervous system affected, cognitive disabilities
60–100	Permanent brain damage

Data from "Air Quality Criteria for Lead," Environmental Protection Agency 600/8-77-017, pp. 13–25.

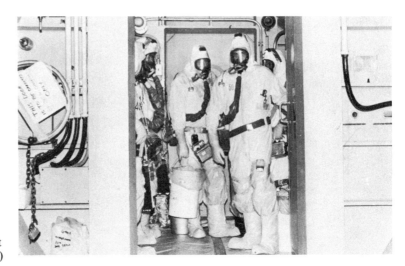

Figure 19-8
Nuclear power plant workers encased in clothing and gear to protect against radiation. (United Press International.)

cause pregnant women share materials in their blood with the developing embryo, babies are sometimes born who are already suffering from lead poisoning.

Although polluted air is the main source for lead entering the lungs and blood, food may also contribute significant amounts of lead, since plants and animals also assimilate lead from the air and soil. Food may add from 50 to 200 micrograms of lead a day to the body.

Lead in the environment is one of the most serious pollution problems facing our society. Elevated blood levels of lead in children may be partly responsible for learning disabilities, hyperactivity, and even mental retardation. Herbert L. Needleman of Harvard Medical School and Sergio Piomelli of New York University Medical Center (1978) have written a report describing and documenting the many health hazards of lead exposure, especially from low levels. They conclude: "Lead in the air is a product of man's activity and can be controlled by man. Rarely do important biomedical problems offer themselves to such available remedy."

Mercury

In 1953, an epidemic of methylmercury poisoning occurred in several villages around Minamata Bay in Japan. Since the first epidemic, mercury poisoning has become known as "Minamata disease," and another outbreak occurred in Japan in 1965. In 1970, high levels of methylmercury were found in Lake St. Clair in Canada, where a chemical plant had been discharging its wastes. In 1970, the U.S.

Food and Drug Administration began to determine which bodies of water in the United States were contaminated by mercury, and as a result of their investigation, fishing limitations were imposed eventually in eighteen states because of unsafe mercury levels in fish.

Mercury poisoning is characterized by muscle weakness, lack of coordination, paralysis, progressive blindness and deafness, and mental retardation. Like many other toxic substances, methylmercury is concentrated as it moves up the food chain. Children and developing embryos are the ones most affected by mercury and lead poisoning because their body and brain cells are still growing rapidly.

Radiation

The cells of the body are continuously exposed to various forms of electromagnetic radiation, such as gamma rays, x-rays, ultraviolet (UV) light, and subatomic particles from nuclear disintegrations—all of which go undetected by any of the senses. These are all forms of ionizing radiation and can cause permanent changes in cells that may result in cancer or an increased risk of birth defects, may destroy molecules, and may affect chemical reactions in living cells. Much of the potentially harmful radiation from the sun and stars is filtered by the earth's atmosphere. However, as anyone who has had a sunburn knows, too much radiation is dangerous.

Electromagnetic radiation and radioactivity result from natural processes, but technologies de-

> The accident at Chernobyl posed more dramatically than ever before the immediate problem of dealing with the known risks of nuclear energy.
> *Medical News*

veloped in recent years have produced a marked increase in people's overall radiation exposure, especially for certain occupational groups such as x-ray technicians and nuclear industry workers.

Radiation hazards tend to remain more localized than those stemming from chemical pollution of air and water. A medical x-ray exposes the patient and persons in the immediate vicinity, such as the doctor or technician. Exposure to radioactivity is usually limited to persons who live or work near radioactive materials, such as those produced in nuclear power plants and those found in uranium mines or in places where radioisotopes are used. However, radioactive materials can also be spread over large areas as a result of radioactive fallout from atomic explosions and from uranium mining. For example, there has been concern that the higher incidence of leukemia reported among children in southern Utah might have been due to atomic test explosions carried out in neighboring Nevada in the 1950s. Finally in 1984, a federal judge ruled, in a suit filed by leukemia victims, that the federal government was liable for damages where the evidence appeared convincing that the leukemia was caused by radioactive fallout. Also, at least seven states in the southwest United States have large areas of land polluted with millions of tons of radioactive debris resulting from uranium mining. The radioactive materials are spread even further by wind and rain, which washes the radioactivity into the rivers.

Any exposure to x-rays or radioactivity carries with it some degree of risk. There is no such thing as a safe dose of radiation. One can argue that the radiation risks are greatly outweighed by the benefits for particular circumstances—taking an x-ray to facilitate setting a fractured bone or using radiation therapy to treat an inoperable tumor. Nonetheless, we should not forget that even the brief radiation exposure from a diagnostic x-ray poses some health risk (Bross, Ball, and Falen, 1979). Some studies have indicated that certain people may be particularly sensitive to low levels of radiation and that children who develop leukemia are often in this "susceptible" group (Bross and Natarajan, 1972). As more data have become available in recent years, the allowable radiation standards established by federal regulatory agencies have been steadily lowered (see Box 19-3).

Each person has the responsibility for minimizing his or her exposure to radiation and radioactivity. You are entitled to a complete explanation from your doctor or dentist as to the necessity for any x-ray diagnosis or radiation therapy that is recommended. You should ask yourself whether you really need a routine annual chest or dental x-ray exam if there are no symptoms present. Many dentists, for example, will routinely take an x-ray with every checkup because it was an accepted practice when they were trained. Many cavities can be detected by a careful visual exam, and if a person has had no cavities for several years, an x-ray is probably unwarranted. Discuss with your dentist the pros and cons of routine x-ray examination. If you are unsatisfied, you may prefer to find a dentist who is more conservative in the use of dental x-rays.

BOX 19-3

ESTIMATING YOUR ANNUAL RADIATION EXPOSURE

The recommended maximum dose of radiation from all sources is 500 millirems per year. Use this chart to estimate your annual radiation exposure.

Source of radiation	Approximate annual dose in millirems
Cosmic rays from space: 40 mrem average at sea level; add 1 mrem for each 100 feet above sea level	_____
Radioactive minerals in rocks and soil: ranges from 20 to 400 mrem; *U.S. average =* 55	_____
Radioactivity from air, water, and food: ranges from about 20 to 400 mrem; *U.S. average =* 25	_____
Medical and dental x-rays and tests: 22 mrem for chest x-ray, 500 for x-ray of lower gastrointestinal tract, 910 for whole-mouth dental x-ray film, 1500 for breast mammogram, 5 million for radiation treatment of a cancer; *U.S. average =* 80	_____
Living or working in a stone or brick structure: 40 mrem for living and an additional 40 for working in such a structure	_____
Smoking one pack of cigarettes a day for one year: 40 mrem	_____
Nuclear weapons fallout; *U.S. average =* 4	_____
Air travel: 2 mrem per year for each 1500 miles flown	_____
TV or computer screens: 4 mrem per year for each 2 hours of viewing a day	_____
Occupational exposure: 100,000 mrem per year for uranium ore miner, 600–800 for nuclear power plant worker, 300–350 for medical x-ray technician, 50–125 for dental x-ray technician, 140 for jet plane crews; *U.S. average –* 0.8	_____
Normal operation of nuclear power plants, nuclear fuel processing, and nuclear research facilities; *U.S. average –* 0.1	_____
Miscellaneous: luminous watch dials, smoke detectors, industrial wastes, etc.; *U.S. average –* 2	_____
Your annual total	_____
Average annual exposure per person in the United States	230

Chart adapted from *Living in the Environment* by G. Tyler Miller, Jr. (Wadsworth, 1984).

Many companies and government agencies require annual chest x-rays. Most companies require new employees to have a chest x-ray as part of their physical exam. If a person changes jobs frequently, he or she may be exposed to several unnecessary x-rays each year. Often companies, doctors, and hospitals will not accept x-rays taken elsewhere, thereby adding to a person's radiation exposure.

Some medical x-ray machines, because they are defective or adjusted improperly, expose patients to unnecessarily high doses of radiation. During x-ray examination or treatment, the reproductive organs should be protected by a lead apron or screen. During pregnancy, no x-rays should be taken unless absolutely necessary for the diagnosis of some serious abnormality of the mother or fetus. By being cau-

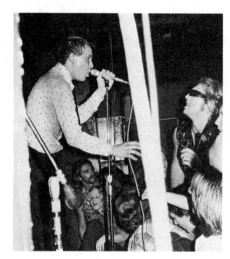 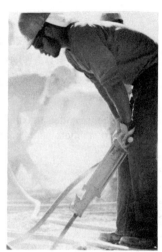

Figure 19-9
Two common sources of loud noises in the environment. (*Left:* Jackie Estrada; *right:* Courtesy Environmental Protection Agency.)

tious regarding your exposure to ionizing radiation over a lifetime, you can help preserve your health and minimize damage to your body's cells.

Other forms of nonionizing electromagnetic (EM) radiation, such as radio, television, radar, and microwaves, are widespread in the environment. Indeed virtually all forms of electronic communication and other aspects of our technological society depend on using low-level EM radiation. Over the years various concerns have been raised regarding possible deleterious biological effects of long-term exposure to this kind of radiation. Despite considerable research into the biological consequences of such exposure, no harmful effects have been consistently observed or documented (Foster and Guy, 1986). However, despite the low risk it probably is advisable to avoid ongoing exposure to powerful transmitters of nonionizing EM radiation.

Noise Pollution

Have you ever been kept awake during the night by a dripping faucet? Do fire and ambulance sirens put you on edge? Does the persistent pounding of rock music affect you? Have you ever found yourself thinking, "If that noise doesn't stop, I'm going to scream"?

Most of us are disturbed daily by some kind of noise. We usually dismiss our annoyance by accepting noise as part of the environment. Yet noise interferes with sleep and causes fatigue, irritability, anger, tension, and anxiety. High levels of noise, such as exposure to high-intensity rock music, jet

planes, and jackhammers, can cause permanent hearing loss as well as physiological changes that are detrimental to health (Figure 19-9).

Sound activates the nervous system and in so doing affects functions of the endocrine, cardiovascular, and reproductive systems (Raloff, 1982). As defined in Chapter 10, noise is a "stressor" and can increase blood pressure, alter hormone levels, constrict blood vessels — in short, can contribute to the development of disease just as do other kinds of stress. Figure 19-10 shows the noise levels in various situations and environments that most people encounter. Many people live and work amidst the din of urban life and tend to forget how necessary to health and how comforting silence can be to one's state of mind. When you have the good fortune to spend time in the woods or mountains, you become aware of the quiet. The human need for stillness was expressed most eloquently in 1854 by Chief Seattle, after whom the modern city is named:

There is no quiet place in the white man's cities. No place to hear the unfurling of leaves in spring or the rustle of insect's wings. But perhaps it is because I am a savage and do not understand. The clatter only seems to insult the ears. And what is there to life if a man cannot hear the lonely cry of the whippoorwill or the arguments of the frogs around a pond at night? I am a red man and do not understand. The Indian prefers the soft sound of the wind darting over the face of a pond, and the smell of the wind itself, cleansed by a midday rain or scented with the pinion pine.

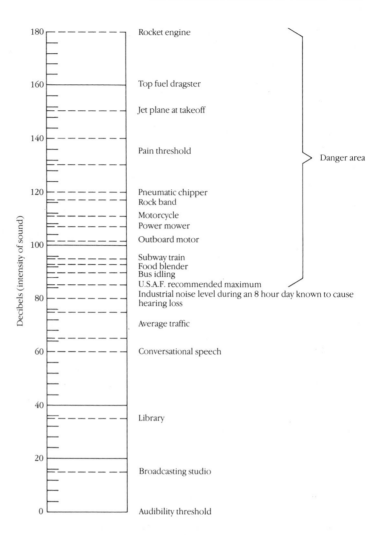

Figure 19-10
The noise level in different environments. Sound intensities are measured in decibels, which are expressed on a logarithmic scale. An increase in sound intensity by a factor of 1000 corresponds to an increase of 30 decibels (log 1000 = 3). For example, the intensity difference between conversational speech (60 dB) and an outboard motor (100 dB) is 40 dB, or 10,000 times. (Adapted from *Our Precarious Habitat* by Melvin A. Benarde, by permission of W. W. Norton & Company, Inc. Copyright ©1970 by W. W. Norton & Company, Inc.)

Nuclear Winter

In 1945 atomic bombs were dropped on the cities of Hiroshima and Nagasaki in Japan. An estimated 140,000 people died in Hiroshima and another 70,000 in Nagasaki from the blasts and fires that resulted. Since then the world's nations and citizens have been concerned with the possibility of nuclear war and the destructive consequences to the environment and life. The term "nuclear winter" was introduced to describe the global destruction that some scientists believe would result from a large-scale nuclear war (Turco et al., 1983).

A nuclear war would cause the social and economic fabric of societies to collapse. Food and water would be contaminated or destroyed. Hunger and starvation would be widespread. Some experts believe that the earth's temperature would change and that the environment could be changed so drasti-

cally that human life might eventually cease to exist. Even if this view is extreme, physicians have predicted dire consequences for human health following a nuclear war (Leaf, 1986). However, even these predictions have been contested by critics who argue that estimates of destruction and problems are overblown. They also argue that discussions of nuclear winter are inappropriate for both scientific and political reasons (Nuclear War Letters, 1987).

Nuclear war and nuclear winter are events that everyone fears and hopes can be avoided. Yet the disturbing reality is that nations (and individuals) have not learned how to resolve differences without violence or the threat of violence. Until people learn how to live and interact without violence, nuclear war and nuclear winter remain as the ultimate threat to the environment. Perhaps the slogan of the peace activists says it more clearly than all the arguments: "No one is right if no one is left."

> ### To subdue the enemy without fighting
> ### is the acme of skill.
> **Sun Tzu**

Accidents

Most people don't think of accidents as health problems, but accidents affect the well-being of millions of people every year (see Figure 19-11). When people think of accidents they usually think of something over which they have no control. Accidents are commonly described as occurring by chance, for no specific reason, or because God made it happen. It is true that the victims of some accidents have no control over the injurious occurrence. They are passengers on a train or airplane that crashes, they eat food or drink water that contains poisons, or they are hurt in a tornado or flood. But the overwhelming majority of accidents are caused by poor judgment, inattention, or confused mental states.

People cause accidents and are also the victims. For example, alcohol abuse is known to be a primary cause for all kinds of accidents. That drinking is responsible for most automobile fatalities has been shown in many studies. A recent sudy in Texas, for example, showed that 72 percent of the drivers killed in auto crashes in Houston had blood alcohol levels over 150 mg per 100 ml of blood (the legal index of intoxication). Psychological tests given to persons who have been involved in an auto accident and survived showed that 76 percent had an alcohol or personality problem, while in a control, nonaccident group, 88 percent of the people were classified as normal by the same psychological criteria. Among

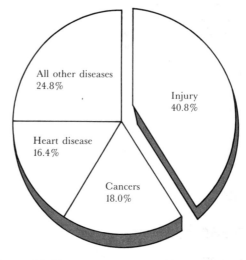

Figure 19-11
Percentages of years of potential life lost before age 65. Injury causes more loss than cancer and heart disease combined. Some facts to remember: injury is the fourth leading cause of death; injury caused 143,000 deaths in 1983; injury causes about half of all deaths in children aged 1–14. Be careful!

young people between the ages of 15 and 24, accidents claim more lives than all other causes of death combined, and automobile fatalities are a major contributor to teenage deaths (see Figure 19-12).

Some authorities single out September 13, 1899, as a memorable day in the history of the automobile. On that day it was reported that Mr. H. H. Bliss was struck and killed by an electric taxi at 74th Street and Central Park West in New York City. Bliss may have been this nation's first automobile fatality, culminating in what has today become a carnage on the highways. Traffic fatalities in the United States have accounted for more deaths than have been recorded in all of the wars that the United States has fought since the country was founded. One drink too many, a moment's inattention, a reckless decision, or simply a brief joy ride can result in a lifetime of regret and pain (see Figure 19-13).

Safety in the broadest sense means being in harmony with oneself and with the environment. Usually when the bread knife slips and cuts a finger or when you stumble and fall, it is because you are upset or angry or distracted in some way that allows the mishap to occur. If a person has been trying to cope with life's problems by using alcohol or drugs, the capacity for judgment, as well as muscle coordination, is impaired and the chances for an accident are significantly increased. People not only endanger their own physical safety and health when they become intoxicated with alcohol or take drugs, they endanger the lives of other people as well. A philosophy of safety that fits in with the ideas of holistic health was expressed 40 years ago in a classic article by Herman H. Horne (1940). His broad view of accidents is that

> the universe of which we are a part, that is, the cosmos, is characterized, so the astronomers tell us, by law, harmony, sym-

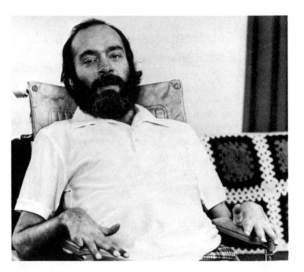

Figure 19-13
"I was a good driver. I had never had a ticket during the two years I'd been driving. I really believed nothing could happen to me. But a five-minute joy ride took away everything I had except my brain. I was 18 and naive. I didn't know what a quadriplegic was until I became one." — Jack Burnett (Reproduced with permission of the American Insurance Association.)

metry, and rhythm and order. Nothing happens in the world at large by chance, everything occurs according to law. Safety for man means only that he is catching step with the universe of which he is a part and which explains his being here at all.

Accidents do not just happen. They are caused. Fatalism is an incorrect philosophy of life. Self-determinism is better. Man himself in his choices is a cause, and in a measure man can control external causes and situations.

Ultimately, health and well-being depend on how people choose to interact with the environment that nurtures and sustains all life. If you strive to establish a harmonious interaction with all of nature, it becomes clear that you cannot tolerate pollution, contamination, noise, or accidents, for they all result from people's negative actions and destructive states of mind. If people are feeling positive and loving, they will not think of throwing a bottle at the earth, much less at another person or animal. So we must find ways to live more gently on the earth. Our health and safety depends on it.

Figure 19-12
Teenage male drivers have the highest percentage of deaths from motor vehicle accidents. Male and female drivers below age 25 have the most accidents and the greatest number of deaths. (Data from the Insurance Institute for Highway Safety.)

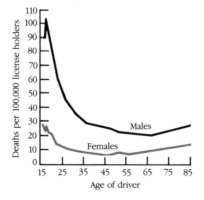

Supplemental Readings

Brodeur, P. *Outrageous Misconduct: The Asbestos Industry on Trial.* New York: Pantheon Books, 1985. Documents how manufacturers of asbestos products knowingly exposed workers for over 50 years while continually denying the lethal hazards of asbestos exposure.

Brown, L. R. *State of the World 1987.* New York: W. W. Norton and Co., 1987. A report of the Worldwatch Institute on the multiple environmental problems facing the nations of the world.

"Chernobyl—An Early Report." *Environment,* June 1986. Explains what happened at the worst nuclear accident in history and some of its consequences.

Christian, John J. "Love Canal's Unhealthy Voles." *Natural History,* October 1983. An article describing the disease and death occurring among small rodents living near Love Canal.

Commoner, Barry. "The Environment." *New Yorker,* June 15, 1987. An insightful examination of the environmental movement in the U.S. over the past 20 years.

Nero, A. V., Jr. "The Indoor Radon Story." *Technology Review,* January 1986. A comprehensive analysis of the risks of radon gas in housing in the U.S.

Raloff, J. "Occupational Noise—The Subtle Pollutant," and "Noise Can Be Hazardous to Our Health." *Science News,* May 22, 1982, and June 5, 1982. Two short articles that discuss the health hazards of noise in the environment.

Samuels, M., and **Bennett, H. Z.** *Well Body, Well Earth.* San Francisco: Sierra Club Books, 1983. Contains useful information on environmental hazards to health and how to prevent them.

Walsh, R. *Staying Alive—The Psychology of Human Survival.* Boulder: Shambala Publications, 1984. A thoughtful discussion of world problems and what individuals can do to help solve them and live healthier lives.

Summary

Environmental pollution constitutes a serious hazard to health. For optimal well-being, people require unpolluted air, water, and food. The air is too contaminated by smog, hydrocarbons, nitrogen and sulfur oxides, lead, and other particles. Drinking water frequently contains heavy metals and poisonous chemicals that can cause cancer and other diseases. The land is becoming increasingly polluted from excessive pesticide use. Many of these chemicals enter the food chain and end up being deposited in people's bodies.

Radioactivity, x-rays, other forms of electromagnetic radiation, and noise are also forms of environmental pollution that can impair health. Ionizing radiation either damages cells and genetic material directly or produces physiological changes that are harmful.

Accidents—the leading cause of death among Americans between the ages of 1 and 38—are caused when individuals are out of harmony with themselves, with other people, and with the environment. Most accidents are not caused by chance; accidents are caused by people who are careless or distraught for some reason. Alcohol abuse and drug-taking are major contributors to accidents.

Each one of us has the responsibility for creating a healthy environment for ourselves and for other people who share the environment with us. Caring for the environment means reducing, in whatever ways we can, air, water, and land pollution; practicing safety at home and at work; and keeping our social environment free of stressful and destructive interactions.

> There is no such thing as an accident. What we
> call by that name is the effect of some cause
> which we do not see.
>
> **Voltaire**

FOR YOUR HEALTH

Reducing Pollution

List the ways that you contribute to environmental pollution. For example, smoking cigarettes; driving a car; throwing away cans, bottles, and paper. Can you find ways to live so that you pollute less? For example, can you walk or ride a bicycle to school or work? Can you recycle materials that you normally throw away?

Avoiding Accidents

Recall the last time you had an accident. Can you remember your mental state? Were you angry or upset? Had you been drinking alcohol or using drugs? Do you think your mental state contributed to the accident? Program your mind to pay more attention to how you feel and how you are functioning at all times so that you can avoid accidents in the future.

UNIT THREE

Life Cycles

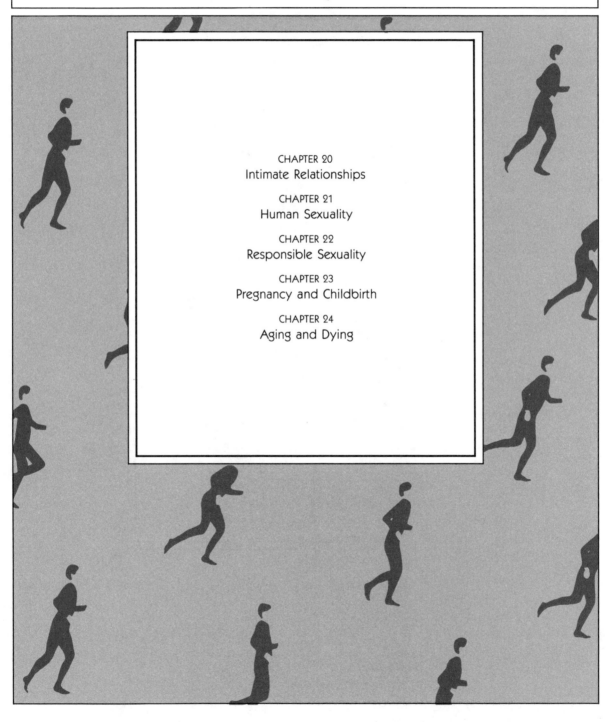

CHAPTER TWENTY

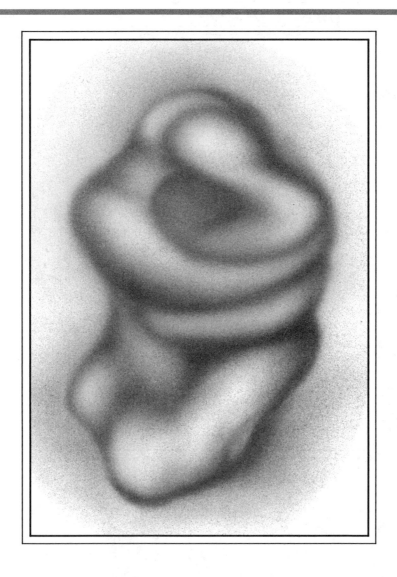

Healthy relationships make for healthy
people.

Intimate Relationships

We all need intimacy—that feeling of closeness, trust, and openness with another person that inspires the confidence that our innermost self can be shared without fear of attack or emotional hurt and the confidence that we are understood in the deepest sense possible.

Intimacies are some of life's most intense experiences. Hence they have an enormous impact on your sense of vitality and well-being. When an intimate relationship is flowing smoothly, it can produce a richness of emotional satisfaction unparalleled by any other experience. Those who are involved in genuinely supportive and caring relationships tend to feel unswervingly confident about the seeming infinite potential of life to be harmonious and beautiful. On the other hand, when an intimate relationship is not going well, the people involved can be overwhelmed by moroseness and are unable to think of anything but their misery. They can be angry, depressed, anxious, or distraught, sometimes to the point of being unable to function at work or at school.

A lack of intimacy in life can adversely affect physical health as well as emotions and feelings. Studies indicate that married people are in better physical health than divorced, separated, and widowed people (Verbrugge, 1979, 1983), possibly reflecting the detrimental effects of the stress of losing an intimate partner. The possible association of intimacy and physical health is suggested as well by the finding that recently widowed people suffer greater mortality during the first few months after the death of their spouse (Parkes, 1972). Apparently, these people do indeed die of a "broken heart" (Lynch, 1977). Such evidence demonstrates the substantial link between emotions and physical health that is so fundamental to the holistic health philosophy.

Recognizing the relationship between the degree of satisfaction with one's intimate life and personal health, we present in this chapter some ideas on the nature of intimate relationships and some thoughts on how to make them as rewarding and as meaningful as possible.

> The image of myself which I try to create in
> my own mind in order that I may love myself
> is very different from the image which I try
> to create in the minds of others in order
> that they may love me.
>
> **W. H. Auden**

What Intimacy Is

Many people mistakenly equate genuine intimacy with sexual intercourse. That happens because love and affection are feelings associated with intimacy, and in our culture there is much confusion about love and sex. But intimacy is a feeling, not an act. It is the *quality* of a relationship between two people — a shared experiencing of their personal lives. People who have an intimate relationship may or may not choose to express their closeness with sex.

Many kinds of intimacies are possible. There are intimacies between marital partners (the term marital partners in this context means people living in marriage-type relationships regardless of whether or not they are legally married), children and parents, members of a family, neighbors, close friends, and even co-workers. Each intimacy has its unique and distinctive quality depending on the people involved, on the extent to which their personal histories are similar, and on the facets of themselves they choose to share with each other.

Yet intimacies possess certain common characteristics. They are relationships of mutual consent. One person cannot be intimate with another unless both agree that that is what they want. Intimacies tend to grow deeper and richer over a period of time; intimates need to share meaningful experiences in order to establish genuine trust and caring. Intimacies also carry the feeling that the personalities of the intimates are interconnected in some complex way. This is not the same as the feeling of having their identities merge so they become "one," but rather that they feel both joined and separate at the same time in some spiritual way.

Pairing Intimacies

There is no question that for the majority of people the most intimate relationships in life are adult partnerships that involve feelings of love and affection, sex, and often the idea of permanence, which usually takes the form of marriage. These kinds of pairing intimacies are the ones to which people devote much time and energy.

Yet what we see around us appears to be an overwhelming number of intimate partnerships that do not last. Data from the National Center for Health Statistics indicate that one-third to one-half of all marriages end in divorce (see Figure 20-1). Of course, many unmarried couples, both homosexual and heterosexual, who "break up" after some time of going together or even living together are never included in official statistics.

Obviously, many people are not finding the emotional satisfaction they seek in marriage and marriage-like relationships. Why not? Of the many possible answers to this question, some of the most commonly offered are the loss of respect for institutions of all kinds, economic affluence, the easy availability of effective contraceptives, and the loss of religious values.

That the percentage of married people is now the highest in our country's history and that the

> We learn only from those whom we love.
>
> **Goethe**

great majority of previously married people remarry indicate that people still want to be involved in stable, intimate partnerships. It appears, however, that many have not learned how to carry on a successful pairing intimacy in these times when people are skeptical of the ideal of permanence, when sexual exclusivity is no longer valued by many, and when people no longer need to be married for economic or social reasons.

A great burden has been put on pairing intimacies at this time in the history of our culture. The marriage of preindustrial America was a partnership established primarily for the dual purposes of economic support and child-rearing. The romantic ideal we consider of paramount importance today

was not inconsequential then, but neither was it of fundamental importance. Large families were considered advantageous and included not only the principal couple and their children but also their brothers, sisters, and even parents.

Industrialization and the movement of masses of people to cities changed that lifestyle for many. As families moved to cities for economic reasons, it became advantageous to have fewer family members to share the wage-earner's pay. Moreover, urban life tended to isolate people from one another, with the consequence that greater demands were placed on the primary relationship to fulfill emotional and support needs that were formerly fulfilled by an extended family and members of the community. One

Figure 20-1

The rising U.S. divorce rate. This rate, measured as the number of divorces per 1000 married woman age 15 and older, has more than doubled in the past 20 years. (Data from *Statistical Abstracts of the United States,* 1984.)

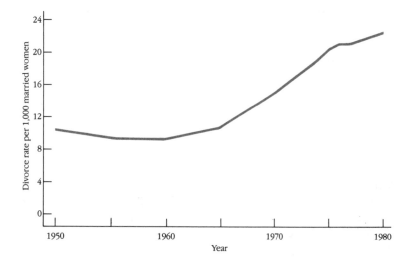

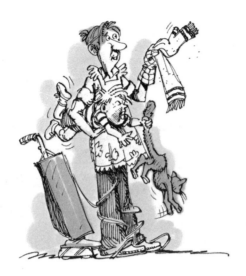

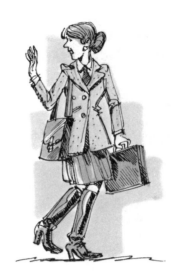

possible reason for high divorce rates is that marriages are now overburdened with too many expectations and demands to supply needed emotional fulfillment.

Today it has become common to expect that intimate relationships will fulfill almost all of a person's emotional needs. This is the message of most "family" television programs, it is the implicit agreement in traditional marriage vows, and it is accepted without much question as a condition of the "ideal relationship." It is possible, however, that intimate partnerships can suffer great harm if burdened with many expectations (Lederer and Jackson, 1968). It has been suggested that relationships flourish and continue when the partners free themselves of preconceived ideas about themselves and their relationship and let their intimacy grow in its own natural way (Rogers, 1972). Acceptance of the other person—as he or she actually *is*—is an essential ingredient of a successful relationship.

Unfortunately, too many people have expectations and ideas about how their intimate relationships *should be* and how their intimates *ought to act,* and they conduct themselves according to how closely their relationships conform to their ideal. If one partner behaves in a way that is not consistent with the other's ideal, then tensions and angers can arise and break up the intimate relationship. If the partners have very different fantasies of how their relationship should be, the stage is set for failure.

Here's a hypothetical example. Joan is a high school English teacher who is also an accomplished amateur tennis player. In addition to her teaching duties, she spends lots of time playing tennis. Joan and Jim (who works in an office) have been going together for a long time and recently decided to live together. What Joan doesn't know is that Jim believes that the woman he lives with should cook all the meals and clean house, just as his mother did. Jim isn't even aware that he may be asking Joan to do something she may not want to do. He merely thinks it's somehow natural—that this is the way intimates live together—and automatically *assumes* that Joan will see it that way, too.

However, Joan considers housework to be an infringement on her time for tennis, and furthermore, she considers it a bore, something that at best is only to be tolerated. She believes that both partners should share cooking and cleaning responsibilities equally. Because she often plays tennis in the evening and because Jim comes home directly from the office, she thinks it might be a good idea for him to prepare many of the meals or for them to eat out often; she'll take care of most of the housework on the weekends when she has more time.

One possible way for Joan and Jim to head off a potential problem is to share with each other, before they begin to live together, their ideas of how each thinks their intimacy is to be, in order to test how closely their fantasies will conform to reality.

Such discussion might include such subjects as cooking and housework, whether and when they might marry or have children, the role of sex in the relationship, economic and social goals, and the kinds of emotional needs they expect each other to fulfill. If their partnership is to survive, Jim and Joan will need to give up some of their views about how a partner "should" or "ought" to be and will

BOX 20-1

WAYS TO DEVELOP INTIMATE RELATIONSHIPS

Most people want their intimate relationships to develop feelings of closeness, positive regard, warmth, and familiarity with the other's innermost thoughts and feelings. This deep knowledge of each other comes from sharing the most important and often secret aspects of one's personality—one's goals, aspirations, strengths, weaknesses, and physical and sexual desires. The sharing of such private information is called **self-disclosure.**

When two people first become attracted to each other, it is highly unlikely that they immediately feel the trust, empathy, and closeness characteristic of intimacy. Most newly formed relationships can be described as superficial, in the sense that little knowledge of the person's "true self" is revealed. As the psychologist Sidney Jourard (1971) points out: "We conceal and camouflage our true being before others to foster a sense of safety, to protect ourselves against unwanted or expected criticism, hurt, or rejection."

When relationships begin, little intimate information is usually disclosed. People talk about the weather, the stock market, or politics. They gossip about professors, students, or other people they know. And they ask each other the classic leading questions: Where are you from? What do you do? What's your major? People face these questions so many times that they become adept at revealing as much or as little about themselves as feels comfortable. It is when they begin to talk about their personal history, current life problems, hopes and aspirations, and fears and personal failures that they begin to disclose important information—important because to disclose it makes them feel vulnerable. Most people discuss their deepest feelings only with those in whom they have developed considerable trust.

Intimacy develops through a progressive, mutual revealing of innermost thoughts. Psychologists Irwin Altman and Dalmas Taylor (1973) compare people's personalities to onions—having many layers

from an outer surface to an inner core. As acquaintances gain more and more knowledge about each other, they penetrate deeper and deeper through the layers of the other's personality, which establishes their intimacy. Another view compares intimate development to the peeling of an artichoke. Resistances and barriers to sharing information about oneself are like the leaves of the artichoke; as intimacy progresses, intimates peel away the leaves to get to the other's "heart."

Self-disclosure leads to the development of intimacy in two ways. First, you tend to be affected either positively or negatively by the information that is disclosed. If you make a positive judgment, you are likely to want to continue interacting with that person, for you believe that future interactions will be equally positive, and perhaps even more so. The same logic applies to negative assessments. If your reaction to what is disclosed is unfavorable, you are likely to terminate the relationship, or perhaps maintain it on a lesser level of intimacy.

The second way that self-disclosure leads to intimacy is the *act* of self-disclosure, regardless of the information offered, often leads to reciprocal self-disclosure by the other. By sharing important information, you communicate that you trust the other person, and usually that person accepts your trust and becomes more willing to disclose information to you. In this way intimacy progresses by a cycle of self-disclosure leading to trust, which brings about self-disclosure, which leads to more trust, and so on.

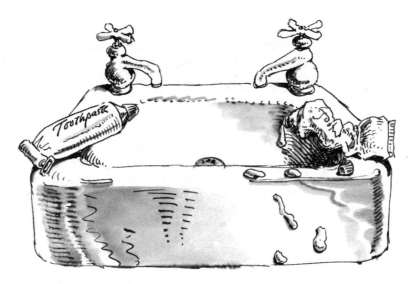

need to be open to doing things in new ways. This is particularly true of ideas about what men are supposed to do in relationships and what women are supposed to do. In our culture, a sex role stereotype has persisted for many years that, in its most simplified form, specifies that men work outside the home for a wage and women work inside the home without pay and that men be concerned about economic and public affairs and women be concerned with children and housework.

Where do people get their ideas about how to carry on an intimate relationship? One strong influence is the example set by parents or others in intimate relationships. People also learn about pairing from religious training, television, books, and movies. In each instance, people are applying rules and suggestions invented by others to their own relationships.

Accepting a model of how to act in a relationship is not necessarily bad. It may be that the model a person chooses to emulate is one that is exceptionally well suited to his or her personality. Problems arise, however, when people accept models, rules, expectations, and roles thrust upon them by parents, church, school, society, or even the intimate partner. In this circumstance, the person runs the risk of sooner or later feeling stifled by the role and of feeling angry at having to fulfill a list of expectations that he or she has not freely chosen.

A useful concept to keep in mind is that of "letting go." Very often when one sets up an imaginary plan of how a relationship is supposed to be, energy gets directed into making the partner try to fulfill the expectations and criteria assigned to the role of "intimate" in the plan. Thus, one cries, shouts, seduces, bribes, cajoles, and argues, trying to manipulate the partner to conform to a prescribed role or to "change." Usually the role is an unspoken one and certainly not one that has been discussed and agreed on.

It is much better idea for intimates to let each other be the person he or she feels comfortable being, rather than a stereotype of the "ideal partner." After all, this is the person who was originally found attractive, so why try to change him or her into someone else with a different set of personality characteristics? Love is "letting go" — allowing the partner to develop his or her personality in ways that he or she deems best. People are not objects, pets, or possessions, and in truth they cannot be manipulated to conform to your wishes. Although you might influence your intimates to behave in certain ways, if such behavior is not "natural" for them, they may some day rebel and leave the relationship.

The idea of conducting intimate relationships without preconceived expectations does not mean that the best relationships have no rules to guide them. Few relationships can be conducted without some rules governing the partners' behavior. The issue is not total freedom versus restricted behavior but rather how the rules governing the relationship are established. This means that presupposed expectations about behavior should be held to a minimum and that intimates should agree on the rules by which they are going to conduct their relationship. When disagreements arise, they should be settled by negotiation, by compromise, and by understanding of the partner's needs. If irreconcilable conflicts and

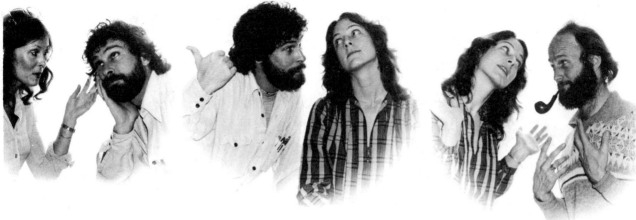

Communication is a mutual understanding of a message passed between people.

disagreements arise, perhaps the goals of the intimacy need to be examined and possibly changed. These ideas are summarized in a poetic way in family therapist Virginia Satir's list of "The Five Freedoms," reproduced below.

For many of us, the love and understanding we want from our intimate relationships is so important that the suggestion that we not try to control them in accordance with some notion of the "ideal relationship" may be difficult to accept. To let go in a situation that is very meaningful seems paradoxical. But the collective wisdom of many psychologists and counselors suggests just that. Apparently, love, like a beautiful flower, thrives when given freedom to grow.

The Five Freedoms

1 To see and hear
what is here
Instead of what should be,
was, or will be.

2 To say
what one feels and thinks
Instead of what one ought.

3 To feel
what one feels
Instead of what one ought.

4 To ask
for what one wants
Instead of always
wanting permission.

5 To take risks
in one's own behalf
Instead of choosing to
be only "secure"
and not rocking the boat.

Virginia Satir

Anger and Fighting Fair

For many the idea of being angry and fighting verbally with an intimate is unthinkable. It seems not to make sense. How can you be angry with someone you love?

Although it may not seem logical to feel anger for a loved one, it does, in fact, often happen. When people are involved in intense relationships and share intimacies, they may find many situations that displease them and make them angry. This may be especially true of people who live together, because ways of common day-to-day living may differ greatly and create tensions and disagreements.

There are situations when anger is highly appropriate. One such situation occurs when an intimate (or anyone) is doing something self-destructive, in which case your anger is justified because you love that person and don't want him or her to suffer or to be hurt. Anger is also appropriate when someone is hurting you. You have a right to stick up for yourself, a duty actually, for that is necessary to be honest and truly intimate in relationships. In fact, you have an obligation to your intimates to tell them when they hurt you—and angrily if that's how you feel—for presumably they love you and are not hurting you intentionally. By telling them "ouch, that hurt!" you give them important information about you, and presumably they will be more solicitous in the future.

Anger can also communicate to an intimate that you care a lot about him or her and that you want to improve things between you. Not being angry can

> Love is a great exaggeration of the worth of one
> individual over the worth of everybody else.
> George Bernard Shaw

communicate indifference, like saying, "This relationship means so little to me it's hardly worth getting worked up over." Suggestions for expressing anger constructively are presented in Box 20-2.

Feeling anger toward an intimate occasionally happens. Rather than feeling guilty or repressing that anger, it is usually better to express it at a suitable time and in an appropriate manner. Such expressions often enhance relationships as they "clear the air" and allow the partners to feel closer.

Threads of Permanence

Most people would like to establish and maintain a joyous, lasting intimacy. Psychologist Carl Rogers (1972), who has worked with couples for many, many years, has summarized his thoughts about achieving meaningful intimacies in terms of four important aspects of any lasting partnership: dedication, communication, dissolution of roles, and becoming a separate self. These are what Rogers calls "threads of permanence."

One of Rogers' fundamental ideas is that once a good relationship is established, it is imperative that the partners *pay attention to it*. An intimate relationship is a growing entity and must be cared for and tended like anything else that grows. In a true intimacy, static roles are dissolved and the people involved give energy to the *process* of their relationship virtually every day.

Rogers also points out that the word "communication" is frequently overused and misunderstood. Most would agree that communication—a mutual

understanding of a message passed between people—is a fundamental aspect of any relationship. When you are communicating, you are both a sender and a receiver. Suggestions for being a good listener are presented in Box 20-3. When you are a sender, it is best to attempt to be as clear as possible about how you are thinking and feeling. It is important to be as sure as you can that whatever you are hoping to communicate to another, either verbally or nonverbally, is an accurate representation of what you want to get across.

There are two steps to that process. The first is to be clear in your own mind about how you feel, and second, to be as adept and sincere as possible at putting your message across. It's also a good idea to solicit feedback from the other person about what he or she heard you say, so that you can judge whether your message was received and understood correctly.

If the message you put out isn't received, either you didn't say what you meant accurately or clearly or the person to whom you're communicating cannot understand your intended meaning because he or she may not be psychologically prepared to accept your point of view. People sometimes listen to, but do not really understand, an attempted communication. Unfortunately, there is little you can do about that. In communication, the best you can do is to be clear about what you say. If your partner chooses not to hear you, that isn't your fault.

How do you get clear about what you want to communicate? The best way is to honestly get in touch with your true inner feelings. When you're aware of the truth inside yourself, you'll experience

BOX 20-2

EXPRESSING ANGER CONSTRUCTIVELY

Disagreements and conflicts are inevitable in any close relationship. The notion that intimates shouldn't have to fight because love makes them see eye-to-eye on everything and the idea that you can't possibly be angry with someone you love are romantic myths. By expressing anger constructively, intimates are fighting for the success of their relationship as well as for their individual needs.

In constructive fighting, there should be no "winner" and no "loser." Fights are efforts of individuals to be heard and to improve the relationship. The best fights occur when the people involved feel that they have gained something.

Here are some suggestions for expressing anger constructively:

1. Try not to let anger and resentment build up over time. Express feelings when you become aware of them.

2. Agree on a time, a place, and the content for fights. It is certainly acceptable to get mad spontaneously if that is how you feel, but it is better to set aside a specific time for the resolution of an issue rather than trying to deal with it when you or your partner may not be psychologically or physically ready to argue. Try not to fight at random times. Try not to ambush someone by attacking with anger when it is least expected. Be sure that the person you are angry with knows what the issue is before the fight.

3. Be specific about what you are angry about and stick to the issue. Don't bring up old hurts. Try not to discuss second and third topics, especially as a means of retaliation.

4. Attack the problem, not each other. Don't take the opportunity to denigrate another's personal qualities. Use "I" statements to communicate resentments. "I" statements tell how you feel. "You" statements are often received as personal attacks. For example, say "It burns me up when you're late. If you can't make it on time, phone and let me know." Don't say, "You're inconsiderate as hell!"

5. Try to resolve the issue with an air of compromise and respect. Try to understand the other's point of view.

6. Know when it is time to stop. Sometimes you can sense that the argument isn't getting resolved. It is OK to acknowledge that and to take a few hours or days to reconsider things and to discuss the issue again. Sometimes emotions are too high and it is not possible to think clearly. That may be a time to stop the fight until tempers cool.

7. Engaging in sex or any other affectionate behavior before an issue is resolved should not be taken as a sign that everything is forgotten. Such behavior shows that the fight fits into the healthy construct of the relationship.

8. Don't hold grudges.

a feeling of solidity and clarity — an internal ring of truth — and if you act on that feeling you're being straight with your partner.

Very often people say things that they think other people want to hear. That's particularly true of intimates. We tell them what we think they want to hear because we think it will make them feel better or be nicer to us. Or, we tell them lies because we want to hide something ugly from them for fear they will stop liking us. Neither is a good idea.

If you tell your partner something that is untrue or dishonest, deep inside that person is likely to know, and he or she may come to distrust your statements and may even come to dislike you. And if you try to protect your partner by not saying how you really feel, you may become increasingly angry and hostile, since the ugly issue you don't want to talk about remains inside you, like a sore that doesn't heal. It is generally better to tell the truth about how you are presently feeling, not necessarily in anger, but always openly and honestly.

That means you have to know something about your true self and also how to accept and appreciate yourself just as you are — even with your faults and doubts and weaknesses. These are all part of being human — of becoming yourself. Self-acceptance is the first step to self-love, the prerequisite of rewarding intimacy.

BOX 20-3

EFFECTIVE LISTENING

Effective communication is what holds close relationships together and enables them (and the people involved) to grow. Many people forget that communication requires both sending *and* receiving—both talking *and* listening. Here are some ideas to help you become a more effective listener.

Give the Sender Your Full Attention

1. Don't fake it. If you can't pay attention because you are tired, hungry, distracted, angry, or whatever, tell the sender how you're feeling and whether it's OK to have the talk at another time. The sender is likely to grant your request if time is not at issue because he or she certainly wants your full attention.

2. Make eye contact. Try to assume similar postures (both of you sitting or both standing) to create a sense of equal status.

3. Just listen. Don't interrupt until you have a signal that the sender is finished or until the sender has asked for a response—unless, of course, you don't understand at all what is being communicated. You can acknowledge that you are actively listening with gestures, nods, and vocalizations such as "Uh-huh," "Yes," and "Go on."

4. Be empathic. Try to "hear" the sender's feelings as well as the words. Be open to receiving the sender's intentions and motivations as well as his or her ideas.

5. Be receptive. Be an open channel for receiving the message. Don't judge or evaluate the sender or the message while the sender is talking. Try not to correct the sender or to defend yourself. Communication is more effective when you understand how the sender thinks and feels about things.

Give Feedback

1. Don't mind-read. Acknowledge that the message has been received and understood or not understood. Ask for clarification if there's something you're not sure about.

2. Paraphrase the message. Repeat the message in your own words ("What I hear you saying is . . . ") so the sender knows that you are getting what is being communicated.

3. Acknowledge feelings. Ask about the sender's feelings if you're unsure: "It seems to me that you're angry. Do I have that right?"

Be Supportive

1. Praise the effort. Acknowledge the sender's efforts for investing the time, energy, and caring to communicate with you. Support the sender's efforts at communicating any difficult thoughts and feelings.

2. Be unconditional. Let the sender know that you think that he or she is respected and liked even if you are uncomfortable with the messages that are being communicated. Assure the sender that you will not become defensive or rejecting or leave the relationship. Indicate that you are willing to negotiate problems and that you are committed to work through difficult feelings.

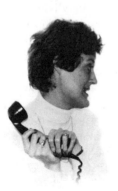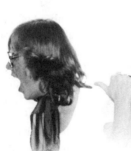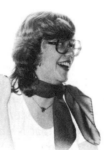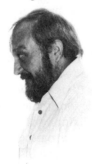

> Language has created the word *loneliness* to express the pain of being alone, and the word *solitude* to express the glory of being alone.
> **Paul Tillich**

Loneliness

Loneliness is a common and pervasive human experience. At some time or another, just about everyone feels the desperation, hopelessness, desolation, emptiness, and nonbelonging that characterize loneliness.

Loneliness is the result of the emotional isolation that comes from lack of intimate ties with a spouse or lover or the social isolation that occurs with lack of a network of close relationships with peers, fellow-workers, and friends (Weiss, 1973). Loneliness is not the same as being alone. People who are surrounded by others virtually all day and all night may often feel lonely, whereas individuals who live and work in solitude may feel lonely infrequently. The distinguishing feature of loneliness is not the quantity of interpersonal interactions but how closely one's relationships match one's needs and expectations for intimacy.

Because our society accords high status to the married (or at least the "paired"), single people can feel worthless and lonely. Unfortunately, marriage is not an absolute haven against loneliness. In fact, the severest feelings of loneliness can be felt in marriage. The reason: people often expect marriage to provide abundant love, understanding, communication, and fulfillment. Sometimes, however, intimate relationships are not blissfully fulfilling, and there

Loneliness can be experienced at any age, but the elderly, who may have outlived family, friends, and job, are particularly susceptible. (Jackie Estrada.)

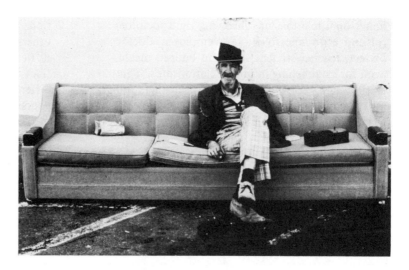

> Honest, open communication—however
> combative—is essential in every
> successful relationship.
>
> **Abigail Van Buren**
> *Dear Abby*

can be problems, tension, and anger that seemingly build a stone wall between partners. This mismatch between the expectation of intimacy and the reality of emotional separation from a loved one can lead to feelings of despair and isolation.

Emotional isolation from the lack of intimate ties with a lover or spouse is not the only cause of loneliness. Ours is a highly mobile society, and this contributes to the prevalence of loneliness (Gordon, 1976). Frequent changes of job or residence (the Postal Service reports that nearly 50 million Americans move each year and that the average number of lifetime relocations is 14) make social networks fragile. People are continually saying good-bye to old friends and having to establish close relationships with new ones.

Another contributor to loneliness is that modern mass society is structured on a variety of impersonal relationships involving rigid sociological and economic roles—boss/employee, doctor/patient, teacher/student—with no built-in mechanism for establishing intimate relationships. Thus, even though people may interact with others during the course of a day, these interactions are often characterized by indifference, superficiality, and expected role behavior.

Some suggestions for dealing with loneliness are:

1. Understand that loneliness has many possible causes, some of which are social and others of which are personal. Try to determine the particular causes of your loneliness. Ask yourself whether you are to blame or whether your loneliness is caused by some situation in your environment. Be certain not to overemphasize personal factors and underestimate social conditions.

2. Avoid thinking negatively about yourself. Telling yourself that you are ugly, stupid, or worthless only leads to social isolation. It is better to like and accept yourself; that often leads to others liking and accepting you.

3. Try to effect a change. Some social conditions may be more difficult to change than others. For example, it may be more difficult to leave a relationship or marriage than to find a new job or transfer to a different school. You can set new goals for yourself that are more attainable in the immediate future rather than trying to accomplish only long-range plans.

BOX 20-4

SHARING YOUR INNERMOST FEELINGS

Sharing your innermost feelings with the people you love is the basis of true intimacy. That is the way to establish trust, understanding, and commitment.

To help individuals improve their ability to share deep feelings with their intimate partners, counselors Philip and Lorna Sarrel (1978) offer these suggestions:

1. *Try not to avoid talking about your feelings.* Many people censor their feelings. Some people do this because they do not believe they should burden their partner with negative feelings such as sadness, anger, fear, or loneliness. To withhold your true feelings deprives your partner of a significant part of you. Think of your feelings as facts that your partner needs in order to participate fully in the relationship. Withholding that information deprives the relationship of much of what it needs to grow and thrive. In some relationships, one partner assumes that the other is not interested in his or her feelings. It's always best to verify such assumptions with a simple discussion at a time when interest in feelings is the principal subject. Such a discussion should not be used as a prelude to a discussion of the feelings themselves. If one partner wants to share inner feelings and the other does not want to hear about them, some compromise must be reached if the relationship is to continue harmoniously.

2. *Try to tell your partner when your feelings have been hurt.* When you do not tell your partner that your feelings have been hurt you are not giving him or her vital feedback about how you truly feel. How is he or she to know you are hurt unless you say "ouch"?

3. *Try to assert your own rights and feelings in an argument with your partner.* Disagreement is natural in close relationships. And when it occurs, the partners can use it to discover more about each other and to become closer. The best way to assert yourself in disagreements is with "I" statements such as "I feel such and such" or "I think that . . . " Avoid using "You always . . . " or "You never . . . " Accusing your partner only puts him or her on the defensive, which stops productive negotiation and resolution of the problem.

4. *Try to take responsibility for your weaknesses and failures.* Everyone has weaknesses and failures. And it is natural to want to make the best impression on your partner and not burden him or her with your troubles. But intimacy means sharing all facets of yourself, both the good and the not so good.

5. *Try to find ways to work out problems together.* Working out problems is a matter of negotiating. Some couples erroneously believe that their closeness and affection for each other means that they will automatically see things identically and have identical preferences. But couples are composed of separate individuals and individuals have different preferences. Most of the time, one person feels less strongly about an alternative, and so it is easier for that person to give in. If each feels equally strong about different alternatives, then one partner may get the choice this time and the other partner chooses next time. If possible, do both.

Supplemental Readings

Bach, George, and **Wyden, Peter.** *The Intimate Enemy.* New York: Wm. Morrow, 1969. Describes the principles and practice of expressing anger and fighting fair with intimate partners.

Gottman, J.; Notarius, C.; Gonso, J.; and **Markman, H.** *A Couple's Guide to Communication.* Champaign, Ill: Research Press, 1976. An excellent how-to book on understanding and improving communication in close relationships.

Lederer, W. J., and **Jackson, Don.** *The Mirages of Marriage.* New York: W. W. Norton, 1968. A discussion of how preconceived expectations about marriage can lead to difficulties between partners.

Miller, S.; Wackman, D.; Nunnally, E.; and **Saline, C.** *Straight Talk.* New York: New American Library, 1982. An excellent guide to improving communication and achieving harmony in close relationships.

Rogers, Carl. *Becoming Partners.* New York: Delacorte, 1972. A renowned psychologist's perceptions about various kinds of partnerships and his suggestions on how to make them successful.

Scarf, Maggie. *Intimate Partners.* New York: Random House, 1987.

Summary

Because everyone needs the feelings of understanding and closeness that intimate relationships bring, people are involved in various kinds of intimate relationships throughout their lives. Although people are involved in parent-child intimacies and close relationships between friends and co-workers, the most intense intimacies are those between adults that often have some kind of permanency as a goal.

Many psychologists suggest that one possible step to forming lasting intimate relationships is for the intimate partners to free themselves of preconceived ideas about how their relationship should proceed. How you behave in intimate relationships and how you expect your partner to behave is influenced by parents, TV, books, movies, and religious training. Sometimes the models suggested by these examples are not totally suitable for your particular individual personalities, and trying to live by them becomes difficult. Moreover, you may not make your partner aware of the principles that guide your intimate behavior, and conflicts may arise because mutually agreed-on goals are not established.

In addition to being free of preconceived expectations about how intimates should act, other features of lasting intimate relationships include being able to express anger at an appropriate time and in a suitable manner, not taking the relationship for granted, and being open in honestly expressing inner feelings.

Loneliness is the empty feeling that comes from the mismatch between one's needs and expectations for intimacy and the nature of one's close relationships. Lifestyle changes and changes in expectations can often reduce feelings of loneliness.

FOR YOUR HEALTH

What You Need from Intimate Relationships

What are the needs you expect to have fulfilled in your intimate relationships? Choose the three most important needs from the list below. If you are involved in an intimate relationship, suggest that your partner choose three items from the needs list. Compare your responses and then discuss them.

I want someone to:

Love me.

Confide in me.

Show me affection.

Respect my ideals.

Appreciate what I wish to achieve.

Understand my moods.

Help me make important decisions.

Stimulate my ambition.

Look up to.

Give me self-confidence.

Stand by me in difficulty.

Appreciate me just as I am.

Admire my ability.

Make me feel that I count for something.

Relieve my loneliness.

Support me and our children.

Accept my need to be self-sufficient and independent.

Reap What You Sow

Verbally expressing love and affection can sometimes be difficult, for it demonstrates a certain degree of commitment and exposes some of your innermost feelings. Nevertheless, telling others what you feel about them can make you feel good. Devote some effort to telling the important people in your life how much you appreciate them. Certainly tell your intimates that you love them, but also tell your friends and co-workers how much you like and respect them.

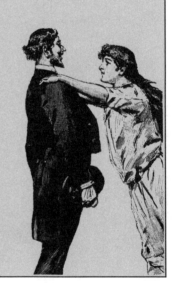

CHAPTER TWENTY-ONE

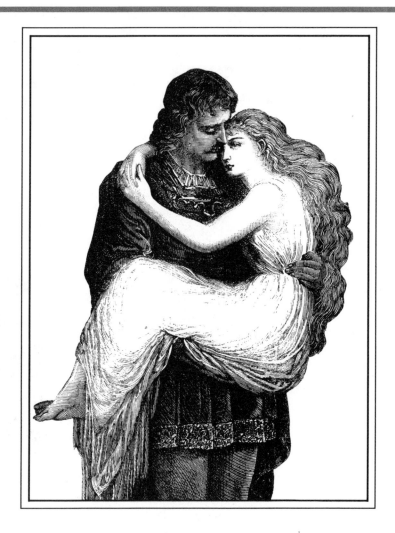

Sexual knowledge makes better
partners and parents

Human Sexuality

Sexuality represents a truly holistic aspect of living, for it involves the simultaneous expression of mind and body—the whole self. Although it is common to find sexuality represented publicly in advertising and other media as having to do solely with physical gratification, most people are aware that sexuality involves much more than the stimulation of the body's sex organs. Sexuality involves feelings and emotions, too. Sexuality is also a powerful form of communication between people.

From the standpoint of personal health, sexuality offers an area of life over which you have considerable individual control. You choose when and with whom you wish to be sexual, and which feelings you wish to express in sexual ways. With some fundamental knowledge of sexual biology, you can conduct your sexual life responsibly, thus avoiding unnecessary illness and exercising a choice of whether and when to have children. This chapter introduces the topic of sexuality and discusses the nature of the sexual self and of sexual expression.

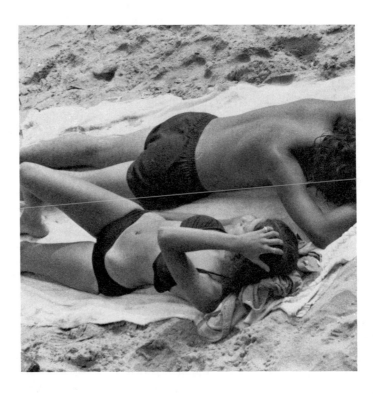

> Some things
> are better than sex,
> and some things are worse,
> but there's nothing exactly
> like it.
>
> **W. C. Fields**

Sexual Values and Decisions

Our culture has traditionally been rather conservative in regard to sexual behavior, with both laws and cultural norms prohibiting nearly all forms of sexual activity except sexual intercourse between legally married heterosexual adults. But many of our culture's traditional sexual values, expectations, and behaviors are becoming less restrictive. For example, in recent years the public has become increasingly tolerant of the showing of sexual activity in feature films. Television, which was once a medium of ridiculous prudery, has become one of society's major purveyors of sex, as characters openly ask each other for sex, carry on (usually complicated and illicit) sexual affairs, and occasionally appear on the screen half-dressed in preparation for sex. It is rare to find a popular magazine that does not contain a story about improving your love life or sex life. One need only observe how much sex is used in advertising to see how tolerant of sex our society has become.

In spite of this bombardment of sexual inducements, many people are reluctant to accept a totally open, laissez-faire attitude about sex. They ask such questions as: With whom do I make love? What does it mean to have sexual relations? What will it mean to my partner if I have sex with someone else? Which kinds of relationships and feelings make sexual relations appropriate and which do not? All these questions require answers before people can be totally comfortable with sharing themselves sexually with another.

In the moral climate of a generation or two ago, a set of socially approved standards for sexual behavior that would help people answer these questions was available. People were rarely confused about what constituted acceptable sexual behavior, even if they did not always follow those dictates. Today, however, people have few clear, socially approved guidelines for sexual behavior; therefore, they must adopt a personal set of values that is appropriate for them. Some people believe that nonmarital sexual interaction is wrong. Others believe that there may be times when sex is morally acceptable outside of marriage, but they face the task of defining the appropriate circumstances.

One possible guideline for sexual behavior is mutual consent. If both partners agree that sex is all right, then presumably such behavior is appropriate. This may not always be the case, however. Many people without regular sex partners complain that they constantly feel socially pressured to seek out and engage in sexual activity, and feel pressures in social situations not to say no to sex, lest they be thought prudish. The set of social values that pressure people to say yes to sex when they don't want to is just as tyrannical as the formerly traditional sexual values that pressure people to say no to sex when they did desire it.

Another possible guideline for appropriate sexual behavior is to determine whether sex actually fulfills your personal needs (see Table 21-1). Sometimes you may feel a need to be physically close but do not necessarily want to be sexual. Sometimes you may just feel like being held. However, the pressures to say yes to sex may prevent you from engaging in relationships that are appropriate in fulfilling your needs. Many women are aware of the difference between wanting sex and wanting simply to be held,

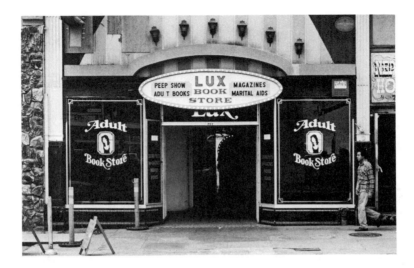

cuddled, or nurtured. Unfortunately, many men are not as aware of their own needs. Because of the stereotypic sex-role image of the man as being in control of his feelings and being the sexual aggressor, many men learn to interpret all of their feelings for love, affection, and closeness in terms of sex (Zilbergeld, 1978). Thus, many men seek emotional expression through sexual intercourse when, in fact, they might better fulfill their emotional needs by having their back rubbed or simply talking meaningfully with a trusted friend.

Although our culture lacks strict rules governing sexual behavior, personal guidelines for appropriate sexual behavior can nevertheless be established. First, you must determine whether sex is your goal or whether some other form of interpersonal behavior is perhaps more appropriate. If you and your partner agree that the proper goal is

Table 21-1
Reasons for Sex

Expressing love, affection, and emotional closeness
Curiosity and adventure
Release of sexual tension
Release of nonsexual anxiety and frustrations
Relieving boredom
Recreation and fun
Duty
Giving and/or receiving comfort and affirmation
Proving one's sexual prowess
Proving one's femininity or masculinity
Enhancing one's social standing or popularity
Desire to feel powerful or exploitive
To mend emotional wounds

sex, you must be fair to each other; you must not exploit each other, and you should ensure that no harmful physical and emotional consequences will result from your mutual decision.

Sexual Biology

In the most fundamental way, your sexuality is defined by your sexual biology, for the primary role of sex for humans, as with other animals, is the continued reproduction of the species. The biological role of the male is to produce reproductively capable **sperm** and to deposit them in the female reproductive tract during sexual intercourse. The biological role of the female is to provide reproductively capable eggs, called **ova,** and to provide a safe, nutrient-filled environment for the embryo to develop in until the infant is born. This she accomplishes by nourishing the developing fetus in her uterus for the nine months of pregnancy.

You have either male or female organs of sexuality and reproduction because at the time of conception you received sex-determining chromosomes from your parents. Your mother contributed an X sex-determining chromosome and your father contributed either an X or a Y sex-determining chromosome. Those who received an XX pair of chromosomes became females, and those who received an XY pair became males.

Once the chromosome pattern is set, the embryonic development of the sexual anatomy follows from the precise instructions of the genes contained in the chromosomes. The particular chromosome set determines whether the as-yet-immature sex cells

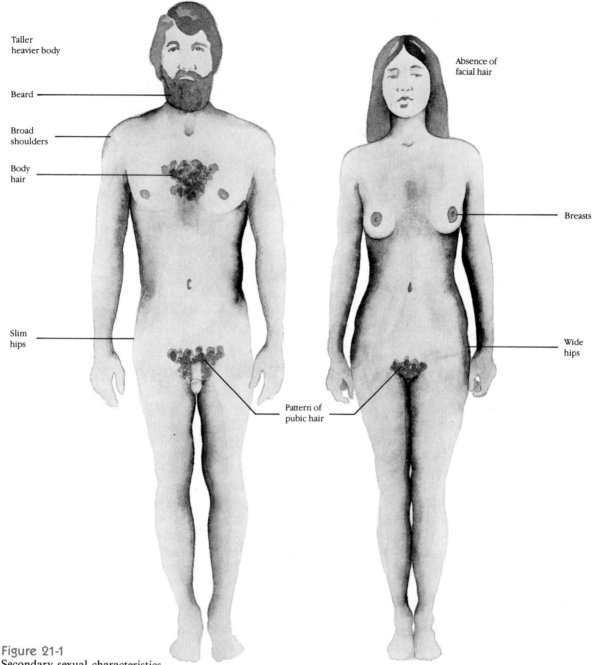

Taller
heavier body

Beard

Broad
shoulders

Body
hair

Slim
hips

Absence of
facial hair

Breasts

Wide
hips

Pattern of
pubic hair

Figure 21-1
Secondary sexual characteristics
of men and women.

that appear at about the fifth week of development will eventually produce sperm or ova. The sex chromosomes determine whether the fetus will ultimately develop the male sexual organs—testes, sperm ducts, semen-producing glands, and a penis—or the female organs—ovaries, fallopian tubes, uterus, vagina, and external female genitals.

The genetic determination of sexual anatomy also specifies the pattern of male or female steroid hormone production, which in turn affects the **secondary sex characteristics** that distinguish adult males and females: the extent and distribution of facial and body hair; body build and stature; and appearance of breasts (see Figure 21-1).

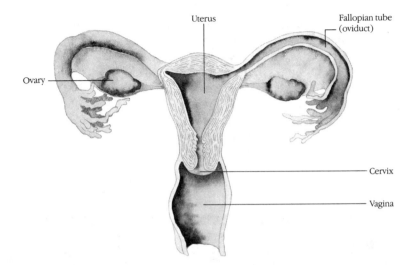

Figure 21-2
The female sexual and reproductive
system.

Female Sexual Anatomy

A woman's internal sexual organs consist of two
ovaries, which lie on either side of the abdominal
cavity, the **fallopian tubes,** the **uterus,** and the **vagina;** together these structures make up a specialized tube that goes from each ovary to the outside
of the body (see Figure 21-2). The function of the
ovaries is to produce fertilizable ova and sex hormones, which control the development of the female
body type, maintain normal female sexual physiology, and help maintain the course of a normal pregnancy. The fallopian tubes gather and transport ova
that are released from the ovaries (about one each
month). The two fallopian tubes connect to the
uterus, an organ about the size of a woman's fist,
which is situated just behind the pelvic bone and
the bladder (see Figure 21-3). The uterus is part of
the passageway for sperm as they move from the vagina to the fallopian tubes to effect fertilization;
after fertilization, it provides the environment in
which the fetus grows. It is the inner lining of the
uterus that is shed each month in menstruation (see
Chapter 23).

The lower part of the uterus is called the **cervix,** which means "neck," and the cavity of the
uterus is connected to the vagina by means of a small
opening called the cervical os. The cervix secretes
mucus, which changes in consistency depending on
the phase of the menstrual cycle. Some women learn
to estimate the time of **ovulation** (ovum release) by
examining their cervical mucus, thus providing a

method of contraception that does not involve pills
or any of the various mechanical contraceptive
devices.

The vagina is a hollow tube that leads from the
cervix to the outside of the body. Normally, the vaginal tube is rather narrow, but it can readily widen
to accommodate the penis during intercourse, a tam-
pon during menstruation, the passage of a baby during childbirth, or a pelvic examination. The vagina
possesses a unique physiology that is maintained by
the secretions that continually emanate from the
vaginal walls. These secretions help control the
growth of microorganisms that normally inhabit the
vagina, and they also help to cleanse the vagina. Be-

Figure 21-3
A side view of the female reproductive and sexual
organs.

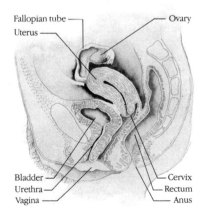

cause the vagina is a self-cleansing organ, it is usually unnecessary to employ any extraordinary cleansing measures, such as douching. Very often douching merely upsets the natural chemical balance of the vagina and increases the risk of developing vaginal infections, called **vaginitis** (see Box 21-1).

A woman's external genitals (see Figure 21-4) consist of two pairs of fleshy folds that surround the opening of the vagina, and the **clitoris.** The smaller, inner pair of folds are called the **labia minora,** and the larger, outer pair are called the **labia majora.** The clitoris, a highly sensitive sexual organ, is situated above the vaginal opening.

The opening of the **urethra,** which is the exit tube for urine, is located at the vaginal region just below the clitoris. The fact that the urethra is only about ½ inch long and located so close to the vagina makes it susceptible to irritation and infection,

---

BOX 21-1

VAGINAL INFECTIONS (VAGINITIS)

Vaginitis is any irritation or inflammation of the vagina. Because one of the most common causes of vaginitis is infestation with the yeast *Candida albicans,* vaginitis is often referred to as a yeast infection. Other types of vaginitis are the result of infection with either *Trichomonas vaginalis,* a protozoan, or the bacterium *Hemophilus vaginalis,* or *Gardnerella vaginalis* as it is now called.

Regardless of the particular organism involved, the symptoms of vaginitis are usually a burning sensation, annoying itching in the vaginal region, and discharge from the vagina. This discharge is not to be confused with the normal vaginal discharge, **leukorrhea,** which is composed of sloughed-off vaginal cells and cervical mucus. The discharge of vaginitis is usually gray, yellow, or greenish in color. It may resemble cottage cheese or it may be foamy, and it may have an unpleasant smell.

Normally, the vagina is populated by bacteria and other microorganisms, including yeast. The relative proportion of these organisms is kept in check by the competition between them for nutrients and a suitable place to live. If something upsets the inter-

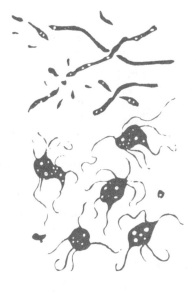

nal environment of the vagina, however, one or another of the organisms can take advantage of the change, their population can increase, and vaginitis results. Many factors can upset the vaginal environment and predispose a woman to vaginitis. Among them are antibiotics, which kill many of the bacteria in the vagina and therefore provide yeast and "Trich" a chance to thrive; pregnancy and birth control pills, which change the internal chemical composition of the vagina;

tight clothing, hot and humid weather, and underwear made of synthetic fabrics, all of which increase the moisture in the vaginal region, thus improving the environment for the growth of microorganisms; obesity, diabetes, and other dietary metabolic problems; and having intercourse with someone carrying the infectious microorganisms.

Vaginitis can be treated by specific drugs after the infecting organism has been identified. Women can try to prevent vaginitis by:

1. Wearing cotton underpants or at least pants with a cotton crotch.
2. Avoiding tight undergarments, girdles, and pantyhose, especially when wearing tight jeans or pants.
3. Avoiding routine douching, feminine hygiene sprays, and bath products that contain chemicals that irritate the vagina.
4. Avoiding oral contraceptives if vaginitis is a persistent problem.
5. Wiping from front to back after urinating to prevent spreading bacteria from the rectum to the vagina.

> I find that the three major
> administrative problems on a campus
> are sex for the students, athletics for
> the alumni, and parking for
> the faculty.
>
> **Clark Kerr**
> **Former president of the University of California**

called **urethritis,** which is characterized by a burning sensation during urination and usually by a frequent urge to urinate. Occasionally, bacteria introduced into the urethra migrate the short distance to the bladder and produce a bladder infection called **cystitis.** The symptoms of cystitis are similar to those of urethritis.

The most frequent causes of urethritis and cystitis are irritation from sexual intercourse and the introduction of bacteria from the anal region into the vaginal region and into the urethra. To prevent

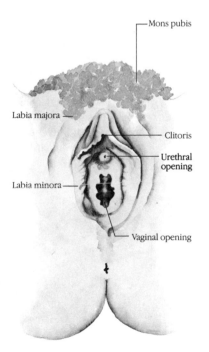

Figure 21-4
External female genitals.

Labels: Mons pubis, Labia majora, Clitoris, Urethral opening, Labia minora, Vaginal opening

urethritis and cystitis, it is recommended that care be taken not to introduce anal bacteria into the vaginal region during sexual activity (manually or with the penis), that a woman urinate immediately after having sex, that a woman wear absorbent cotton underpants or underpants with a cotton crotch, and that women wipe the urethra in the front-to-back direction after urinating.

If a woman develops a mild case of urethritis or cystitis, she can often eliminate the irritating bacteria by drinking a lot of fluids to wash the bacteria from the urinary tract and by trying to kill the bacteria by making the urine more acidic, either by taking high doses of vitamin C or by drinking acidic fruit juices. It is also advisable not to drink alcohol and ingest caffeine or spices, for these substances may irritate an already inflamed urinary tract. If pain is severe or if there is blood in the urine, a physician should be consulted.

A woman's secondary sex characteristics include the **breasts**—a network of milk glands and milk ducts embedded in fatty tissue. The variation in breast size among women is due to the differing amounts of fatty tissue within the breasts. There is little variation among women in the amount of milk-producing tissue; thus, a woman's ability to breast-feed is unrelated to the size of her breasts.

The breasts are supplied with numerous nerve endings, which are important in the delivery of milk to a nursing baby. These nerves also make the breast highly sensitive to touch, and many women find certain forms of tactile stimulation to be sexually pleasurable. Sexual arousal, tactile stimulation, and cold temperatures can cause small muscles in the nipples to contract, resulting in erection of the nipples.

BOX 21-2

A CONVERSATION WITH A WOMAN GYNECOLOGIST ABOUT THE GYNECOLOGICAL EXAM

Q: What is the purpose of the gynecological exam?

A: The gynecological exam, or GYN exam, is a whole-person exam for women. The GYN exam includes a pelvic exam, which gives information about a woman's internal health from an examination of her external anatomy. It also includes an examination of the breast, and frequently other parts of the body. The GYN exam can be reassuring that everything is normal or can help solve problems a woman may have, such as abnormal secretions, an infection, discomfort or problems with intercourse, diagnosis of pregnancy, and concerns about birth control.

Q: How often should a woman get a GYN exam?

A: It depends on the stage of a woman's life. A young woman may want a GYN exam to be sure she is capable of intercourse and having children, or to seek advice about expressing her sexuality. The next stage, other than for pregnancy or illness, is mid-30s and older. During this time the GYN exam should take place yearly to check for cervical cancer (done with a Pap smear), and the possibility of other problems. The next stage is premenopause. This is when a woman has to deal with physiological changes and possible emotional difficulties about sexuality and changes in life patterns.

Q: How can a woman best prepare herself for a GYN exam?

A: First, a woman should take the attitude that the exam is for her, and she should attempt to participate as much as possible. In the ideal case, the GYN exam is an opportunity for a woman to learn about her body. She can ask to feel what the examiner is feeling and also watch with a mirror. Before coming to the exam she should not douche or clean up any problem she has. The physician needs to see the full extent of the symptoms. She should bring with her a list of questions and concerns, the names of medications she is taking and how long she has been taking them, and the dates of past surgeries. If she uses a diaphragm, she should bring it to be sure it still fits and is OK. She should be an active patient, which means asking questions, and she should decide beforehand that her GYN exam will be a positive experience.

Q: What happens in a GYN exam?

A: First, there's a conversation to find out if there are any problems or concerns. Then the physician obtains the woman's medical history and her family medical history. After that, usually a brief physical exam, including listening to the heart, and recording of height, weight, and blood pressure. The breasts are checked, and the examiner will probably discuss the breast self-exam, too. The pelvic exam includes examination of the vagina to determine the nature of the vaginal secretions, and inspection of the vagina and cervix. Then there's a bimanual exam, in which the examiner feels the length of the vagina and the mobility of the cervix, and the shapes, sizes, textures of the woman's uterus, ovaries, and fallopian tubes. Several tests may be carried out, including a Pap smear, a urine test, and a blood test for iron deficiency. If a woman is anxious about the possibility of venereal disease or is pregnant or planning to get married, a test for gonorrhea may be done as well.

Q: What is a **Pap smear?**

A: A Pap smear is a screening test for cancer of the cervix. A few cells are taken from the surface of the cervix with a soft swab and observed for any abnormality. Precancer cellular changes can be detected and more serious trouble prevented. Most women probably ought to obtain Pap smears every year or two.

Q: What about self-exams?

A: Self-exams are better than no exams, but there are problems. For example, it is not easy to do a proper Pap smear yourself. Also, it's just easier for someone else to make all the necessary observations. When a woman reaches her thirties, she should examine her breasts every month for lumps or changes (described in Appendix B). If a woman has concerns about her sexuality, marital life, or problems with intercourse, a gynecologist can be a helpful counselor.

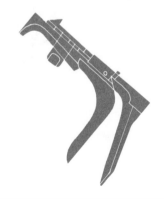

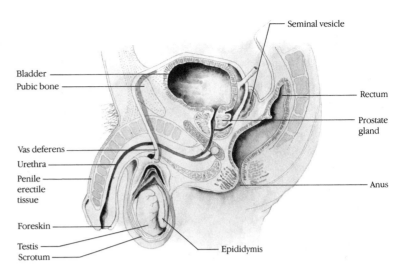

Figure 21-5
The male sexual and reproductive system.

Male Sexual Anatomy

The principal reproductive role of male sexual organs is to make numerous viable sperm cells and to deliver them into the female reproductive tract during sexual intercourse. The male sexual and reproductive system consists of two **testes,** the sites of sperm and sex hormone production; a series of connected sperm ducts that originate at the testes, course through the pelvis, and terminate at the urethra of the penis; glands that produce seminal fluid; and the **penis,** the organ of copulation (see Figure 21-5).

The testes are located in a flesh-covered sac, the **scrotum,** that hangs outside the man's body. In the embryo, the testes develop inside the body, but just before birth they descend into the scrotum. Inside the scrotum the testes are kept at a temperature a few degrees cooler than the internal body temperature, a condition that is apparently necessary for the production of reproductively capable sperm. One testis is usually a little higher than the other.

Sperm are deposited in the female reproductive system during sexual intercourse or copulation. At that time, the male and female reproductive tracts are joined and form an uninterrupted passageway for sperm to travel from the testes to the fallopian tubes, where fertilization of the ovum takes place. When a man ejaculates, sperm are propelled through the sperm ducts and out of the penis by contractions of the smooth muscles that line the ducts and the muscles of the pelvis, which contract during orgasm. As they make their way out of the male body,

the sperm mix with secretions of seminal fluid from the seminal vesicles, prostate gland, and Cowper's glands to form semen. The semen, which is the gelatinous milky fluid that is emitted at ejaculation, contains a mixture of about 300 million sperm cells and about 3 to 6 ml of seminal fluid. The seminal fluid contributes 95 percent or more of the entire volume of semen.

The penis is normally soft, but when a man becomes sexually aroused, its internal tissues fill with blood and the penis enlarges and becomes erect. All men are born with a fold of skin, the **foreskin,** that covers the end of the penis. For centuries, Jewish and Moslem families have surgically removed the foreskin from male children for religious reasons. Nowadays, **circumcision,** as this procedure is called, is often carried out routinely on newborn males regardless of religion. Although there is no clear medical indication that circumcision is beneficial, removal of the foreskin does eliminate the buildup of **smegma,** a white, cheesy substance that can accumulate under the foreskin. Although some scientists have suggested that smegma may contribute to the development of penile and cervical cancer in a few individuals, Edward Wallerstein (1980) points out that the scientific evidence does not support this point of view. The belief that circumcision leads to an increase in sexual arousal because it exposes the glans, and the related belief that circumcision produces an inability to delay ejaculation have been shown to be incorrect (Masters and Johnson, 1966). For most men, circumcision has no effect on sexual arousal and sexual activity.

There is no reason why physical
intimacy with men should always consist
of foreplay followed by intercourse and male
orgasm; and there is no reason why intercourse
must always be part of heterosexual sex. Sex
is intimate physical contact for pleasure.
There is never any reason to think
that the "goal" must
be intercourse.

Shere Hite

Gender Identity and Sex Role

Although anatomy and physiology provide the biological bases of human sexuality, most people's sexual experiences also involve beliefs, thoughts, feelings, and social behaviors. Even if a person knows little about his or her reproductive biology, he or she is aware of the socially approved behaviors for males and females. The awareness of being either a male or a female is called **gender identity,** and gender-specific behaviors are referred to as the **sex role.**

How individuals come to think and behave sexually is almost entirely a product of what they learn as children about the gender to which they belong and the kinds of behaviors that are expected of members of one sex or the other. Studies of psychosexual development indicate that the development of gender identity and the subsequent expression of sex-specific behaviors begins with the **sex typing** of newborn infants (Hampson and Hampson, 1961; Money and Ehrhardt, 1972). When a child is born, almost the first thing noticed is its biological sex as determined by the appearance of its external genitals. If the infant is born with a penis, virtually everyone attending the birth will exclaim "It's a boy!" Similarly "It's a girl!" follows the observation of a newborn's female external genitals.

Having been sex typed at birth, the infant is thereafter treated by adults in a manner they think is appropriate for a child of that gender, and eventually the infant incorporates into its self-image the awareness of being a male or a female. By about the age of 2 years, a child's gender identity is fixed for life (Hampson and Hampson, 1961). How the child comes to act on the self-knowledge of its maleness or femaleness depends on the interrelationship of a variety of factors. Children learn attitudes and behaviors by modeling after adults such as parents, teachers, celebrities, and fictional characters, and they are also trained by reward and punishment. Whatever the sources of information and influence, children learn early in life which attitudes and behaviors are appropriate for males and which are appropriate for females. By the age of 3, children are capable of citing a long list of behaviors that are characteristic of one gender and not the other.

Exactly which attitudes and behaviors are deemed appropriate for both sexes depends on the culture in which people live. In some societies, sex role behaviors are strictly defined, and little deviance from the expected sex role stereotype is allowed. Our culture possesses a set of traditional stereotypic sex role behaviors, which include economic role, dominance or submissiveness in social relationships, responsibilities for home and child care, mode of dress, personal appearance, and the mode of expression of emotions. There is little evidence to indicate that our culture's traditional sex role stereotype was ever the predominant behavioral pattern, except perhaps on television shows and in romantic fiction. Today the American sex role stereotype is certainly a myth, because approximately 50 percent of the labor force consists of women, couples in increasing numbers are sharing the responsibilities of fam-

> We are men and women,
> but first we are human beings
> and have human roles to play
> as human beings rather than
> as males or females.
>
> **Mary S. Calderone**

ily care, women are becoming more assertive about their needs and wants, and men are becoming freer to express their feelings and display emotion.

Another aspect of our cultural sex role stereotype is that people should be sexual only with members of the opposite sex, and that same-sex (homosexual) relationships are wrong, illegal, immoral, or indicative of psychological illness. In our culture there is a strong bias against same-sex rela-

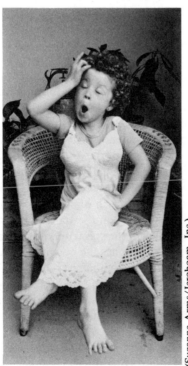

(Suzanne Arms/Jeroboam, Inc.)

tionships, although in some cultures homosexuality in some degree is condoned (Ford and Beach, 1951).

In spite of this bias, it appears that many people have had at least one sexual experience with someone of the same sex (Kinsey et al., 1948, 1953). Only about a third of the population is thought never to have had a same-sex experience. About 5 percent of the population is exclusively homosexual. The rest have had at least one same-sex experience, which probably occurred in childhood, when sexual experimentation is common. As adults, many of these people now define themselves as exclusively heterosexual.

The fact that many people have had some homosexual experience and that many admit to being erotically aroused by individuals of the same sex, even if they do not act on their feelings by having sex with them, supports the idea that homosexuality is not an illness. Moreover, attempts to find some genetic, hormonal, or metabolic explanation of homosexual inclinations have had no success. Psychological explanations proposing some form of psychopathology are also not accepted. The lack of evidence to support the contention that homosexuality is an illness is summed up by the official position of the American Psychiatric Association: "Homosexuality by itself does not necessarily constitute a psychiatric disorder. Homosexuality *per se* is one form of sexual behavior and, like other forms of sexual behavior which are not themselves psychiatric disorders, it is not listed (as one of the) mental disorders."

> Homosexuality
> is assuredly no advantage,
> but is nothing to be ashamed of,
> no vice, no degradation,
> it cannot be classified as an illness;
> we consider it to be a variation
> of the sexual function.
>
> **Sigmund Freud**
> "Letter to an American Mother"

There is such a strong bias that heterosexuality is somehow natural and homosexuality unnatural that people often wonder why some people are homosexual at all. In light of the lack of evidence that homosexuality is a psychological disorder and because there apparently is no biological explanation for homosexuality, the question is not what makes someone homosexual but rather what factors determine sexual orientation, whether heterosexual, homosexual, or bisexual (preference for members of either sex). Some people believe that humans are, in fact, inherently bisexual and that any preference for sexual partners of one sex or the other is determined by early learning experiences, as are most other forms of sexual behavior.

Sexual Arousal and Sexual Response

In recent years an enormous amount of scientific information about the biology of human sexual response has been accumulated. This information has helped to dispel the destructive attitude that sexuality is immoral, dirty, or unnatural. These studies provide ample proof that sexual responsiveness is a natural part of being human, as natural as any other physiological or behavioral response.

By observing the responses of volunteer human subjects to various conditions of sexual arousal, William Masters and Virginia Johnson (1966) showed that regardless of the specific form of sexual stimulation, whether self-stimulation or sex with a member of the opposite sex or the same sex, the body's physiological response is similar in both men and women. Masters and Johnson called this patterned response the **sexual response cycle** (see Figure 21-6).

The sexual response cycle consists of four phases: (1) the **excitement phase,** in which the person experiences sexual arousal from any source; (2) the **plateau phase,** characterized by more intense sexual arousal, (3) **orgasm,** the release of sexual tensions built up in the first two phases of the response cycle, and (4) the **resolution phase,** a return to the nonstimulated physiological state. It should be noted that although the sexual response cycle seems to be characteristic of human biology, there is nevertheless considerable variation in the extent and duration of the sexual response among males and females. There is even variation in the nature of the response cycle in the same person, for not every sexual encounter is identical to every other.

The first phase of the response cycle, the phase of excitement, can be initiated by a variety of situations and events. The way another person looks or talks may trigger a rush of sexual excitement, and most people will respond sexually to being touched in certain ways. In the spectrum of human activity, just about anything has the potential to be sexually stimulating and just about everything is. The variety of stimuli that can produce sexual arousal demonstrates that the brain is really the primary sex organ, for it decides what is regarded as sexually stimulating.

Not only does the brain set the stage for sexual activity by interpreting situations as sexy, but it also

> The only unnatural sex act
> is that which you cannot perform.
> **Alfred Kinsey**

regulates the body's physiological responses that make intercourse possible. When a person becomes sexually aroused, the brain and nervous system prepare the body for sexual activity. Impulses from the brain are transmitted by the spinal nerves to various parts of the body, which cause physiological changes. These changes include tightening of many skeletal muscles; the congestion of blood in certain body regions, particularly the pelvis; increase in heart rate, blood pressure, and respiration; and an increase in the general level of excitement. Constriction of certain blood vessels and dilation of others in the pelvic area lead to the accumulation of blood in that region, which causes the most obvious initial physiological responses to sexual arousal: erection of the penis, lubrication of the vagina, and

tumescence of the clitoris. These responses occur within seconds after a person becomes sexually aroused in any way.

If a person feels comfortable with the idea of sex, and if the time, the place, and the circumstances are appropriate, the initial sexual response can be followed by more intense sexual activity. Often this involves engaging in sex with a partner or using self-stimulation (**masturbation**). Increasing the level of sexual arousal and response usually involves touching and/or kissing the sexually sensitive parts of the body, particularly the genitals, and may include sexual intercourse. The increase in sexual arousal marks the plateau phase of the response cycle.

With continued sexual stimulation, the level of sexual excitement reaches a peak, and the accumu-

Figure 21-6
The sexual response cycle.

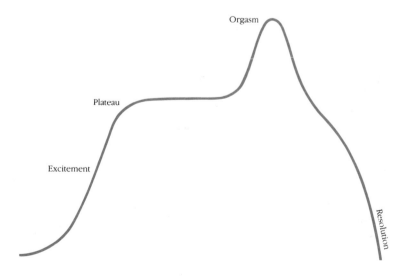

> It is very important to realize
> that masturbation is a normal mode of
> sexual behavior. There are numerous myths that
> masturbation can cause acne, sterility,
> impotency, insanity, and so forth.
> Masturbation produces no
> harmful physical effects.
> **James M. Tolan**

lated physiological sexual tensions are released in a form known as a climax, or orgasm. The orgasmic response is characterized in both men and women by rhythmic contractions of the pelvic muscles, tightening of the muscles of the face, hands, and feet, and feelings of intense pleasure. Most commonly, men ejaculate during orgasm, although it is possible for some males to experience orgasm without ejaculating (Jensen and Robbins, 1977). Women do not ejaculate at orgasm. However, some women may express fluid from the urethra at orgasm, which may seem like the counterpart of male ejaculation. There is a controversy over whether this fluid is urine or a product of the Graffenberg spot (**G-spot**), a region in the vagina that some researchers claim is a site of sexual sensitivity and possibly a homologue of the male prostate (Ladas, Whipple, and Perry, 1982).

With the release of accumulated sexual tension by orgasm, and without further sexual stimulation, a person's body physiology usually returns to its prestimulated state. This is referred to as the resolution phase of the response cycle. Masters and Johnson (1966) noted that after ejaculation most men experience a period during which they cannot be sexually stimulated, which is called the **refractory period**. The refractory period can last minutes, hours, or days, depending on the man and the situation. There seems to be more variation in the resolution phase of women than in the resolution phase of men. Some women apparently do not experience a refractory period; they are capable of repeated epi-

sodes of sexual arousal and repeated orgasm. Other women have a refractory period, often characterized by the clitoris and external genitals being too sensitive to be stimulated any further without discomfort. This refractory period can last from a few seconds to several minutes.

Relating Sexually

Our society is highly achievement oriented. From childhood on, many people are instilled with the value that success (however it is defined) is one of the most important goals in life, and that they must work hard to obtain the highest level of success. Unfortunately, it has become common to apply measures of success to lovemaking. For example, many people believe that success in lovemaking is determined by how frequently the woman partner achieves orgasm during sexual intercourse. By this standard, a "successful male" is someone who can delay ejaculation until his partner has experienced at least one orgasm, and preferably more. The same standard of success applied to women calls for them to have several orgasms in every sexual encounter. Men and women who cannot achieve these standards of success may be erroneously thought of as inadequate.

With the emphasis on the attainment of orgasm, many of the pleasurable aspects of sex—touching, kissing, and the expression of love and affection—are lost. By focusing on the product of

> It's always been acknowledged
> that women have the right to say no, but it
> has not been acknowledged that men can say no,
> too. A man should be able to say no to spending
> the night. He should be able to say,
> "I like you but I'm not ready
> for sex yet."
> **Bernie Zilbergeld**

sexual activity, the many different pleasures associated with the process are often overlooked. As Philip Slater (1973) points out:

> Most sex manuals give the impression that the partners in lovemaking are performing some sort of task; by dint of great cooperative effort and technical skill (primarily the man's), an orgasm (primarily the woman's) is ultimately produced. The bigger the orgasm the more "successful" the task performance . . . Leisurely pleasure-seeking is brushed aside, as all acts and all thoughts are directed toward the creation of a successful finale.

When people become overly concerned with whether they are succeeding or performing well, they can become psychologically detached from the activity and become a spectator rather than a full participant (Masters and Johnson, 1970). Rather than abandon themselves completely to the sexual experience, they withdraw their attention and judge their actions by some measure of performance. **Spectatoring,** as this is called, can lead to worry and anxiety—"I wonder how I'm doing?"—which is one of the principal ways that the natural mind-body interactions that lead to truly enjoyable sex are inhibited. Spectatoring also cheats the partner of being with someone who is completely present in the moment.

In addition to inducing spectatoring and performance anxieties, emphasis on achieving orgasm

arbitrarily tends to limit the definition of sex to sexual intercourse. In the words of psychologist Lonnie Garfield Barbach (1975):

> Intercourse is only one of a number of ways to give and receive sexual pleasure. Sexual relationships and sexual feelings extend far beyond the act of intercourse. To make intercourse the goal of sex does grave disservice to many enjoyable ways of touching . . .
>
> The term sex includes anything that turns you on and gives you sexual pleasure. It doesn't have to include a partner, but it can. It doesn't have to include orgasm, but that's a possibility. It doesn't have to include any genital touching—it could be just fantasy.

To enhance sexual experience by relieving the pressure to achieve orgasm these recommendations are offered by psychologist Carol Ellison:

1. Make sure time is set aside for sex—time that is free of intrusions and distractions. Disconnect the phone, lock the door to the bedroom (or wherever) to ensure privacy, and do not limit your activity with time deadlines.

2. Make yourself an open, effective channel for sexual arousal energy before sexual activity begins. Sex is not a mechanical activity involving only bodies. Satisfying sex is a blending of mind-body energies. To prepare your mind-body system for sex, remove

> Unsatisfactory sexual relations are a
> symptom of marital discord,
> not the cause of it.
>
> **William Lederer and Don Jackson**

sources of sex-negative arousal (hunger, fatigue, anger, distraction) and focus your energies into sex through deep breathing exercises or perhaps some other relaxing activity.

3. Be aware of any differences between you and your partner in the state of readiness for sexual activity. Try to synchronize your states of sexual arousal (through talking, light touching, massage, and so on) before beginning sexual activity.

4. Address concerns about birth control and the possibility of contracting a sexually transmitted disease.

5. Go about your lovemaking slowly; take your time.

6. Communicate likes and dislikes to your partner either verbally or nonverbally. Try to be positive and supportive by saying something such as: "I like it a lot when you . . . " rather than putting the partner down with "Don't do it that way!" If you find it hard to communicate your feelings with words, simply move your partner's hand or face to guide him or her to do what you like.

7. Forget about orgasms. Learn to appreciate the many sexual sensations from touching traditionally nonerotic body regions (face, back, arms, legs, and feet) as well as the genitals and breasts. Sometimes a total body massage is tremendously pleasurable and sensual. Notice how good it can feel to do the touching—to feel your partner's skin.

How you express yourself sexually is a choice that reflects your personal values about sexuality and its role in human relationships. By being aware of the influence of our culture's success ethic about sexual relations and the arbitrary distinction of sex as only sexual intercourse, individuals can become more responsible and satisfied sexual beings.

Sexual Difficulties

It is not uncommon for people to experience occasional dissatisfaction with their sex lives or even to experience the inability to engage in sexual activity. Illness, injury, infection, depression, anger with the sex partner, worry about being an "adequate" lover, or intense stress can limit a person's desire for sex and can alter the body's capability of responding sexually. The sexual and reproductive mechanisms are extremely susceptible to interference by internal and external influences. People can experience difficulty becoming sexually aroused; men can have problems getting and maintaining erections; women can have problems producing enough vaginal lubrication to make sex enjoyable; both men and women can come to orgasm so rapidly that it produces dissatisfaction with sex; some men and women are unable to experience orgasm; and some people experience painful intercourse (see Box 21-3).

The reasons people have sexual difficulties are many and varied. Although some problems are the result of physical disabilities, most often sexual difficulties stem from fears, anxieties, and negative attitudes about sex (Renshaw, 1978; Ficher, 1978).

BOX 21-3

COMMON SEXUAL PROBLEMS

Impotence

The inability of a man to get and maintain an erection is called impotence. Although it can sometimes be caused by injury or disease of the nervous system or by the ingestion of too much alcohol, drugs such as heroin, or medications to control high blood pressure, impotence is most often caused by fear, anger, anxiety about one's sexual performance, or dislike for the sex partner.

Rapid Ejaculation

How long intercourse should last depends on the needs and desires of the people involved. Therefore, it is impossible to say precisely what constitutes "rapid" or "premature" ejaculation. Rather than trying to define rapid in quantitative terms of so many seconds or so many thrusts, it is more useful to define the condition as the absence of voluntary control over ejaculation.

Dyspareunia

Dyspareunia is painful sexual intercourse. Although it is usually thought of as a woman's problem, men can suffer from painful intercourse, too. The major causes of dyspareunia in women are vaginal infections, insufficient production of vaginal lubrication during sexual activity (usually the result of not being sexually aroused), and anxiety-produced spasms of the muscles surrounding the vagina, which makes penile penetration difficult and painful. Another source of painful intercourse that is sometimes found in both men and women is a deep, aching sensation in the pelvis and male scrotum that sometimes comes after a sexual episode. This pain is caused by the congestion of blood in the pelvic structures, which would normally be relieved at orgasm. If orgasm does not occur, however, the blood remains and causes pain.

Difficulty Reaching Orgasm

Some people have difficulty reaching orgasm. This is true of both men and women. Male difficulty in reaching orgasm is also called **retarded ejaculation.** It is not a frequent complaint. Failure to achieve orgasm is probably the most frequent female sexual complaint, however. It can be overcome by learning to appreciate one's body, by assuming positive attitudes about sexual expression, and by learning the ways one's body best responds to sexual stimuli.

Fears include fear of being unable to please the partner, of losing control over the body, and of being unable to orgasm or to withhold orgasm. Anxieties may be about the possibility of pregnancy, the adverse effects of contraceptives, contracting a sexually transmitted (venereal) disease, or being discovered and punished. Negative thoughts range from feeling that sex is dirty to anger, dislike of the partner, or unresolved interpersonal conflicts.

According to Helen Singer Kaplan (1974), sexual difficulties can arise when people:

1. Avoid or fail to engage in sexual behavior that excites and stimulates both partners.
2. Fear they will fail in meeting their own or their partner's expectations.
3. Create perceptual and intellectual defenses against erotic pleasure.
4. Do not communicate their genuine feelings, wishes, and responses openly and without guilt and defensiveness.

The human sexual response consists of a complex series of physiological responses that work best if you are free from anxiety and if the process is left alone and not consciously controlled. Because sexual responsiveness is a natural part of being human, the elimination of sexual difficulties often means "giving up" some learned value, belief, attitude, or behavior that inhibits the natural flow of sexual activity. Sometimes, early negative sexual learning experiences must be replaced by more positive experiences. Many self-help books and various therapeutic procedures exist to help people discover and eliminate sexual difficulties and increase sexual enjoyment.

BOX 21-4

A CONVERSATION WITH A SEX THERAPIST

Q: What is sex therapy?
A: It's a type of therapy specifically designed to deal with sex problems. There's a problem with calling it only sex therapy, however, because often a sex problem is not simply a sex problem but is part of a larger problem within a relationship.

Q: How do people know if they need a sex therapist?
A: If someone is not functioning physically as he or she would like to; or if there is a feeling that if sex were better, the relationship would be better. It's sometimes hard to separate out a purely sexual problem from whatever else is going on in a relationship.

Q: How do people locate a reliable sex theraist?
A: They should be certain to go to someone who has had supervised training in working as a counselor or therapist, such as a psychologist, clinical social worker, or licensed marriage and family counselor, and who has also had special training in sex therapy. Therapists should be asked about their training, if they have the required licenses, if they belong to professional societies, and how long they've been doing therapy.

Q: Is there one approach to sex therapy that is best?
A: It's probably best to find someone whose therapy involves not only talking about the problem but also giving assignments to work on at home. To just talk about sex problems is not as helpful as learning new ways of doing sex.

Q: What happens in sex therapy?
A: It depends. Sometimes the therapists works with couples and sometimes with individuals. Some therapist work with groups of people, all of whom have a similar problem, such as preorgasmic women. In some instances, couples work with a man-and-woman therapy team. At the beginning of therapy, the therapist and clients agree on the nature of the problem and set goals for the therapy. Then the therapist gives clients assignments to do at home to try to realize the goals of the therapy. In the next session, the therapist and clients discuss what happened at home, and new assignments are given. This continues until the goals of the therapy are reached.

Q: How long does sex therapy usually last?
A: The time of therapy varies a lot, but the average is about three

months. Often sex therapy is just a matter of learning new ways of making love, which may not take much time at all. Other times the relationship may need work. The couple may need to open up new ways of communicating or express long-held angers. That might take several months.

Q: What causes sexual difficulties?
A: Some people have physical problems from disease, but that's rare. Most of the problems come from the fact that most people learn about sex by trial and error. Unknowingly, they may fall into bad habits, which eventually causes a problem. That's just a learning pattern, and people can easily learn to do sex differently. Another cause of sex problems is performance anxiety. People get caught up in standards of performance that come from who knows where, instead of just enjoying each other. They are concerned with "How am I doing?" rather than just enjoying themselves. Some sex problems are caused by people not being comfortable with their bodies or having negative feelings about sex.

Q: How can sex problems be prevented?
A: If people could learn to communicate so that partners would not emotionally wound each other, if they could learn to ask for changes in their relationships, if they could learn to negotiate issues of disagreement without hurting each other, there would be fewer sex problems. Another way is to teach people how to create sexual pleasure—not just the mechanics of how to do sex, but also how to create intimacy.

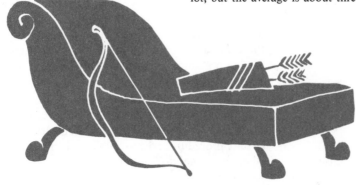

Supplemental Readings

Barbach, Lonnie G. *For Yourself.* New York: Doubleday, 1975. An excellent guide for understanding and expressing female sexuality. The book is beneficial for men as well as women.

Boston Women's Health Book Collective. *New Our Bodies, Ourselves.* Rev. Ed. New York: Simon & Schuster, 1985. A complete discussion of all aspects of human sexuality, including sexual anatomy and sexual relationships. Although written primarily for women, its information is helpful to men.

Kaplan, Helen S. "No-Nonsense Therapy for Six Sexual Malfunctions." *Psychology Today,* October 1974. A noted sex therapist discusses some of the causes and treatments of common sexual difficulties.

Slater, Phillip. "Sexual Adequacy in America." *Intellectual Digest,* November 1973. An analysis and condemnation of the success ethic in sexual relations.

Zilbergeld, Bernie. *Male Sexuality.* Boston: Little, Brown, 1978. A helpful and insightful analysis of male sexuality in America.

Summary

Sexuality involves the simultaneous expression of the total self — body, mind, and spirit. How you choose to express your sexuality depends on your personal code of sexual values. Our culture has not replaced the strict Victorian code of sexual behavior with a set of guidelines applicable to everyone. You have to formulate your own personal standards of sexual behavior, which should emphasize fairness, lack of exploitation, and regard for preventing physical or psychological harm.

In addition to sexual values, a person's sexuality is determined by biological and psychological factors, including genetic makeup (the XX chromosomes of females or the XY chromosomes of males), the female or male set of sexual and reproductive organs, and gender-specific behavior, which is learned early in life.

Sexual relations involve a four-phase physiological process called the sexual response cycle. The first phase involves becoming sexually excited; the second phase involves a continuation of sexual arousal until a third stage is reached, that of climax or orgasm. The fourth stage is one of resolution, when the body physiology returns to its nonstimulated state.

Many phychological and physiological factors can lead to sexual difficulties, most of which can be overcome by increased sexual knowledge and evaluation of one's personal attitudes toward sex.

FOR YOUR HEALTH

Learning Sexual Attitudes

Much of our adult behavior is shaped by early learning experiences and attitudes that become programmed into our minds. Set aside some time to reflect on your earliest learning experiences about sexuality. Were they open and positive experiences, or were they shrouded with secrecy and shame? How have these learning experiences influenced your present sexual attitudes and behaviors? If you are dissatisfied with your mental programs about sexuality, you can utilize any of the mental relaxation techniques discussed in Chapters 2 and 3 to reprogram your mind. In a state of deep relaxation, imagine yourself undergoing your first sexual learning experiences, and in your imagination recreate these situations in ways that change negative experiences into positive ones.

Sexual Context

Make a list of situations and relationships in which sexual expression is permissible for you personally. Would your list be different for your son or daughter?

CHAPTER TWENTY-TWO

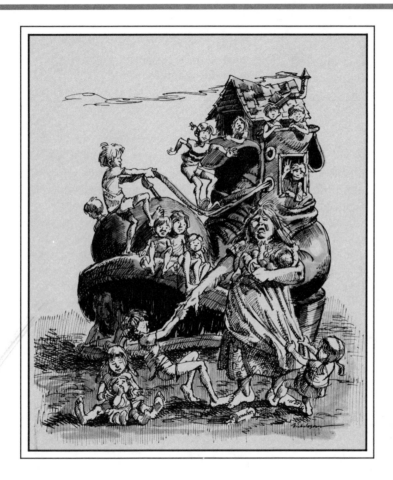

How to keep sexual relationships
healthy and happy.

Responsible Sexuality

Perfection of moral virtue does not wholly take away the passions, but regulates them.

Aquinas

To be aware of the many facets of human sexuality—sexual values, the structure of sexual anatomy, aspects of sexual identity and sexual behavior, and sexual responsiveness—is the first step toward attaining a healthy and fulfilling sex life. Because sexual activities nearly always involve others, our sexual decisions must also involve concern for the health and well-being of the partner. In this chapter, we discuss responsible sexual decision making as it pertains to the avoidance or termination of unintended pregnancy and the prevention of sexually transmitted (venereal) diseases.

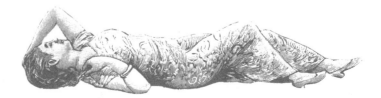

Birth Control

Nearly 66 million Americans engage in a total of between 1 and 6 billion acts of sexual intercourse each year for reasons other than to produce children.* Instead of procreation, people often have sex because it is pleasurable and a way to express love and affection. Given the choice, most persons would prefer to separate nearly all of their sexual experiences from conception. People have many reasons for practicing birth control (Table 22-1) and,

fortunately, modern biotechnology has produced highly effective aids for preventing unplanned pregnancies.

Throughout history hundreds of methods of birth control have been advocated, including the administration of different kinds of potions, elixirs, vaginal inserts (pessaries), and douches made of assorted plant and animal substances; having the woman jump or sneeze after intercourse to try to dispel semen from the vagina; and will power. However, at no time in the past have people had available to them as many safe, reliable methods of birth control as they have today. Unlike the ancient methods, which were rooted in superstition and folklore, today's birth control methods are based on scientific knowledge of human reproductive biology.

*This estimate was derived by assuming that the number of sexually active, fecund American women who wish to avoid pregnancy each year is 33 million (Dryfoos, 1982) and that their frequency of intercourse is between 15 and 100 times per year (Trussell and Westoff, 1980).

Table 22-1
Some Common Reasons for Birth Control

Reason	Explanation
Enhancing sexual pleasure	Anxiety about the possibility of pregnancy can divert a person's attention from the sexual experience and interfere with the flow of sexual feelings. Also, worry during intercourse can cause difficulties with erection and ejaculation in men, and with vaginal lubrication and orgasm in women.
Family planning	Safe, reliable birth control affords couples the opportunity to plan the size of their family and the timing of their children's births. Couples can have children when the family's financial resources are sound and the parents' relationship is ready for raising a child or children.
Increasing women's life choices	Birth control allows women to choose when to devote time and energy to various life pursuits, including parenthood. In the not-too-distant past, when birth control methods were unreliable, it was difficult for a woman to integrate her personal goals with parenthood because she had little control over the timing of the births of her children.
Health considerations	Birth control helps couples reduce the risk of passing a hereditary disease to children. Birth control also is advantageous for women for whom pregnancy and childbirth may be a significant health risk. Birth control can prevent pregnancy in teenagers, who experience more pregnancy-related problems than older women.
World overpopulation	Some couples keep their families small because they want to take some responsibility for limiting the growth of the human population. At the current rate of growth, the world's population is doubling about every 30 years, which means that by the end of this century it will total almost 8 billion. Some people fear that overpopulation will create pressures for food, water, living space, energy, and other resources.

Table 22-2
Use Rate of Contraceptives in Sexually Active, Fecund U.S. Women, Ages 15 to 44 (1982)

Method	Use rate (percent)		
	Age 15–24	Age 25–34	Age 35–44
Pill	48.2	25.7	6.4
Tubal ligation	2.4	19.6	35.4
Vasectomy	1.6	13.6	26.2
Condom	15.1	12.2	9.2
IUD	5.1	8.2	4.9
Diaphragm	5.1	7.0	2.8
Spermicides	4.6	3.7	3.9
Withdrawal	3.8	2.3	1.6
Fertility awareness	0.8	1.4	2.5
None	12.8	5.9	7.0

Data from J. D. Forrest and S. K. Henshaw, "What U.S. Women Think and Do About Contraception," *Family Planning Perspectives*, 15 (1983), p. 157.

Some of the modern birth control techniques are **preconception methods** (contraceptives). They work by preventing the development or union of sperm and ova. Other techniques are **postconception methods.** They inhibit in various ways the development of the fertilized ovum or embryo. The most frequently used methods of contraception are listed in Table 22-2.

When you consider the several methods of birth control, keep in mind that sex without intercourse is a highly effective way to prevent pregnancy. Genital (penis-in-vagina) intercourse is not the only way to give and receive sexual pleasure. Touching, kissing, and stroking can bring intense sexual enjoyment and even orgasm to both partners.

Withdrawal

The withdrawal method of birth control (**coitus interruptus**) requires that the man withdraw his penis from the vagina before ejaculation. In theory, withdrawal prevents sperm from being deposited in the vagina and subsequently fertilizing an ovum. However, the withdrawal method is relatively ineffective. One reason is that the male must exercise great control and restraint in order to withdraw the penis in time. Withdrawal is also risky because a small sperm-containing emission may occur prior to ejaculation. Even if no sperm are actually deposited in the vagina, pregnancy is possible if sperm are released near the vagina and enter later, perhaps inadvertently through body contact.

In addition to its lack of effectiveness, withdrawal can diminish a couple's sexual pleasure. When the man must concentrate on withdrawing and the woman is concerned about whether he will withdraw in time, neither is free to fully experience the pleasure of sexual intercourse. Despite its disadvantages, withdrawal can *sometimes* be a suitable method of birth control, especially if it is used in conjunction with another method, such as fertility awareness (to be described later in this chapter).

Hormonal Contraception: The Pill

In 1960, the U.S. Food and Drug Administration (FDA) approved the use of oral hormonal contraceptive agents for women. Today, approximately 10 million women in the United States are "on the Pill." Worldwide, the number of users is thought to exceed 150 million. In the United States, the Pill is the most popular reversible method of birth control, accounting for 27 percent of contraceptive use among all women and nearly 50 percent of contraceptive use among women younger than 25.

The reasons for the Pill's popularity include its convenience, its low cost, its reversibility, its tolerable side effects (to most users), and, most significantly, its effectiveness. The Pill is nearly 100 percent effective in preventing conception when used correctly.

The most commonly used hormonal contraceptives contain a combination of two synthetic hormones that in many ways mimic the actions of a

> Why birth control? There are two reasons. The first is a personal reason: one simply does not want to have a child (or another child) at this time, under these conditions. The second reason we might call a community reason: birth control is needed to achieve population control. Each year there are 70 million more people on the limited spaceship we call Earth.
>
> **Garret Hardin**
> **Biologist**

woman's naturally occurring ovarian hormones. One of the synthetic hormones is similar to the natural hormone estrogen, and the other synthetic hormone is similar to the natural hormone progesterone. The progesterone-like compound is called a progestogen or progestin. In addition to the combination-type oral contraceptives, a progestin-only pill is available. This is the so-called "minipill." The mechanisms by which the synthetic hormones are thought to prevent pregnancy are presented in Table 22-3.

Over forty different brands of birth control pills are available. Many have similar ingredients in identical dosages but are produced by different manufacturers. Combination pills generally contain between 20 and 80 micrograms of estrogen and 0.3 and 3 mil-ligrams of progestin. Progestin-only minipills contain 0.35 milligrams of progestin or less. Some combination pills have an iron supplement to help prevent iron-deficiency anemia. In some brands of pill, the amounts of estrogen and progestin vary in order to mimic the natural ovarian hormonal cycle.

Regardless of brand or of the dose of synthetic hormones, the method of taking the combination oral contraceptives is the same. The pills come in a package that contains twenty-one or twenty-eight pills. In the twenty-one-pill packets, all the pills contain a prescribed mixture of the two synthetic hormones. In the twenty-eight-pill packets, twenty-one of the pills contain hormones; the other seven pills are inert or contain iron and serve as a way to keep track of the days that no hormone is to be taken.

Table 22-3

Mechanisms of Action of Estrogens and Progestogens Used in Oral Contraceptives

Hormone	Mechanisms of action
Estrogens	1. Inhibition of ovulation by suppressing the release of pituitary hormones FSH and LH.
	2. Inhibition of implantation of the fertilized egg.
	3. Acceleration of transport of the ovum in the fallopian tube.
	4. Accelerated degeneration of the corpus luteum, which secretes progesterone, and consequent prevention of normal implantation of the fertilized ovum.
Progestogens	1. Production of thick cervical mucus, which blocks sperm transport from the vagina to the uterus.
	2. Change in the character of cervical mucus such that sperm are less able to effect fertilization.
	3. Deceleration of ovum transport in the fallopian tubes.
	4. Inhibition of implantation.
	5. Interruption of the hormonal regulation of ovulation.

> Fully one-third of all girls between
> 15 and 20 years of age have at least
> one unwanted pregnancy.
> *Science* magazine news report

The pills with the hormones are usually a different color than the inert, iron-containing tablets. The first pill in a packet is taken on a predetermined day, and one pill is taken each day until the packet is used up. Approximately two days after the last active pill is taken, a menstrual period should occur. Minipills come in twenty-eight-day packets; each pill contains active hormone. One pill is taken each day for an entire pill cycle, even during menstruation.

Pill users are encouraged to associate taking their daily pill with some routine activity, such as eating a meal, brushing their teeth, or going to bed. Taking the pill at the same time each day increases its effectiveness and decreases the likelihood of forgetting to take a pill. If a woman forgets to take one pill, she should take the missed pill as soon as possible and take the next day's pill at the regular time. If she misses taking two pills, she should take two pills as soon as she remembers and two the next day. In either case, it is wise to use another birth control method, such as the condom or foam, during that cycle. If three pills are missed, a woman should discontinue taking that packet of pills and begin a new packet the following Sunday even if she is having a menstrual period. During the next pill cycle she should use an alternative method of birth control.

Approximately half of the women who use oral contraceptives experience unwanted and unintended side effects. Most of the time the side effects present little long-term risk to health, and often they disappear after several cycles on the Pill. The more common of the less serious side effects are nausea, weight gain, breast tenderness, mild headaches, spotty bleeding between periods, decreased menstrual flow, an increased frequency of vaginitis, increased depression, and a lowering of the sex drive. Some other frequent side effects of the Pill are considered by many women to be beneficial. Among these are decreased and even absent menstrual cramps, a decreased number of menstrual bleeding days, and absolute regulation of the menstrual cycle, which can be important for travelers and athletes. Studies indicate that Pill use may help prevent certain diseases (Ory, 1982). Women who take birth control pills have about one-third the chance of developing pelvic inflammatory disease, one-half of the chance of developing benign (noncancerous) breast disease and ovarian cysts, nearly complete protection against ectopic pregnancy, and one-half the risk of developing iron-deficiency anemia (probably because of diminished blood loss at menstruation). Data also indicate that the Pill may reduce the occurrence of rheumatoid arthritis, endometrial cancer, and ovarian cancer.

There is no evidence that fertility is affected by taking the Pill, even after many years of use, although some women experience several months of not having periods after discontinuing the Pill, which may affect their ability to become pregnant soon after discontinuation. There are some data to indicate that a small number of former Pill users (less than 1 percent) may experience an increased risk of spontaneous abortion and stillbirth during their first pregnancy after discontinuing the Pill. However, studies indicate that there is no association between Pill usage and the possibility of birth defects in children born to former Pill users (Linn et al., 1983).

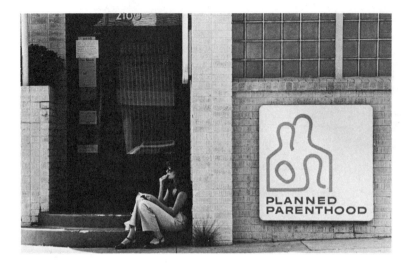

For a small percentage of women, using oral contraceptives presents a severe health risk. Several studies have shown that the risk of fatal blood clots and heart attack is greater for women who take oral contraceptives than for those who do not (Rosenfield, 1978). Women most at risk are those who are over 30 years old and who smoke cigarettes (see Figure 22-1). These women should consider using a birth control method other than the Pill. Any Pill user who experiences severe abdominal pain, chest pain, headaches, unusual eye problems (blurred vision, flashing lights, blindness), or severe calf and thigh pain should consult a physician promptly. The risk of developing liver disease, gallbladder disease, high blood pressure, and stroke is also greater for Pill users. Recent studies show that Pill usage carries *no* increased risk of developing breast cancer (Lipnick et al., 1986).

Because the side effects and health risks associated with the use of combined oral contraceptive pills are almost totally due to the presence of the synthetic estrogen in the pills, some women favor taking the progestin-only oral contraceptive, or minipill. Compared to the combined oral contracep-

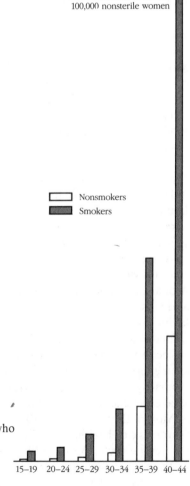

Annual number of deaths/ 100,000 nonsterile women

Nonsmokers
Smokers

15–19 20–24 25–29 30–34 35–39 40–44

Figure 22-1 ▶

Smoking and taking the Pill. The risk of death among Pill takers who smoke cigarettes increases with age. (Data from H. Ory, "Mortality Associated with Fertility and Fertility Control," *Family Planning Perspectives,* 15 [1983], p. 60.)

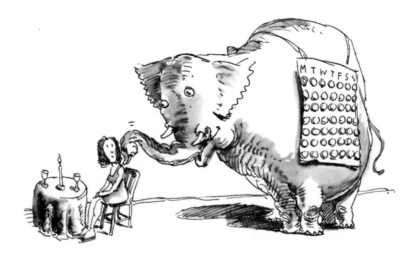

tives, the progestin-only pills are somewhat less effective in preventing pregnancy, but users are often willing to accept that potential drawback in favor of eliminating the side effects and health risks of the combination pills. In many countries it is possible to obtain a long-acting progestin-only implant that is placed under the skin at monthly or even yearly intervals. This method has not met with FDA approval, however, and is not available in the United States.

Another type of hormonal contraceptive is the so-called "morning-after pill." If a woman who has had intercourse believes that she may become pregnant, she can obtain (from a doctor or a family planning agency) a large dose of synthetic estrogen, which renders the reproductive tract unable to support a pregnancy. The major drawback to morning-after contraceptives is that they may cause nausea and vomiting, and although they are very effective, they are too inconvenient to rely on for long-term contraceptive protection. Another potential drawback to postcoital contraception is the possible adverse effect of the hormone on the development of a fetus should the contraceptive action fail and the pregnancy continue.

Although oral contraceptives are extremely effective and considered by many to be simple to use, the potential risks to health and the side effects in using them (nausea, weight gain, interference with normal sexual functioning) signal that couples need to be fully aware of their contraceptive choices before deciding on one or another method.

The Intrauterine Device (IUD)

The **intrauterine device (IUD)** is a small plastic object placed inside the cavity of the uterus to prevent pregnancy. The placing of objects in the uterus to prevent pregnancy is apparently an ancient practice. Nomadic desert tribesmen once put stones in the uteri of their camels to prevent pregnancy during long treks across the desert. Humans use small plastic devices, which are extremely effective. After the Pill, the IUD is the most effective nonsurgical type of contraceptive.

During the 1960s and 1970s several different kinds of IUD were available. By early 1986, however, all but one of the major types of IUD had been withdrawn from the U.S. market. Over the years medical research indicated that IUDs could be quite dangerous—complications associated with IUD use include an increased risk for pelvic inflammatory disease, uterine perforations upon insertion, and an increased risk of ectopic pregnancy should pregnancy occur with the device in place. **Pelvic inflammatory disease (PID)** can damage the fallopian tubes sufficiently to make a woman infertile or to increase the likelihood that a pregnancy will take place in one of the fallopian tubes instead of the uterus (known as an **ectopic pregnancy**). IUDs were removed from the market because hundreds of users claimed that they had been harmed by the device and brought lawsuits against the manufacturers. The manufacturers, in turn, chose to withdraw IUDs from the U.S. market rather than face

Table 22-4
A Comparison of Various Contraceptive Methods

Method	How it works	Effectiveness	Advantages	Disadvantages
Withdrawal	Man withdraws penis from vagina before ejaculation	Low	Causes no health problems	Requires considerable control on the part of the male; may decrease sexual satisfaction
Fertility awareness	Intercourse only on a woman's "safe" days	Moderate if used consistently and conscientiously	Causes no health problems Little if any religious objection	Sometimes difficult to predict "safe" days May require long periods of abstention from sexual intercourse
The Pill	Prevents the release of eggs from the ovaries	High	Easy to use Does not interfere with sexual activity	May cause unintended physiological effects (weight gain, breast tenderness) May cause serious health problems
IUD	Prevents implantation and first stages of pregnancy	High	Always available when needed Does not interfere with sexual activity	May cause heavy menstrual bleeding and cramps May increase the chance of pelvic infection
Diaphragm	Blocks sperm from reaching egg; kills sperm	High if used consistently and correctly	Causes no health problems	Must be used with each incidence of intercourse Must be fitted by a clinician
Contraceptive sponge	Kills sperm; blocks sperm from reaching egg	Moderate if used consistently and correctly	Can be obtained without a doctor's prescription; can be inserted several hours before intercourse	May irritate the vagina Risk of toxic shock syndrome
Vaginal foam or creams	Kills sperm	Moderate if used consistently and correctly	Causes no health problems Can be obtained without a doctor's prescription Protects against sexually transmitted diseases	Must be used before each incidence of intercourse Found messy by some couples
Condom	Prevents sperm from entering vagina	High if used consistently and correctly	Causes no health problems Can be obtained without a doctor's prescription Helps prevent spread of sexually transmitted diseases	May detract from sexual pleasure May break or tear

Table 22-4
(continued)

Method	How it works	Effectiveness	Advantages	Disadvantages
Vaginal foam and condom together	Prevents sperm from entering vagina and kills any sperm that accidentally enter	High	Causes no health problems Can be obtained without a doctor's prescription Helps prevent spread of sexually transmitted diseases	Same as for condom alone and foam alone

lawsuits and large financial settlements. So costly were the damages brought against the maker of one IUD, the Dalkon Shield, that the manufacturer declared bankruptcy.

In 1982 approximately 7 percent of women using contraceptive methods were using IUDs. Now, however, because of the perceived health risk and lack of availability, it is estimated that only a small number of women will choose the IUD as their method of birth control.

Barrier Methods

Because conception involves the union of a sperm cell and an ovum, one way to prevent conception is to place a barrier between these two cells. Several contraceptive methods work on this principle, including the diaphragm; the cervical cap; the contraceptive sponge; spermicidal foams, jellies, and creams; and the condom.

The **diaphragm** is a dome-shaped, latex contraceptive that is placed in the back of the vagina before intercourse takes places. In this position it covers the cervix and therefore prevents the passage of sperm from the vagina to the uterus. The effectiveness of the diaphragm as a physical barrier to sperm movement is greatly increased by coating the rim and dome of the diaphragm with a spermicidal ("sperm-killing") cream. In fact, it may be that the effectiveness of the diaphragm has little to do with the physical barrier but may be almost entirely due to the presence of the spermicides—the device being an efficient way to place and retain the spermicide where it can act most effectively.

One of the great advantages of the diaphragm is that there are no major side effects or long-term health risks associated with its use. Perhaps the only reason someone might not be able to use a diaphragm is that she is allergic to the latex or the spermicide. The great disadvantage of the diaphragm is that it must be inserted each time inter-

Figure 22-2
Procedure for inserting a diaphragm.

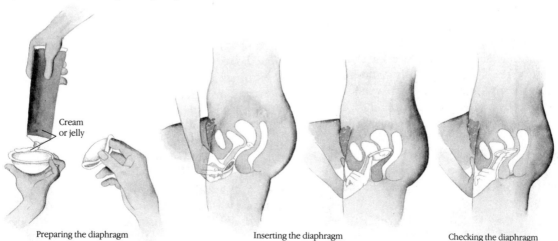

Cream or jelly

Preparing the diaphragm   Inserting the diaphragm   Checking the diaphragm

> For the past two decades, birth control devices have been reflecting the social and political statements of the times.
>
> **Merilee Kernis**

course takes place, which means its effectiveness is highly dependent on the motivation of people to use it correctly *every time* they have sex. Correct usage involves:

1. Being sure that the diaphragm is the right size. Women are not anatomically identical, so each woman must be fitted (by a family planning professional or physician) with a diaphragm that is the right size for her. A woman should not use another woman's diaphragm, because the fit may be wrong.

2. Inserting the diaphragm properly and with a liberal application of the spermicide (see Figure 22-2). This can be done up to 2 hours before intercourse, which means that a couple does not have to interrupt sexual activity to deal with birth control. If a diaphragm is inserted several hours before sexual activity, however, it is advisable to put an additional amount of spermicidal jelly or cream into the vagina before intercourse.

3. Leaving the diaphragm in place for at least 6 hours after intercourse. Early removal increases the risk that some sperm will survive and be able to effect fertilization. The diaphragm can remain in the vagina for up to a day without harm. If intercourse occurs again before the 6 hours have elapsed, the diaphragm should not be removed, but additional spermicide should be put into the vagina.

4. Checking the fit of the diaphragm if there is any change in overall body size from a gain or loss of several pounds, or if there has been a pregnancy or pelvic surgery.

5. Washing the diaphragm after each use with a mild soap and warm water, rinsing it thoroughly, and drying it in air or with a towel. Perfumed talcum powders, petroleum jelly, or scented creams should not be used with the diaphragm. Occasionally the rubber darkens, but this generally does not impair effectiveness. Periodically the diaphragm should be held against a light to check for tiny holes and weak spots (where the rubber buckles). With proper care the diaphragm will last a year or two.

The **cervical cap** is a cup-shaped rubber device that snugly covers the cervix in much the same way that a thimble fits on a finger. Like a diaphragm, a cervical cap is coated with spermicide, but unlike the diaphragm, it can remain in place for several days. When cervical caps were first introduced several decades ago, they were made of silver or copper and were left in place for three or four weeks. Now, however, the rubber caps are removed each week or so, principally to replace the spermicide. Cervical caps come in several sizes and must be fitted for each individual woman.

The principal advantages of the cervical cap are safety and convenience. Once the cap is inserted, sexual activity can take place spontaneously without having to be concerned about birth control. The major disadvantages of the cervical cap are difficulty with insertion and removal, occasional discomfort during intercourse, and occasional dislodging during intercourse. At this writing cervical caps

> When activity is freed of tension and superfluous effort, the resulting ease makes for greater sensitivity.
>
> **Moshe Feldenkrais**

are approved only for use in clinical trials of the method's safety and effectiveness.

The **contraceptive sponge,** which became available in the United States in mid-1983, is made of a compressible plastic and is shaped like a mushroom cap. The sponge is designed to fit in the vagina with its concave side against the cervix. The sponge is impregnated with a spermicide and hence works as a contraceptive in three ways: by destroying sperm, by absorbing ejaculate, and by blocking the entrance to the uterus.

Because the sponge hasn't been in general use for very long, its effectiveness and risks to health have not been completely evaluated. Preliminary tests of efficacy indicate that the sponge is slightly less effective at preventing pregnancy than the diaphragm but more effective than spermicidal agents alone. The most common health problems associated with using the sponge are allergies to the device or spermicide and vaginal (and occasionally penile) irritation and soreness. Some authorities have expressed concern that using the sponge might increase the risk of cervical cancer; however, there are no data to support this contention. Use of the sponge is associated with a slightly higher-than-expected (although still very low) incidence of toxic shock syndrome. The risk can be lessened by not leaving the device in place for longer than 24 hours and not using it during menstruation. The sponge's package insert contains considerable information on proper use and also on toxic shock syndrome.

It is possible to obtain significant contraceptive protection from spermicidal agents alone. These can be obtained (without a doctor's prescription) in the forms of foams, creams, or jellies (like those used with a diaphragm), or a vaginal suppository or tablet that releases the spermicidal chemical after being placed in the vagina. When using any of these spermicidal methods, it is important that they be placed far back in the vagina so the spermicide will cover the cervix and prevent sperm from entering the uterus. It is also important to apply a fresh application *before each act* of intercourse to ensure the highest possible protection. As with the diaphragm, the only complications that arise from using these spermicides are related to allergies to the chemicals in them.

A major advantage of vaginal spermicides is that they are available without a doctor's prescription and can be purchased in pharmacies and many supermarkets. Another advantage is that the spermicidal chemicals decrease the likelihood of transmitting most sexual diseases. Spermicides can also augment vaginal lubrication. The effectiveness of spermicides as birth control agents increases to nearly 100 percent when a spermicide is used simultaneously with a condom.

A disadvantage of vaginal spermicides is that some couples find them messy. Also, this method can be a deterrent to oral-genital sex. Disadvantages of vaginal suppositories include having to wait the prescribed time to allow a tablet to melt and possible discomfort and irritation if intercourse takes place before the tablet has dissolved completely. Concern that the use of spermicides near the time of conception might cause birth defects has not been validated (Scholl et al., 1983).

The **condom,** or rubber, is a sheath that covers the penis and prevents ejaculated sperm from entering the vagina. Many types are available. Some

> Whenever I hear people discussing birth control,
> I always remember that I was the fifth.
>
> **Clarence Darrow**

are lubricated, ribbed, or colored—accoutrements that add nothing to the contraceptive effectiveness of the condom but that are intended to increase their sales appeal. Condoms can be purchased in just about any pharmacy without a prescription, and they are also available through mail order advertisements found in magazines and newspapers.

Using the condom requires that the device be unrolled over the erect penis and that about ½ inch of space be left at the tip to collect the emitted sperm. Some condoms are manufactured with a special tip for semen collection. After intercourse, the condom should remain on as the penis is withdrawn to be sure it does not come off in the vagina. Condoms should be used only once. The contraceptive effectiveness of the condom is greatly increased if it is used in conjunction with one of the vaginal spermicides, such as foam.

In addition to use as a contraceptive, the condom is helpful in preventing the transmission of sexually transmitted (venereal) diseases, such as trichomonas (vaginitis), gonorrhea,, chlamydia, syphilis, herpes, and the AIDS virus.

Fertility Awareness

Fertility awareness, or "natural" birth control ("natural" because it uses no devices, chemicals, or pills), attempts to determine the days in a woman's menstrual cycle when she is fertile—that is, when an ovum is capable of being fertilized. Because the day of ovulation in any given menstrual cycle can-

not be predicted, fertility awareness methods of birth control either *estimate* when ovulation is most likely to occur or indicate that ovulation has already taken place.

Knowing when ovulation is likely to occur or that it has already occurred tells a couple which days in the menstrual cycle not to have unprotected intercourse. These are referred to as the "unsafe" days; the rest are called the "safe" days. On the unsafe days a couple should abstain from intercourse or use an alternative method of birth control.

Calendar rhythm is the most traditional of the fertility awareness methods. This method estimates the most likely fertile, or unsafe, days in a woman's menstrual cycle by assuming that:

1. Ovulation takes place 14 days (plus or minus 2 days) prior to the onset of the next menstrual cycle.
2. An ovum is capable of being fertilized for 24 hours.
3. Sperm deposited in the vagina remain capable of fertilization for up to 3 days.

Thus, in a 28-day cycle the unsafe days for unprotected intercourse range from day 10 to day 17, and the safe days range from day 1 to day 9 and from day 18 to the last day of the menstrual cycle. These intervals are determined by assuming that ovulation is likely to occur between day 12 and day 16, that an ovum could be fertilized anytime between day 12 and day 17 (since an ovum can survive one day), and that sperm in the vagina after day 9 could possibly fertilize an ovum released on day 12.

The unsafe days in a menstrual cycle of any length are estimated in the following way:

1. The first fertile day of the cycle, which is the first unsafe day, is estimated by subtracting 18 from the length of the cycle. Thus, if a cycle were 31 days, the first fertile day would be day 13. The number 18 takes into account that ovulation could take place as early as 16 days before menstruation and that sperm deposited in the vagina 2 days before then could still be capable of fertilization.

2. The last fertile day, or the end of the unsafe interval, is estimated by subtracting 11 from the length of the cycle. This accounts for the possibility that an ovum could be released 12 days prior to menstruation and that an ovum can survive for one day.

The contraceptive sponge is available without a doctor's prescription and is extremely easy to use. Once inserted, it can be left in the vagina for up to 24 hours regardless of the number of times a woman has intercourse. After intercourse the sponge is left in the vagina for at least 6 hours and is then discarded.

A woman wishing to use calendar rhythm must take into account the variation in the lengths of her menstrual cycles. This is done by recording the lengths of at least eight cycles and preferably twelve. The length of each cycle is calculated by taking the first day of menstrual bleeding as day 1 and the day before the onset of the next menstrual period as the last day of the cycle.

For women whose menstrual cycles are of the same length, the calculation of safe and unsafe days is straightforward. However, women whose cycle lengths vary by more than a day cannot be sure at the start of any given cycle how long it will be. Table 22-5 helps estimate the first and last fertile days in any cycle from knowledge of the shortest and longest menstrual cycles.

In order to improve the reliability of calendar rhythm, one can try to determine by more direct methods the actual days ova are present in the reproductive tract. Two such methods exist, both of which are related to hormonally based changes in a woman's physiology associated with ovum production. One involves the monitoring of the basal body temperature (BBT), which changes during the menstrual cycle (see Figure 22-3), and the other involves watching for changes in the consistency in cervical mucus. Monitoring the change in BBT is referred to as the **temperature** method of contraception, while evaluating changes in cervical mucus is referred to as the **mucus** method. Monitoring both body temperature and cervical mucus is call the **symptothermal** method.

Table 22-5
Calendar Rhythm Method of Contraception

If your shortest cycle has been (no. of days)*	Your first fertile (unsafe) day is	If your longest cycle has been (no. of days)	Your last fertile (unsafe) day is
21	3rd day	24	13th day
22	4th	25	14th
23	5th	26	15th
24	6th	27	16th
25	7th	28	17th
26	8th	29	18th
27	9th	30	19th
28	10th	31	20th
29	11th	32	21st
30	12th	33	22nd
31	13th	34	23rd
32	14th	35	24th

*Day 1 = first day of menstrual bleeding.
Data from R. A. Hatcher et al., *Contraceptive Technology, 1980-1981.* © 1980 by Irvington Publishers, Inc. Reprinted by permission.

Figure 22-3
The basal body temperature method of contraception. A woman's body temperature rises about one degree during the days following ovulation. Once the BBT has risen for 3 consecutive days, it can be assumed that ovulation has taken place and that the rest of the days in that menstrual cycle are safe for unprotected intercourse. To use the BBT method, a woman must record her basal body temperature each morning before engaging in *any* activity. Thus, it is advisable to prepare to record the body temperature before going to sleep. Temperature measurement should last at least 5 minutes.

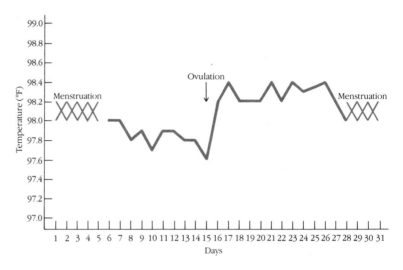

Sterilization

Sterilization is the surgical process of permanently altering the reproductive system to prevent pregnancy. For people who are certain that they do not want children, or, as is more often the case, no more children, surgical methods that render the person sterile but that have no effect on ability to engage in or enjoy sex may be the most desirable form of contraception. Indeed, for couples over 35 years of age, "permanent birth control" (sterilization of either the male or female partner) has become the chosen method of contraception.

The sterilization of a man is called **vasectomy**. This procedure involves the cutting and tying of each of the two vasa deferentia, the tubes that connect the testes (where sperm are made) to the penis (see Figure 22-4). When these tubes are cut, sperm are no longer emitted upon ejaculation because their passage is blocked. Because the cut is made upstream from the organs that produce seminal fluid, a man still ejaculates, but the semen contains no sperm cells. And since the sperm cells make up only a small percentage of the total volume of the semen, neither a man nor his partner is aware of any change in their sexual life, except that no other form of contraception need be used.

Although vasectomy should be considered a permanent form of contraception, it is sometimes possible to reverse the condition by rejoining the cut ends of the vasa. The success of vasectomy reversal as measured by the ability to have children again is about 50 percent, although some surgeons claim much higher reversal rates.

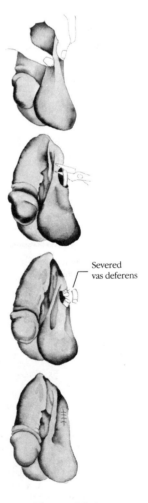

Severed
vas deferens

Figure 22-4
Vasectomy.

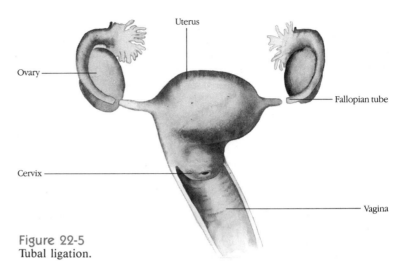

Figure 22-5
Tubal ligation.

One of the reasons vasectomy is such a popular method of contraception is that it is uncomplicated and produces few problems. The procedure is usually carried out in a doctor's office with a local anesthetic in about 15 to 30 minutes. Within a week after the operation, most men have returned to their regular activities, including sex. About one-half to two-thirds of vasectomized men develop antibodies to sperm, but there is no evidence to suggest that this is harmful. Although studies with laboratory animals indicate that vasectomy may be related to the development of atherosclerosis (the disease that causes many heart attacks and strokes), so far there is no indication that this happens in humans.

The principal sterilization procedure for women is **tubal ligation,** the blocking of the fallopian tubes (see Figure 22-5). Blocking can be accomplished by cutting and tying the tubes, by sealing the tubes (cautery), or by closing them with clips, bands, or rings. Most tubal ligations can be performed under local anesthesia in about 20 minutes in a clinic or a doctor's office, and the woman can usually go home the same day or the day after. The incidence of postoperative complications is very low.

Most tubal ligations are "band-aid" surgeries, so-called because the operation requires only one or two inch-long incisions to be made. The incisions allow the surgeon to enter the abdominal cavity and locate and block the fallopian tubes. Entry to the abdominal cavity can be through an incision in the back of the vagina or an incision in the lower abdomen. Vaginal tubal ligation is called **culpotomy.** There are two types of abdominal tubal ligations, **minilaparotomy** and **laparoscopy.** The main

difference between the two is the way the fallopian tubes are visualized. With minilaparotomy, the doctor exposes the tubes to direct view, whereas in laparoscopy the tubes are visualized with a cylindrical viewing device (the laparoscope), which is placed in the abdominal cavity through a small surgical incision.

Although tubal ligation is intended to be a permanent form of birth control, accidental pregnancies occur because a blocked tube spontaneously reopens. In about half of the cases of unintended pregnancy, the pregnancy is ectopic. Surgical reversal of tubal blocking is possible if a woman later decides that she wants to have children, but the success rate is only 50 to 70 percent.

Another female sterilization technique is **hysterectomy,** the surgical removal of the uterus. Most experts do not recommend hysterectomy solely for sterilization purposes because, when compared to tubal ligation, the chances for postoperative complications are 10 to 100 times greater, the operation is more expensive, and the negative psychological impact may be greater.

Choosing a Contraceptive

It is perhaps unfortunate that none of the presently available contraceptive methods possesses all the qualities of the perfect contraceptive. No one method is simultaneously 100 percent effective, 100 percent free of side effects, 100 percent safe, and 100 percent reversible. Without the availability of a perfect contraceptive, sexually active people who wish

Table 22-6
Theoretical and Actual Effectiveness of Various Contraceptives: Number of Pregnancies per 100 Nonsterile Women During First Year of Use

Method	Theoretical effectiveness	Actual use effectiveness	Method	Theoretical effectiveness	Actual use effectiveness
Abstinence	0	?	Condom	2	10
Hysterectomy	0.0001	0.0001	Diaphragm (with spermicide)	2	10
Tubal ligation	0.04	0.04	Spermicidal foam	3–5	15
Vasectomy	0.15	0.15	Penile withdrawal	16	20–25
Oral contraceptive (combination)	0.50	2	Rhythm (calendar)	2–20	20–30
			Lactation for 12 months	25	40
Condom + spermicidal agent	Less than 1	5	Chance (sexually active)	90	90
Low dose oral progestin (minipill)	1	2.5	Douche	?	40
IUD	1.5	4			

Data from R. A. Hatcher et al., *Contraceptive Technology*, 1984–1985. © 1984 by Irvington Publishers, Inc. Reprinted by permission.

to avoid unwanted pregnancies must weigh the benefits and risks of every method and attempt to choose the one that best suits them.

Most users of birth control are principally concerned with two questions: How well does the method work, and is it safe? The efficacy of a birth control method can be evaluated in terms of both theoretical effectiveness and actual effectiveness. The *theoretical* effectiveness is how well the method performs if it is used as intended and consistently. The *actual* effectiveness is a measure of how well a method performs in actual use in a population. Measures of actual effectiveness take into account improper and careless usage. A summary of the theoretical and actual effectiveness of the principal birth control methods is presented in Table 22-6.

Considerations of the safety of birth control methods must take into account the risks to health of using a particular method. Thus individuals should consider any dangers associated with using the method, such as serious illness, the possibility of infection and its consequences, the risk of death, the risk of being unable to have children in the future, any effects on unborn children, and undesirable and unhealthful changes in the body.

The evaluation of a birth control method's safety should also include an assessment of the physical and psychological consequences of an unintended pregnancy. These include the risks associated with terminating the pregnancy with an abortion and the risks associated with carrying the pregnancy to term. Factors such as a woman's age, her physical health, whether she has had previous children,

and her capacity to care for another child also need to be evaluated.

Of course, the most serious risk associated with the use of any contraceptive is the risk of death. Table 22-7 shows the number of yearly deaths associated with various contraceptive methods and with abortion. Also presented is the number of deaths that occur if no contraception is used and women become pregnant. Note that except for Pill use by women over 35 years old who smoke, no contraceptive method carries a greater risk of mortality than pregnancy.

The Responsibility for Birth Control

Most people engage in sexual activity because they want a joyous, rewarding experience. Because an unintended pregnancy can cause enormous hardship, birth control is an important part of every sexual relationship. Denying the possibility of pregnancy by assuming "it can't happen to me" is just gambling against the odds. Couples who have intercourse for one year and who use no birth control have a 90 percent chance of becoming pregnant.

The responsibility for birth control has two components. First, a method of birth control must be chosen, taking into consideration the nature of an individual's sexual activities or a couple's sexual relationship, the frequency of intercourse, future plans regarding having children, and personal and

Table 22-7

**Annual Number of Deaths Associated with Contraception
per 100,000 Nonsterile Women by Method and Age**

	Age group					
Contraceptive method	15–19	20–24	25–29	30–34	35–39	40–44
None*	7.0	7.4	9.1	14.8	25.7	28.2
Abortion	0.5	1.1	1.3	1.9	1.8	1.1
IUD	0.8	0.8	1.0	1.0	1.4	1.4
Pill, nonsmoker	0.3	0.5	0.9	1.9	13.8	31.6
Pill, smoker	2.2	3.4	6.6	13.5	51.1	117.2

*Birth related deaths.

Note: There is no risk of mortality from using the condom, diaphragm, spermicidal agents, and fertility awareness, except that which accompanies either pregnancy or abortion in the event that the method fails.

Data from H. W. Ory, "Mortality Associated with Fertility and Fertility Control: 1983," *Family Planning Perspectives*, 15 (1983), p. 60.

religious values. Second, the chosen method must be used consistently and correctly.

For both technological and sociological reasons, there has been a tendency to associate the responsibility for birth control with women. But as the women in the Boston Women's Health Book Collective (1976) point out, expecting women to take total responsibility for birth control is both unfair and detrimental to relationships:

Total responsibility for birth control is a burden for [women]. We must make arrangements, see a doctor, get examined, go to the drugstore, and usually pay for the supplies. With the pill or IUD, it is our bodies that feel the side effects, and, more seriously, our bodies that take whatever risks are involved. Total responsibility means that if we don't have some kind of birth control and we are pressed to have intercourse, it is up to us to say no; if we have sex without birth control it is our fault if we get pregnant. Our total responsibility for birth control often means that the man can relax more than we can in lovemaking. Total responsibility often creates angry and resentful feelings that can't help but get in the way of loving feelings.

There are a number of ways couples can share the responsibility for birth control (see Box 22-1). The most important is to discuss it. Partners who share the responsibility for birth control are more likely to use their chosen method properly, which

makes birth control more effective, reduces the fear of pregnancy, and makes sex more enjoyable.

Despite their desire not to become pregnant, approximately one-fourth of sexually active individuals use no birth control or at best use some method irregularly. Several of the reasons that people are poor contraceptors include (Miller, 1986):

1. *Low motivation.* People who know that they want children soon, who are ambivalent about avoiding pregnancy, or who do not care about becoming pregnant are less motivated to use birth control.

2. *Incorrect perception of risk.* Some people erroneously believe that that they are not fertile ("It can't happen to me") or that pregnancy isn't possible if a woman has an orgasm or if she urinates after intercourse. Or they believe that the method they are using is more effective than it really is.

3. *Negative attitudes about birth control.* Some people believe that birth control is immoral, a hassle, unromantic, or harmful.

4. *Ambivalence about being sexual.* Some people are unable to "plan ahead" with respect to birth control because they cannot admit to themselves and others that they are choosing to be sexually active.

5. *Irregular sexual activity.* Couples with irregular sexual contact—either because of geographical separation or relationship problems—and individuals with several sexual partners may not establish a birth control regime.

BOX 22-1

THE MALE ROLE IN FAMILY PLANNING

Millions of couples successfully use condoms as their primary method of contraception, and millions more are free of any form of contraceptive use because the male has had a vasectomy. Yet, males in our culture are stereotyped as having little or no interest in contraception and family planning. Myths persist that men are sexually irresponsible, that they "only want sex," and that they are unfeeling about pregnancy and abortion.

But the truth is that many men feel excluded from the contraceptive decisions that affect them and their partners. They are confronted with the attitude that because it is the female who gets pregnant, she should have the primary responsibility for contraception. This attitude is abetted by the greater number of contraceptive methods for women as opposed to those for men, and also by the activities of family planning agencies, which traditionally promote their services only to female clientele.

The fact is that men are involved in family planning, even if the female is the principal contraceptor. The male often influences the choice of contraceptive method that the couple will use. He may support or interfere with his partner's choice and use of a particular method. And he usually influences whether the chosen method is properly used. If an unwanted pregnancy occurs, most men want to be involved in the decision about what course of action to take.

Thus, the male role in family planning extends beyond the use of a particular contraceptive method. This means that couples need to discuss their methods of contraception. And such discussions have an additional benefit: they are conducive to better sex. Not only do they help reduce the fear of unwanted pregnancy, they also foster more open communication about sexual matters, which in turn can bring about a more harmonious sexual relationship.

Abortion

Abortion is the termination of pregnancy by medical or surgical means, preferably within 8 to 12 weeks after conception. Although not considered a contraceptive method, abortion nevertheless is used as a method of family planning by many women. Since 1973, when the United States Supreme Court ruled that abortions were legal in the United States, approximately 15 million have been performed.

The principal method of abortion is **vacuum curettage,** which involves removing the products of conception from the uterus by suction within the first 12 weeks of pregnancy. The procedure can be carried out in an office setting with local anesthesia, and the risks of postoperative complications, such as infection and severe blood loss, are low. The risk of death is also low if the procedure is carried out before the eighth week of pregnancy (Center for Disease Control, 1977). Another abortion method is **dilatation and curettage** (D and C), which involves dilating the cervix and removing the uterine contents with a scraping instrument (the curette).

Between 12 and 20 weeks of pregnancy, abortion procedures include saline, urea, or prostaglandin (a hormone) infusion, which bring about expulsion of the uterine contents, or dilatation and extraction, which is physical removal of the products of conception. The risks of injury to the woman's reproductive organs, of postabortion complications, and of death are greater for D and C abortions and for abortions later in pregnancy than for vacuum curettage.

Despite the fact that abortion is legal, many people have mixed feelings about it. Because there is no universally acceptable scientific definition of when life begins, some individuals question the morality of abortion. Some opponents of abortion believe that it encourages irresponsible sexual behavior, leads to haphazard use of birth control methods, and is a threat to family life. Proponents of abortion argue that women have the right to control their bodies and that abortion is needed if contraception fails, if a woman is pregnant because of rape or incest, if the fetus is diagnosed as having a birth defect, or if the woman's life or health is jeopardized by pregnancy and childbirth.

Results from a 1982 National Opinion Research Poll showed public approval rates for legal abortion in various situations:

> We should not rely on definitions of fertilization and the ambiguous term conception in reaching moral judgments and legal decision on abortion.
>
> **John D. Biggers**

Ninety-two percent of those polled approved of legal abortion if a woman's health were seriously endangered by the pregnancy.

Eighty-seven percent approved of abortion if a woman were pregnant because of rape.

Eighty-four percent approved of abortion if there were a strong chance of a serious birth defect in the baby.

Fifty-two percent approved of abortion if the family had a very low income and could not afford any more children.

Forty-nine percent approved of abortion if an unmarried woman did not want to marry the father.

Forty-nine percent approved of abortion if a married woman wanted no more children.

Forty-one percent approved of abortion for any reason.

Sexually Transmitted Diseases

There are several kinds of contagious infections and infestations of the genital and pelvic regions that are passed from person to person by sexual contact. Traditionally, these diseases have been called **venereal diseases** (VD), but concern about the negative connotations of that terminology, and an attempt to identify their etiology more clearly, has led to replacing that traditional usage with the term **sexually transmitted diseases,** or STD.

The reason for this change in classification is not insignificant, for the negative feeling people have for VD is the principal reason that an epidemic of STD exists in the United States. The total number of reported cases of sexually transmitted diseases exceeds that of all other infectious diseases except the common cold. No one is embarrassed to admit to having a cold, but discovering one has gonorrhea can lead to mortification and even panic. In spite of our society's professed openness about sexual matters, there are aspects of sexuality that are still thought of as "dirty" or "sinful," including sexually transmitted disease. That is why people do not seek diagnosis and treatment when they suspect that they have an STD; they fear ridicule and accusations of being immoral. That is why infected people do not tell their sexual partners of their problem; they fear rejection and being thought irresponsible.

Because there are no vaccinations for the bacterial and viral infections that cause the common sexually transmitted diseases, the only way they can be prevented is for people to assume responsibility for eliminating their propagation. Sexually active people, particularly those with several sexual partners, should become aware of the first signs of STD and make a commitment to themselves to seek professional diagnosis and immediate treatment if such signs occur. The fact that many infected people show no signs of infection makes it a good idea for people with more than one sex partner to obtain periodic (say, every six months) examinations for STD, particularly gonorrhea and chlamydia. Many family planning agencies routinely check for STD in their clients receiving contraceptive services, and most states still require premarital blood tests for syphilis. For most of us, dealing directly and

Table 22-8
Common Sexually Transmitted Diseases (STDs)

STD	Symptoms	Treatment
Gonorrhea	Usually within 2 weeks: discharge from the penis, vagina, or anus; pain on urination or defecation or during sexual intercourse; pain and swelling in the pelvic region; genital and oral infections may be asymptomatic	Antibiotics
Syphilis	Usually within 3 weeks: a chancre (painless sore) appears on the genitals, anus, or mouth; secondary stage—skin rash—appears if left untreated; tertiary stage includes diseases of several body organs	Antibiotics
Herpes genitalis	Usually within 2 weeks: painful blisters appear on site(s) of infection: genitals, anus, cervix; occasionally itching, painful urination, and fever	None; acyclovir relieves symptoms
Trichomoniasis	Yellowish green vaginal discharge with an unpleasant odor; vaginal itching; occasionally painful intercourse	Metronidizole
Moniliasis	Thick, cheesy discharge from the vagina and intense itching of the genital region	Nystatin
Gardnerella	Yellow-green vaginal discharge with an unpleasant odor; painful urination; vaginal itching	Metronidizole
Chlamydia (Nongonococcal urethritis, NGU)	Usually within 3 weeks: infected men have a discharge from the penis and painful urination, women may have a vaginal discharge, but often are asymptomatic	Antibiotics
Pubic lice	Usually within 5 weeks: intense itching in the genital region; lice may be visible in pubic hair; small white eggs may be visible on pubic hair	Gamma benzene hexachloride
Genital warts	Usually within 1 to 3 months: small, dry growths on the genitals, anus, cervix, and possibly mouth	Podophyllin

responsibly with STD is not easy. We have to overcome a lot of negative programming. However, we owe it to the people we love and care for to do so. Table 22-8 outlines the major STDs, including their symptoms and treatment. Table 22-9 offers guidelines for "safer sex" methods for preventing STDs.

Gonorrhea

Gonorrhea, also known as "the clap," is responsible for about 1 million infections a year. The disease is the result of infection of the mucous membranes of the genital tract by the bacterium *Neisseria gonorrhoeae.* Its preference for moist, dark regions of the body means that this organism is capable of living in nongenital parts of the body, including the throat, the anus, the rectum, and the eyes. Therefore, people can transmit gonorrhea by oral-genital and anal sex, and it can be passed to newborns as they pass through the vagina at childbirth. That is why in most states antibiotics or several drops of silver nitrate are put into the eyes of newborns. These agents kill the gonorrhea bacteria and prevent possible blindness. The fact that the organisms live in moist regions means that they

cannot survive on toilet seats, doorknobs, bedsheets, clothes, or towels. They must be passed directly from one body region to another.

One of the reasons gonorrhea infections are so prevalent is that many infected people have no symptoms to indicate to them that infection has occurred. About 80 percent of women are asymptomatic, as are about 20 percent of men. When symptoms do occur, they usually appear within a week to 10 days after contact, and they most frequently include painful urination and a yellowish discharge in men, and a vaginal discharge and painful urination in women. There may also be pain in the groin, abdomen, and testes. If symptoms occur, or if contact with an infected person is suspected, a simple test for the presence of gonorrhea organisms can be obtained from a public health clinic, a Planned Parenthood clinic, or a physician. If the test confirms the presence of gonorrhea, treatment with antibiotics will eradicate the disease in a few days. Left untreated, the infection can spread into the reproductive organs and cause painful pelvic infection and/or sterility. The body does not build up any immunity to gonorrhea, which means that people are susceptible to reinfection whenever they have contact with other infected people.

Table 22-9
Guidelines for "Safer Sex"

Method	Explanation
Telling a partner	Many people do not tell their sexual partners that they have an STD, for fear of rejection, humiliation, and possibly loss of the relationship. If an STD is suspected or known, telling a partner is the only responsible thing to do. When telling a partner, it's best to be straightforward and honest. Be prepared for anger and resentment, and be willing to discuss your partner's feelings. Certainly refrain from sexual contact until you know that an infection is no longer present.
Periodic exams	Sexually active people who are not in an exclusive sexual relationship with one partner should have professional exams for STD every 3 to 6 months.
Discuss with a first-time partner	Ask first-time sexual partners about their personal histories with STDs. Be sure they know you are concerned about protecting yourself. If you have been exposed to herpes, admit that first, perhaps by saying something like, "Before we have sex, there's something that we should talk over."
Use contraceptives that offer protection	Condoms and spermicidal creams, foams, and tablets help to prevent the spread of many STDs.
Wash the genitals	Washing the genitals before and after sex, and urinating after sex, can remove infectious organisms from the body.

Syphilis

Syphilis, like gonorrhea, is a bacterial infection, only in this instance the infecting organism is a spiral-shaped bacterium called *Treponema pallidum,* which is often simply called a **spirochete.** Like the gonorrhea bacteria, spirochetes can be transmitted not only to the genitals but also to the mouth and anus. They can enter the body and bloodstream through almost any break in the skin.

The first noticeable sign of a syphilitic infection is the appearance of an open, painless ulcer or sore, called a **chancre** (pronounced "shanker"), on the infected region. The chancre can appear anytime between the first week and the third month after infection. If the disease is not treated within that time, the chancre will go away by itself, although the person is still infected. Within about six months, the so-called "secondary stage" of syphilis then appears. It is characterized by a skin rash, especially on the palms of the hands and the soles of the feet; the loss of hair; and the appearance of round, flat-topped growths on the moist areas of the body. If the disease remains untreated, these secondary symptoms of syphilis will disappear. The disease then enters

a latent stage in which there are no obvious symptoms but during which the organisms are infecting many of the organs of the body, including the heart, brain, and abdominal organs. Infection of the heart can result in early death, and infection of the brain can lead to psychosis and senility.

Syphilis can be successfully treated with any number of antibiotics. As with gonorrhea, the body builds no immunity against these organisms, so reinfections an occur.

Herpes Genitalis

Herpes genitalis is an infection of the genitals caused by the herpes simplex virus. Strains of this virus cause cold sores on the mouth. Other varieties produce cold-sore-like lesions on the penis, the vagina, the vaginal labia, and the skin of the genital, pelvic, and anal regions. A herpes lesion usually appears within 2 to 20 days after exposure to the virus, which almost always comes from contact with an active herpes sore (mouth or genital) on another person's body. (Transmission of the virus on clothing, bed linen, towels, and toilet seats or in public

> Sex education without the concept of love
> and responsibility is like a piece of pie that's
> all crust and no filling.
>
> C. Everett Koop
> U.S. Surgeon General

spas and pools is highly unlikely.) The principal symptom of a herpes infection is the presence of one or more painful open sores on the skin that last about 2 or 3 weeks. Herpes is extremely contagious when a sore is present, and people with about-to-open sores or open sores on their mouth or genitals should not kiss or have sex until the lesions disappear.

Each year between 500,000 and 1 million people are newly infected with herpes. As many as 50 million Americans may already be infected. There is no cure for herpes infections, although the antiviral drug **acyclovir** is often helpful in reducing symptoms. Infected people can minimize the discomfort caused by the ulcer by not wearing tight clothes and by keeping the area clean. As with cold sores, it is possible to experience recurrent flare-ups of herpes in the same region even if no reinfection has occurred, because the viruses remain in the body cells in a dormant condition. Any kind of stress or anxiety, improper nutrition, or even sunlight can bring on a flare-up of herpes. Usually, the severity of the symptoms decreases with time.

Because the virus remains in nerve cells near the site of the original infection, and because sores can reoccur, some people with herpes (and their potential sex partners) believe that they have to refrain from sexual interaction altogether. This attitude causes unnecessary emotional hardship. People with herpes can learn to manage their condition and can continue to be sexual. The principal thing to remember is not to have sex when active lesions are present. Some people with herpes can tell when a flare-up is about to happen. They get a tingling sensation,

itching, pain, or numbness at the site of the initial infection. It is uncertain, although possible, that condoms and spermicides may decrease the likelihood of transmitting herpes. If there is any doubt about transmission, these contraceptives should be used.

Women with herpes are advised to have annual Pap smears to check the condition of the vagina and cervix. Pregnant women should notify their doctors of past herpes infections to avoid complications resulting from passing the infection to their newborn child.

Pubic Lice

Pubic lice, also known as "crabs," are small insects that can inhabit the genital-rectal region. These tiny organisms attach themselves to skin hairs and feed on blood taken from tiny blood vessels in the skin. Some people are highly sensitive to the bites and may experience intense itching when infested with pubic lice. Itching is often the only symptom of an infestation. Although they are tiny, the lice can be seen. They look like small freckles. Their eggs, which are called "nits," are small white pods that can be seen attached to hair shafts. Transmission of pubic lice is accomplished by physical contact and also by contact with objects on which eggs might have been laid, such as towels, clothes, and bedsheets. Eradication of pubic lice is accomplished by shampooing with a special soap that contains the disinfectant gamma benzene hexachloride, or with other medications designed to eradicate such infestations.

> The basic impulse to propagate our race has propagated a lot of other things as well.
>
> G. C. Lichtenberg

Vaginal Infections

Although not often regarded as sexually transmitted diseases, vaginal infections such as trichomoniasis and moniliasis (see Box 21-1) are transmissible. The microorganisms responsible for these conditions usually produce symptoms only in women, but they can survive in the urethra of the penis or under the penile foreskin. A man who harbors these organisms can infect other sexual partners and even reinfect his usual partner. Sometimes a woman with a vaginal infection will successfully undergo treatment only to be reinfected by her partner, who was originally infected by her. Often it is necessary for both sexual partners to be treated in order to completely cure a vaginal infection.

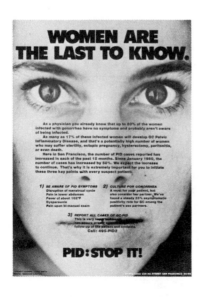

Chlamydia

Chlamydia, an infection caused by the bacterium *Chlamydia trachomatis,* produces symptoms similiar to gonorrhea—that is, painful urination, urethral discharge (usually in men), and vaginal discharge. Chlamydia (formerly called nongonococcal urethritis, NGU) now surpasses gonorrhea as America's most frequent cause of sexually transmitted disease. An estimated 3 million people are infected each year. Because the infection is often asymptomatic, especially in women, some authorities estimate that as many as 10 million people are infected each year, most of them unaware of the presence of the disease. Chlamydia can be treated successfully with antibiotics. Left untreated, chlamydia infection can cause pelvic inflammation and sterility in both sexes, and it can cause permanent eye damage in newborns who come into contact with the organisms at birth.

Genital Warts

Genital warts are hard, often cauliflower-like growths that appear on the genitals and anal region. Genital warts are caused by a virus and usually appear on the body about three months after contact. They are usually treated by applying a liquid material containing podophyllin, which dries up a wart and causes it to fall off. Additional treatment may be required for large or persistent warts. Genital warts are a nuisance and can be dangerous. Studies indicate a link between the occurrence of genital warts and cervical, vulvar, and penile cancer.

> Sex is a drive where there are many accidents
> due to careless drivers.
>
> Evan Esar

 ## Supplemental Readings

Belcastro, P. *The Birth Control Book.* Boston: Jones and Bartlett, 1986. An objective and comprehensive resource on present and future birth control methods.

Boston Women's Health Book Collective. *New Our Bodies, Ourselves.* Rev. Ed. New York: Random House, 1985. One of the best guides to female sexuality, with a comprehensive discussion of birth control.

Connell, E. B. "The Crisis in Contraception." *Technology Review,* May/June 1987. Discusses how political pressures are preventing contraceptive sales and research.

Corsaro, M., and **Korzeniowsky, C.** *STD: A Commonsense Guide to Sexually Transmitted Diseases.* New York: Holt, Rinehart and Winston, 1980. A practical and useful reference that describes thirteen common sexually transmitted diseases.

Hamilton, R. *The Herpes Book.* Los Angeles: J. P. Tarcher, 1980. A holistic, sensible approach to dealing with herpes infections.

Hatcher, R. A., et al. *Contraceptive Technology 1984–85.* New York: Irvington Publishers, 1984. A comprehensive report on all aspects of family planning.

Summary

Healthy sexuality involves responsible sexual decision making, including taking measures to avoid unwanted pregnancy and preventing sexually transmitted diseases.

There are many ways to prevent unwanted pregnancy, including oral contraceptives (the Pill), intrauterine devices (IUDs), diaphragms, condoms, vaginal foams and creams, fertility awareness, sterilization, and abortion. Every couple must weigh the suitability of any given contraceptive practice based on their needs, the method's theoretical effectiveness, its risk to health (if any), and their own motivation to use the method properly. They should choose only contraceptive methods they will use.

Sexually transmitted diseases (formerly called venereal diseases or VD) are infections and infestations passed from person to person most frequently by sexual contact. Some common sexually transmitted diseases are gonorrhea, syphilis, genital herpes, vaginal infections, chlamydia, and pubic lice. Although most sexually transmitted diseases can be treated successfully (as yet, herpes cannot), the best way to deal with the high incidence of these diseases is for sexually active people to take care not to pass them to their sex partners.

FOR YOUR HEALTH

Choosing the Best Contraceptive

Which contraceptive practices do you think are best? Rate the contraceptives in the list below and list the reasons for your choices.

Method	Very suitable	Suitable	Not suitable	Reasons
Abstinence	☐	☐	☐	_____
Hysterectomy	☐	☐	☐	_____
Tubal ligation	☐	☐	☐	_____
Vasectomy	☐	☐	☐	_____
The Pill	☐	☐	☐	_____
Condom	☐	☐	☐	_____
IUD	☐	☐	☐	_____
Diaphragm	☐	☐	☐	_____
Spermicidal foam	☐	☐	☐	_____
Rhythm	☐	☐	☐	_____

The Abortion Issue

How would you counsel a friend involved in an unwanted pregnancy if she were considering getting an abortion? Add to this list of reasons for and against abortions.

Reasons for:

1. When pregnancy endangers the life of the mother.
2. A woman has the right to decide the fate of her body.
3. . . .

Reasons against:

1. Encourages sexual irresponsibility.
2. Abortion is murder.
3. . . .

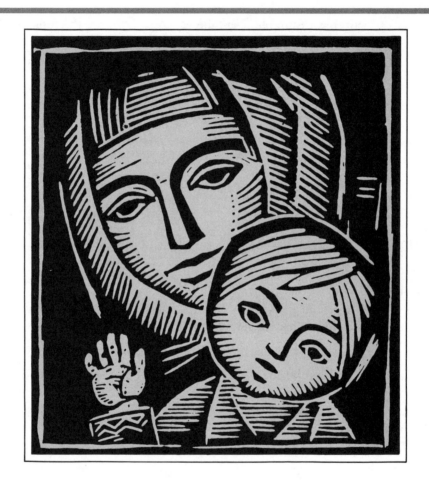

CHAPTER TWENTY-THREE

The health of our children
will determine the future health
of our society.

Pregnancy and Childbirth

Your children are not your
   children
They are the sons and
   daughters of
Life's longing for itself.
They come through you but
   not from you,
And though they are with
   you yet
they belong not to you.

Kahlil Gibran

This chapter is about one of the most profound of all of life's experiences: having a baby. Many people are overwhelmed by the idea that the union of one of your body's cells with one from your mate brings forth a unique human being whose life and happiness are highly dependent on the physical and emotional foundations you provide. There is a tremendous sense of responsibility in being the best kind of parent so that you, your child, and society will all benefit.

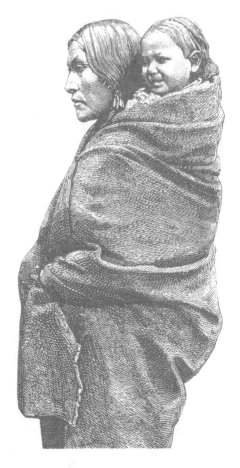

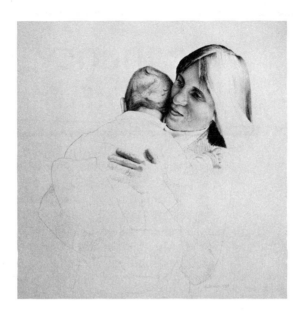

The Decision to Parent

From the time of childhood, almost everyone, and particularly most women, is instilled with the expectation that to have a child is the fulfillment of the purpose of life. Many people never question their role as parents or parents-to-be. They simply assume that they will have children just as their parents did, as if it were as natural a process as breathing. It is common for people to believe that parenting is a special and rewarding part of life and that it would be a mistake not to experience it. Some may see having a child as a way to leave a legacy of themselves to the world—a way of achieving a kind of immortality.

Not everyone is suited for parenthood, however. Many people are becoming aware that in spite of our society's pronatal values, having a child is not what they consider best for them or for an already overpopulated world. They may see parenthood as an infringement on their career goals or perhaps as an unnecessary or unwanted addition to their intimate partnership. Perhaps they have doubts about their psychological or economic abilities to nurture and support a child. Some people refrain from parenthood because they know or suspect that their child might inherit a genetic disease.

Giving birth to and raising a child is an enormous responsibility for both father and mother, and it often requires major adjustments in their personal lives. It certainly requires a change in the way family resources—time, energy, physical space, and money—are distributed. It may involve a change in the career plans of one or both of the parents. Decisions about how leisure time is spent will often be changed. Travel in some instances, for example, will be more difficult. As Joan Ditzion and Dennie Wolf of the Boston Women's Health Book Collective (1978) point out:

> The decision to parent cannot be taken lightly. As soon as we've decided to become parents through pregnancy, adoption, or step-parenting, we find ourselves confronted with new emotional decisions. We want to develop a strong bond with our child and at the same time maintain our partnership, our adult friendships, as well as our involvements with the outside world. What we discover even before we have a baby is that our lives are thrown off balance once we become parents and we need time to establish a new equilibrium.
>
> The period of parenting is an intense one. Never again will we know such responsibility, such productive and hard work, such potential for isolation in the caretaking role, and such intimacy and close involvement in the growth and development of another human being.

Our children do not ask to be born into the world. We make that decision for them. And so we must be as certain as we can that our decisions to parent are appropriate for our life goals and that we have the means for caring for our children.

Becoming Pregnant

For most people, becoming a parent involves pregnancy—a 40-week period during which a fetus grows inside the mother's uterus and the mother's body undergoes considerable change to nurture the child developing within her. Every pregnancy begins with **fertilization,** the fusion of a father's sperm cell with a mother's ovum to form the first cell of their child, called the fertilized egg or **zygote.** When a man ejaculates during sexual intercourse, millions of sperm cells are released into the vagina. Propelled by the swimming motion of their long tails, these tadpolelike cells make their way through the uterus and into the fallopian tubes, the usual site of fertilization (see Figure 23-1). Only one of the many sperm cells actually fertilizes the egg. After fertilization, the zygote moves to the uterus, where it implants in the inner lining and proceeds to develop.

Soon after the zygote implants in the uterus, a unique hormone of pregnancy is secreted into the mother's bloodstream. That hormone, called **human chorionic gonadotropin,** or **HCG,** functions to change the production of estrogen and progesterone in the mother's ovaries (see Figure 23-2). Under the influence of HCG, the ovaries release increasing amounts of these two hormones, which in turn bring about the first noticeable signs and symptoms of pregnancy: absence of the next menstrual period,

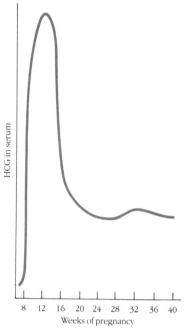

Figure 23-2
The pattern of human chorionic gonadotropin (HCG) secretion during pregnancy.

occasional nausea and vomiting referred to as "morning sickness," enlarged and tender breasts, increased frequency of urination, and enlargement of the uterus. Very often the appearance of these signs and symptoms will convince a couple that the woman is pregnant, but actual proof of pregnancy depends on confirmation of the presence of a fetus in the uterus. This information is most often initially obtained by analyzing the mother's urine for the presence of HCG (a test that women can now administer to themselves with home pregnancy kits—see Box 23-1). After the fetus has grown in size, it is possible to feel it moving around, to hear its heartbeat, or to visualize it with diagnostic ultrasound. Visualization of the fetus with x-rays should be avoided except in highly unusual cases, as the x-rays can cause birth defects.

Fertility and the Menstrual Cycle

Human males are fertile and females are capable of conception after they become sexually mature at puberty, which almost always occurs during adolescence. From the time of physical sexual maturity,

Figure 23-1
The joining of sperm and egg in fertilization. After fertilization, the zygote travels down the fallopian tube to the uterus. Implantation of the multicelled organism begins approximately six days after fertilization.

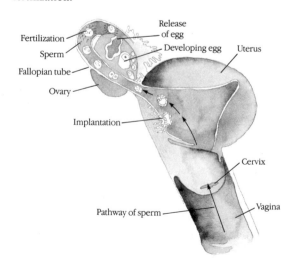

BOX 23-1

HOME PREGNANCY TESTING

When a woman wants to know whether she is pregnant, she can consult a physician or go to a family planning or public health clinic. Or, she can administer a pregnancy test to herself. Several home pregnancy testing kits are now available without prescription. They cost between $10 and $15 and are relatively easy to use.

Virtually all chemical tests for pregnancy—those carried out in clinics and the self-test kind—analyze a woman's blood or urine for the hormone of pregnancy, human chorionic gonadotropin, HCG. In some home pregnancy tests, a woman puts a few drops of her first morning urine (it contains the highest concentration of HCG) into a test tube, adds the test chemicals, and waits 1 or 2 hours. A brown ring appearing at the bottom of the test tube indicates that she is pregnant. In other tests a chemically coated test stick is used to detect HCG in urine. A change in the test stick's color signals the presence of HCG.

The home pregnancy tests are not 100 percent accurate. Only rarely (about 3 times in 100) does the test indicate pregnancy when the woman is not pregnant. A "false positive" is likely to be discovered when the woman seeks prenatal care.

The home test for pregnancy is wrong about 20 percent of the time when it indicates that a woman is not pregnant when in

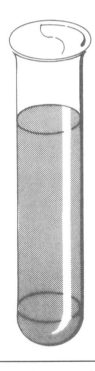

fact she is. About half of these "false negatives" occur because the test has been administered too early in the pregnancy. About half of the "false negatives" are corrected if the test is re-administered in about a week. However, about 10 percent of women who are pregnant still get the inaccurate test result that they are not pregnant. This is one of the most serious drawbacks of home pregnancy tests, for the risk of complications in pregnancy and abortion rise the longer in pregnancy a woman waits to obtain professional care.

In spite of the possibility of inaccuracy, many physicians and family planning consultants believe home pregnancy testing to be useful. It enables women to take a more active part in their own health care, and it may help women who "would rather not think about it" confront the possibility that they are pregnant. Home pregnancy testing may protect the privacy of women who may not want it known that they are sexually active. And it may help women with irregular menstrual periods relieve what may be frequent anxiety about the possibility of being pregnant.

---

men are capable of producing a continuous supply of sperm cells—about 150 million a day—for many years. Women, on the other hand, are not fertile on a daily basis like men. Neither do they remain capable of producing ova for as long a time as men are capable of producing sperm. From the time of sexual maturity, women usually produce only one fertilizable ovum each month, and ovum production stops altogether for most women usually between the ages of 40 and 55.

The fact that fertilizable ova are produced on a near monthly schedule is the basis of a woman's **menstrual cycle.** During each period of ovum production, a woman's body undergoes several hormonally induced changes that prepare her body for pregnancy if the ovum is fertilized. One of these changes involves the thickening of the lining of the uterus, called the **endometrium,** which enables that organ to nurture a fertilized ovum and to support the first stages of pregnancy. In addition to the

> Most of us become parents long before
> we have stopped being children.
>
> **Mignon McLaughlin**

thickening of the endometrium, certain blood vessels in the uterus increase in size. Their role is to bring maternal nutrients to the fetus via the placenta if a pregnancy occurs. If the ovum is not fertilized, however, the enlarged endometrium and the blood vessels within it become unnecessary and are shed. This produces a loss of about 25 to 60 cc (about two or three tablespoons) of blood and tissue debris, which leaves the body through the vagina over the course of 3 to 6 days. This periodic discharge is called **menstruation.**

The length and regularity of the menstrual cycle varies from woman to woman. Most women experience menstrual cycles of approximately 28 days, with cycle lengths between 24 and 35 days being most common. Shorter and longer cycle lengths are possible, and so too, are irregular cycles that occur nearly monthly but in which the number of days between menstruations varies from cycle to cycle. Irregular cycles are typical when women first begin to menstruate and also when they stop producing ova later in life. Eventually a woman's menstrual cycle ceases completely, which is referred to as the **menopause.**

The menstrual cycle is controlled by a number of hormones (see Figure 23-3). Hormones from the hypothalamus in the brain, called **releasing factors,** are secreted and influence the release of other hormones from the pituitary gland. These pituitary hormones are called gonadotropins; their function is to induce the production of a mature ovum in the ovary and to stimulate the production of the hormones estrogen and progesterone in the ovary. These ovarian hormones circulate throughout the woman's bloodstream and induce changes necessary to support pregnancy. The preparation of the lining of the uterus for pregnancy is but one function of estrogen and progesterone (see Table 23-1). The menstrual cycle is regulated in such a way that if fertilization does not occur, the hormonal support of tissue growth in the uterus stops, and the uterine tissue is lost in a menstrual discharge.

For some women, menstruation may be accompanied by unpleasant symptoms. For example, it is estimated that 50 percent of women experience abdominal pain, commonly referred to as "cramps" and medically referred to as **dysmenorrhea,** usually during the first day or so of menstrual flow. Although psychological, anatomical, and hormonal factors can contribute to menstrual cramps, in most cases the likely cause is the induction of strong, frequent uterine contractions by naturally occurring substances called **prostaglandins.** The prostaglandins are formed when the uterine lining breaks down at the time of menstruation. Their likely function is to produce uterine contractions so that the menstruate will be completely removed from the uterus. Women who suffer from menstrual cramps tend to produce high levels of prostaglandins during menstruation. In many instances, the severity of cramps is reduced or eliminated if no ovum is released during a cycle. This is why many women have no cramps when they take birth control pills but do have them when they are off the Pill. The severity of menstrual cramps is sometimes lessened if a woman's body is flexible. Physical exercises can help increase body flexibility, and relaxation through meditation, autogenic training, image visualization, or any of the

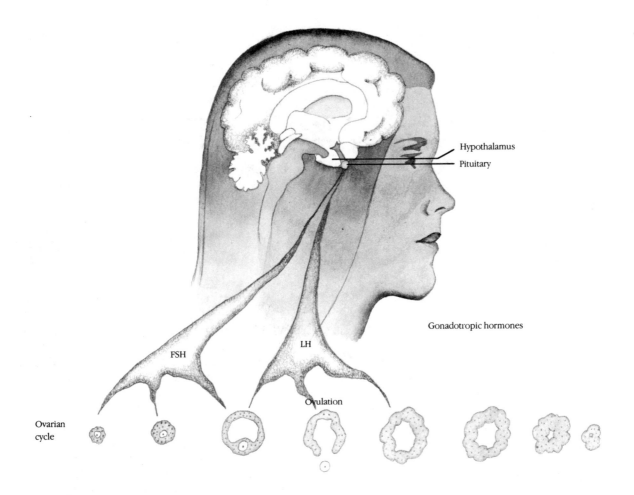

Hypothalamus

Pituitary

Gonadotropic hormones

FSH

LH

Ovulation

Ovarian cycle

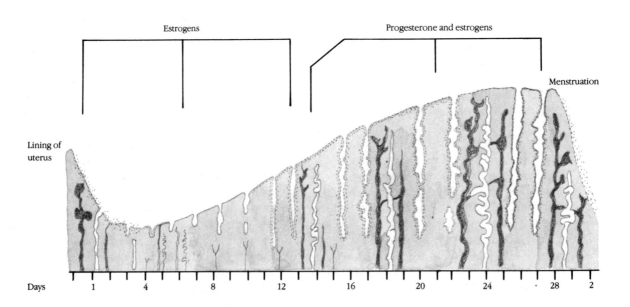

Estrogens

Progesterone and estrogens

Menstruation

Lining of uterus

Days

Table 23-1
Functions of Estrogen and Progesterone

Organ	Effect of estrogen	Effect of progesterone
Ovary	Increases sensitivity to gonadotropins	
	Stimulates growth in ovarian cells	
Fallopian tubes	Increases motility and secretion	Decreases motility
Uterus	Stimulates proliferation of blood vessels	Increases secretory activity of endometrium
	Increases size of muscle cells	Decreases contractions in uterine muscle
	Stimulates production of cervical mucus	Causes changes in viscosity of cervical mucus
Vagina	Stimulates growth and changes in vaginal cells	Causes changes in cells of vagina
	Maintains vaginal secretions	
Breasts	Stimulates growth and development of nipple and milk ducts	
Secondary sex characteristics	Stimulates feminine pattern of hair growth	
	Stimulates feminine pattern of fat distribution	

several relaxation techniques discussed in previous chapters of this book may also relieve menstrual discomfort. Medications that reduce the effects of prostaglandins can also help relieve cramps.

Another frequent problem with menstruation is changes in feelings and disposition as the time of menstruation approaches and during the first day or two of menstrual flow. Although reliable statistics are unavailable, it is possible that near the time of menstruation approximately half of all women experience distressing physical, psychological, and behavioral changes, collectively known as **premenstrual syndrome** (PMS). These changes may include headache, backache, fatigue, feeling bloated, breast tenderness, depression, irritability, unusually aggressive feelings, and social withdrawal. With the onset of menstruation, most sufferers of PMS report prompt relief from the symptoms, although many also experience dysmenorrhea (cramps) as menstruation ensues.

Whether PMS is the result of changes in hormone levels or is the manifestation of negative attitudes and experiences with menstruation is uncertain (Parlee, 1982). A number of hypotheses regarding the biological basis of PMS have been proposed, including progesterone insufficiency, vitamin B_6 (pyridoxine) insufficiency, fluid retention, hypoglycemia, and abnormal changes in endogenous opiate peptides (endorphins) in the late phases of the menstrual cycle (Reid and Yen, 1983). So far, however, none of these hypotheses has been proven by scientific evidence. However, a number of private clinics have been established to treat PMS, often with high doses of progesterone or vitamins. The efficacy of these treatments is uncertain; the greatest benefit may be going to clinics that charge high fees for administering to women with PMS (Eagan, 1983; Heneson and Strain, 1984). Many physicians treat the symptoms of PMS with diuretics, tranquilizers, antidepressants, and other drugs, which often only make the symptoms worse (Reid and Yen, 1983).

Still another common menstrual difficulty is the unexpected interruption or cessation of menstrual periods, called **amenorrhea**. The most frequent reason that periods stop is pregnancy, but the list of factors that can interfere with normal menstruation is quite long. It includes any kind of psychological stress, such as grief, depression, trauma, marital or sexual problems, excess fatigue, and even the fear of pregnancy. Other reasons that menstrual periods may stop are nutritional abnormalities (including crash diets), obesity, ingestion of drugs such as chlorpromazine or heroin, or taking the Pill.

Although there may be a physiological basis for some menstrual disorders and discomforts, often the

◄ Figure 23-3
(Opposite) Hormonal control of the menstrual cycle. Hormones from the hypothalamus control the release of hormones from the pituitary gland, which in turn regulates the production of the ovum and sex hormones from the ovaries. Note how the rise and fall of the hormones is related to the building up and sloughing off of the uterine lining.

Hold your baby, stroke and cuddle,
Talk while rocking to-and-fro;
Solace, trust, good health, and pleasure
Are the treasures you bestow.
Milton Hildebrand

problems have a psychological origin. Impressionable young girls are often told what the "curse" will be like by sisters or other relatives; they may be told that having a menstrual discharge is unclean, or that they will feel uncomfortable and irritable when "on the rag."

The hormones and functioning of the reproductive system are particularly sensitive to a woman's mental state and beliefs about menstruation. Often a reexamination of any negative programming stemming from childhood or adolescence can release some fear and tension that may be associated with menstruation. Positive, comfortable suggestions given to oneself during relaxation exercises and mentally visualizing the menstrual cycle as a natural, biologically normal process can sometimes reduce and perhaps even eliminate cramps and other menstrual problems.

A woman can also try to ameliorate menstrual distress by attending to her diet and exercise patterns near the time of menstruation. To help reduce fluid retention, she can limit salt intake. To help maintain emotional stability, she can cut down on or eliminate the use of caffeine and sugar, especially in large doses. Vigorous exercise can promote endorphin release, which may modulate any tendency toward mood swings and possibly relieve physical discomforts.

Menopause

At some point in a woman's life she will stop menstruating altogether. This is the **menopause,** otherwise known as "the change of life." It is a time when the ovaries stop producing ova and the ovaries' production of hormones wanes considerably. Therefore, the two principal biological consequences of the menopause are that a woman no longer is capable of becoming pregnant and that her body may undergo some changes from the diminished production of ovarian hormones. The average age at which menopause occurs is about 50. It is thought that the age at which menopause occurs may be affected by hereditary, social, and nutritional factors. There is no relation between the age at which menopause occurs and the age at which a woman first begins to menstruate.

Some people, both men and women, have negative feelings about menopause. They see it as a time of rapid degeneration of a woman's body and the onset of a prolonged time of emotional instability or "crotchetiness." They may also have the mistaken idea that because menopause signifies the end of reproductive capacity that it necessarily means the end of a woman's sexual interests and abilities. None of these beliefs has a factual basis, but in this case, too, what is believed may have a powerful effect on changes in physiology. We have ample evidence all around us that age is no barrier to living a fulfilled and enjoyable life. Women who accept menopause as a natural part of their life process need not slow down. They can continue to be active and healthy and can continue to have enjoyable sex. Some women are relieved that menopause means that they no longer have to bother with contraceptives or to worry about pregnancy. One problem that women of any age may have, but that may occur more frequently after menopause, is difficulty with adequate vaginal lubrication during sex. This may happen be-

> For everything its season and for every
> activity under heaven its time.
>
> **Ecclesiastes**

cause the hormone levels are low. A remedy is the use of a water-soluble vaginal lubricant. Water-insoluble lubricants such as petroleum jelly should not be used, since they can harm the vagina.

Menopause can be a time of difficulty for some women and their families. Women who have devoted much of their lives to caring for and raising children may begin to feel that life is meaningless as their children move away from home to establish homes of their own. A woman's parents may now need her to assist them with problems of old age or her husband may need psychological support to cope with his midlife changes. Indeed, the change of life is oftentimes an apt description of the menopause for reasons that have nothing to do with physiology.

Any dramatic change in a person's life situation is likely to produce some kind of emotional distress, anxiety, depression, confusion, and even stress-related physical illnesses. This is natural. Unfortunately, many people look upon stress as an illness in need of medical treatment. They demand services from physicians, who often prescribe tranquilizers, sleeping pills, and (for women experiencing menopause) estrogen replacement pills. There is enormous controversy over the advisability of prescribing such medications for distressed older people. Tranquilizers and sleeping pills provide little help in adjusting to a life change and estrogen therapy can carry with it an increased risk of uterine cancer (Gambrell, 1982). As with any unsettling life change, menopause can be taken as an opportunity for growth and development—a chance to seek out and discover new experiences, relationships, and ways of being.

Infertility

Approximately 10–15 percent of couples who want to have children have difficulty doing so. These couples may be **infertile,** particularly if they have not been able to achieve a pregnancy after a year of trying without using a contraceptive. About half of these infertile couples can eventually conceive if the reason for infertility is discovered and if there is some way to overcome the problem. Occasionally, couples are unsuccessful in achieving pregnancy simply because they are not having intercourse frequently enough at the time when an ovum is most likely to be in the fallopian tubes. The same techniques used for the rhythm method of contraception (calendar rhythm, recording of the basal body temperature, or observation of cervical mucus) can also be used to pinpoint the time of ovulation, and a couple can use this knowledge to help the woman get pregnant. Infertility may also result if one or the other partner is in ill health. Diabetes, hepatitis, chronic alcoholism, malnutrition, anxiety, stress, and fatigue can lessen one's reproductive capabilities. Fortunately, medical management of a problem or a change in lifestyle can often restore fertility.

In about 40 percent of infertile couples, the specific problem stems from the inability of the male partner to produce or deliver into the vagina a sufficient number of reproductively capable sperm cells. From the time of puberty, when a man becomes sexually and reproductively capable, he can produce about 150 million sperm cells daily, unless there is some problem. Injury, disease, drug and alcohol abuse, stress, and genetic or developmental problems can reduce the number of healthy sperm cells a man

BOX 23-2

NEW WAYS TO OVERCOME INFERTILITY

At the moment of her birth in the summer of 1978, Louise Brown became an instant celebrity, not because her parents were famous but because Louise was the first "test tube baby"—the first child to be conceived outside the mother's body. Like millions of other couples, Louise's parents are infertile. The revolutionary medical procedure that helped bring Louise into the world, called *in vitro* fertilization, is only one of several unprecedented methods that infertile couples are using, or soon will use, to have children.

In vitro fertilization is an alternative when a woman's fallopian tubes are physically obstructed. The woman can produce eggs, but the blocked tubes prevent the meeting of egg and sperm. To overcome this problem, a doctor removes eggs from the woman's ovaries and places them in a laboratory dish (the "test tube"), where they are bathed with sperm donated by the husband. Fertilization takes place in the dish. Then the fertilized egg is inserted into the mother's uterus, where it develops into a baby in the normal way.

Hundreds of children who were conceived in "test tubes" have already been born. And many more are likely to be as more medical specialists learn the complicated procedure of *in vitro* fertilization. Already the few specialists who have been successful with it are being deluged with pleas for help from hopeful infertile couples.

Whereas *in vitro* fertilization raises some ethical dilemmas for a few, most people seem to be enthralled with rather than worried about it. Such acceptance of new medical technologies for overcoming infertility may allow the application of more unusual methods for dealing with the problem.

For example, when a woman cannot have a normal pregnancy, she and her husband can hire a "surrogate" mother to have the child for them. A woman is chosen from a group of consenting candidates to be artificially inseminated by the husband's sperm. The surrogate receives a fee for carrying and giving birth to the couple's child.

Another possible way for surrogates to be used is to combine *in vitro* fertilization with surrogate motherhood. That is, the infertile couple donates egg and sperm, which are brought together in the laboratory to form a fertilized egg. But instead of putting the embryo back into the donor's uterus, it is implanted in the surrogate's uterus, where it develops into a child.

Yet another possibility is "prenatal adoption." An egg donated by a surrogate is fertilized *in vitro* with the husband's sperm. The resulting embryo is then placed inside the wife's uterus, thus allowing a woman who cannot produce eggs to experience pregnancy and childbirth.

Couples who overcome their infertility problem, whatever the procedure, are grateful that they can have children. Those who donate eggs and sperm to others, or who serve as surrogate mothers, usually feel special in that they are helping to give life and are helping others to fulfill important life goals. As for the children brought into the world with these unusual techniques, most experts believe that a child's well-being is determined not by where conception takes place, or by who carries the baby to term, but by the quality of the love and care they receive after birth.

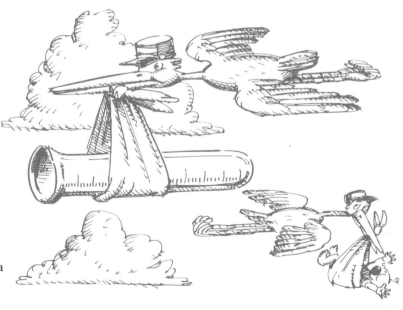

> Yesterday I went to the grocery store. I had filled up the cart and was halfway through the check stand before I realized I had shopped for the whole family. The last child left two years ago. I don't know what got into me.
>
> **From *Voices***
> **by Susan Griffin**

produces to the point that too few sperm capable of fertilizing an ovum are emitted on each ejaculation. It is thought that conception is highly improbable unless about 20 million healthy sperm are deposited in the vagina. Difficulty in getting and maintaining an erection or ejaculating in the vagina can also inhibit fertility.

The number of infertile couples in which the problems stem from the female partner is about equal to those in which the problem is due to the male. The most frequently encountered female factor in infertility is the preventing of the sperm from meeting the ovum. In some instances a benign growth or tumor in the uterus or cervix will block sperm movement to the fallopian tubes. Sometimes cervical mucus is too thick and/or voluminous to allow sperm entry into the uterus. Infections of the female reproductive tract, especially untreated

gonorrhea and chlamydia, can cause permanent scarring that blocks the tubes. And there are a variety of hormonal imbalances that can upset the growth, development, and release of reproductively capable ova. In some cases, either surgery to remove physical blocks to the movement of sperm and ova or hormone therapy can overcome the problem, and the couple will be able to conceive.

Health Habits During Pregnancy

Every child deserves to be born as healthy as possible. It is only fair to the unborn child—who did not ask to be conceived—that all the genetic potential to develop a healthy body and mind be given the opportunity to be fully expressed. Few of us are as

Louise Brown, the first "test tube baby." (United Press International.)

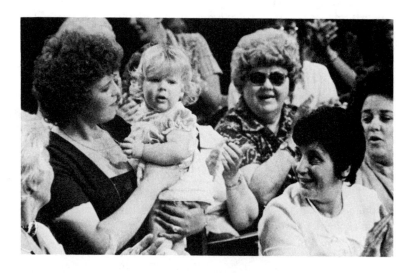

> Perhaps like cigarette packs, labels of all alcoholic beverages should contain a warning such as "The Surgeon General has determined that alcohol can cause damage to unborn babies of pregnant women."
>
> Jonathan Fielding and
> Alfred Yankauer

careful about maintaining proper health habits as we could be. Most people live with whatever risk might be associated with nonhealthy behaviors and are presumably willing to accept the consequences of those behaviors. But when a woman is pregnant, disregarding fundamental health practices endangers her child as well as herself, and perhaps more so, because the developing baby's body and mind are extremely vulnerable to damage. It is extremely important that a mother-to-be make every effort to practice good health habits. If her developing baby could talk, he or she might say, "Mom, my lifelong health and well-being are in your hands now. I know nine months is a long time to have to be concerned about what you eat and drink, but it's important to me that you do the right things for both of us. Not only will that give me the chance to become the best person I can be, but will also keep you healthy so we can share a lot of good times after I'm born." The factors that deserve a pregnant woman's attention to ensure her own health and that of her baby are proper nutrition, obtaining professional prenatal care, getting enough exercise, refraining from smoking or consuming alcohol or other drugs while pregnant, and accepting and dealing with emotional and sexual feelings that may be different from those experienced when not pregnant.

Nutrition

Throughout pregnancy, the fetus' cells and physiological capacities are developing. Perhaps more than at any other time of life, an ample supply of nutrients is required so that the making of new cells and the developing of organs proceeds optimally. All of the fetus' nutrients come from the mother via the placenta. Therefore, a pregnant woman directly influences the nutritional status of her baby, and she must be aware that she must "eat for two," meaning that she must be sure her diet contains adequate nutrients for herself and for her baby. Mothers-to-be who eat highly nutritious diets during pregnancy are more likely to give birth to healthy babies than are mothers whose diets are nutritionally poor. It is recommended that pregnant women increase their intake of essential nutrients and calories (see Table 23-2). Some women are advised to supplement a generally well-balanced diet with extra iron and folic acid.

Many pregnant women are concerned with the amount of weight they gain. There was a time in the not-too-distant past when most doctors severely restricted the weight gained by the pregnant women in their care because they felt that gaining too much weight caused a serious high blood pressure disease of pregnancy, **toxemia.** While it is never good to weigh too much, current obstetric practice allows a mother-to-be to gain a reasonable amount of weight, about 22 to 26 pounds by the end of pregnancy, most of which comes in the last two-thirds of pregnancy. About 7 of these pounds are contributed by the fetus. The enlarged uterus accounts for another 2 pounds and the placenta and amniotic fluid contribute 1 pound each. About 4 to 8 pounds of fluid are added to the maternal system as extra blood and extracellular fluid. And the mother may gain about 4 pounds of body fat. It was once considered good

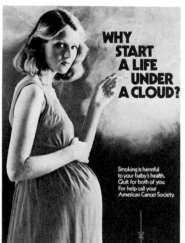

obstetric practice to prescribe diuretic drugs (to reduce water in the body) and appetite suppressants (amphetamines) to reduce a mother's body weight and thereby to try to prevent certain diseases that are characteristic of pregnancy. This is no longer recommended.

Prenatal Care

Pregnancy involves several profound biological changes. Not only does the fetus develop from a single cell to a 7- or 8-pound newborn infant composed of many millions of cells, but also the mother's body undergoes a number of anatomical and physiologi-cal changes in order to support fetal development. Moreover, the fetal-maternal relationship is maintained by the placenta, an organ that develops only during pregnancy and is expelled from the mother's uterus after the baby is born. Any rapidly changing system is vulnerable to errors and problems, and so it is with pregnancy and fetal development. That is why it is recommended that mothers-to-be receive professional prenatal care. A number of studies have shown that the more prenatal care a pregnant woman receives, the fewer will be her problems during pregnancy and childbirth and the more likely that her infant will be born healthy and well. By obtaining professional prenatal care, a mother-to-be can avoid the consequences of a number of pregnancy-specific illnesses, such as toxemia, diabetes of pregnancy, and infection. These illnesses can threaten both the mother's health and the proper development and delivery of her baby. Professional prenatal care can also help manage problems resulting from a malfunctioning placenta and can educate a mother with regard to proper nutrition during pregnancy and advise her on how smoking at any time during pregnancy can adversely affect her baby's development, as can regular consumption of alcohol (King and Fabio, 1983). Maternal infections that are harmful to the fetus, such as rubella (German measles), syphilis, gonorrhea, toxoplasmosis, and herpes, can be detected and managed. Another reason for prenatal care is to be sure the maternal and fetal blood cells are immunologically (Rh factor) compatible (discussed in Chapter 9).

Table 23-2
Recommended Daily Dietary Allowances for Nonpregnant, Pregnant, and Lactating Women, Ages 23–50

	Nonpregnant	Pregnant	Lactating		Nonpregnant	Pregnant	Lactating
Protein (g)	44	74	64	Folacin (mg)	400	800	500
Vitamin A (mcg)	800	1000	1200	Vitamin B_{12} (mcg)	3	4	4
Vitamin D (mcg)	5	10	10	Calcium (mg)	800	1200	1200
Vitamin E (mg)	8	10	11	Phosphorus (mg)	800	1200	1200
Vitamin C (mg)	60	80	100	Magnesium (mg)	300	450	450
Thiamine (mg)	1	1.4	1.5	Iron (mg)	18	*	*
Riboflavin (mg)	1.2	1.5	1.7	Zinc (mg)	15	20	25
Niacin (mg)	13	15	18	Iodine (mcg)	150	175	200
Vitamin B_6 (mg)	2	2.6	2.5				

*Supplementation of 30–60 mg of iron per day is recommended.
Data from Food and Nutrition Board, *Recommended Dietary Allowances* (Washington, D.C.: National Academy of Sciences National Research Council, 1980).

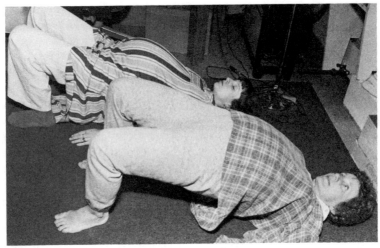

(© Irene Kane.)

Physical Activity and Exercise

People who are physically active look and feel good and are healthy. Pregnant women are no exception, and there are even special benefits to being physically active during pregnancy. Some women feel very lethargic during pregnancy. In just a few weeks their bodies take on unfamiliar proportions and they have to carry up to 20 percent more weight than when they are not pregnant. They may feel uncomfortable, unattractive, and clumsy. Through movement and exercise, a pregnant woman can become accustomed to the temporary changes in her body and can learn to accept pregnancy as a positive and fulfilling time of her life. Physical activity also helps prepare the mother's body for childbirth, which is often physically demanding. By keeping active, a pregnant woman can improve her circulation and thereby reduce swelling and formation of varicose veins in the lower legs, which are quite common in pregnancy. Perhaps the greatest benefits from phys-

ical activity during pregnancy is maintaining the habit of being active. That way, after the baby is born, the mother can lose body fat gained during pregnancy and return her body to a firm nonpregnant state.

The degree of physical activity a pregnant woman engages in depends on her desires and abilities. Some women who are very athletic engage in their sports almost to the day of delivery. Women who are not routinely athletic are wise to begin an exercise program early in pregnancy that involves exercises to maintain correct posture, strengthen the abdominal muscles, and improve breathing and ability to relax muscles (see Figure 23-4).

Emotional Well-being

Pregnancy can be a time of intense feelings, not only for the mother-to-be but also for her partner and

Figure 23-4
Some recommended exercises during pregnancy. (Data from P. Shrock, *Clinical Obstetrics,* vol. 2.)

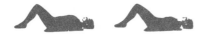

Pelvic tilt
Lie on back with both knees bent and feet on the floor, 18 inches apart. Press small of back to the floor for a count of four, then relax. Repeat ten times.

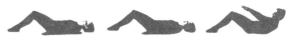

Universal toner
Same position as pelvic tilt. Press small of back to floor and lift head and stretch right arm to left knee, hold a few seconds, then relax. Repeat stretching left arm to right knee.

> ### The most powerful way to forge a strong bond between mother and infant is through breast-feeding.
> **John Kennell**

others who are close to her. Enthusiasm, excitement, anticipation, fear about the baby's condition, uncertainties about one's suitability as a parent, a desire for more love, affection, and sex, or a desire for less love, affection and sex, are all natural. To recognize that intense feelings are normal in pregnancy and to accept them with patience and understanding are the keys to having a rewarding pregnancy experience.

Perhaps the best way to deal with intense feelings at any time in life, including pregnancy, is to take time each day to quiet the mind and body with meditation, yoga, or other relaxation methods. Massage is also beneficial, and it fulfills some of the desires of those who feel more sensual during pregnancy. Some couples feel an increased desire for sexual intercourse during pregnancy, which is all right unless the woman has a medical problem that would be worsened by sex. In that event couples can engage in the many forms of pleasuring that do not involve sexual intercourse.

Childbirth

Few human events are as dramatic as childbirth. We can only surmise what each new baby feels while negotiating the mother's birth canal during the several-hour-long journey from the protective confines of the uterus to the outside world (see Figure 23-5). Whether he or she would describe it as painful, frightening, or exhilarating, anyone who could recall the birth experience would probably agree that it was intense. For parents, childbirth brings exaltation and relief that the nine months of pregnancy and waiting are over. For onlookers and family members, childbirth elicits wonder, sometimes reverence, and concern for the condition of the mother and baby. Childbirth, with its nakedness, blood, mess, effort, sweat, and tears of both pain and joy exposes our primal humanness like nothing else.

The release of intense emotions in childbirth is heightened by the inherent risk of danger to both mother and baby. Although they occur only in a

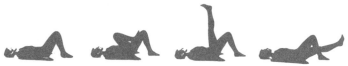

Hip-knee-ankle toner
Lie on back or on side. Upon exhalation, bend right leg, bringing knee to chest. Then stretch leg straight, trying to touch ceiling with heel. Slowly lower leg to floor. Repeat twice for both legs.

Neck and shoulder toner
Sit with back straight. Slowly drop chin to chest and gently circle to left in a large arc, making a complete circle. Repeat in other direction.

small percentage of births, certain life-threatening complications occasionally do arise during the birthing process. Mothers can bleed extensively, infection may occur, or the baby's oxygen supply can be cut off as it makes the transition from the aquatic environment of the amniotic fluid to air. If the air supply is cut off for too long, brain damage and even death can result. Thus, the goal of childbirth is to make the emotional experience as rewarding as possible and also to make the entire event safe.

Not many years ago, many expectant mothers and their families feared childbirth. They knew it could be painful, that the baby could be stillborn, and that the mother could even die. The high risks to maternal and child health led to the development of a specialized type of medical practice—obstetrics—dedicated to eliminating the harmful complications of pregnancy and childbirth. With the advent of anesthesia, antibiotic therapy, identification of high-risk mothers, techniques of fetal monitoring, and trained birth attendants, the degree of maternal and infant mortality and the incidence of maternal and infant illness is presently quite low (see Figure 23-6). Serious complications arise in about 500 out of 10,000 unaided pregnancies and childbirths. With modern obstetric help, however, the complication rate is about 1 or 2 in 10,000.

In the recent past, nearly all births were carried out the same way, which we see portrayed in part in old movies and on TV shows: Mother begins to experience rhythmic uterine contractions and stoically tells her husband it's time to go to the hospital. He is overcome with excitement and rushes her to the hospital where she is taken to a room to deliver. The husband then goes to a waiting room to pace nervously, to absent-mindedly accept a cigar from a man whose wife has just delivered, and to be reassured by an older man whose wife has already had several children. The baby is born and put in a small crib in a nursery filled with other newborns. Father, disheveled and ecstatic, looks at all the babies in the nursery from behind a glass partition, trying to determine which is his. A gowned nurse holds one up and father smiles. He then passes out cigars to the other waiting fathers as he is led to his wife, who looks a little fatigued, but whose hair is perfectly coiffed.

Some of the real-life action that the movies and TV shows do not usually show include the mother being "prepped" for labor by being given an enema and perhaps being given a tranquilizer, a pain-killing drug, or an injection of an anesthetic drug in the

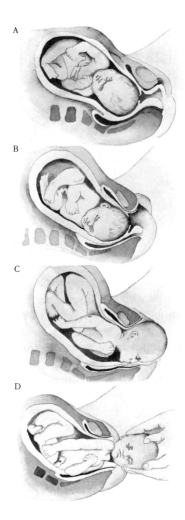

Figure 23-5
Childbirth.

pelvic region to eliminate all pelvic sensations during childbirth. When the baby is about to emerge, the mother is transferred to a delivery room where her doctor and the nursing attendants assist with the remainder of the birth. It is likely that the doctor will perform an **episiotomy,** a surgical incision between the vagina and the anus that helps prevent tears to the vagina and perineum by enlarging the vaginal exit. In many births, the mother holds the baby immediately after it is born. The baby is then taken to a nursery, and mother is taken to a recovery room.

One of the characteristics of the traditional hospital birth is that the families have little control over the procedure. Once the obstetrician is selected, virtually all decisions about how the birth is carried out are left to the doctor and the obstetrical assist-

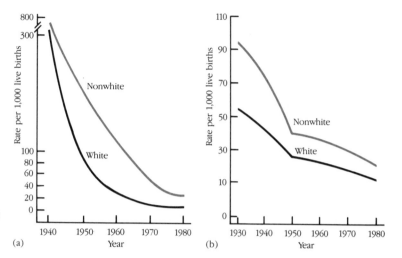

Figure 23-6
(a) Incidence of maternal mortality in the United States, 1940–1980.
(b) Incidence of infant mortality in the United States, 1930–1980. (Data from National Center for Health Statistics.)

ants in the hospital. Many families appreciate this, for they trust the doctor and hospital staff to make decisions that they feel unqualified to make. Other families, however, want to participate in the birthing experience. For example, they might find a traditional hospital setting too formal and cold for what they feel is a joyous, warm occasion, and consequently may want to have their baby in an "alternative birth center" or at home. Because unforeseen medical emergencies can occur during childbirth, the alternative birth center — a hospital-based delivery room with a homelike atmosphere where the entire family can be together to participate in the birth — is preferable to birthing at home, where no medical backup is immediately on hand.

Couples may want to make other decisions about the birth experience in addition to choosing the birth setting. They may want the father present in the room and assisting the mother's labor. Friends, other family members, and even siblings of the newborn child may be present as well. They may want the mother to be awake and in full control of her body, which means that she receives no anesthesia or only minor pain relief. The mother may not want to have an episiotomy unless the birth is difficult. The couple may want the lighting in the birthing room low and perhaps have soft background music to make the mother more comfortable, and also presumably to make the actual experience of birth less traumatic for the baby (Leboyer, 1975).

Several programs and organizations teach families how to prepare for childbirth. These prebirthing courses are called "natural childbirth," or Lamaze classes, after a French doctor who developed what has become a popular program. Almost all the childbirth preparation courses teach the parents the basic biology of pregnancy and childbirth, and they also teach breathing and relaxation exercises to help make the actual delivery of the baby proceed smoothly. While attending the 6- to 8-week courses, parents-to-be meet other expectant couples with whom they can share normal anxieties and experiences. It is in the class that couples learn of the many choices they have about their childbirth experience and can find the setting and professional birth assistant to work with them.

Breast-feeding

After the baby is born, the mother will have the choice of whether or not to breast-feed her infant. A survey of breast-feeding conducted in 1980 by the U.S. Centers for Disease Control showed that 51 percent of white mothers and 25 percent of black mothers breast-fed their babies. These percentages represented a nearly threefold increase in the incidence of breast-feeding since 1969. Apparently, more and more women are becoming aware of the many benefits of breast-feeding as compared to bottle-feeding:

1. Breast-feeding provides maternal antibodies and immunological cells that provide immunity to the newborn and that also stimulate the infant's own immune defenses.

2. Breast milk promotes the maturation of the infant's digestive system as both a food processor and a barrier to infectious agents.

3. Breast-feeding improves the psychological attachment between mother and infant—so called "bonding"—which some believe to be a factor in the future psychological well-being of both mother and child.

4. Breast-fed babies have fewer infections, less diarrhea, and fewer allergies.

5. Breast milk contains the proper amount and composition of fat, cholesterol, and amino acids.

6. The hormones involved in milk production and release contribute to the mother's psychological well-being after childbirth and also help the uterus return rapidly to its normal size.

7. Breast-feeding can act as a natural contraceptive if infant suckling is frequent (Short, 1984).

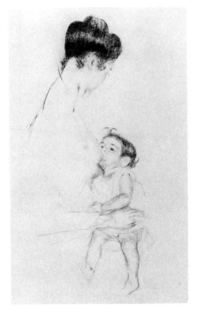

(Mary Cassatt, "Mother Louise Nursing Her Child," 1899, Minneapolis Institute of Art.)

All the advantages of breast-feeding should not be taken to suggest that bottle-feeding is bad. There are many healthy, well-adjusted people who were bottle-fed infants. Some mothers choose not to breast-feed their children because career and other responsibilites make it inconvenient. Breast-feeding in public is still not acceptable in many communities. Some babies are such vigorous feeders that breast-feeding becomes too painful and mothers stop. An organization devoted to helping mothers learn about breast-feeding is the La Leche League. Perhaps the most important factor in feeding an infant is an abundance of contact and loving.

Supplemental Readings

Boston Women's Health Book Collective. *Ourselves and Our Children.* New York: Random House, 1978. An excellent account of all aspects of parenting.

Hotchner, Tracy. *Pregnancy and Childbirth.* 2nd ed. New York: Avon, 1984. A comprehensive guide to all aspects of pregnancy and childbirth.

Kitzinger, Sheila. *Your Baby Your Way.* New York: Pantheon, 1987. Discusses all of the choices pregnant couples must make in preparing for childbirth.

La Leche League. *The Womanly Art of Breastfeeding.* 3rd ed. New York: New American Library, 1981. A thorough and sensitive discussion of all aspects of breast-feeding, produced by an organization devoted to the dissemination of information about this natural practice.

Leboyer, Frederick. *Birth Without Violence.* New York: Alfred A. Knopf, 1975. A description of a delivery method that proposes to make the birth experience as untraumatic as possible for the child.

Shapiro, Jerrold Lee. *When Men Are Pregnant.* San Luis Obispo, CA: Impact Publishers, 1987. Discusses pregnancy and childbirth from a male perspective.

Summary

Becoming a parent can be one of life's most rewarding experiences, but the decision to be a parent cannot be taken lightly. Raising a child is a demanding responsibility, requiring psychological and physical preparation so that the child can enter a family able to provide the best child care.

Pregnancy is a 40-week period during which a fetus develops inside the mother's body. Every child begins life as a single cell, formed by the union of a sperm cell from the father and an ovum from the mother. The male continually produces sperm cells, but a woman produces only one ovum each month or so. The monthly cycles of ovum production are called menstrual cycles. If a pregnancy does not occur during a menstrual cycle, a small amount of blood and tissue debris is discharged from the uterus via the vagina. The cessation of the menstrual cycle later in life is called the menopause.

Some couples are infertile, which means that they are unable to conceive a child after many months of trying. Many times the causes of infertility can be determined and corrected and the couple can achieve pregnancy.

During pregnancy, a mother-to-be must be aware that whatever she puts into her body may possibly affect her unborn child. She should endeavor to eat properly and avoid consuming drugs, including alcohol and tobacco, which are known to harm the fetus. Mothers-to-be can make their pregnancy and post-pregnancy adjustment go more smoothly if they exercise, give special attention to maintaining emotional well-being, and seek professional prenatal care.

Childbirth, although it is a natural process, can sometimes be difficult for mother and baby, so parents are advised to investigate all the aspects of the birth process and choose a birthing situation they are comfortable with, whether it be a traditional hospital delivery or a home-style birth in an alternative birth center. Mothers are encouraged to breast-feed their infants for optimal development and health.

FOR YOUR HEALTH

Managing Menstrual Difficulties

If you or a friend suffers from menstrual difficulties, utilize a relaxation or visualization technique (see Chapters 2 and 3) just before or during the menstrual period in order to relieve symptoms and to improve the experience. Relaxation and visualization can also help when medications are being taken. The mind can prepare the body to accept the healing actions of medications.

Parenthood and You

Are you planning to have children? Which of the following motivations for parenthood do you hold most strongly? Can you add others to the list?

1. To have a child who looks like me.
2. To have a child who will carry on my admirable qualities.
3. To have a child who will be successful.
4. To have someone who will carry on my name.
5. To have someone to inherit money or property.
6. To have someone who will regard me very highly.
7. To do something I know I could do well.
8. To feel pride in creating another human being.
9. To keep me young at heart.
10. To help me feel fulfilled.
11. To make my marriage happier.
12. To make me feel masculine/feminine.
13. To please my family and society.
14. To teach someone about the beauty of life.
15. To help someone grow and develop.

CHAPTER TWENTY-FOUR

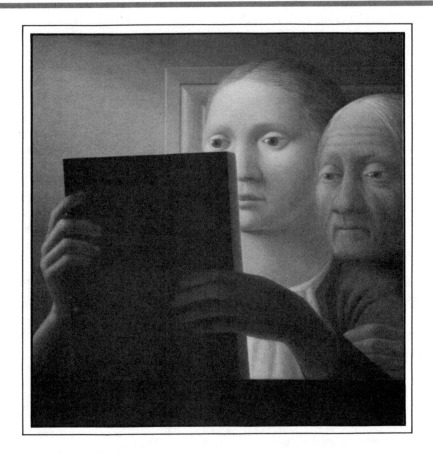

Acknowledging the processes of
aging and dying as natural enables us
to live healthful and satisfying lives.

Aging and Dying

As a boy I was rather sickly, and my parents have told me that it was predicted I would die young. This prediction has been proven completely wrong in one sense, but has come profoundly true in another sense. I think it is correct that I will never live to be old. So now I agree with the prediction. I believe that I will die *young.*

Carl Rogers

Human beings have long sought the means to slow down aging processes and to postpone the inevitability of death. Over the centuries, magic, herbs, alchemy, and modern drugs and scientific technology have been employed to prevent aging and death. In the sixteenth century the Spanish conquistador Ponce de Leon sought the legendary "fountain of youth" in the Americas, which was supposed to restore the health and youth of anyone who drank from it. More recently, people have contracted to have their bodies frozen by cryogenic (cold storage) techniques and preserved in a frozen condition until some future time when science presumably will have learned how to cure fatal illnesses or prolong life indefinitely. (This tactic is based on the dubious assumption that the human organism can survive long periods of deep-freezing.)

Everything in the universe—plants, animals, mountains, planets, stars and galaxies, even atoms and subatomic parti-les—undergoes changes with time, which is what is meant by an aging process. The earth we live on is aging and will eventually die, its volcanic processes will cease, and its biosphere of life will disappear. The stars will burn out and come to an end, often with violent explosions that produce novas and supernovas. Human beings are born, become old, and eventually die. The mechanisms and time scales of aging are different for stars than for people. But the end result for both is the recycling of matter that is continually reused in the birth of new stars and new people.

Many people in the United States today view old age as a time of sickness, disability, loneliness, and inactivity. They believe that death is something to be avoided at all costs—even though everyone knows that death is unavoidable. Until quite recently, old age and death were taboo subjects and old people were regarded as being fundamentally different from people who were not old. Such negative, unhealthy views of old age and death are false, and fortunately, these ideas are changing. In many other cultures and societies, in fact, old people are venerated, and their accumulated knowledge and wisdom is recognized and respected by younger members of the society.

But in America many myths about aging are still promulgated by movies, magazines, television soap operas, and advertising. The ideal American is portrayed as eternally young, active, and wrinkle-free. Aging is viewed as being synonymous with

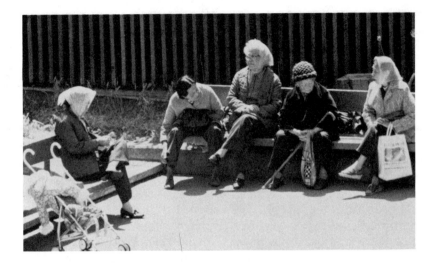

poor health. Advertisements exhort people to feel young, to act young, and to stay young by drinking diet sodas, by using face creams and dyes to mask graying hair, by dressing in the latest youthful fashions, by taking vitamins and elixirs, or by driving the latest sports car.

Aging is not a sickness. Neither can the normal processes of aging be avoided or prevented by any means yet devised. Aging is a continuous life process. It begins at birth and progresses throughout life. The noticeable effects of aging result from wear and tear on the body's essential cellular functions that gradually change and become less efficient over the years. The body wears out even as the best-designed and well-cared-for machine wears out. But with care and an understanding of physical limits, a person's mind and body can remain active and healthy until the very end of life.

In this chapter we discuss the biological and psychological aspects of aging and dying. The period of life we call old age can be a time of further learning and enjoyment of new activities. Health and joy are not restricted to the young; they are for all ages. Even death is a natural part of life. All of us need to understand death and come to accept it as we do other life changes.

The Human Life Span

As a group, people undergo a predictable aging process, although individuals within the group age at different rates. **Senescence** refers to the process

of aging. The study of the biological mechanisms that cause aging is the branch of science called **gerontology.** If one measures the number of persons surviving in a population as a function of age, as shown in Figure 24-1, it is apparent that there exists an **absolute human life span,** the age at which there are no survivors. Such data can also be used to define the **mean life span,** the age at which one-half of the individuals in the population have died. Data such as these are used by insurance companies to calculate the death risks for various populations of people and to determine what premiums are necessary in order to pay the survivor benefits.

Figure 24-1
Survival as a function of years in an idealized aging population.

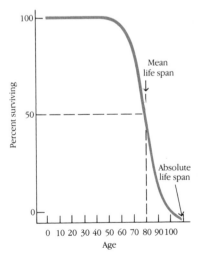

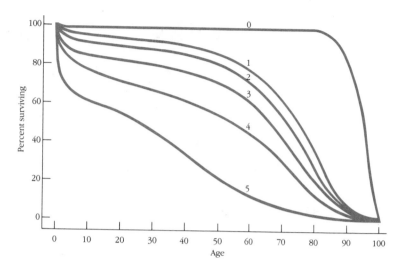

Figure 24-2

Actual survival curves for various human populations. (0) Idealized survival curve, (1) New Zealand, 1934–1938, (2) U.S. whites, 1929–1931, (3) Italy, 1930–1932, (4) Japan, 1926–1930, (5) India, 1921–1930. (Data from Comfort, 1956.)

In the idealized situation all individuals that were born would survive to an age close to the theoretical maximum (somewhere between 110 and 140 for humans), and thereafter the number of survivors would decrease rapidly. In reality, no population ages in quite such a simple fashion. Some actual human population survival curves are shown in Figure 24-2. Childhood diseases and accidents may take a heavy toll on human life. In India in the 1920s, about 40 percent of children died before the age of 10 and only a very few individuals survived to old age. In the United States and New Zealand there was considerably less childhood mortality and about half the population survived to age 40. In recent years in the United States and in many other countries,

more and more people are surviving to advanced ages largely as the result of improved nutrition and health care.

One consequence of our improved living conditions and medical care is that overall, the American population is becoming increasingly older, so that by the year 2030 it is estimated that there will be approximately 50 million Americans over 65, or about 20 percent of the population. The dramatic rise in the number of older people in the U.S. population projected in the near future is shown in Figure 24-3.

The burgeoning population of older people is primarily the result of a greatly increased life expectancy. Since 1900 the average life expectancy in the

Figure 24-3

Percentage of the American population age 65 and older from 1900 to 1984, with projected percentages to 2030. (Data from U.S. Census Bureau.)

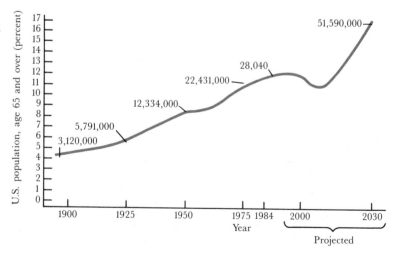

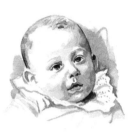

1900
Life expectancy 47 years

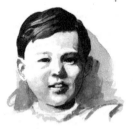

1929
Life expectancy 57 years

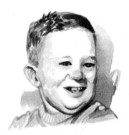

1950
Life expectancy 68 years

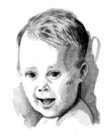

1984
Life expectancy 70.7 years (males)
78.3 years (females)

Figure 24-4
Increase in life expectancy in the United States, 1900 to 1984.

United States has increased by almost 30 years (see Figure 24-4). Factors contributing to this dramatic extension of life expectancy are better nutrition and medical care (especially treatment of infectious diseases), fewer accidents, improved sanitation and hygiene, and healthier lifestyles.

College students reading this book today will be among that older group of Americans 40 or 50 years from now. Therefore, it is especially important to initiate positive, healthy lifestyles now, so that when you become old (a thought that is almost incomprehensible when one is young), you will still be creative, healthy, and able to participate in and enjoy all aspects of living (see Box 24-1). It is also important while you are young to dispel myths and fears about old age and death that you may have.

BOX 24-1

THE FUTURE IS WHAT YOU MAKE IT

Is a person's health status in the later years affected by health practices and behaviors earlier in life? Judging from a study by Richard Benfante, Dwayne Reed, and Jacob Brody (1985), the answer is yes. During a 12-year period they collected extensive physical, psychological, and social data on approximately 5000 men aged 46–69 of Japanese ancestry living in Hawaii. All of the men were disease-free at the beginning and over 1600 were still disease-free at the end of the study. The lifestyles of the healthy men were compared to the lifestyles of 3400 men who became ill during that time to determine factors that contribute to health status in later life.

The analysis showed that poor health in later life was associated with earlier-in-life systolic blood pressures greater than 130 mm Hg; high rates of cigarette and alcohol consumption; overweight; and high serum levels of triglyceride (fat), glucose, and uric acid. Interestingly, men who had lived for several years in Japan (in most cases to attend school while young) were healthier in later life. The investigators hypothesize that men who spent their early years in Japan were exposed to the traditional Japanese lifestyle, which includes a low-fat, high-carbohydrate diet and high levels of physical activity.

While findings from the study of one particular group may not apply equally to other groups, nevertheless the study does show the factors associated with a healthier later life are the same ones associated with overall better health when people are young. It also demonstrates that infirmity and illness are not inevitable in later life.

Consider the 101-year-old man who went to the doctor complaining that his right leg hurt. The doctor told him he had to expect that at his age. The man replied that his left leg was the same age as his right, yet it did not hurt.

Robert N. Butler
Director, National Institute of Aging

Ageism: A Harmful Prejudice

The maxim "you're as old as you feel" expresses a great deal of truth. As with all other aspects of health, what you believe about your old age can profoundly affect your physical and psychological well-being as your body begins to age. If you believe that infirmity, decrepitude, and senility are the inevitable consequences of old age, your mind has the power to produce the destructive changes in physiology that lead to these afflictions. As one prominent gerontology researcher, K. Warner Schaie, has put it, "The expectation of a decline is a self-fulfilling prophecy. Those who don't accept the stereotype of a helpless old age, but instead feel they can do as well in old age as they have in other times in their lives, don't become ineffective before their time." As we noted in Chapter 9, mental depression, negative attitudes, and a loss of interest in life will lower immunological defenses, reduce vitality, and increase the likelihood of disease and incapacitating illness. If one believes that retirement from work at age 65 is the end of a useful, productive life, such a belief may indeed become a self-fulfilling prophecy.

The way that our society regards aging and the elderly exerts a powerful effect on how each of us thinks about old people and what it must be like to be old. Here is how Alex Comfort (1976), an expert in gerontology, describes the stereotype of the aged American:

He or she is a white-haired, inactive, unemployed person, making no demands on anyone, least of all the family, docile in putting up with loneliness, rip-offs of every kind, and boredom, and able to live on a pittance. He or she, although not demented, which would be a nuisance to other people, is slightly deficient in intellect and tiresome to talk to, because folklore says that old people are weak in the head, asexual, because old people are incapable of sexual activity, and it is unseemly if they are not. He or she is unemployable, because old age is second childhood and everyone knows that the old make a mess of simple work.

These sorts of views on aging have no basis in fact. Yet many older people are forced by family and society to conform to this ridiculous stereotype. Views on how elderly people should live and act are gradually changing, but much prejudice is still found in family relationships, in nursing homes, and even among health professionals.

This age-related prejudice is called **ageism** and has been defined by Robert N. Butler, director of the National Institute on Aging, as "a systematic stereotyping and discrimination against people because they are old, just as racism and sexism accomplish this in relation to skin color and gender" (Butler and Lewis, 1977). Butler also emphasizes that senility is *not* a part of the normal aging

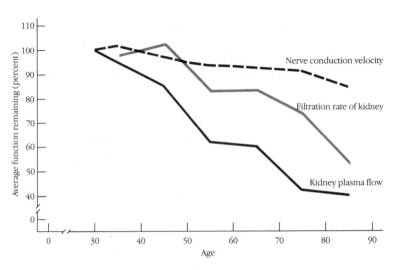

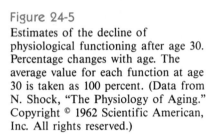

Figure 24-5
Estimates of the decline of physiological functioning after age 30. Percentage changes with age. The average value for each function at age 30 is taken as 100 percent. (Data from N. Shock, "The Physiology of Aging." Copyright © 1962 Scientific American, Inc. All rights reserved.)

process; senility is a sign of disease and affects only a small proportion of the population.

More and more older people are asserting themselves and demanding that they be treated with respect and accorded the same opportunities as younger people. This represents a healthy change in our society. More and more older people choose to remain active and involved with all the aspects of living they enjoyed when younger. Maggie Kuhn (1979), founder of an organization called the Gray Panthers, which fights for the rights of older people, says:

> To get from the airport to my home in Philadelphia, I have to pass a junkyard where old cars are thrown on a heap, left to rust and disintegrate, and finally smashed to smithereens by a society that wants everything shiny new. The junkyard haunts me because America does the same thing to people. When we turn 65, we are trashed. Well, I don't want to be dumped on the scrap heap. I don't want to be isolated from mainstream living or from the companionship of people of all ages.

Older people can and should continue to be active physically, sexually, and emotionally. Awareness of the biological changes that occur as we age can help keep the mind and body functioning optimally at all stages of life. Just because a person may not be as strong or have as much endurance as he or she had when young does not mean he or she must become inactive or unfeeling.

The Biology of Aging

Although it should be apparent from the preceding discussion that some of the health changes that begin to be manifested as we become older are caused by societal prejudice, environmental pressures, and emotional stress, there are, nevertheless, certain biological changes that everybody experiences as he or she grows older. Loss of hair or change in hair color, wrinkling of the skin, loss of muscle tone and physical stamina, less efficient immune response, and reduced lung capacity are some of the changes that occur in almost everyone as he or she becomes older. Figure 24-5 shows several characteristic changes observed in essential body functions as people age. A false belief that has been held for many years by doctors and medical scientists is that the heart inevitably pumps less blood in older persons as compared to young people and that this restricts the activities of older people. However, recent experiments conducted by scientists at the National Institute of Aging show that, if the heart is free of disease, blood is pumped just as efficiently in a 90-year-old as in a young adult. The aging heart apparently compensates for a slower rate of pumping in older people by enlarging, thereby increasing its capacity to pump more blood through the veins and arteries with each heartbeat. The lungs of healthy old people have about one-half the maximum breathing capacity of young people. Aging processes cause a decrease in bone mineral content, resulting in increased brittleness of the bones (see Box 24-2), and cause an increase in blood levels of

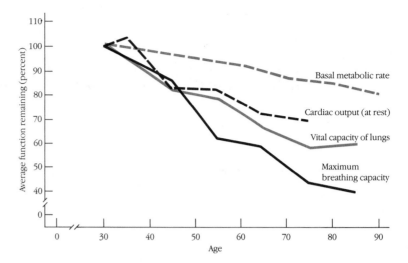

Figure 24-5
(continued)

cholesterol and glucose, which may contribute to cardiovascular disorders and diabetes. The sensory organs involved in seeing, hearing, tasting, touching, and smelling lose some acuity and sensitivity with age.

The basic human developmental stages are usually described as infancy, childhood, adolescence, early adulthood, and mature adulthood. Each of these life stages is accompanied by new capacities; physical, mental, and emotional maturation; and personal growth. The changes that accompany early developmental stages are regarded positively—as being useful, beneficial, and necessary to human development. Yet once people approach middle age, a different view prevails. At that time people are regarded as entering a stage of decline, of losing functions and abilities and of beginning to deteriorate both mentally and physically. Development is viewed in negative terms. Each change after the middle years is regarded as making a person less able to participate fully in life. Physical changes are often viewed as something to be disguised or ignored.

Each stage of life affords opportunities for creative, joyful living. Older people have more time and freedom to read, to travel, and to engage in activities they had no time for when they were younger. They have usually raised their children. Material needs and the time devoted to earning a living are usually less. As long as attitudes toward aging remain positive and healthy, the normal biological changes associated with aging are not likely to interfere with people's capacities to engage in enjoyable activities.

Theories of Aging

Why do people, and all living organisms for that matter, age and die? What are the mechanisms of aging? There are no final answers yet to these questions, but there are a number of hypotheses. In general, the hypotheses fall into two classes: those that ascribe aging to some biological mechanism within us, and those that view aging as the consequence of external factors. It is likely that normal aging results from many factors, both internal and external. Your genetic endowment undoubtedly plays a part in the aging process. For example, in **progeria,** an exceptionally rare genetic disease, individuals age prematurely—children with this disease have gray hair, often develop atherosclerosis and eye cataracts, and usually die in their early teens.

Different species of animals age at very different rates. A fruit fly is old at 2 weeks, a mouse at 1.5 years, a dog at about 13 years, a horse at 25 years, and a human at 70 years. Since each animal species seems to have a fixed maximum life span, it is reasonable to assume that there must be a biological aging clock. In the same way that all biological functions are ultimately regulated by the genetic information in cells, it is reasonable to suppose that the cells' genetic information also causes cells to age in a predetermined way for each species.

Evidence supporting the idea of a "cellular aging clock" comes from studies in which cells from different animals are grown *in vitro* (in glass dishes or test tubes) to determine how long cells from different animal species can continue to grow and

---

BOX 24-2

THE OSTEOPOROSIS CONTROVERSY

Recent medical studies indicate that a substantial number of postmenopausal women suffer from **osteoporosis,** a process that results in bone loss such that remaining bone becomes thin, porous, and brittle. This brittleness in turn leads to the bones fracturing under the least bit of stress. It is estimated that of about 6 million spontaneous fractures occurring in the United States each year, approximately 5 million occur in postmenopausal women.

Osteoporosis, while technically not a disease, begins when the rate of bone breakdown exceeds the ability of the body to make new bone. Because bone formation is strongly dependent on adequate dietary calcium, if the body's stores of calcium are depleted or insufficient, bone repair and bone replacement are hindered. Thus, the level of calcium in the blood appears to play an important role in osteoporosis.

The osteoporosis controversy is over what to do about bone loss, especially in older women who are its major victims. The medical establishment and the drug companies support the view that decreased estrogen production after menopause is the primary cause of osteoporosis. They recommend long-term maintenance doses of estrogen or a combination of estrogen and progestogen hormone therapy. Women's groups such as the National Women's Health Network believe that estrogen therapy for osteoporosis creates unwarranted risks for the development of cancer and other diseases. They think that women are being victimized by the medical-pharmaceutical industry because of the enormous profits that are to be made from the prescribing of hormones to millions of women.

Many women and health professionals argue that osteoporosis can be prevented by improved nutrition and by implementation of healthy lifestyles, which include regular exercise and minimal use of tobacco and alcohol. A sound nutritional approach to the prevention of osteoporosis would seem to be more prudent than lifelong estrogen therapy. Increased consumption of foods rich in calcium such as hard cheeses, milk, and yogurt, is recommended. Diet supplementation with calcium carbonate is also helpful in preventing osteoporosis. Adequate amounts of vitamin D are essential to bone formation, but excess phosphorus in the diet should be avoided as it encourages bone loss by reducing the supply of calcium.

---

divide. Table 24-1 shows that the greater the maximum life span for a species, the greater the number of divisions a cell will undergo before growth stops. These data suggest that the cells in the body may be biologically programmed to grow and divide for a certain number of generations and then lose capacity for further growth. It is interesting to note that aging and death are characteristic of normal cells. Cancer cells can grow indefinitely *in vitro* and so have lost the capacity to age. Cancer cells also exhibit chromosomal changes and other changes in the expression of genetic information (see Chapter 17).

Other hypotheses about aging propose that it occurs as the result of accumulated genetic and cellular damage. For example, the longer you live, the more radiation and chemicals your body is exposed to, and eventually some essential cellular functions may be damaged. Human cells possess a variety of enzymes that can repair damage to chromosomes and other vital cellular structures. If one or more of these enzymes were to become defective, it is possible that accumulated genetic and cellular damage could not be repaired and that essential cellular functions would begin to fail. This has been called the "error catastrophe" hypothesis. Damage to cellular genetic information by mutation may be one of the causes of the aging process.

Nobel-prize-winning immunologist F. M. Burnet (1976) has proposed that the decline in immune system functioning may play the key role in the aging process, perhaps because the production of immune

Table 24-1

Generations of Growth of Embryonic Cells from Different Animals

Species	Approximate number of cell doublings	Approximate maximum life span (years)
Galapagos turtle	108 ± 18	175
Human	50 ± 10	110
Chicken	25 ± 10	30
Mouse	21 ± 7	3.5

Data from Leonard Hayflick, "The Cell Biology of Human Aging," *New England Journal of Medicine* (December 2, 1976), p. 1302.

cells is particularly sensitive to mutational damage. As pointed out in Chapter 9, a decline in the functioning of the immune system results in increased susceptibility to all kinds of disease, including atherosclerosis and cancer, because the body can no longer recognize and eliminate damaged cells efficiently. In addition, autoimmune diseases, such as some forms of arthritis, are more common in older people.

The thymus gland plays an important (although little understood) role in the production of immunologically competent cells. As people grow older, the thymus gland atrophies and the production of one of its hormones, **thymosin,** declines markedly (see Figure 24-6). The significance of the age-related decrease in thymus-dependent immunity on the normal aging process has yet to be determined, but it may be that the thymus gland regulates the biological aging clock.

The most that can be said for all the hypotheses and guesses about aging is that it results from multiple internal and external factors that interact in a complex way and that vary from person to person. There is no cure for aging. Neither is there any scientific breakthrough lurking on the horizon that will be able to prevent normal human aging or death. What all persons should strive for is the retention of their mental and physical health throughout all stages of life.

It is interesting to calculate what the maximum human life span would be if all the major diseases and disease-related causes of death were to be eliminated (see Table 24-2). If *all* forms of vascular and heart disease were to disappear from our society, people could expect to live, on the average, an additional 18 years. People would still die, of course, but more and more people would live longer. More surprising is the relatively small gain in maximum life

Figure 24-6

Atrophy of the thymus gland with age and the decrease in production of the hormone thymosin. (Data from A. L. Goldstein et al., in A. Cherkin, ed., *Physiology and Cell Biology of Aging,* Vol. 8, 1979. Used by permission of Raven Press, New York.)

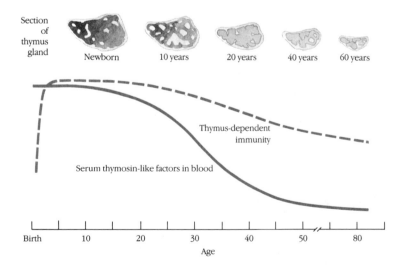

Table 24-2
Gain in Life Expectancy If Various Causes of Death Were Eliminated

Cause of Death	Gain in expectation of life if cause were eliminated (years)	
	At birth	At age 65
Major cardiovascular-renal diseases	10.9	10.0
Heart diseases	5.9	4.9
Vascular diseases affecting central nervous system	1.3	1.2
Malignant neoplasms	2.3	1.2
Accidents, excluding those caused by motor vehicles	0.6	0.1
Motor-vehicle accidents	0.6	0.1
Influenza and pneumonia	0.5	0.2
Infectious diseases (excluding tuberculosis)	0.2	0.1
Diabetes mellitus	0.2	0.2
Tuberculosis	0.1	0.0

Data from life tables published by National Center of Health Statistics. U.S. Public Health Service & U.S. Bureau of Census, "Some Demographic Aspects of Aging in the United States," February 1973.

expectancy that would result from the conquest of cancer or diabetes. If cancer were to be conquered, only about 2 years would be added to the average human life span, while a cure for diabetes would add only 2 or 3 months.

There is much more to the prevention or elimination of disease, however, than merely extending the human life span by a few months or years. The relief of human suffering, improvement in the quality of life, and a reduction in the cost of hospital and medical care are but a few of the important consequences of disease prevention or disease cure. The absolute number of years of life is not nearly so important as the capacity to live actively, joyfully, and creatively for all the years of life, however many they may be.

Charlie Smith, who in 1972 was officially recognized as the oldest person in the United States, worked on a citrus farm until he was 113. He then worked in a store in Barstow, Florida, until he was 133, when he officially retired. Charlie Smith died of "old age" at 137. When asked for the secret to his longevity Smith replied, "I smoked, I drank, I chased women. If I'd known I was going to live so long, I'd have taken better care of myself."

Fear of Aging

When people are young, they rarely think about getting old. In their teens and twenties, many individuals think of anyone over the age of 40 as old.

Young people expect old people to act, think, and live differently. Old people are "straight." Old people don't have fun. Old people are serious and cranky. Old people don't enjoy sex. Old people are always talking about how things used to be in the good old days.

As pointed out earlier in this chapter, our society holds many false ideas about aging and about old people. Old age has been a subject people avoid talking about, yet nearly everybody has fears and worries about what it is like to grow old. Most young people see old age as a time of becoming physically unattractive, of losing sexual vigor, and of becoming mentally dull. Rarely do you see a TV or magazine advertisement showing old people displaying sexual desires or even showing physical love or affection.

Many drug advertisements that appear in the medical journals emphasize the distressful conditions and debilities of being old. Old people are portrayed as apathetic, disturbed, confused, disruptive, insecure, temperamental, or out of control. Naturally, the advertisements promote the use of drugs to relieve all of these symptoms. Other TV, newspaper, and magazine advertisements urge people to use cosmetics, face-lifts, vitamins, and rejuvenating elixirs to stop or reverse the aging process. It is small wonder that most people are afraid of becoming old. Most people do not look forward to old age positively or optimistically because their minds have been programmed since childhood with negative attitudes and fears of aging.

> I don't believe in aging.
> I believe in forever altering
> one's aspect to the sun.
> **Virginia Woolf**

Fear of aging can cause many aging problems and the anxieties and stress may hasten the aging process itself. Some people look much older than their years, while others seem to age very little. A few of the many fears people associate with aging

Figure 24-7
Reported current sexual activity in Americans age 50 and older. (Data from Edward Brecher, *Love, Sex and Aging,* Boston: Little, Brown, 1984.

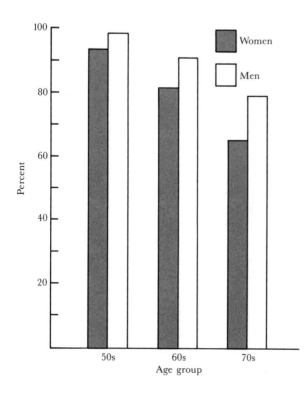

are ill health, poverty, being attacked or victimized, falling or being hurt while alone, loss of dignity, failure of memory, and sexual inadequacy. Most of the fears of old age are not well founded. For example, very few old people live in institutions—only about 4 percent of all those over the age of 65. Old people have about half as many acute illnesses as young people, although they do suffer from more chronic relatively minor health problems.

As for the fear of loss of sexual capacities, gerontologist Alex Comfort (1976) states categorically, "In the absence of two disabilities—actual disease and the *belief* that the old are or should be asexual—sexual requirement and sexual capacity are lifelong" (see Figure 24-7).

Another fear perpetuated by myth and misunderstanding is that of senility. Old people can become emotionally disturbed and depressed by problems, as can anybody else. Because of dissatisfaction with their lives, many older people turn to alcohol and medications for relief of their emotional distress. Old people are often the victims of addicting drugs prescribed by doctors to sedate and tranquilize them so that they won't be a bother. Thirty percent of all prescriptions written by physicians are for people 65 and older (Thompson et al., 1983). Peter Bourne (1979), former director of the President's Office of Drug Abuse, points out that

not only do older people take a disproportionate percentage of manufactured drugs, they are also more physically susceptible to their effects than younger people. They are

> As a society, how much are we willing to spend (sacrifice) to prolong life? The easy answer is any amount, but that answer is neither true nor feasible.
>
> **Lester Carl Thurow**
> **Professor, Massachusetts Institute of Technology**

less capable of metabolizing most drugs and more susceptible to direct, side, and interactional effects of drugs. Nearly one-fifth of the patients entering the geriatric service of one general hospital displayed disorders directly attributable to the effects of prescribed drugs. Most often this is due to a failure to recognize that many older people require smaller quantities of most drugs and hence are prescribed amounts in excess of their needs.

Of even more concern is the prescribing of drugs for elderly people confined to nursing homes. Often medication is not given to benefit the patients but to keep them subdued so that they create a minimum of disturbance for the staff. The rights of patients in nursing and convalescent facilities have been established by the U.S. Social Security Administration. These rules require that all patients be informed of their rights and privileges.

People should not accept the unwarranted notion that their intellectual faculties must deteriorate with age. As long as life is stimulating, as long as you remain curious and eager to enter each day, and as long as general good health persists, your mental faculties will remain intact.

Alzheimer's Disease and Senile Dementia

Approximately 15 percent of people over age 65 have some loss in cognitive functioning—what is medically referred to as **senile** (associated with aging)

dementia (loss or impairment of mental powers). About half of these individuals have a particular type of disorder called **Alzheimer's disease,** a condition characterized by progressive loss of many cognitive functions, including memory, use of language, perception, learning ability, problem-solving ability, and the ability to make judgments.

The disease is named for Alois Alzheimer, a German physician who in 1907 first described abnormal microscopic structures in the brain tissue of women who died of senile dementia. Alzheimer's findings at autopsy revealed what are still the diagnostic criteria for the disease: (1) the presence of bundles of tangled fibrils in certain nerve cells, (2) the presence of a specific protein (amyloid protein) concentrated in abnormal structures called neuritic plaques, and (3) the presence of amyloid protein in blood vessels of the brain. Alzheimer's disease is also associated with loss of a neurotransmitter, acetylcholine, in certain areas of the brain. How all these changes affect brain function or how they are involved in the disease process are unknown.

Some evidence suggests that developing Alzheimer's disease in old age is hereditarily determined to some degree. This idea is supported by the recent isolation of a gene on human chromosome 21 that codes for the synthesis of the amyloid protein. However, since presumably everyone has the gene but only a small number of people develop Alzheimer's disease, other factors must be involved. Some of the environmental factors that have been suggested as "triggering" agents for the disease are accumulation of aluminum or silicon in brain tissue, infection by a special class of viruses, or severe head injury.

As yet there is no treatment or cure for Alzheimer's disease. Depending on the severity of the illness, afflicted individuals, who currently number about two million, may require support and care that exceed the personal and financial resources of their families. About one-fourth of patients in nursing homes suffer from Alzheimer's and the cost to society is estimated at $10–$20 billion annually. People are living longer. The fastest growing segment of the U.S. population is the post-70-year-olds, the group at highest risk for Alzheimer's disease. Because the "graying of America" is likely to continue, treatments for this disease are urgently needed.

Death and Dying

Fear of the unknown invariably produces anxiety in people. Entering into a new relationship, traveling to a foreign country, starting a new job, leaving home, or thinking about death—all involve movement into the unfamiliar and create apprehension and stress (the health consequences of stress are discussed in Chapter 11). Most people fear serious illness and death. Many deal with their fears by ignoring them or by pretending that death is something that only happens to other people. Avoidance of contemplating death, which, after all, is the inevitable natural consequence of living, only makes the fear worse when death becomes imminent. Just as they become more comfortable after having been in a foreign country or in an unfamiliar place for a while, people can become comfortable with the ideas of dying and of their own death by facing their fears.

Elisabeth Kübler-Ross (1969), a noted physician, has devoted years to talking and working with patients who are dying and who are trying to come to grips with the reality that they soon will cease to exist in the world. Kübler-Ross herself has spent countless hours discussing and thinking about death and dying. She writes about the origins of the fear of death:

> The ancient Hebrews regarded the body of a dead person as something unclean and not to be touched. The early American Indians talked about the evil spirits and shot arrows in the air to drive the spirits away. Many other cultures have rituals to take care of the "bad" dead person, and they all originate in this feeling of anger which still

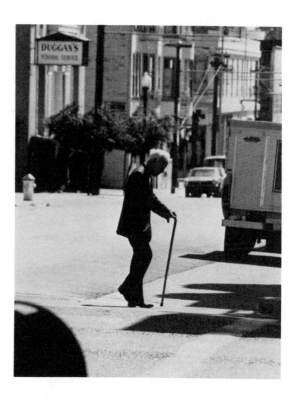

exists in all of us, though we dislike admitting it.

People have many different attitudes towards dying. Most people, however, generally go through a number of stages after being told that they have an incurable disease or are going to die soon. Kübler-Ross has observed and described five distinct stages in the process of dying: (1) denial and isolation, (2) anger, (3) bargaining, (4) depression, and (5) acceptance. Not all people go through all these stages. Neither do all people come to accept their death.

Almost everyone would like to live a full, active, satisfying life right up to the moment of death. Still, some people will experience lingering illnesses consisting of a prolonged period of disability, suffering and dependence on others for many physical and emotional needs. Modern medicine and scientific technologies often have the means to prolong life beyond the point when the dying person is able to function or can responsibly guide the course of his or her own life. The use of extreme medical measures to sustain and prolong life is defended by some people and decried by others (Wanzer, 1984). Some physicians and patients are beginning to openly discuss the ethical dilemmas surrounding the decision of allowing a debilitated aged person to die.

> Death is no threat
> to people who are
> not afraid to die.
> **Lao-tzu**

Dr. David Hilfiker (1983) expresses the distress many physicians feel:

> We have been forced into the role of God, yet we hardly seem to have recognized it. For my part, the underlying irrationality of my decisions has gnawed at me; the life-and-death importance of my actions has kept me awake at night; the guilt and depression of never really knowing whether I have acted properly have been overwhelming.

Some people are more concerned about the quality of their lives and are less concerned about its duration. For these people it is not how long they live that matters but rather *how* they live. These people do not want to lose control over their lives. Neither do they want to let other people make decisions about whether they should live or die. Such people may decide to fill out a living will and carry it with them (see Figure 24-8). This document conveys to physicians and family their wishes with regard to the medical measures they wish to be taken in case they are seriously incapacitated and unable to participate in decisions concerning their health and survival.

There are many ways to deal with the fears and insecurities associated with the idea of one's death. Many people turn to their religious beliefs for comfort and as a source of inner strength. Many people find the concept of returning to God or to a state of bliss and peace a source of great solace, especially after a life of struggle and suffering. Other people believe in reincarnation or some form of life after death, which allows them to see a continuity to their existence. What follows death is beyond the realm of scientific investigation yet is something that all people think about. Eventually people come to a decision about it that feels right for them.

Elisabeth Kübler-Ross (1975) writes and lectures widely on issues related to death and dying. She expresses her personal view of death in the following way:

> There is no need to be afraid of death. It is not the end of the physical body that should worry us. Rather, our concern must be to *live* while we're alive — to release our inner selves from the spiritual death that comes with living behind a facade designed to conform to external definitions of who and what we are. . . . It is the denial of death that is partially responsible for people living empty, purposeless lives; for when you live as if you'll live forever, it becomes too easy to postpone the things you know that you must do.

Because questions about death and dying make us feel uncomfortable, most people will defer thinking about such issues until they are forced to. Yet you may have no deep inner peace until you do confront and resolve your feelings about death. Because death is a part of life, you are not completely free to fully enjoy life until you deal with the reality of

---

A LIVING WILL

TO MY FAMILY, MY PHYSICIAN, MY LAWYER, MY CLERGYMAN
TO ANY MEDICAL FACILITY IN WHOSE CARE I HAPPEN TO BE
TO ANY INDIVIDUAL WHO MAY BECOME RESPONSIBLE FOR MY
HEALTH, WELFARE OR AFFAIRS

Death is as much a reality as birth, growth, maturity and old age—it is the one certainty of life. If the time comes when I, _____, can no longer take part in decisions for my own future, let this statement stand as an expression of my wishes, while I am still of sound mind.

If the situation should arise in which there is no reasonable expectation of my recovery from physical or mental disability, I request that I be allowed to die and not be kept alive by artificial means or "heroic measures." I do not fear death itself as much as the indignities of deterioration, dependence, and hopeless pain. I, therefore, ask that medication be mercifully administered to me to alleviate suffering even though this may hasten the moment of death.

This request is made after careful consideration. I hope you who care for me will be morally bound to follow its mandate. I recognize that this appears to place a heavy responsibility on you, but it is with the intention of relieving you of such responsibility and of placing it upon myself in accordance with my strong convictions, that this statement is made.

Date_____   Signed _____

Witness _____   Witness _____

Copies of this request have been given to:

_____   _____

_____   _____

Figure 24-8
Some states have passed laws ensuring the legality of living wills such as this one.

your own death. The removal of fear—any fear, but especially the fear of death—can powerfully enhance your health and enjoyment of life.

The Hospice Movement

The term **hospice** was originally applied to Christian hospitals set up to care for the poor, the aged, and the sick, as well as to provide refuge for people on religious pilgrimages. Providing physical necessities, medical care, and spiritual comfort was the primary goal of the early religious hospices.

Today, there is a growing hospice movement (about 1200 facilities in the U.S.) that is organized to provide extended care for a dying person and his or her immediate family. The goals of the hospice staff are to meet the total health needs—physical, psychological, and spiritual—of the patient who has only weeks or months to live. Medications are given to ease pain and suffering—not to cure. If possible, the patient is attended to and allowed to die at home in familiar surroundings. Patients requiring additional care may spend their last days in the hospice itself. The companionship of family, children, and pets is encouraged. Patients are encouraged to en-

> The hour of departure has arrived and we go our
> ways—I to die and you to live. Which is better,
> God only knows.
>
> **Socrates**

gage in activities. The atmosphere in the hospice is positive, warm, cheerful, and supportive.

With almost 800,000 cancer cases diagnosed annually in the United States, many of which are terminal illnesses, the need for hospices is growing. Hospitals provide space while a patient is being treated and while there is still the possibility of a cure. Nursing homes provide care for the elderly and for people recuperating from illnesses. However, people in the last stages of their life have special needs and need special attention. Edward Dobihal

(1974), chairperson of Hospice, Inc., states that "hospice means a community of people with a common goal—to care for travelers on the way. We chose the name because it is most appropriate for the person resting and finding refreshment and renewal in concluding the journey of life."

Hospice care provides for the spiritual as well as the medical needs of the terminally ill. Death with dignity and family support should be provided to all those who choose to experience their death in this fashion.

 ## Supplemental Readings

DuBois, Paul M. *The Hospice Way of Death.* New York: Human Sciences Press, 1980. Describes the growth of the hospice movement in the United States.

Fettner, A. G., and **Weintraub, P.** "Elixirs of Youth." *Omni,* October 1986. A pop version of what researchers are cooking up so that we can stay young.

Hilfiker, D. "Allowing the Debilitated to Die." *New England Journal of Medicine,* 308 (1983), 716. A physician's honest statement concerning the agony of making life-or-death medical decisions for the aged.

Levine, Stephen. *Who Dies? An Investigation of Conscious Living and Conscious Dying.* New York: Anchor Books, 1982. A sensitive discussion of how to die with dignity and awareness.

Masters, W. H. "Sex and Aging—Expectations and Reality." *Hospital Practice,* August 15, 1986. A report from a famous sex expert on the changes that occur in sexual functions as we get older.

Rowe, J. W., and **Kahn, R. L.** "Human Aging: Usual and Successful." *Science,* July 10, 1987. Discusses recent research on aging and makes recommendations on how to age successfully.

"Why We Age Differently." *Newsweek,* October 20, 1986. Discusses the social and psychological factors that affect how we age.

Wurtman, Richard J. "Alzheimer's Disease." *Scientific American,* January 1985. Describes what is known and unknown about this disease.

Summary

Aging and dying are natural stages of living that all people will experience. By facing fears and worries concerning aging and dying, individuals are able to live more healthful and satisfying lives. People should strive to remain physically, emotionally, and sexually active throughout their lives.

Although there are physiological changes that occur as a consequence of the aging process, they need not be incapacitating or debilitating. Many people's fears of aging are encouraged by movies, TV, and advertising. Old people tend to be over-medicated for problems that might be eliminated by an improvement in relationships and in the living environment. If people think young, they may re-main young in spirit and may actually retard the bi-ological processes of aging.

Death is an experience that every person even-tually faces. People experience their dying in a ser-ies of stages: denial, anger, bargaining, depression, and acceptance. A living will can ensure that a per-son is not kept alive beyond the point where all con-trol over living is lost. The most important aspect of coping with aging and dying is confronting and eliminating fear. Hospices provide an alternative way of dying for people with terminal illnesses, in which death can be experienced with dignity and with the spiritual support of family and friends.

FOR YOUR HEALTH

Here are some suggestions for helping you examine how you think and feel about aging and dying.

1. Can you remember the death of a close friend or relative? What were your thoughts and feelings at the time? Were you confused, sad, fright-ened, angry? What are your feelings now about that person's death? Ask yourself why feelings change with the passage of time. Is it possible that your own feelings about dying will change as you become older?

2. Make a list of all the things that con-cern you the most when you think about becoming old and dying. For example, are you afraid of becoming sexually inactive, of losing physical vigor, of becoming unattractive, of possible pain and suffering, and so on? After you have made your list, think about each item in an objective manner. Are such fears realistic or have you been *taught* to fear some of things on your list?

3. Examine your beliefs and fears con-cerning death. Were these beliefs programmed into your mind by par-ents, teachers, and religious training? For example, do you believe in hell or punishment after death because of personal knowledge or because you were taught that such things exist? If such ideas cause you anxiety, perhaps you can find ways to dispel such no-tions from your mind.

Seeking Help

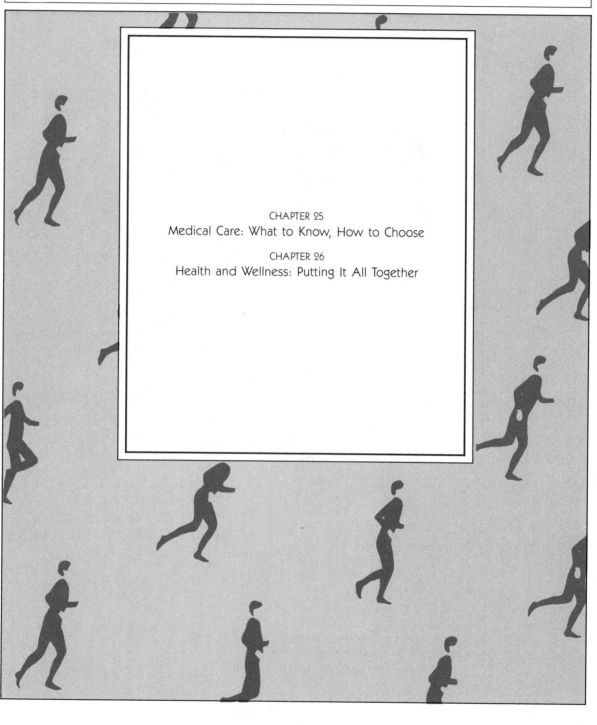

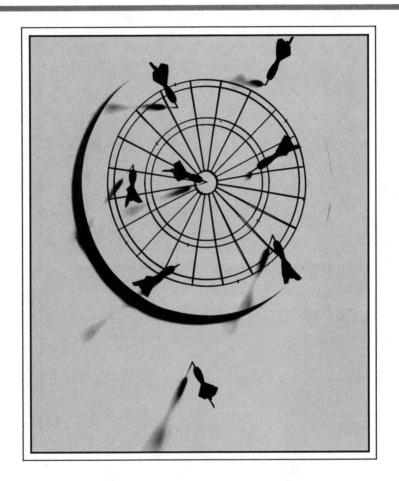

CHAPTER TWENTY-FIVE

The best medical care comes from a
knowledgeable and informed
consumer.

Medical Care: What to Know, How to Choose

The secret of the care of the patient is caring for the patient.

Francis Peabody

Everyone needs medical care at some time or another. People need to go to a physician for vaccinations, checkups, and advice and healing help when they feel sick. Sometimes people need to be hospitalized for a serious illness, for diagnostic tests, or for surgery.

It is generally conceded that medical care in the United States is of the highest quality, perhaps higher than anywhere else in the world. But increasing numbers of people in this country—perhaps as many as half according to some surveys—are dissatisfied with the medical care they receive. Even if their original complaint has been taken care of, many may complain later about how poorly they were treated by hospital personnel, how much they suffered, all the things that were wrong with the treatment, and how much they were overcharged for services.

One of the reasons for the many criticisms of the medical care people receive is that few people have a complete understanding of what the medical profession, and their physicians in particular, can or cannot do for them. Although most people expect a doctor or hospital to "fix them up," they nevertheless enter a physician's office or a hospital with considerable apprehension because they do not know what to expect. Neither do they know how to find out. Too often, people know little or nothing of their rights and responsibilities as patients or how to aid their own healing processes.

Surely most medical professionals care deeply about helping the sick and the infirm. Yet, as with any service, the quality of medical care can vary. The wise consumer of medical care finds out the risks and benefits of a particular diagnostic test, treatment, or surgery before accepting it. Understanding your rights as a patient and learning how to communicate your concerns to the health professionals whose services you seek can help ensure that you receive quality medical care.

This chapter discusses aspects of seeking medical care that we hope will help you receive the kind of care you desire and need.

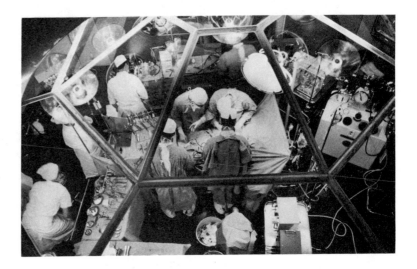

Figure 25-1
Examples of extremes in medical care.
(*Left*) Open-heart surgery being
performed by a team of medical
experts in a modern hospital. (*Right*)
What surgery is like in an African
village. (Courtesy World Health
Organization.)

Some Problems with Modern Medical Care

The following discussion focuses on some of the problems of modern medical care so that as a consumer of that care you will be able to select services that help maintain your health and that most effectively heal you when you become sick.

Underemphasis of Disease Prevention and Wellness

Many physicians and critics of the U.S. medical care system believe that conventional medical care in the United States needs to be radically changed. Perhaps the most outspoken and harshest critic of medical care is Ivan Illich (1976). The analysis of the present U.S. medical care system, presented in his book *Medical Nemesis,* begins with the statement: "The medical establishment has become a major threat to health." Some consider this an extreme position, but other voices of criticism have been raised. Physician Steven Jonas' (1978) view of the problems of medical care in the United States is: "The most important failing of the health care delivery system is failing to prevent preventable disease." And Arnold S. Relman (1987), editor of *New England Journal of Medicine,* has said: "It is a paradox of health care in the U.S. that even as it is becoming ever more sophisticated, it is also becoming ever more inequitable."

To a considerable degree, the problems of modern medical care are the result of adverse doctor-patient relationships. Patients and doctors are both aware of the problems, but solutions are not readily apparent. In a recent article advocating a more humanistic approach in the education of physicians, Richard Gorlin and Howard Zucker (1983), who work at the Mount Sinai Medical Center, point out:

> Something has gone wrong in the practice
> of medicine, and we all know it. It is ironic
> that in this era, dominated by technical
> prowess and rapid biomedical advances, pa-
> tient and physician each feels increasingly
> rejected by the other. . . . High technology
> tends to dehumanize care, and third-party
> regulations, paperwork, and malpractice
> threats distract the doctor.

Because of the many problems associated with medical care, it behooves each person to understand how to prevent diseases and how to best use the medical care system when it is needed.

For the most part, today's physicians are not trained to deal with disease prevention and the promotion of wellness. For example, traditionally, medical students have learned little about the relation of nutrition to disease prevention and wellness, although that situation is now changing. Unfortunately, nearly all of the physicians in practice today did not receive adequate nutrition education when they were in medical school. The same holds

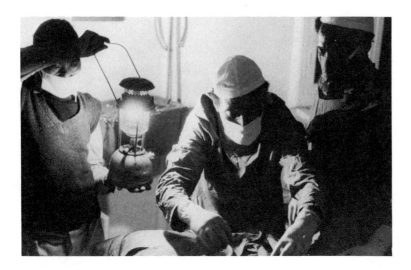

true for the psychological and social aspects of disease. As we discussed in Chapter 2, psychological factors are often the most important in the attainment of wellness and in the healing of illness.

Scientific medical care began with the teachings of the ancient Greek physician Hippocrates, and the practice of medicine still tries to adhere to the principles of Hippocrates as codified in the **Hippocratic Oath**. These principles can be summarized as:

1. Human health and well-being is affected by all environmental factors—the quality of food, air, water, living conditions, and social interactions. Understanding the effects of the environment on human health is the fundamental basis of the art of healing.

2. Health results from a harmonious interaction between the person and the environment. The Greeks thought of this harmonious balance as dependent on the four basic humors—blood, phlegm, yellow bile, and black bile. The ancient Chinese expressed the need for harmony as a balance between Yin-Yang forces. Today we would say that achieving a harmonious balance depends on emotional and spiritual health.

3. The mind affects the body's functions and the health of the body influences the mind. Mind and body are inseparable and health depends on proper functioning of both.

4. The physician should utilize rational therapies to restore a harmonious balance to the mind and body. Above all, the practice of medicine implies a reverence for the human condition and must be based on strict moral and ethical conduct.

It is apparent from these Hippocratic principles that the practice of medicine is both a science and an art. Nowadays, there is increasing emphasis in medical education and in governmental health agencies on preventive medicine and on alternatives to conventional health care such as are embodied in the ideas of holistic medicine. These include adopting some simple health habits, improved nutrition, stress reduction, more physical activity, and increased self-responsibility for one's health. Some insurance companies have even incorporated premium reductions and other financial incentives in their health plans for people who reduce their need for medical care.

A report issued by the U.S. Surgeon General (1979) concluded that "improvements in the health of the American people can and will be achieved—not alone through increased medical care and greater health expenditures—but through a renewed national commitment to efforts designed to prevent disease and promote health." It is likely that physicians in training today will adopt more preventive and health-oriented attitudes, which in turn will contribute to the improvement of the health of the population.

> ### God heals, and the Doctor takes the fee.
> **Ben Franklin, 1744**

High Medical Costs

Traditionally, the medical profession in this country has enjoyed a high degree of public confidence. In 1966, a Harris poll showed that 72 percent of the population had confidence in their physicians. By 1973, however, this number had declined to 57 percent, and the downward trend may be continuing. Part of people's dissatisfaction rests with the dramatic increase in medical care costs in recent years. Physicians' fees have increased sharply, hospital costs have skyrocketed, and the total health costs to the nation are approaching 11 percent of the gross national product. In 1985 that came to $425 billion. Much of the increased cost of medical care comes from expensive diagnostic procedures, joint and hip replacements, and organ transplants (see Table 25-1).

The number of organ transplants performed is limited principally by the availability of organs. The American health care system will soon have to weigh the costs of medical procedures that add a few months or years to an individual's life against other pressing national health problems such as the AIDS epidemic or the rapidly increasing health costs of the aged. The amount of money allotted to health care cannot increase indefinitely.

Technological advances in CAT (computerized axial tomography), NMR (nuclear magnetic resonance), and PET (positron emission tomography) scans are estimated to cost billions of dollars and add significantly to medical care costs as these expensive pieces of equipment are increasingly used for diagnostic purposes. Also, physicians' earnings contribute appreciably to medical costs. In 1986 the average income of U.S. physicians was $120,000, up 6.5 percent from the previous year. In that same year the average income of radiologists rose 17 percent to $168,000.

The questions raised by the costs of medical care are not easily answered. Who is to decide when to transplant an organ or when to let a person die, when to exhaust all diagnostic procedures and when to say enough is enough? Physicians agonize over these questions just as their patients do (Engelhardt, 1984).

Table 25-1
Organ Transplants and Costs in 1984

Organ	Average cost	Number	Potential number
Heart	$100,000	175	10,000
Liver	$135,000	160	5,000
Pancreas	$50,000	200	10,000
Kidney	$40,000	6,000	12,000

> Some patients, though conscious that their condition is perilous, recover their health simply through their contentment with the goodness of the physician.
>
> **Hippocrates**

Disappearance of the Family Physician

Even as the costs of medical care have risen dramatically, people have found it more and more difficult to find a physician that they can consult concerning their everyday health worries, aches, and minor illnesses. This sort of service used to be provided by the family physician, but the general practitioner that most people relied on for advice is almost as threatened by extinction as the whales. And finding general practitioners in poor rural areas or in city slums where they are most needed is even more difficult than finding them in economically affluent regions. For example, New York State has an average of 228 physicians per 100,000 residents, but some sections of New York City have fewer than 50. The state of Mississippi has only 82 physicians per 100,000 residents, and few of those practice in rural areas.

In recent years, a new medical specialty has arisen called family practice, which is an attempt to fill the gap created by the decline in general practitioners. Nurses who assist in family practice clinics are usually referred to as nurse practitioners. Both family practice physicians and nurse practitioners spend much more time than usual in helping patients prevent disease and improve the healthful aspects of their lives. They also devote time to listening to patients' complaints and problems, and many already practice holistic medicine without calling it that. If serious illnesses are detected, patients are referred to specialists for additional diagnostic tests and treatments.

Consumer Misuse of the Medical System

Most people do not realize how much control they have over their own health. Neither are they aware of the many health choices available. Instead, they leave issues of health and wellness in the hands of the doctor. Unfortunately, this attitude leads to considerable overuse and misuse of the medical care system.

Most people who go to a physician have minor complaints or go for a routine checkup or consultation (see Table 25-2). Sidney R. Garfield (1970), founder of the Kaiser Permanente hospitals in California, distinguishes four categories of patients: (1) those who think they are well and go to a physician for confirmation, (2) those who think they are well but actually are sick, (3) those who think they are ill and are, and (4) the "worried well" who are concerned about their health and are seeking reassurance. This last group of patients may constitute 30 to 50 percent of all patients who go to see a physician.

Statistics show that 15 percent of office visits are for a routine consultation or physical exam. Although many physicians still encourage annual checkups, privately they concede that frequent exams for basically healthy people are unnecessary. How often you should see a physician or get a physical checkup is a matter of personal choice and personal responsibility. The National Center for Health Statistics estimates that Americans make approximately 600 million office visits each year. Doctors rate more than half of these visits as "nothing serious," "no problem," or "nonsymptomatic." It is clear

> The time has passed when the American taxpayer
> can promise full coverage of health benefits to
> the victims of known, self-destructive behavior
> without asking some contribution from them.
> **Anne R. Somers, M.D.**

that people are asking for more from their doctors than just medicines.

If people are more actively involved in promoting their own health and wellness rather than delegating that responsibility to physicians, hospitals, or government agencies, it is likely that they would be healthier, medical care costs would decrease, and medical services would improve because physicians would have more time to devote to the healing of serious disease.

Unnecessary Surgery

The United States has about twice as many surgeons per capita as there are in England and Wales, and twice as many operations are performed per capita in this country. In areas of Maine that have the highest number of surgeons, the number of gallbladder operations is more than double the number performed in other parts of the state where there are fewer surgeons. These kinds of data suggest that operations may be recommended to patients for reasons other than necessity for health (Wennberg and Gittelsohn, 1982).

Children are frequently the victims of unnecessary surgery. Studies show that in different areas of Vermont, the rate at which tonsils and adenoids were removed varied between 4 and 41 cases per thousand children—a tenfold difference. The inescapable conclusion is that removal of children's adenoids and tonsils bears little relation to sickness or health but depends on other factors that influence the de-

Table 25-2
The 20 Most Common Complaints, Problems, or Symptoms for Doctor Visits

Rank	Complaint	Number of visits (thousands)	Percent of all visits	Rank	Complaint	Number of visits (thousands)	Percent of all visits
1	Progress visits	75,673	11.7	11	Gynecological exam	13,154	2.0
2	Physical exam	26,117	4.0	12	Visit for medication	13,103	2.0
3	Pain, etc.—lower extremity	25,944	4.0	13	None	13,043	2.0
4	Pregnancy exam	25,942	4.0	14	Headache	12,314	1.9
5	Throat soreness	20,726	3.2	15	Fatigue	11,768	1.8
6	Pain, etc.—upper extremity	18,956	2.9	16	Pain in chest	11,350	1.8
7	Pain, etc.—back region	18,824	2.9	17	Well-baby exam	10,699	1.7
8	Cough	18,347	2.8	18	Fever	9,822	1.5
9	Abdominal pain	16,418	2.5	19	Allergic skin reaction	9,458	1.5
10	Cold	13,460	2.1	20	All other symptoms	279,776	43.7

Data from *Monthly Vital Statistics Report,* July 14, 1975, Supplement 2.

Stay away from doctors and stay out of hospitals.
An extraordinary proportion of the people in
hospitals are quite ill, so obviously they are not
suitable places for people who wish to be well.
Reuel A. Stallones
Dean, Texas School of Public Health

cision of the physician. Leon Eisenberg (1977), professor of psychiatry at Harvard Medical School, is outspoken in his criticism of these operations. He writes:

> Consider, for example, the fact that about 1 million tonsillectomies and adenoidectomies are done each year in the United States; T and A's make up 30 percent of all surgery on children . . . Current mortality has been estimated at one death per 16,000 operations. Yet this procedure (whose origins are lost in antiquity) continues at epidemic rates though there is *no evidence* that it is effective except in a few uncommon conditions.

In the past few years the rate of T and A operations has declined dramatically. However, operations for removal of the prostate, gallbladder, appendix, and uterus are still performed at a high rate and may differ by as much as a factor of four from one area of the country to another. Table 25-3 lists the most common surgical procedures performed in the United States. It is dismaying that the second, third, sixth, ninth, and eleventh most common surgical procedures have to do with the female reproductive system or breasts. Not on this list are about 150,000 cosmetic breast operations that are performed each year.

Many hysterectomies — the surgical removal of all or part of the uterus — are performed for such minor complaints as chronic lower back pain or fear of pregnancy, and the frequency of hysterectomies varies widely in areas of the United States. More than twice as many hysterectomies are performed in the United States as are performed in Great Britain on a per capita basis, yet there is no medical evidence that the uteruses of American women are more diseased than the uteruses of English women. Complete hysterectomies — removal of ovaries and uterus — are still the most frequent major surgical procedure in this country.

Even the delivery of babies has become increasingly a surgical matter. In 1984 approximately one baby in five was delivered by cesarean section, more

Table 25-3
The Most Common Surgical Procedures in the United States (1975)*

1. Biopsy (microscopic examination of a small piece of tissue — most often to detect cancer cells).
2. Dilation and scraping of the uterus.
3. Hysterectomy (removal of the uterus).
4. Tonsillectomy (removal of the tonsils).
5. Repair of hernia in the groin.
6. Removal of the ovaries.
7. Removal of the gall bladder.
8. Dental surgery.
9. Female sterilization.
10. Repair of muscles and tendons.
11. Removal of a breast.

*Data exclude delivery of babies or circumcision.

Data from Steven Jonas, *Medical Mystery* (New York: W. W. Norton, 1978), p. 106.

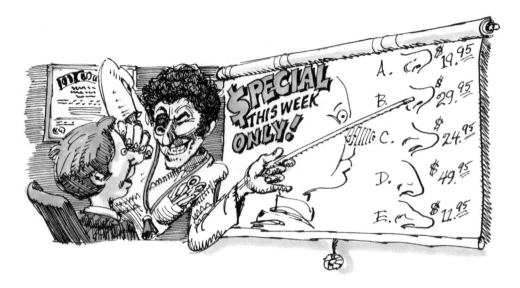

than in any other industrialized country. In Japan about one baby in twelve is delivered by cesarean section. Authors Nancy Cohen and Lois Estner (1983) believe most cesarean deliveries are unnecessary:

> In our culture, women often come to birth frightened, anxious, malnourished, uninformed, and unsupported. . . . We believe that birth is not a medical circumstance. We believe that birth is a safe passage for both mother and child, and that both are fully equipped for the journey.

Liposuction is now the most frequent type of plastic surgery in the United States. Thousands of liposuctions are performed at costs ranging from $500 to $5000. Liposuction is relatively safe (even if costly and unnecessary for health), but another popular operation advertised as a cure for nearsightedness (myopia) is far from safe. **Radial keratotomy** involves cutting the outer lens (cornea) of the eye to flatten it and correct the focusing problem. Since almost all nearsightedness can be corrected with glasses or contact lenses, a surgical procedure that can result in numerous visual complications makes no sense whatsoever. Indeed most ophthalmologists do not recommend it. Why is radial keratotomy becoming popular? As Perry S. Binder, an ophthalmologist at the University of California, San Diego, Medical School sees it: "The practice of medicine today has shifted to one of marketing, not only for radial keratotomy but to all aspects of health-care delivery."

Millions of Americans suffer low back pain every year. Low back pain and upper respiratory infection are the leading causes of absence from work. Until quite recently "ruptured disc" was the usual diagnosis for low back pain and the disc surgery (laminectomy) was recommended. In 1978 almost half a million disc operations were performed. Today bed rest of two to three weeks is advised before surgery is considered. However, a recent study showed that many persons with acute lower back pain were able to return to work after only two days of complete bed rest (Deyo et al., 1986).

Advertising, entrepreneurism, and plain old hustling have pervaded the medical profession. Arnold S. Relman (1985), editor of *New England Journal of Medicine,* describes the problem:

> Practicing physicians now have financial interests in diagnostic laboratories, radiologic imaging centers, walk-in clinics, ambulatory surgery centers, dialysis units, physical therapy centers, and other facilities. In most of these business ventures, the investing physicians' profits depend, at least in part, on referral of patients to these facilities . . .

In this new climate of medical free enterprise, people seeking medical advice and assistance need to be more questioning and cautious in accepting recommended procedures, especially those involving invasive tests or surgery.

We present this view of surgery not to argue that all operations are unnecessary or that surgery is not beneficial. Surgery can save lives. There are many

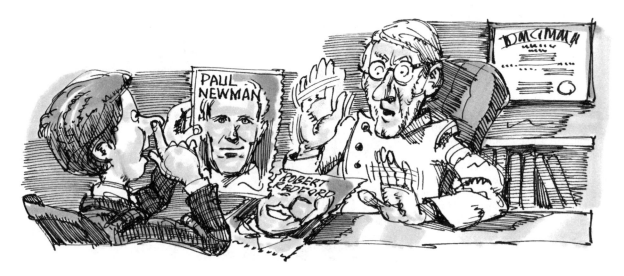

instances where surgery to remove cysts and tumors, to stop internal bleeding, to repair broken bones and torn muscles, and to correct congenital defects is vital to a person's well-being. Removal of an infected appendix before it ruptures or replacement of a defective heart valve can save a person's life. However, wholesale removal of uteruses, tonsils, adenoids, gallbladders, ovaries, breasts, and vertebral disks, without compelling medical reason, must be condemned.

Your body belongs to you. Your well-being is your responsibility. Before allowing some part of your body to be removed, explore all the alternatives. You cannot rely solely on the advice of a particular surgeon. We recommend, whenever possible, that you obtain the advice of at least two physicians before undergoing surgery, especially elective surgery. In fact, many health plans now require a second opinion.

It is important to remember also that the diagnosis and advice you receive from your physician is separate and distinct from any agreement you make regarding treatment. In any illness, there are two important choices to be made: first, realizing that you are ill and finding out what's wrong, which is the diagnostic process; and second, deciding on the best course of treatment after the diagnosis is made. For example, suppose you have had lower back pain for some time, which is diagnosed as a dislocated disk. An orthopedic surgeon might recommend an operation to repair or remove the damaged disks in the vertebrae. A chiropractor might recommend manipulation and exercise. A

practitioner of holistic medicine might recommend medication or relaxation exercises to stretch and strengthen back muscles and perhaps recommend changes in the diet to facilitate weight loss. It is your responsibility to decide on the kind of treatment that is best for your condition and general health.

Diagnosis and Treatment

A physician is trained to diagnose the disease that is causing a patient's symptoms or suffering and to recommend appropriate treatment. Since the nineteenth century, a vast medical technology has arisen to assist the physician in diagnosing disease. At the turn of the century, all a physician had was the thermometer, the stethoscope, and the microscope. On a house call, all the physician's tools could be carried in a little black bag. Today there are x-ray machines, electrocardiographs (ECGs), electroencephalographs (EEGs), devices that can be inserted into every human orifice, hundreds of biochemical tests for blood, sputum, and urine, and even computerized axial tomography machines (see Figure 25-2).

However, this increased dependence of medicine on technology has also decreased the communication and empathy between physician and patient that is essential to the healing process. Increased technology can assist but can never replace the physician's own medical judgment and intuition. Andrew Weil (1983), a physician who has explored and written about the usefulness of alternative therapies

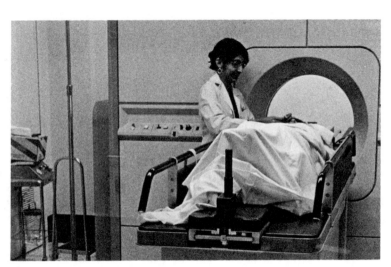

Figure 25-2

(*Left*) A patient being examined by computerized axial tomography (CAT). (*Right*) The CAT display for this patient's brain scan. The computer integrates a series of x-ray exposures of the head so that doctors can examine the brain from many angles. Tumors, broken blood vessels, and other brain abnormalities can be detected. (Courtesy Mount Zion Hospital and Medical Center, San Francisco.)

and the shortcomings of traditional medicine as it is practiced today, describes the true art of medicine as "the ability of a practitioner to select and present to individual patients those treatments most likely to elicit healing from within."

It could be argued that medicine could not be practiced at the high level of competence upheld in this country without sophisticated instrumentation and laboratory tests. However, an alternate view is provided by a diagnosis made by a Buddhist physician and priest, Yeshe Dhonden, while visiting an American hospital. Richard Selzer, himself a renowned surgeon, decribes in Box 25-1 how this remarkable diagnosis was made without laboratory tests or modern technology.

It's true that we live in a different culture and a different place from that in which Buddhist physicians practice. Yet, it is also important to remember that the practice of medicine at the highest level of competence involves not only knowledge of science and technology but utilization of human sensitivity and intuition as well.

Even if one acknowledges that diagnosis of disease is as much an art as it is a science, what about the treatment or cure that is recommended? Is it necessary for physicians to rely almost exclusively on drugs and surgery to effect a cure? A physician can assist and initiate the healing process, but it is the person's mind and body that does the healing, that repairs tissues, organs, and bones. A surgeon can set a broken bone, but it is the person's own internal healing processes that mend the break. One person might be able to mend the bone and tissue completely in 2 weeks, whereas another person might require 2 months. You can encourage heal-

ing by developing, in your mind, images of healthy tissues being formed. As described in Chapter 2, positive thoughts, the use of mental imagery, and freedom from anxiety are invaluable aids in healing.

The Buddhist priest Chogyam Trungpa (1977) carries these ideas even further and believes that

the role of the doctor is to cut through your tendency to see disease as an external threat, and not just to cure you. By providing companionship and some kind of sympathy, the doctor creates a suggestion of health or underlying sanity that tends to undermine our naive conception of disease. It is not the sickness that is the big problem, but the psychological state behind it, which must be cured.

Self-healing is important even in the case of infectious diseases. The physician may prescribe an antibiotic for strep throat or gonorrhea that will destroy most of the bacteria. But the final cure—the removal of all pathogenic organisms and the repair of tissue—is accomplished by the person's mind and body. In the introduction to his book *The Healer's Art,* Eric Cassell (1976) vividly describes how he came to learn about self-healing:

Many years ago, while in residency training at Bellevue Hospital in New York City, I had a midnight call from the psychiatric ward: an old woman was having difficulty breathing. I found the patient gasping for air, her skin blue from lack of oxygen; she had full-blown pulmonary edema (water in the lungs) resulting from a blood clot in her

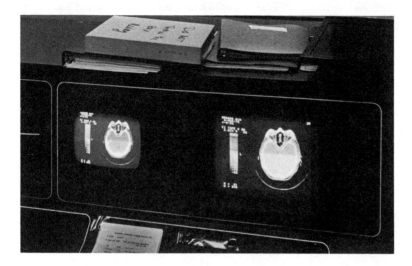

lung. I stood at the bedside feeling impotent, but the old woman's face and her distress pleaded for help. So I began to talk calmly but incessantly, telling her why she had the tightness in her chest and explaining how the water would slowly recede from her lungs, after which her breathing would begin to ease bit by bit and she would gradually feel much better. To my utter amazement that is precisely what happened.

What all of us need to understand as patients, and what the essential point of this chapter really is, is how to actively participate in your own healing process when you are sick and need medical help. You need to understand how to assist in the healing process to make any treatment that may be undertaken more effective.

The Office Visit

About 80 percent of all health care visits are to physicians in private practice. Clearly, a lot of people's satisfaction or dissatisfaction with their medical care occurs in the physician's office. The quality of medical care depends in large measure on the interaction that takes place between the physician and patient. You can greatly increase the chances of a positive result of your encounter with your physician if you have a clear understanding of what you want from the visit, how to help with the diagnosis and treatment, how to communicate effectively, and how to remain positive through the entire medical procedure.

Many medical observers have pointed out that poor communication and misunderstanding between physician and patient are causes for mutual dissatisfaction. A study of the various concerns voiced by patients and physicians (see Box 25-2) shows how stressful and unhealthy a visit to a physician's office may be to a patient, as well as being disturbing to the physician. Here are some guidelines to keep in mind the next time you have to go to a physician's office or to a hospital.

1. The physician you choose should be someone you trust and in whose medical skills and advice you have complete confidence. Don't choose a physician you don't like or who makes you feel uncomfortable. Trust your own judgment and take time in choosing a physician. He or she should be someone in whom you feel you can confide and with whom you can talk honestly and openly regarding your health concerns. Community hospitals are often less frightening than large city, county, or university hospitals and may also be closer to home so friends and family members can visit. Your physician may be able to give you a choice of hospitals.

2. Clear communication between you and the physician is of the highest priority. You should understand what your medical problems are and what the different opinions are in order to make a responsible health decision. You are entitled to *all* the information regarding your condition. Your

BOX 25-1

MEDICAL DIAGNOSIS AS ART

On the bulletin board in the front hall of the hospital where I work, there appeared an announcement. "Yeshi Dhonden," it read, "will make rounds at six o'clock on the morning of June 10." The particulars were then given, followed by a notation: "Yeshi Dhonden is Personal Physician to the Dalai Lama." I am not so leathery a skeptic that I would knowingly ignore an emissary from the gods. Not only might such sangfroid be inimical to one's earthly well-being, it could take care of eternity as well. Thus, on the morning of June 10, I join the clutch of whitecoats waiting in the small conference room adjacent to the ward selected for the rounds. The air in the room is heavy with ill-concealed dubiety and suspicion of bamboozlement. At precisely six o'clock, he materializes, a short, golden, barrelly man dressed in a sleeveless robe of saffron and maroon. His scalp is shaven, and the only visible hair is a scanty black line above each hooded eye.

He bows in greeting while his young interpreter makes the introduction. Yeshi Dhonden, we are told, will examine a patient selected by a member of the staff. The diagnosis is as unknown to Yeshi Dhonden as it is to us. The examination of the patient will take place in our presence, after which we will reconvene in the conference room where Yeshi Dhonden will discuss the case. We are further informed that for the past two hours Yeshi Dhonden has purified himself by bathing, fasting, and prayer. I, having break-fasted well, performed only the most desultory of ablutions, and

given no thought at all to my soul, glance furtively at my fellows. Suddenly, we seem a soiled, uncouth lot.

The patient had been awakened early and told that she was to be examined by a foreign doctor, and had been asked to produce a fresh specimen of urine, so when we enter her room, the woman shows no surprise. She has long ago taken on that mixture of compliance and resignation that is the face of chronic illness. This was to be but another in an endless series of tests and examinations. Yeshi Dhonden steps to the bedside while the rest stand apart, watching. For a long time he gazes at the woman, favoring no part of her body with his eyes, but seeming to fix his glance at a place just above her supine form. I, too, study her. No physical sign nor obvious symptom gives a clue to the nature of her disease.

At last he takes her hand, raising it in both of his own. Now he bends over the bed in a kind of crouching stance, his head drawn down into the collar of his robe. His eyes are closed as he feels for her pulse. In a moment he has found the spot, and for the next half hour he remains thus, suspended above the patient like some exotic golden bird with folded wings, holding the pulse of the woman beneath his fingers, cradling her hand in his. All the power of the man seems to have been drawn down into this one purpose. It is palpation of the pulse raised to the state of ritual. From the foot of the bed, where I stand, it is as though he and the patient have entered a special place of isolation, of apartness, about which a vacancy hovers,

and across which no violation is possible. After a moment the women rests back upon her pillow. From time to time, she raises her head to look at the strange figure above her, then sinks back once more. I cannot see their hands joined in a correspondence that is exclusive, intimate, his fingertips receiving the voice of her sick body through the rhythm and throb she offers at her wrist. All at once I am envious—not of him, not of Yeshi Dhonden for his gift of beauty and holiness, but of her. I want to be held like that, touched so, *received*. And I know that I, who have palpated a hundred thousand pulses, have not felt a single one.

At last Yeshi Dhonden straightens, gently places the woman's hand upon the bed, and steps back. The interpreter produces a small wooden bowl and two sticks. Yeshi Dhonden pours a portion of the urine specimen into the bowl, and proceeds to whip the liquid with the two sticks. This he does for several minutes until a foam is raised. Then, bowing above the bowl, he inhales the odor three times. He sets down the bowl and turns to leave. All this while, he has not uttered a single word. As he nears the door, the woman raises her head and calls out to him in a voice at once urgent and serene. "Thank you, doctor," she says, and touches with her other hand the place he had held on her wrist, as though to recapture something that had visited there. Yeshi Dhonden turns back for a moment to gaze at her, then steps into the corridor. Rounds are at an end.

(Continued on next page.)

BOX 25-1 (Continued)

We are seated once more in the conference room. Yeshi Dhonden speaks now for the first time, in soft Tibetan sounds that I have never heard before. He has barely begun when the young interpreter begins to translate, the two voices continuing in tandem—a bilingual fugue, the one chasing the other. It is like the chanting of monks. He speaks of winds coursing through the body of the woman, currents that break against barriers, eddying. These vortices are in her blood, he says. The last spendings of an imperfect heart. Between the chambers of her heart, long, long before she was born, a wind had come and blown open a deep gate that must never be opened. Through it charge the full waters of her river, as the mountain stream cascades in the springtime, battering, knocking loose the land, and flooding her breath. Thus he speaks, and is silent.

"May we now have the diagnosis?" a professor asks.

The host of these rounds, the man who knows, answers.

"Congenital heart disease," he says. "Interventricular septal defect, with resultant heart failure."

A gateway in the heart, I think. That must not be opened.

Through it charge the full waters that flood her breath. So! Here then is the doctor listening to the sounds of the body to which the rest of us are deaf. He is more than doctor. He is priest.

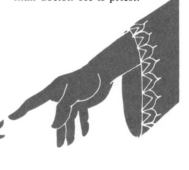

* From Richard Selzer, *Mortal Lessons: Notes on the Art of Surgery.* New York: Simon and Schuster, 1976. Copyright © 1974, 1975, 1976 by Richard Selzer. Reprinted by permission of Simon and Schuster, a division of Gulf & Western Corporation.

physician should take the time to discuss the results of tests, explain simply and clearly what they mean, answer your questions, and allay any fears you may have. You should feel confident enough to share with your physician any particular stresses you may be under, any worries that you may have, and any other concerns about your health. A physician who says to you, "Just you leave everything to me," is treating you like a child. You have an obligation to insist firmly and courteously on obtaining all the information you need to feel reassured. If you are upset for any reason with what is going on, the art of healing is not being practiced.

3. Many people are apprehensive about going to a physician, especially if they suspect something is seriously wrong with their health. Fear and anxiety are destructive to health, as we have pointed out in other chapters. As a patient, you have the responsibility for dealing with your fears. The physician can help by explaining things and by being reassuring, but you have to learn how to relax your mind and body. Fear produces tension, makes communication difficult, and itself may cause illness. Before going to a physician's office and while waiting in the office, it is useful to practice meditation or to visualize a relaxing place in your mind or to use any other relaxation technique that helps calm you.

4. Always remember how suggestible and programmable your mind is during a medical consultation. What the physician *says* about your condition—sometimes called the "physician placebo effect"—can be as important as the treatment. In discussing your illness with you, the physician should impart confidence and expectation of a cure and a return to good health. If the physician is positive and encouraging, the likelihood of cure increases.

The negative side of the placebo effect is just as powerful and you must be careful not to mentally accept destructive statements made by the physician. Statements regarding complications, adverse effects of the treatment, side effects of drugs,

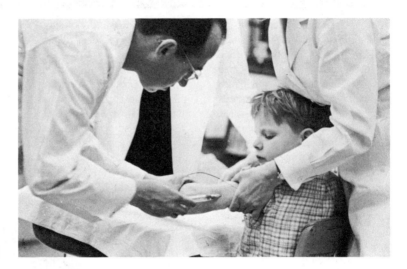

Diagnosis and treatment of disease varies greatly from culture to culture. (Courtesy World Health Organization.)

chances of permanent disability, probable duration of the sickness, and other nonhealing oriented comments can actually cause additional sickness and health problems. For example, Elizabeth Loftus and James Fries (1979) of the Center for Advanced Study in the Behavioral Sciences point out that subjects in a drug study who received a placebo injection suffered from severe, self-induced side effects such as vomiting, nausea, dizziness, and depression. They argue that explicit suggestions of adverse effects of treatments actually cause subjects to experience these effects. Thus, you should become more aware of negative health suggestions in any medical situation and let your mind accept only positive, healing statements.

The Hospital Stay

For most people, admission to a hospital is a confusing and frightening experience. Yet it happens to more and more people every year in the United States. A survey done in 1980 showed that about 10 percent of the population was admitted to a hospital in that year. This means that most people will enter a hospital at some time or other during their lifetime. Willard Gaylin (1973), president of the Institute of Society, Ethics, and the Life Sciences, describes the hospital experience:

> A stay in a hospital exposes an individual to a condition of passivity and impotence unparalleled in adult life, this side of prison. You are dressed in an uncomfortable garment, leaving you exposed and ludicrous;

told when you must sleep and when you must rise, informed of what you may eat and when you have to eat it; notified as to when you can have visitors, who they shall be, and how long they can stay. You are discussed in the third person in your presence as though you were some idiot child or inanimate object. If you are unfortunate enough to have an interesting case, you will be presented to a group of strangers who may take the invasion of your privacy as their privilege.

Since many people will be confronted with this unpleasant reality at some time or other in their lives, it is advisable to understand what a hospital patient's rights and obligations are.

On admission to a hospital, a patient is required to sign a consent form. By signing it, the patient is delegating all decisions regarding his or her care to the hospital and physicians. In most instances, physicians will obtain informed consent for any invasive procedure, either diagnostic or therapeutic, before proceeding. But the amount of information that is given and the extent to which a patient understands what the treatment involves usually depend on many factors affecting communication between the patient and the physician. In 1973, the American Hospital Association published a Patient's Bill of Rights covering the situations and questions most often encountered by patients in a hospital, and most hospitals should be able to supply you with the list. You are entitled to ask the hospital administrator for a list of patients' rights in that hospital.

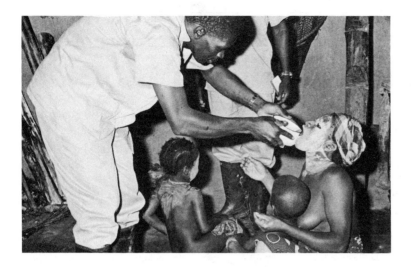

The most frustrating and anxiety-producing situations for a patient are not understanding what is going to happen and, even worse, not knowing what is happening while being subjected to unfamiliar and painful procedures (see Figure 25-4). Except in the case of a life-threatening emergency that demands immediate action, you have a right to be fully informed of all medical procedures and the reasons for them. As a patient, you have the responsibility for deciding what you want done. Once you have made that decision, you should understand how to cooperate fully to gain the most benefit. Visualizing a positive outcome of the treatment and anticipating a full recovery will often facilitate healing processes.

Medical Alternatives

Although most people will elect to visit a physician when they are sick, there are many alternatives to conventional, or **allopathic,** medicine. All licensed physicians (medical doctors, M.D.s) are trained to practice allopathic medicine. The guiding principle of allopathic medicine is quite sound and simple: if the functioning of the body deviates from normal—that is, is diseased—some counteracting measure should be employed. In principle this makes good sense. But in practice it has often led to extraordinarily harsh and harmful medical practices. For example, irritants of all sorts have been used

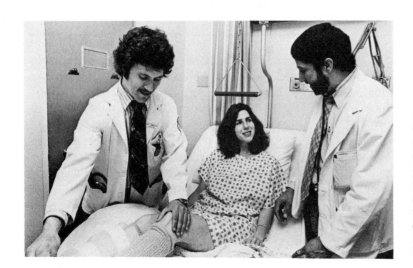

Figure 25-3
The stress and anxiety produced by a hospital stay can be reduced by treating the patient as a person and providing psychological as well as physical care. The patient helps by asking questions about her disease and treatment and by sharing her fear or concerns. (Courtesy Mount Zion Hospital and Medical Center, San Francisco.)

BOX 25-2

PATIENT-PHYSICIAN COMPLAINTS—WHO'S RIGHT?

Patient's Complaints

Doctors are never available when I need them. I had to wait weeks for an appointment, even though I'm sick right now. If I'm well and just want to discuss my problems, they don't want to see me at all. I have to wait until a crisis has occurred before I can get to see my doctor.

The costs of medical care are ridiculous. I was in there for two minutes and it cost thirty dollars. I just wanted my prescription renewed and it cost me twenty dollars. I can't afford to be sick.

The doctor won't take the time to listen to me. I don't think he even knows who I am. Sometimes he doesn't even remember what my disease is, even though he should have a record of it.

Doctors just want to get patients in and out as fast as possible. They really don't treat people anymore. We're just machines to them and I get serviced like a car.

There's no human interaction anymore. It's all fancy equipment and expensive tests. And after all that, they still don't know what's wrong.

Doctors treat patients like little children. They don't take the time to explain what's happening and act like I'm too dumb to understand. And that upsets and aggravates me.

Doctors are insensitive and detached. They're interested in some part of my body and act like I wasn't even there. And if I ask a question, they act like it's none of my business.

I have to sit in the waiting room for hours sometimes. Doctors act like my time isn't worth anything. And the nurses scowl if the kids get noisy and restless.

Physician's Complaints

I've been trained as a physician — not to be a psychologist or a counselor. Patients expect too much from me.

Patients are often demanding and discourteous. They don't real-ize how busy I am or the pressure I'm under.

Patients aren't responsible. They won't take care of themselves. They don't take my advice anyway and often won't do what I prescribe.

Patients don't appreciate all the things a doctor has to do. I'm usually swamped with phone calls, reports to write up, and insurance forms to fill out. I hardly have time to practice medicine.

Patients think I charge too much but they don't understand how much it costs to run an office and pay all the people who work for me. Not to mention the thousands of dollars I spend in malpractice insurance. I'm still trying to pay off the money I borrowed to get through medical school.

Patients expect miracles. They expect things that we cannot do. There are many diseases that medicine can do very little about. I can only do what's possible — I'm not God.

---

* Adapted from D. A. Tubesing, *Wholistic Health—A Whole Person Approach to Primary Health Care.* New York: Human Sciences Press, 1979.

(and are often still used) to purge the body. Bleedings, cuppings, leechings, enemas, and emetics (vomit inducers) were all used freely in the past. They generally weakened the patient and interfered with the process of self-healing.

While one would like to conclude that all harmful medical practices are a thing of the past, controversy still surrounds the use of such conventional therapies as whole-body radiation and chemotherapy in the treatment of certain cancers and radical mastectomies in the treatment of breast cancer (see Chapter 17); coronary bypass surgery for mild heart disease (see Chapter 16); gastric bypass surgery in which part of the stomach is surgically removed or tied off to treat obesity; and electroconvulsive therapy (ECT), which is used to treat depression and other mental and emotional disorders.

Allopathic medicine has become more and more technologically oriented and impersonal. Often the tests and diagnostic procedures are painful and increase patients' suffering and apprehensions. As a reaction to the real and perceived shortcomings of modern allopathic medicine, many people are turning to alternative healing techniques for relief of

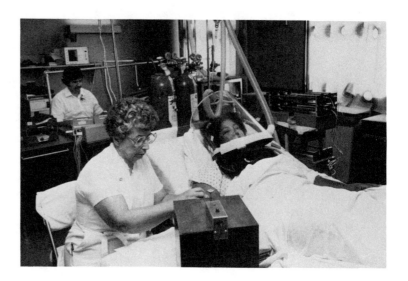

Figure 25-4
Modern hospital procedures involve
sophisticated technology and may seem
strange and frightening. (Courtesy of
the National Institutes of Health.)

pain and suffering and for cures for their diseases.
The same injunction holds true for alternative therapies as for allopathic medicine: understanding the
strengths and weaknesses of various healing alternatives is essential to making a wise choice. To this
end we have included a discussion of some of the
more readily available alternative therapies (see Table
25-4).

Homeopathy

Homeopathy emerged in the eighteenth century
largely in reaction to the heroic and abusive treatments of allopathic medicine—cuppings, leechings,
bleedings, forced vomitings, and so on. The principles of homeopathy were developed by Samuel
Hahnemann, a doctor and pharmacologist who was
born in Saxony in 1775. Hahnemann believed that
tiny doses of a substance (a drug) that evoked dis-
easelike symptoms could somehow stimulate the
body's natural defenses and promote healing. According to Hahnemann, homeopathy is based on
four principles:

1. The law of similars, which says that substances that produce the same symptoms in
   an individual as the disease does will cure
   him.
2. Only a single dose of the substance is required.
3. Smaller doses are more potent than un-
   diluted solutions.

4. Vital forces must be released in the individual that will result in reestablishing
   body harmony or homeostasis.

Homeopathic practitioners are trained to attend
to the patient's physical, mental, and emotional
state—in other words, to treat holistically. In addition to dispensing a substance that the homeopath
determines is specific for the disease, the practitioner
will also recommend exercise, nutritional changes,
relaxation techniques, and so on.

Table 25-4
**A Partial List of Alternative Healing Methods
and Techniques**

Physical and nutritional	Mental and spiritual
Rolfing	Hypnosis
Massage	Autosuggestion
Feldenkrais technique	Progressive relaxation
Alexander technique	Meditation
Reflexology	Biofeedback
Kinesiology (Touch for Health)	Cocounseling
Acupressure	Psychodrama
Shiatsu	Rebirthing
Yoga	Scientology
T'ai chi ch'uan	EST training
	Primal scream therapy
	Psychic healing
	Psychic surgery
	Past lives therapy
	Christian Science
	Encounter groups

> Those who flow as life flows know they need no other force. They feel no wear, they feel no tear, they need no mending, no repair.
>
> **Lao-tzu**
> *The Way of Life*

Perhaps the most controversial aspect of homeopathy is its reliance on doses of drugs that frequently are so dilute that the solutions contain little or none of the active substance that is supposed to mimic the symptoms and produce a cure. Certainly administering such dilute solutions can do the patient no harm; on the other hand, doing so does not seem to make any sense scientifically. One explanation for homeopathic cures is that they result from placebo effects (see Chapter 3); in some cases, cures occur spontaneously. However, homeopaths staunchly maintain that their dilute drug solutions do produce a real effect and are responsible for curing many different diseases.

Since it was founded in 1846, the American Medical Association (AMA) has vigorously opposed homeopathy. According to the AMA's code of ethics, physicians are prohibited from consulting with "practitioners whose practice is based upon a specific dogma." This particular edict was specifically designed to isolate homeopaths. By 1855 the AMA directed all state affiliates to expel all homeopaths from their membership. (In 1878 a physician was expelled from the AMA for consulting with a homeopath—his wife.) Despite persistent AMA attacks between 1850 and 1900, homeopathic practitioners increased in number. In 1900 there were about 15,000 homeopaths in the United States and twenty-two homeopathic colleges (Hahnemann founded the first homeopathic college in Philadelphia in 1836).

After 1900, the number of homeopaths gradually declined, particularly as allopathic medicine became more scientific and more successful in treating diseases. Today homeopathy is having a mild resurgence. This again may be due to the excesses of modern medical treatments or the failure of physicians to deal effectively and humanely with patients. Homeopathy still cannot be regarded as "scientific," yet for many people it seems to work.

Naturopathy

Naturopathy comprises a potpourri of healing strategies that include nutrition therapy, hydrotherapy, color therapy, herbalism, acupuncture, and massage. Naturopaths are trained to deal with all aspects of health and to tailor their treatments to the individual's needs. The basic principles of naturopathy are (1) all diseases have the same fundamental cause—namely, accumulation of toxic waste substances in the body; (2) disease is caused by the body's attempt to rid itself of these toxic substances; and (3) the body contains the power to heal itself.

Naturopaths teach their patients how to detoxify themselves by fasting, by restricted diets, and by other purifying techniques that frequently use water both internally and externally. Patients are also taught how to rejuvenate their body's vital energies. Many naturopaths work at spas or water resorts and include mineral baths and saunas as part of their treatments. At present only a few states license naturopaths, so the consumer has to be knowledgeable and careful in choosing one. Since most naturopathic techniques are gentle and self-administered, there is little danger to the patient. Most persons will experience some benefit from an

> You cannot teach a person anything. You can only help him to find it for himself.
>
> **Galileo**

occasional fast, a soak in a warm bath, or a massage to relax tense muscles.

A fad among some naturopaths is the use of hair shaft analyses to diagnose biochemical abnormalities in the person's body. A strand of hair can be analyzed for many nutrients and minerals that, in principle, might indicate biochemical abnormalities in the body. Computer printouts that may appear scientific and impressive to naturopathic practitioners and patients actually contain little or no useful health information. First, there is no evidence to indicate that hair chemistry reflects body chemistry to any significant degree. For example, a high level of lead in hair does not mean that blood serum levels of lead are also high. In addition, analyses of hair samples vary markedly from hair to hair and from laboratory to laboratory. Generally speaking, hair shaft analyses produce income for laboratories and practitioners that use them; no other benefits have been documented.

Chiropractic

Chiropractic was founded by Daniel David Palmer (1845–1913), who had no scientific training but who felt throughout his life that he had a "calling" to heal people. At age 50, Palmer cured a man of deafness by manipulating his spine. After several other cures by spinal manipulation, Palmer concluded that virtually all diseases are caused by subluxed (misaligned) vertebrae. Palmer coined the name "chiropractic" (literally, "done by hand") to describe his new healing technique, and he opened the Palmer School for Chiropractic in Davenport, Iowa, in 1895. In 1906, father and son (Bartlett Joshua, better known as B. J.) were arrested for practicing medicine without a license. The father was tried and jailed; the son's case never came to trial.

B. J. Palmer took over chiropractic and turned it into a multimillion-dollar business. B. J. was a genius at commercializing chiropractic; he invented the concept of mail-order diplomas and he advertised widely and effectively. His philosophy of chiropractic was summed up in his description of the spine: "The principal functions of the spine are to support the head, to support the ribs, and to support the chiropractor."

Eventually, chiropractic split into two groups with different philosophies about chiropractic. One group, "the straights," adhere to the original ideas that almost all diseases are caused by subluxation of the vertebrae and that diseases can be cured by spinal manipulation. The other group, "the mixers," take a more holistic approach and, while practicing spinal manipulations to correct subluxations, also dispense advice on nutrition, relaxation, exercise, and other techniques.

The spine consists of twenty-four movable vertebrae (disks) that should flex and move freely. Chiropractors define a **subluxation** as a vertebra that is partly displaced from its correct position and a **fixation** as the restricted movement of one or more vertebrae. Chiropractors are trained to diagnose subluxations and fixations of the spine by studying a person's posture, by touching the spine, and by x-ray exams. The purpose of chiropractic is to realign the vertebrae so that normal nervous system functions

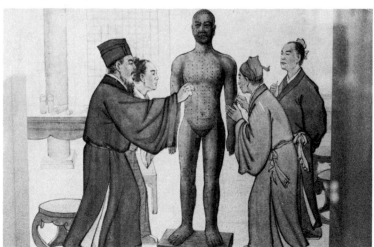

Figure 25-5
Traditional acupuncture. Chinese medical students practiced acupuncture by sticking needles into life-size models. The statue was filled with water and the correct acupuncture points were filled with wax. If the student pierced the right spot, a tiny jet of water emerged. (Courtesy World Health Organization.)

are restored, which, in turn, should alleviate the symptoms and cure the disease.

The American Association of Chiropractors defines chiropractic as "that science and art which utilizes the inherent recuperative powers of the body, and deals with the relationship between the nervous system and the spinal column, including its immediate articulations and the role of this relationship in the restoration and maintenance of health." Today, chiropractors receive extensive scientific training that is comparable to medical school education in many respects. Musculoskeletal disorders, which include not only back aches, pains, and muscle spasms and arthritis but also headaches, allergies, and digestive disorders, are often cured or relieved by chiropractic. A comprehensive government study in New Zealand (Commission of Inquiry, 1979) concluded that chiropractic was an effective, sophisticated therapy for many disorders. The study recommended that chiropractic be supported by government funds in New Zealand, that it be recognized by the country's medical association, and that patients have equal access to both medical and chiropractic care. Some doctors are beginning to refer patients to chiropractors in this country, but many physicians still adhere to the outdated belief that chiropractors are quacks. Chiropractors are licensed to administer any legitimate therapy except surgery and prescription drugs.

Osteopathy

Osteopathy is basically treatment by manipulation of the spine and body. While it is mostly useful for musculoskeletal disorders, psychosomatic illnesses also respond to manipulation. Osteopathic medicine was founded by Andrew Taylor Still, who was born in Virginia in 1828. His father was a preacher-physician and Andrew was a sensitive and observant learner who taught himself the art of healing.

The aim of osteopathic medicine is to restore harmony within the body, as well as between the individual and the environment. While manipulation is the principal therapeutic technique, osteopathy also stresses the importance of hygiene and nutrition. There are more than 15,000 osteopathic physicians and over 500 osteopathic hospitals in the United States. Osteopathic physicians (doctors of osteopathy, or D.O.s) have all the medical rights and privileges accorded to allopathic physicians, and osteopathic medical training is considered to be as comprehensive as that for M.D.s.

Acupuncture

Acupuncture is an ancient Chinese healing art that dates back to 2500 B.C. According to Chinese philosophy, the forces of nature work in harmony

> The only two mammals to remove blood
> regularly from other mammals are
> vampire bats and humans.
>
> **John F. Burnum, M.D.**

with man. Human vital energy is in the form of *chi,* whose balance in the body is maintained by the forces of Yin and Yang (see Chapter 3). Human disease results from a disruption of the harmonious energy balance, which can be corrected by the insertion of very thin needles at specific energy points on the surface of the body (see Figure 25-5). Once inserted, the needles can be twirled, heated, or used to pass electrical currents into the body's energy points to restore a harmonious balance and effect a cure.

In China, acupuncture has been used for pain relief (major surgery is sometimes performed using only acupuncture as an anesthetic) as well as for the cure of various diseases. The basis for the healing effects or for pain relief by acupuncture is not scientifically understood. Most of the pain relief that people report from acupuncture may be due to the patient's belief in acupuncture (a placebo effect). Experiments have demonstrated that every person can synthesize hormonelike substances in the brain called endorphins or enkephalins (see Chapter 3) that affect the perception of pain. The insertion of the acupuncture needles may activate the nervous and endocrine systems in ways we do not yet understand to modify pain and change physiology.

Many Western-educated physicians have traveled to China and Japan to learn the techniques of acupuncture and the philosophy of Chinese medicine. In China, Western medicine is practiced along with the more traditional acupuncture. In the West, a small number of physicians include acupuncture among their choice of treatments, and in the United States acupuncturists who are not physicians are licensed to practice in some states, such as California. In other states, acupuncturists practice with a physician's guidance and supervision.

Although acupuncture is supposed to relate specific points on the body's surface to particular internal organs (see Figure 25-6), no evidence exists that supports the physical reality of acupuncture points or their physiological connections with the organs of the body. Felix Mann (1983), a British doctor who has devoted over 25 years to the study and practice of acupuncture, states in his most recent book on the scientific basis of acupuncture that "acupuncture points do not exist, meridians do not exist, and most of the laws of acupuncture are laws about nonexistent entities. Yet acupuncture works; indeed, I practice it nearly 100 percent of my time." Acupuncture is more accepted and more successful in China and among Chinese than among more skeptical Western patients. As with all healing techniques, the placebo effect may play an important role in acupuncture treatment, particularly in relief of pain, for which it is especially effective.

> Getting obsessed with your health so that it interferes with your life is not normal.
>
> **Charles V. Ford, M.D.**
> **Professor of psychiatry**

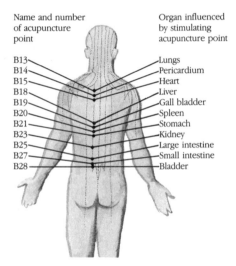

Figure 25-6
Acupuncture points supposedly influence the functions of internal organs.

Herbal Medicine

Herbal medicine uses many plant materials in the treatment of disease. Herbs and plant materials have been used in healing for thousands of years, and many of our most important drugs (ephedrine, digitalis, atropine, reserpine, quinine, and so forth) are derived from plants. Generally, a number of herbs are used in a mixture, so often it is difficult to determine whether any curative effects are due to a single herb, to the combination of herbs, or simply to a placebo effect resulting from the patient's belief in the efficacy of the remedy.

Most of the dangers regarding the use of drugs also apply to herbs (see Chapter 12). The active ingredients in herbal remedies *are* drugs, although the amounts and kinds are more difficult to determine, and many plants contain toxic compounds in addition to the pharmacologically useful substances. Some simple herbal remedies are given in Table 25-5.

Medical Quackery

In the broadest sense, any therapy based on scientifically unproven remedies is quackery. A number of federal agencies such as the Food and Drug Administration, the Federal Trade Commission, and the U.S. Postal Service try to expose false claims and prevent the sale of useless products. However, when people become seriously ill or disenchanted with the medical care and advice they are receiving, they often turn to worthless remedies and fraudulent practitioners (quacks) who profess to be able to cure them. Unfortunately there are many unscrupulous quacks who prey on people's fear and ignorance. According to a leaflet put out by the Postal Service:

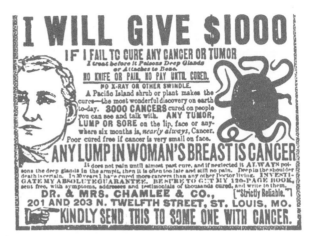

Figure 25-7
Quacks with herbal remedies for diseases such as cancer and arthritis take advantage of people who are sick, afraid, and in search of a magical "cure."

Unlike the pitchman who hawked "magic cures" from the back of a horse-drawn wagon, today's quacks are highly sophisticated salespeople who use widespread deceptive advertising to offer "miracles" they can't produce. The advertising is directed at the unfulfilled desires and vanities we all share to some degree. It promises with little or no effort what it can't deliver—health, beauty, vitality, and happiness.

Anything that sounds "too good to be true" probably is not true. Remedies based on "secret formulas" or that promise quick, painless cures are quack remedies. At present there are no cures for many serious diseases such as arthritis, asthma, psoriasis, AIDS, and many cancers. As a result, people with these serious ailments, as well as those with lesser complaints such as overweight or baldness, are often victims of quackery. Learn to recognize the many forms of medical quackery and do not buy unproven potions, lotions, and gadgets.

Holistic Medicine—The Future

In this book we have been emphasizing the principles that provide the foundation for health. Medical care is slowly changing, both in the way it treats people and in its emphasis on wellness and prevention of disease. Donald A. Tubesing (1979), director of the Institute for Whole Person Health Care in Duluth, Minnesota, has this vision:

Medicine of the future will not look only for a one-to-one correspondence between an individual and a disease, will not separate body, mind, and spirit, will not only find broken parts and mend them, and will not be an isolated approach. Medicine of the future will treat the person in context—in the context of environment and social and cultural atmosphere. It will take the will and the belief system seriously.

Table 25-5
Herbal Remedies for Common Ailments

COLD   Munch on a clove of garlic; drink peppermint tea.
COUGHS   Make a tea of ginger and honey.
CONSTIPATION   Mix equal parts aloe vera and honey, and take a teaspoon before meals.
GAS   Drink peppermint tea to soothe the stomach.
HEADACHE   Chew willow bark or make it into a tea.
SORE THROAT   Drink camomile tea (avoid if allergic to ragweed).
STOMACHACHE   Drink camomile tea or caraway seed tea.

As more and more people demand this kind of healing and approach to curing disease, more change will happen. Medicine is both a science and an art. It is up to you, the consumer, to utilize the best that medical technology and physicians can provide. At the same time, you should remember the power that your mind and body have in maintaining health and promoting healing.

Supplemental Readings

Easterbrook, G. "The Revolution in Medicine." *Newsweek,* January 26, 1987. Decribes how medical costs and care are changing.

Engelhardt, H. T., Jr. *The Foundations of Bioethics.* New York: Oxford University Press, 1986. A thoughtful discussion of the ethical dilemmas in medicine and the new techniques in biology and genetics.

Inglis, B., and **West, R.** *The Alternative Health Guide.* New York: Knopf, 1983. A comprehensive description of over fifty alternative therapies.

Roemer, M. I. *An Introduction to the U.S. Health Care System.* New York: Springer Publishing, 1986. Describes the history, structure, and operation of the U.S. health care system and suggests changes for the future.

Spiro, H. M. *Doctors, Patients, and Placebos.* New Haven: Yale University Press, 1986. A good discussion of the use and appropriateness of placebo therapy in medicine.

Weil, A. *Health and Healing.* Boston: Houghton Mifflin, 1983. A personal view of conventional medicine and alternative therapies by a physician who has tried most of them. A well-balanced overview of pros and cons.

Summary

Medical care is vital to health because nearly everyone is going to require medical assistance at some time or another during life. Even though medical care in the United States is generally regarded as the best in the world, many people are dissatisfied with the care they receive. People complain about being charged high fees, being treated without sensitivity, and not being fully informed about their condition and the recommended treatments.

Many people are overmedicated with drugs, especially when the symptoms and complaints are minor. Thousands of operations are performed annually for conditions that could be treated more conservatively by other, less drastic techniques. People have to assume more responsibility for their health, especially when dealing with hospitals and health professionals. They should insist on all possible information pertaining to the illness and the reasons for the recommended treatment. Having complete trust and confidence in one's physician is of utmost importance. Positive statements and healing suggestions can be a powerful aid in the cure. Conversely, negative, discouraging statements can interfere with recovery.

Most medical office visits involve minor symptoms and illnesses. Indicate to your physician that you would prefer to deal with the symptoms without drugs or surgery if possible. Be open to trying the techniques of holistic medicine, which include relaxation, positive mental imagery, diet improvement, and exercise. Always remember that your health and what is done to your body are your responsibility.

There is no more contradiction between the science of medicine and the art of medicine than between the science of aeronautics and the art of flying.

Francis W. Peabody

FOR YOUR HEALTH

Positive Medical Interactions

Try to remember the times that you have had medical attention in the past. Make a list of the things that you feel helped your recovery and your return to health. Then make a list of those things that made you upset with your medical care or that you felt were not helpful to your recovery. Use this list the next time you need medical attention. Try to increase the number of positive interactions and reduce those things that upset you.

Understanding Your Illness and Care

If you have a medical problem now, ask yourself whether you fully understand the illness and diagnosis and the treatments that have been recommended. Are you satisfied with the progress you are making toward becoming well again? Do you fully understand what causes your symptoms or illness? Do you understand all the alternatives that are available to help you with your problem? Discuss any questions or concerns you have with your doctor or health professional.

Visualization for Surgery

If you should have to undergo surgery (even the extraction of a tooth), you can help the healing process by performing visualization exercises for several days before the surgery. For example, if the surgery is for removal of a growth, visualize the tissues healing rapidly and completely in a short period of time. Visualize the area returning to normal functioning and feeling comfortable. If the surgery is to repair damaged bones or muscles, visualize yourself being able to do all the things you used to do before the injury or illness. Notice that there is no sign of weakness or discomfort.

CHAPTER TWENTY-SIX

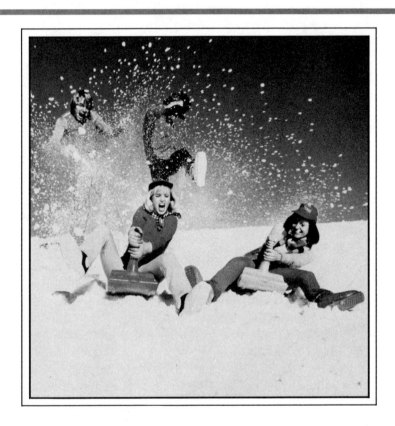

Health and Wellness: Putting It All Together

My granary has burned down—
Now I can see the sun.

Japanese proverb

Good health and wellness are things most people take for granted until health suddenly vanishes. One morning you may wake up feeling really sick. The more serious the illness, the more abruptly all the other worries, thoughts, obligations, and pleasures disappear from your mind. Being in love may be the most exciting and important part of a person's life at one moment, yet a bout of flu with the accompanying aches and fever can refocus all the mind's attention on the importance of being well for the enjoyment of all aspects of living.

You can strive to accomplish all your life's goals, to have enough money to enjoy all the things you want to do, and to feel important and respected. Yet what do the successes and rewards amount to if you become serously ill or if you discover one day that you have cancer? Your perspectives and values may suddenly change when good health is lost and even more so when life is threatened by serious disease. This is but one of many reasons for striving to stay well. But even an illness can be endured as long as you still find meaning in your life and in living.

Throughout this book, we have emphasized a holistic view of health—that health and wellness mean living in such a way that you minimize the risk of illness—but even more, living in a way that emphasizes good relationships with other people and with the environment, that shows concern about what foods and drugs you put into your body, and that has a feeling of joy and satisfaction in the daily tasks and adventures of living. In this final chapter we attempt to broadly outline a philosophy of living, or lifestyle as we have called it, that is healthy and that can help to promote health. We are not presenting any golden rules. Neither do we intend to moralize about how any person ought to live. We are simply presenting some health guidelines that we hope will seem like plain common sense. These guidelines follow logically from the principles that we have discussed regarding how the mind and body are organized and function (see Chapters 2 and 3), the principles regarding the importance of good nutrition and physical activity (see Chapters 4, 5, 6, and 7), and how destructive habits and certain lifestyles can lead to physiological changes that may result in sickness (see Chapters 10 through 15).

> More than any other time in history,
> mankind faces a crossroads. One path leads
> to despair and utter hopelessness. The other, to
> total extinction. Let us pray we have the wisdom
> to choose correctly.
>
> **Woody Allen**

Lifestyle—The Key to Health

In this country there are basically two opposing, and perhaps in a practical sense, irreconcilable views of how to achieve the most health for the American people. The first view advocates that every person is entitled to medical care and should be protected financially so that everyone can afford the medical care he or she needs. This view also advocates frequent medical consultations, routine physical exams, and treatment with drugs and surgery for any diseases that are discovered. This approach to health care places most of the responsibility for health squarely on the shoulders of the health care industry—physicians, nurses, hospitals, pharmaceutical companies, insurance companies, and government agencies. This view of health accepts the idea that the responsibility for maintaining health lies outside ourselves. This view maintains additionally that health can be purchased, legislated, and delivered in the form of medical products and medical care. The principal fault of this view is that it primarily deals with disease *after* sickness has occurred.

The other view emphasizes that a person's health is primarily the responsibility of the individual and that the goal is the prevention of disease and sickness. This does not mean that the first view is wrong—even if you accept the idea that each person has the primary responsibility for maintaining his or her health, individuals still require medical insurance to pay for medical care when they become sick. Medical checkups can sometimes be beneficial, and people should utilize to the fullest the best medical advice and health services that are available when sickness does occur.

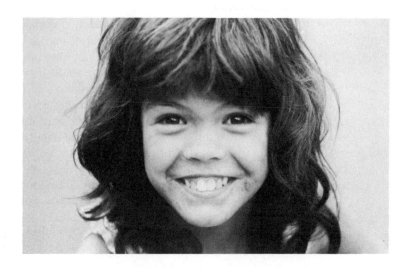

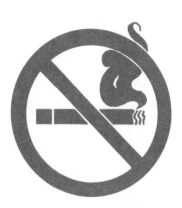

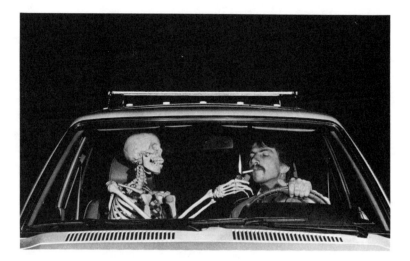

However, much sickness in America today does not come from causes that can be dealt with medically; it results from destructive personal habits and lifestyles that make people more susceptible to disease and sickness. Your personal lifestyle is also what you have the most control over and can do the most to change. As stated in the U.S. Surgeon General's Report on Health Promotion and Disease Prevention in 1979:

> Collectively smoking, misuse of alcohol and other drugs, poor dietary habits, lack of regular exercise, and stress place enormous burdens on the health and well-being of many Americans today . . . Although helping people to understand the need for and to act to change detrimental lifestyles cannot be easy, the dramatic potential benefits clearly make the effort worthwhile.

We will try to summarize the major lifestyle areas in which everyone has considerable freedom of choice and the best chance for improving and maintaining lifelong health.

Avoid Destructive Habits

Smoking tobacco and drinking excessive amounts of alcoholic beverages are two of the most destructive habits in our society today as far as maintaining health and preventing accidents, suicides, and disease are concerned. Humans are the only animals on this planet who choose to breathe smoke instead of fresh air and who choose to drink quantities of alcohol that impair physiology even to the point of death, either directly or by causing accidents. It is

obvious that the responsibility for preventing death and disease resulting from excessive smoking and drinking does not lie with the medical profession, rather, it is the personal responsibility of each person. No one really knows why so many people in our society smoke and drink to excess even when they know how destructive these substances are. Some explanations that have been offered are stress reduction, the need to escape from worries, persistent and persuasive advertising by manufacturers of tobacco and alcoholic products, and social pressures. There are probably hundreds of factors involved and dozens of explanations that could be offered. However, when all the arguments and counterarguments have been presented, the fact remains that the *decision* to smoke tobacco or drink alcohol is made by each individual. Each person can decide that his or her health is more important than the need to smoke or drink.

Most people growing up in our culture will have many occasions to engage in smoking and drinking, and many people will experiment with other kinds of recreational drugs, such as marijuana, LSD, or cocaine. Millions will become habituated or addicted to legal drugs—tranquilizers to reduce anxiety, amphetamines to provide energy, and aspirins and sedatives for pain and sleep. A few experiences with any of these substances, legal or illegal, will not destroy a person's health. However, repeated or excessive use or the inability to stop using any chemical or drug becomes a dangerous habit, which eventually can result in loss of health and in sickness. Destructive habits should not be started; once they are started, every effort should be made to stop them.

> ## Life is what happens
> ## while you're making other plans.
> **Tom Smothers**

Develop Sound Nutritional Habits

Each of us is responsible for getting sufficient amounts of the essential nutrients and chemicals we need to keep us functioning optimally under all conditions of living—that is, to maintain our health. Intellectual capability, emotional satisfactions, energy, and stamina all depend on proper biochemical functioning of all the body's cells and organs. Nutritional deficiencies, as well as nutritional excesses of some substances, can lead to gradual loss of health and increased susceptibility to sickness.

Most people in America have access to adequate amounts of food. In fact, many Americans consume an excess of many kinds of food. The millions of overweight people in this country testify to the fact that many people do not wisely choose the foods they eat—either in kind or amount. Many people eat a great deal more than their bodies need; hence they become overweight and generally are less healthy than people of normal weight. Other people do not eat excessively but rely on relatively few foods for most of their food intake; these persons may suffer from nutritional imbalances or deficiencies of essential nutrients. Many people in this country have acquired unhealthy dietary habits that include eating quantities of foods containing large amounts of sugar or large amounts of fats in the form of meats, dairy products, and fried foods.

Eating reasonable amounts and varieties of fresh, natural foods is vital to maintaining a high level of wellness throughout life. Bodies are chemi-

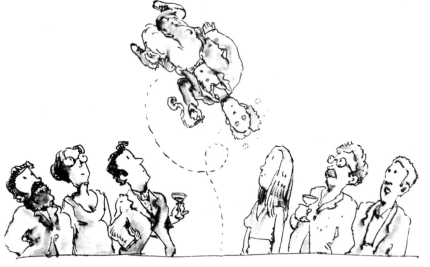

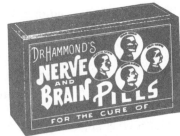

> It's all right to have a good time.
>
> That's one of the most important messages of enlightenment.
>
> **Thaddeus Golas**
> *The Lazy Man's Guide to Enlightenment*

cal factories that operate right up to the moment of death and that require a constant supplying of essential chemicals to the body's cells. What you choose to eat is your responsibility. How often have you seen an ad for fresh fruit or vegetables on TV? How many ads do you see for cheese or nuts or whole-wheat bread? Remember that all food and drug advertisements are designed to make money, not to encourage health and well-being. Do not rely on advertising for information on what is best to eat or drink. Natural foods—those that are not canned, frozen, or manufactured—are generally the best for you.

Be Physically Active

All animals need to move around. Most animals other than humans spend most of their energy moving around looking for food. Humans are animals too, and until quite recently either had to rove continually in search of food or had to work hard to raise the food needed to survive. Humans are designed to be physically active, yet our culture today is organized so that most of us are sitting most of the time. We sit at our jobs, we sit at school, and we sit during recreational activities such as watching TV, reading, or even going to concerts or to the theater.

Find ways to be physically active. Jog. Run. Swim. Hike. Participate in sports. Don't just watch others being active. Stretch your body's muscles with yoga exercises, or try dancing. Plant a garden, walk in the woods, roll in the leaves, throw snowballs—remember to play a little every day. Watch how much fun and pleasure children have running, climbing, rolling, jumping, and just being active. As people grow older they often forget to be active and forget to play during each day, and their health declines as a result of the lack of physical activity.

Choose a Healthy Environment

Many people make choices about where they want to live and work. Americans live in a mobile society. People change jobs frequently, as well as the places where they live. Some work and living environments are healthier than others. Living in areas of high stress, being exposed to constant noise, breathing polluted air, or drinking water contaminated with chemicals day after day can affect health adversely over a period of years. Choices about work and where to live can often be difficult. But remember to ask yourself how your health will be affected before you decide where to live and work.

Aaron Wildavsky (1976), of the University of California, estimates that as much as 90 percent of the difference in health between individual Americans is determined not by medical care but by factors of lifestyle—eating habits, smoking, exercise, and pollution encountered in the work and living environments. He also believes that health is a matter of personal responsibility and says that our national health policy is pathological because

> we are neurotic and insist on making our government psychotic. Our neurosis consists in knowing what is required for good health

> He who feels punctured
> must have been a bubble.
> He who feels unarmed
> must have carried arms.
> He who feels belittled
> must have been consequential.
> He who feels deprived
> must have had privilege.
>
> **Lao-tzu**
> *The Way of Life*

(Mother *was* right: Eat a good breakfast! Sleep eight hours a day! Don't drink! Don't smoke! Keep clean! and Don't worry!) but not being willing to do it. Government's ambivalence consists in paying coming and going: once for telling people how to be healthy and once for paying their bills when they disregard this advice. Psychosis appears when government persists in repeating this self-defeating play.

Ask yourself whether the things you are doing are beneficial to your well-being or whether they are destructive to your health. Do you really need to smoke? Is the convenience of frozen TV dinners and canned foods worth the risk of poor nutrition? Is being angry or depressed a lot of the time really worth it if you know that these states of mind increase the risk of illness? Do you really enjoy what you're doing and how you're living? If the answer to any of these questions is no, why not consider ways in which your lifestyle could be changed for the better?

The Importance of Positive Mental States

If there is a single factor that affects health the most strongly, either for good or for ill, that factor is the mind. The human mind controls all the body's essential functions and activities. The mind is the source of thoughts, fears, beliefs, faith—everything that, taken together, gives each person his or her unique talents, ideas, and lifestyle.

Most people instinctively realize that they need to be careful about what they eat—that their health depends on the substances they put into their bodies. People usually try to select things to eat and drink that supply their body's needs, that will not poison or harm them, and that taste and smell good. Yet most people fail to realize—because it has never been explained to them—that their health also depends on what they put into their minds. Some thoughts, memories, and images make us feel good and are relaxing, which stimulates health. Other thoughts make us feel bad; they cause feelings of worry or fear that are destructive to health. Obviously, it's better to increase the pleasure-producing, positive thoughts and images in the mind. In the same way that you would not eat or drink something offensive, you need not permit your mind to be programmed by offensive images or by statements that you know make you feel uncomfortable or anxious. Be as concerned about what you allow to enter your mind as you are about what enters your body.

As for the fears that already exist in your mind—and everyone has fears—one of the important tasks of living is to find ways to eliminate fears that have been acquired from unpleasant experiences. Real personal freedom comes when the mind is free of fear. Then, and only then, are you able to live in harmony within yourself and to interact in a loving and caring manner with other persons in your environment. A mind that is free of fear and worry is healthy, and it will generate health in all the parts of the body under its control.

> There are two ways of being disappointed in life. One is not to get what you want and the other is to get it.
>
> **George Bernard Shaw**

Acceptance May Be Healthy

Health does not necessarily mean the same thing to everyone. There is no absolute measure of health. Perfect health to a professional athlete may mean something quite different from what it means to a librarian or office worker, because the physical demands on their bodies are different. An airline pilot requires a different degree of health than a postal clerk. For example, a fainting spell or heart attack could have disastrous consequences in one case but not the other. The health that people are satisfied with when they are young is usually quite different from the health they are satisfied with when they get older.

Individuals need to decide what good health means to them and what kinds of habits, beliefs, and lifestyles produce the kind of health that they desire for themselves. People know in their minds how they feel—what the general state of the body, mind, and emotions are. You known instinctively whether you feel sick or feel great. You can train your mind to pay attention to this inner self-knowledge about your state of health. Listen to what your mind tells you to do to improve your health or what to change in your lifestyle. Do the things that make you feel better and chances are your well-being will improve. Avoid doing things that make you feel bad.

Sometimes, even when a person has made all the possible adjustments in habits, diet, activities, and living conditions that can be made to improve his or her health, sickness, accident, or disease still may occur. Unfortunately, there is no law of nature

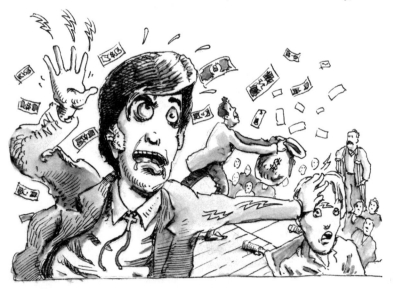

> Every gun that is made, every warship launched,
> every rocket fired, signifies, in the final sense a
> theft from those who hunger and are not fed,
> those who are cold and are not clothed.
>
> **Dwight D. Eisenhower, 1953**

that says that life is fair or predictable. Nobody knows who will get cancer or who will be hit by a car.

At some point in your effort to construct a healthy, responsible life, you will probably realize that there are many aspects of existence that simply must be accepted. Acceptance of unpleasant or unfortunate events in one's life does not mean giving up or refusing to strive toward important goals. Acceptance is best expressed in metaphysical or spiritual terms. To successfully cope with the problems and pressures of living you need to learn to flow with life. Learn when to struggle to overcome obstacles and when to accept the fortunes or misfortunes that occur in your life. There is more to living than either winning or losing. *Learning* from each life experience is also a satisfactory outcome.

Life in our society has become increasingly complex, and for many people, more difficult to understand. Ethical and cultural values change rapidly, even within the space of a single generation. Automobiles, airplanes, and space travel are all inventions of this century, as are computers and nuclear energy. Political ideas, sexual values, and religious beliefs have undergone radical changes within the last generation. Other changes are reflected in the kinds of music people listen to, the clothes they wear, and even the popular hairstyles.

Biologically, humans are not well adapted to the pace and demands of modern living. The human body and brain are more adapted to coping with simpler, slower, less complex modes of living. Yet we all must adapt in some measure to the culture and times we live in or our health suffers and we become anxious and upset. That is the value of learning acceptance—of ourselves and of the differences of others. Acceptance means adapting to what cannot be changed in order to maintain internal harmony—homeostasis in physiological terms, or a balance between Yin-Yang as described in Chinese philosophy.

It does not help to agonize over the reasons why sickness and death may occur at any point in life. There is absolutely no rational basis for believing that sin is responsible for birth defects or serious illness, or that death is a form of God's punishment. That even Jesus recognized this is evident from the biblical passage in John 9:1–3: "As Jesus went along, he saw a man who had been blind from birth. His disciples asked him, 'Rabbi, who sinned, this man or his parents, for him to have been born blind?' 'Neither he nor his parents sinned,' Jesus answered, 'he was born blind so that the words of God might be displayed in him.'"

Anybody can catch a cold or become seriously ill. There is no reason to feel guilty about becoming sick. Neither does it help the healing process to punish oneself for being sick. All human beings are subject to the laws of nature and to the whims of chance.

Life as a Quest

People can learn to endure severe illness. And their lives can still retain meaning and happiness. Steven Hawking, a famous British physicist, provides an

> Life is not a matter of holding good cards, but of playing a poor hand well.
>
> **Robert Louis Stevenson**

example of acceptance and of overcoming severe handicaps.

Hawking is regarded by many other scientists as the most creative, brilliant physicist since Einstein. Some compare his insights into the structure of the universe with those of Einstein. While still in college he became afflicted with a degenerative neurological disease and is confined to a wheelchair, unable to move on his own and barely able to speak intelligently. Despite these handicaps, he is married, has fathered three children, and carries on his research from a wheelchair. Despite his affliction, his life and his work have intense meaning: "One goal of my work has been to understand whether the universe has a meaning, and what our role is in it. I've always wanted to know why the universe exists at all, and what was there before the beginning . . . As human beings, we need the quest."

We have chosen to end this book on this note. Life is a quest for each one of us, each following a unique path. We believe that wellness and lifelong good health play a vital role in the quest for a meaningful, joyful life. We hope that you, the reader, have found and will continue to find ways to change and to improve your health. May you experience harmony and wellness throughout your life.

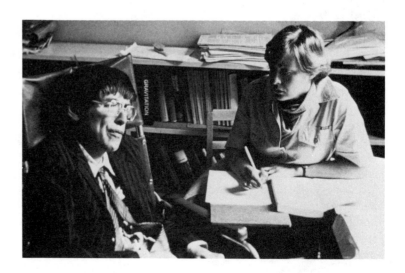

Physicist Stephen Hawking, incapacitated by a neurological disease, performs mathematical calculations mentally and dictates the results to his secretary. (Magnum Photos, Inc.)

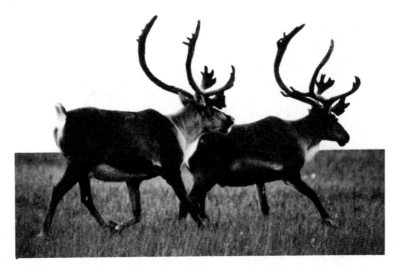

The first peace,
which is the most important,
is that which comes from
within the souls of men when they
realize their relationship,
their oneness, with the universe
and all its powers,
and when they realize that
at the center of the universe dwells
Wakan-Tanka, and that
this center is really everywhere,
it is within each of us.
This is the real peace, and the others are
but reflections of this.
The second peace is that which is
made between two individuals,
and the third is that
which is made between two nations.
But above all you should
understand that there can never be peace
between nations until there is
first known that true peace which . . .
is within the souls of men.

Black Elk
The Sacred Pipe

Appendix A

Nonprescription Medicines: Things to Remember

Pain Relievers
Cold Remedies
Cough Remedies
Antacids
Laxatives
Sleep Aids

Pain Relievers

Pain-relieving drugs that can be obtained without a prescription (over-the-counter) are called mild analgesics. These include aspirin, acetaminophen (Tylenol, Datril, Liquiprin, Tempra), and a variety of products that contain aspirin or acetaminophen. Although there are many different kinds of nonprescription pain relievers available, nothing relieves pain and reduces inflammation better, faster, or longer than an adult dose of plain aspirin: two tablets each containing 5 grains (about 300 mg). "Extra strength" or "combination" preparations, which contain one and a half to two times as much analgesic in each tablet or capsule, have succeeded in increasing manufacturers' profits but do not have greater therapeutic effectiveness. Aspirin substitutes may be preferable for those who are allergic to aspirin or who experience uncomfortable gastrointestinal upset after ingesting aspirin.

Aspirin Dos and Don'ts

1. Always take aspirin with food, milk, or a full glass of water.

2. Do not take more than 15 grains (two or three tablets) at a time; take no more than ten to twelve tablets in a 24-hour period. People with arthritis are an exception and should follow a physician's advice.

3. Individuals with a history of stomach ulcers or gout or who take oral anticoagulant medication ("blood thinners") should consult a physician before taking aspirin.

4. Prolonged use of aspirin for chronic conditions is unwise; consult a physician.

5. Children's doses generally should not exceed 1 grain (60 mg) per year of age, every 4 hours, up to a maximum of 5 grains.

6. Be aware that many medications that are frequently administered with aspirin (such as cough and cold mixtures) already contain aspirin. Be mindful not to overdose, especially with children.

7. Inexpensive "house brands" are equivalent to more expensive and heavily advertised brand names. All adult tablets contain 5 grains of aspirin or acetaminophen.

Cold Remedies

The common cold is a short-term viral infection of the upper respiratory tract. There is no cure. Cold remedies are drugs that provide temporary symptom relief while the cold runs its course. It takes the body's defenses 4 to 7 days to inactivate the viruses and to repair the cells and tissues damaged by them.

Many drug products sold for relief of cold symptoms are unscientific mixtures of several drugs, some of which are ineffective. These products unnecessarily expose individuals to drug side effects while doing little or nothing to alleviate the cold sufferer's miseries. In many cases symptom relief is due more to a placebo effect than to the drugs.

Nasal Decongestants

Decongestants constrict small blood vessels in the nose, thereby stopping the accumulation of fluid (congestion) and the leaking of fluid (runny nose). Common decongestants in sprays and inhalers are phenylephrine and oxymetazoline. Common decongestants in tablets, capsules, and liquids are ephedrine, pseudoephedrine, phenylephrine, and phenylpropanolamine.

Antihistamines

Antihistamines block the action of histamine, a natural substance produced by certain cells that causes inflammation, swelling, and secretion. Although effective against the symptoms of hay fever (runny nose, sneezing, airway obstruction, and itchy eyes), antihistamines have not been proven effective against cold symptoms. Nevertheless, they remain one of the principal ingredients in cold remedies. Common antihistamines are pyrilamine, chlorpheniramine, phenindamine, and pheniramine.

Anticholinergics

Anticholinergics inhibit glandular secretion in the respiratory tract and thus dry up a runny nose. They are almost always mixed with antihistamines in cold remedies. Atropine and other belladonna alkaloids are the most common types of anticholinergic drugs.

Pain Relievers (Analgesics)

Analgesics are included in cold remedies to relieve headache, body aches and pains, and malaise that accompany a cold. Some analgesics are also effective in reducing fever.

Caffeine

Caffeine, a mild stimulant, may relieve some of discomfort of a cold and may also counteract the sedative effects of some other agents used in cold remedies.

Cough Remedies

Coughing is a reflex action controlled by a "cough center" in the brain, which responds to irritation in the respiratory tract. Coughing is essential for clearing the respiratory airways of foreign matter. Coughs are most frequently associated with the common cold and are usually self-limited, are of brief duration, and do not require any therapy for relief. You should see a physician about any cough that persists longer than 7 to 10 days.

Suppressants (Antitussives)

Cough suppressants reduce the activity of the brain's cough center; they are recommended when a cough is persistent, dry, and hacking. Common cough suppressants include codeine (available only with a doctor's prescription; also a pain reliever) and dextromethorphan, the ingredient found in most nonprescription cough suppressants.

Expectorants

Expectorants increase the flow of respiratory tract secretions, thereby facilitating the removal of irritating substances and soothing the irritated tissues. Expectorants are recommended when a cough is congestive and produces considerable fluid. Common expectorants are quaifenesin, ammonium chloride, and terpin hydrate.

Demulcents

Demulcents provide a protective coating for irritated respiratory tissues and are useful with any cough. Hard candy and cough drops are examples of demulcents. Inhaling moist air, produced by either a cool mist humidifier or a hot steam vaporizer, is an effective demulcent for both adults and children.

Combination Products

Many cough products are unscientific mixtures of a specific cough medication with several other drugs, such as a pain reliever, an antihistamine, a decongestant, and in some cases up to 25 percent alcohol (50 proof). In some instances, an added drug works against the cough remedy or may induce unnecessary side effects, such as drowsiness.

Antacids

Antacids are substances that neutralize stomach acid. They are generally obtained without prescription for relief of "heartburn," sour stomach, and acid indigestion. Their use in the management of peptic ulcers should be monitored by a physician.

Antacids containing combinations of aluminum and magnesium salts are preferable to other types. Products containing calcium carbonate are effective, but excessive use can cause neurological and kidney problems from calcium overdose.

Sodium bicarbonate (baking soda) is the least preferable antacid. It can change the acidity of the the blood, and when taken with milk can cause nausea, vomiting, headache, and other symptoms. Sodium bicarbonate in the stomach liberates carbon dioxide gas, contributing to additional stomach acid secretion as well as to intestinal "gas." Furthermore, people who restrict their intake of sodium should avoid sodium bicarbonate antacids.

Laxatives

Occasional constipation and irregular bowel movements are not a symptom of illness and, contrary to advertising claims, do not require treatment with laxatives.

In most situations, the best preventive measure against constipation is a diet containing adequate fiber or roughage. The safest and most effective commerical laxatives tend to mimic the laxative effects of food.

Bulk-forming laxatives absorb water and expand into a gel that facilitates passage of soft stools. These products contain such substances as methylcellulose, carboxymethylcellulose, psyllium, and karaya. These are the safest of all laxatives.

Stimulant laxatives irritate the lining of the intestine and thereby increase bowel emptying. Major stimulant laxatives are bisacodyl, danthron, phenolphthalein, castor oil, senna, and casanthranol. These products act rapidly and may produce cramps, diarrhea, and depletion of body fluids.

Stool softeners enable intestinal fluids to penetrate feces and soften stools. The major types of stool softeners all contain sulfosuccinate compounds. Although these preparations do not corret the causes of of constipation, they do relieve it.

Lubricant laxatives soften feces and lubricate intestinal walls. The major lubricant laxative is mineral oil. Regular use may prevent the absorption of fat-soluble vitamins into the body.

Saline laxatives draw large amounts of water from the body into the intestine to facilitate defecation. Examples are magnesium citrate, magnesium hydroxide, magnesium sulfate, and phosphate preparations. Excessive use can cause dehydration.

Sleep Aids

Nonprescription sleep aids contain substances that may cause drowsiness and thus help an individual fall asleep. Over-the-counter sleep aids are designed for only occasional use. Thus, people with chronic insomnia should not take nonprescription sleep aids on a continual basis. Instead they should consult a physician or a sleep disorder clinic.

Nearly all sleep aids contain the antihistamine pyrilamine. Some also contain scopolamine, usually in doses insufficient to induce sedation but sufficient to augment the sedative effects of other agents. Because therapeutic doses of scopolamine are highly toxic, it is probably best to avoid sleep aids with scopolamine unless advised by a physician to use them.

Ingredients such as passion flower extract, thiamine (vitamin B_1), niacin, and niacinamide are not sedatives and their inclusion in sleep aids is unwarranted.

The use of nonprescription sleep aids for daytime sedation for "simple nervous tension" or "tension due to everyday stress or strain" is neither safe or effective.

Sleep difficulties that are not due to a medical problem are often related to improper living habits. Most occasional incidents of insomnia are related to irregular times of going to bed and arising, night work, daytime naps, a completely sedentary daytime routine, overuse of caffeine, nicotine, or other stimulants, and chronic use of tranquilizers, sleeping pills, or alcohol.

Activities that relax the mind and body, such as regular exercise, meditation, and other relaxation methods, are the best sleep inducers.

Appendix B

Body Care

Caring for Teeth and Gums
Caring for Hair and Scalp
Care of Skin
Back Care
Breast Self-exam

Caring for Teeth and Gums

Proper care of the teeth and gums involves preventing the buildup of food particles, sugars, and acids on the teeth. This is accomplished by thoroughly brushing the teeth after eating, by regular daily flossing, and by avoiding sugar-laden foods.

Tooth Brushing Technique

Experts vary on whether teeth should be brushed with a horizontal or vertical stroke. All experts agree, however, that thorough brushing is more important than the particular brushing technique.

Whether using an up-and-down motion or a back-and-forth motion, be sure to:

1. Massage the gums with the toothbrush while brushing.
2. Brush one tooth at a time with several strokes.
3. Move the brush in several directions over the ridged surfaces of the chewing (back) teeth.
4. Use the front part of the toothbrush in an up-and-down motion to clean the front and rear surfaces of the front teeth.

Tooth Brushing Devices

1. Use a soft toothbrush to avoid injuring gums.
2. Replace a toothbrush when it becomes worn.
3. The head of the toothbrush should be small enough to allow easy brushing of every tooth.
4. Electric toothbrushes found acceptable by the American Dental Association (check package label) are effective and may be especially useful for the handicapped.

Toothpaste

1. Toothpaste and toothpowders are equally effective.
2. Fluoridated toothpaste is superior to non-fluoridated toothpaste. Fluoride has been shown to prevent cavities, especially while teeth are forming.
3. Toothpaste and toothpowders proven effective in preventing dental caries (tooth decay) by the American Dental Association are designated as "acceptable" on the product carton or tube.

537

Flossing

Flossing removes food particles and debris from between the teeth and gums, where a toothbrush cannot reach. All flossing products—floss or tape, waxed or unwaxed—are equally effective. The key to successful flossing is regularity.

Tips on flossing:

1. Use about 18 inches of floss each time.
2. Wind the floss around the first or middle fingers of each hand, leaving 1 inch of floss free.
3. With your thumb and forefinger, guide the inch of floss between the two back teeth on the upper left (or right, if you prefer) side of your mouth.
4. Gently move the floss up and down the sides of the teeth. Move the floss gently but firmly below the free margin of the gums (the space between the gums and teeth) until you meet resistance.
5. Gently remove the floss from between the teeth and move on to the space between the two teeth next in the row.
6. As the floss becomes soiled, free a clean inch from what is wrapped around your fingers.

Caring for Hair and Scalp

Hair grows from tiny depressions beneath the skin called follicles. The average healthy scalp contains about 100,000 hair follicles. At any given time, about 90 percent of the follicles are actively making hair; the others are in a resting stage. Normally about 75 to 100 hairs are lost from the scalp per day, usually from resting follicles. Except in cases of pattern baldness or disease, these hairs are replaced when the follicles become active again.

Proper hair care involves regular washing to remove the normal buildup of dirt, oils produced by skin glands, hair spray, dead skin cells, and other materials. Excessive combing and brushing can harm hair, as can pulling, curling, and "teasing." Frequent permanents and dye treatments can also harm hair, as can vigorous scalp massage.

Shampooing Hair

Although both soap and shampoo are effective hair-cleansing agents, people generally prefer shampoo to soap because, unless it is used in soft water, soap tends to leave a dull film on hair. Of the more than 600 shampoos on the market, all contain water, foaming agents, fragrances (which are added to mask the odors of other ingredients), and various amounts of detergent. Shampoos for oily hair have more detergent than shampoos for nonoily hair. Good shampoos are nonalkaline (pH balanced or slightly acidic).

Detergents make hair lose body and become unmanageable. Therefore, manufacturers may limit the amount of detergent in shampoos so that hair is not completely stripped of oils, or they may add "conditioners," which remain on hair even after rinsing.

Advertisers claim protein shampoos give hair bounce and body and can repair split ends. Protein does not repair hair or hair cells, although it may temporarily "glue" ends together.

Dandruff

Dandruff is caused by the scaling of scalp tissue. Most people have dandruff to some degree. It is not a disease, nor is it a mild form of seborrhea or psoriasis, which are true skin diseases. Dandruff is caused by a continual sloughing of dead scalp cells. The bits of dead skin tend to be large, and they may mix with oils and bacteria.

There is no way to prevent dandruff completely; it is controlled best by frequent cleansing of the hair and scalp. Use of shampoos containing either selenium sulfate or zinc pyrithionate can decrease the rate of sloughing of scalp tissue, and agents such as salicylic acid and sulfur reduce the size of dandruff flakes to facilitate removal.

Agents containing antibacterial or antifungal agents do not decrease dandruff.

Care of Skin

The major cause of skin dryness is a lack of water in the outermost layer of the skin. When the skin moisture level is less than 10 percent, the skin becomes chapped, brittle, rough, itchy, and dry. In addition, dry skin is more prone to bacterial invasion and inflammation. Healthy skin contains a natural moisturizing factor (NMF), which attracts moisture and holds it in the skin.

Dry skin may be caused by low humidity in the environment (below about 60 percent), high external temperatures, exposure to cold, and wind. Contact with substances that damage the skin cells and thereby impair their ability to retain water (chemical solvents, detergents, and so on) can also produce dry skin.

Treating Dry Skin

In conditions of low humidity, humidifiers can improve a dry skin condition. But simply adding water to the skin without the skin being able to retain it is not beneficial. Soaking in water will moisturize the skin, but the skin must be coated with an occlusive substance to prevent the water from evaporating. For this purpose bath oils are not as effective as moisturizing creams that contain NMF or sodium pyrrolidone carboxylic acid. Emollients (skin softeners), such as animal and vegetable oils and lanolin, provide an occlusive barrier that prevents evaporation of moisture from the skin surface, and they may also lubricate the skin and prevent chapping.

Suntans and Sunburns

Moderate exposure to sun's ultraviolet rays increases the skin's production of the pigment melanin, which is the basis of suntanning. The skin's ability to manufacture melanin each day is limited, so only a certain degree of tanning can be achieved with any given exposure. Thus, initial sun exposure should be limited to a maximum of 15–45 minutes; the following day's exposure time can be increased by an additional 15–30 minutes. When 60 minutes of exposure can be tolerated, all-day exposure is probably all right.

Too much sun is hazardous. It can cause severe sunburn, dry skin, premature aging of the skin (wrinkles and a tough, leathery look), and in some instances skin cancer.

Proper skin care in the sun involves limiting exposure to the sun's strongest ultraviolet rays:

1. Unless a suntan is desired, cover the skin when feasible.
2. Sunbathe as little as possible; acquire your tan gradually.
3. Don't sunbathe in the middle of the day (between 10:00 a.m. and 3:00 p.m.) when the sun is strongest.
4. Be aware that ultraviolet rays bounce off clouds, sand, fog, water, snow, patio decks, and other surfaces, thus increasing the dose of radiation you receive.
5. Sun reflectors expose the most delicate facial areas (under the chin, eyelids, earlobes). Don't use them.

Sunscreen products contain ingredients that protect a person from sunburn; they also limit tanning. Effective sunscreen agents, include paraaminobenzoic acid (PABA), cinoxate, digalloyl trioleate, ethylhexyl, p-methoxy-cinnamate, glyceryl p-aminobenzoate, oxybenzone, padamate, phenylbenzimidazone, and methylanthranilate. The amount of protection afforded by a particular sunscreen product is designated by its Sun Protection Factor (SPF), which is a number from 2 to 30 listed on the product label. A product with a low SPF offers the least sunburn protection; products with an SPF of 30 afford the maximum protection from sunburn and permit only limited tanning.

Sunblock products contain titanium oxide, red petrolatum, or zinc oxide. They block 100 percent of the sun's rays and therefore prevent tanning.

Suntanning products include baby oil, cocoa butter, coconut oil, mineral oil, and olive oil. The agents promote suntanning and do not protect against sunburn.

Chemical tanners (quick tan or indoor tan) contain dihydroxyacetone, which stains the skin, usually in a blotchy fashion. Such products offer no protection against sunburn.

Back Care

Emotional tension, strenuous activities, and poor posture when standing, sitting, or lying down can strain muscles and ligaments in the back and cause low back pain. To check your posture:

1. Stand with your back to a wall. Press your heels, rump, shoulders, and head against the

wall. If you feel any space between the small of your back and the wall, your back is arched too much.

2. Move your feet forward and bend your knees so that your back slides a few inches down the wall. Now, tighten your abdominal and buttocks muscles so you can flatten your lower back against the wall.

3. Hold this position and "walk" your feet back so that you slide up the wall.

4. Standing straight, walk away from the wall and around the room.

5. Return to the wall and back up to it to make sure you've kept proper posture.

Back Care Exercises

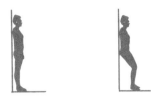

1. *Pelvic tilt.* Lie on a padded floor. Tighten your abdominal and buttocks muscles to press your lower back flat against the floor. Hold for a count of five. Repeat three times; work up to twenty. Begin exercise with your knees bent; advance to straight leg.

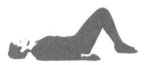

2. *Single-knee raise.* Lie on a padded floor. Lift one knee to chest. Tighten your abdominal and buttocks muscles to press the curve out of your lower back. Hold this position for a count of five. Repeat three times for each leg; work up to ten repetitions for each leg.

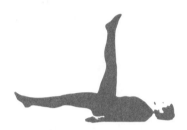

3. *Double-knee raise.* Follow the procedure for single-knee raise.

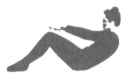

4. *Single-leg raise.* Raise your leg as far as possible without pain, keeping your back flat against the floor. Begin with three repetitions for each leg and work up to ten. Do not do this exercise if you have sciatica ("down-the-leg" pain).

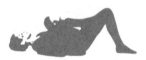

5. *Sit-up.* Begin with partial sit-ups — raising your head, neck, and shoulders and extending your hands to your knees — and work up to full sit-ups. Work up to ten repetitions.

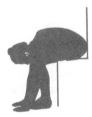

6. *Sitting bend.* While sitting in a chair with feet flat on the floor, bend no farther than is comfortable, reaching your hands to the floor. Repeat three times at first; work up to ten.

Standing Properly

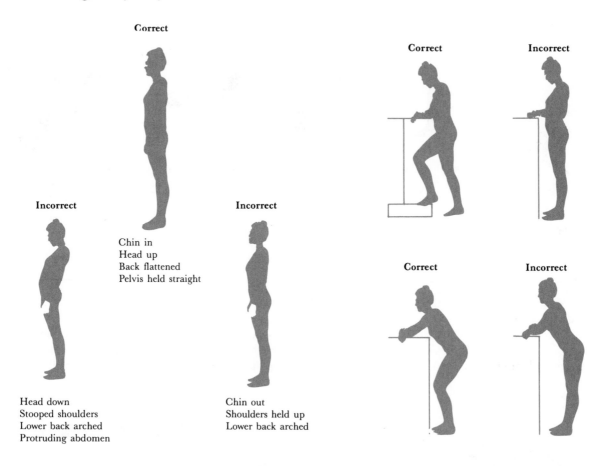

Correct

Chin in
Head up
Back flattened
Pelvis held straight

Incorrect

Head down
Stooped shoulders
Lower back arched
Protruding abdomen

Incorrect

Chin out
Shoulders held up
Lower back arched

Correct   Incorrect

Correct   Incorrect

Lifting and Carrying

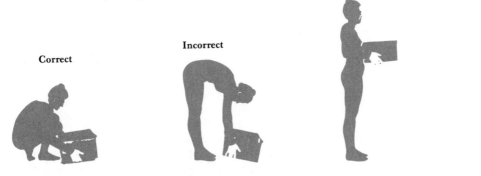

Correct   Incorrect   Correct   Incorrect

To lift an object:
1. Face the object fully.
2. Bend your knees and hips, not your waist.

3. Hold the object close to your body.
4. Use your large thigh muscles for lifting, not your back muscles.

To carry an object.
1. Hold the object close to your body.
2. Avoid carrying unbalanced loads.

3. Do not lift the object higher than your waist.
4. Avoid sudden movements and twisting your torso.

Sitting Correctly

Correct

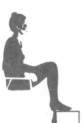

Correct

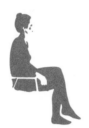

Correct

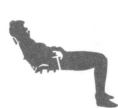

Correct

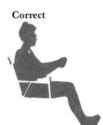

Incorrect   Correct

When you sit, your lower back should be flat or slightly rounded outward. Your knees should be slightly higher than your hips, with both feet firmly on the floor.

A footrest can help keep knees at proper height.

Crossing your knees relieves strain from sitting too long.

Slumping strains your neck, shoulders, and back.

In automobile seats, do not lean forward; sit close enough to reach pedals comfortably without stretching your legs. Use a backrest to keep your back firm and flat. Use a seatbelt or harness.

Lying Down

Firm sleeping supports are better than soft ones or hard ones such as the floor. A standard waterbed or a bed with at least a 720-coil "orthopedic" mat- tress and box spring distribute body pressure evenly. These make the best beds for general use. Too-soft sleeping surfaces can be supported with a bedboard.

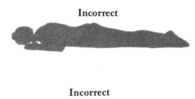

Incorrect

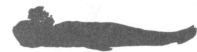

Incorrect

Correct

Incorrect

The recommended position for sleeping is lying on your side (to keep your back flat) with your body partially curled. Lying flat on your

back, using a high pillow, or sleeping face down exaggerates swayback.

Breast Self-exam

Breasts come in all sizes and shapes, just as women do. One woman's breasts are not the same as any others. Nor will her own breasts remain the same throughout her adult life. The monthly menstrual cycle, menopause, childbirth, breastfeeding, age, weight change, birth control or other hormone pills, and even nutrition may change the shape and size of her breasts.

In addition, many women develop one of a va- riety of noncancerous breast conditions, which, as a group, are referred to as "benign fibrocystic dis- ease." Among themselves, women often call them "lumpy breasts." If a woman has one of these con- ditions, lumps or nodules are "normal" for her.

Breast self-examination is done once a month so that a woman becomes familiar with the usual appearance and feel of her own breasts. Familiarity makes it easier to notice any changes in the breast from one month to another. Early discovery of a change from what is "normal" is the whole idea behind BSE.

For a menstruating woman, the best time to do BSE is at the end of her period, when her breasts are least likely to be tender or swollen. A menopausal or postmenopausal woman may find it helpful to pick a particular day, such as the first of the month, to remind herself it is time to do BSE.

If a woman discovers anything unusual—such as a lump, discharge, dimpling or puckering—she should see her physician at once. Eight out of ten breast lumps are *not* cancer, and there are other causes for changes in the breast's appearance. But any change is best diagnosed by a physician.

From "How to Examine Your Breasts" by the American Cancer Society.

How to Examine Your Breasts

1. In the shower: Examine your breasts during bath or shower; hands glide easier over wet skin. Fingers flat, move gently over every part of each breast. Use right hand to examine left breast, left hand for right breast. Check for any lump, hard knot, or thickening.

2. Before a mirror: Inspect your breasts with arms at your sides.

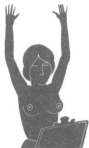

Next, raise your arms high overhead. Look for any changes in contour of each breast, a swelling, dimpling of skin, or changes in the nipple.

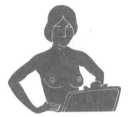

Then, rest palms on hips and press down firmly to flex your chest muscles. Left and right breast will not exactly match—few women's breasts do.

Regular inspection shows what is normal for you and will give you confidence in your examination.

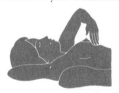

3. Lying down: To examine your right breast, put a pillow or folded towel under your right shoulder. Place right hand behind your head —this distributes breast tissue more evenly on the chest. With left hand, fingers flat, press gently in small circular motions around an imaginary clock face. Begin at outermost top of your right breast for 12 o'clock, then move to 1

o'clock, and so on around the circle back to 12. A ridge of firm tissue in the lower curve of each breast is normal. Then move in an inch, toward the nipple, keep circling to examine *every part of your breast,* including nipple. This requires at least three more circles. Now slowly repeat procedure on your left breast with a pillow under your left shoulder and left hand behind head. Notice how your breast structure feels.

Finally, squeeze the nipple of each breast gently between thumb and index finger. Any discharge, clear or bloody, should be reported to your doctor immediately.

Appendix C

Fitness, Sports, and Relaxation

Determining Your Fitness Index
Determining Your Flexibility Index
Principles of Aerobic Conditioning
Tips for Joggers
Massage

Determining Your Fitness Index

The Harvard Step Test is a standardized measure of cardiorespiratory fitness. To carry out the Harvard Step Test, you need to be comfortably dressed (athletic clothes are best), you need a chair, stool, or bench 12–18 inches high, a stopwatch or clock with a second hand, a pencil and paper, and a metronome or some other method to produce a rhythmic 100–120 beats per minute, such as a recording of a march or some disco music. Once all this is assembled, you can begin.

1. Make a 15-second recording of your resting pulse and multiply by 4 to obtain your rate per minute.
2. Start the metronome or music; 120 beats per minute.
3. Step completely up on the bench with the left leg first, followed by your right leg, then step back down with the left leg first, followed by the right. The stepping should be done on a four-count: up-up-down-down; up-up-down-down . . .

Fitness Index	Rating
above 90	Excellent
80–89	Good
65–79	Good
55–64	Low Average
below 55	Poor

Harvard Step Test Data Record

Time	Heartbeats per 15 seconds		Heartbeats per minute
At rest	_____	× 4 =	_____
15–30 sec.	_____	× 4 =	_____
60–75 sec.	_____	× 4 =	_____
120–135 sec.	_____	× 4 =	_____
180–195 sec.	_____	× 4 =	_____
240–255 sec.	_____	× 4 =	_____
300–315 sec.	_____	× 4 =	_____

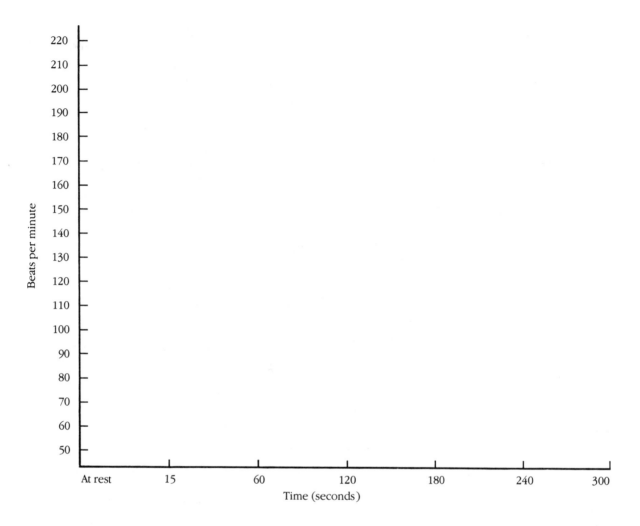

4. Continue the exercise for 3 minutes unless you are over 30 years old and have been rather inactive for more than six months. In that case, do the test for only a minute or two, whichever you think you can do. If you are sure you cannot do the test for even a few seconds, don't.

5. When the 3 minutes of exercise are through, immediately take your pulse. Record the number of heartbeats between 15 and 30 seconds after exercising. Make another heart rate measurement between 60 and 75 seconds; another between 120 and 135 seconds; another between 180 and 195 seconds; another between 240 and 255 seconds; and a final measurement between 300 and 315 seconds.

6. Multiply each of the 15-second heart rates by 4 to give the beats per minute. Record your data on a graph.

7. Compute your Fitness Index: Add the per-minute heart rates for the first 3 minutes after exercise. Then divide that number into 30,000.

Determining Your Flexibility Index

Body flexibility is a fundamental aspect of feeling good and keeping your body young. Use this simple YMCA test to determine your degree of body flexibility, and continue to use it to determine your progress in becoming more limber.

1. Warm up with some stretching before the test.
2. Sit on the floor with your legs extended and feet a few inches apart.
3. With a piece of adhesive tape, mark the place where your heels touch the floor. Your heels should touch the near edge of the tape.
4. Place a yardstick on the floor between your legs and parallel to them. The beginning of the yardstick should be closest to you and the 15-inch mark should align with the near edge of the tape.
5. Slowly reach with both hands as far forward as possible. Touch your fingers to the yardstick to determine the distance reached. Do not jerk to increase your distance—this may cause damage to your leg muscles.
6. Repeat the exercise two or three times and record your best score.

Inches reached		Rating
Men	Women	
22–23	24–27	Excellent
20–21	21–23	Good
14–19	16–20	Average
12–13	13–16	Fair
0–11	0–12	Poor

You can consult a wide variety of exercise and yoga books to find exercises that will help you improve your flexibility.

Principles of Aerobic Conditioning

The five basic principles of aerobic conditioning are:

1. Frequency: you should exercise at least three times a week.
2. Intensity: you should exercise within 65–75 percent of your maximum work capacity, known as your **target zone** (see opposite).
3. Duration: you should exercise within your target zone for 30 minutes each time.
4. Type of exercise: appropriate exercises are rhythmic, are continuous, and utilize the large muscles of the legs and hips. Such exercises include walking, jogging, bicycling, swimming, cross-country skiing, and aerobic dancing.
5. Warm up and cool down; you should do 10 minutes of slow, smooth stretching before exercising and 5 minutes of walking and some stretching after exercising.

Finding Your Target Zone

Your target zone is the level of activity that leads to maximum conditioning. Activity below the target zone conditions little; activity above the target zone may be dangerous for some people.

The target zone is conveniently monitored by the heart rate. After your warm-up period and 10 minutes of activity, take your pulse and compare it to the heart rate for your target zone level of activity. If you are below your target zone heart rate, increase your activity. If above, slow down. To compute your target zone heart rate:

1. Subtract your age from 220. (*EXAMPLE,* for a 20-year-old person with resting heart rate of 80 beats/min.: 220 − 20 = 200.)
2. Subtract resting heart rate from number obtained in step 1. (200 − 80 = 120.)
3. Multiply the result once by 0.65 and once again by 0.75. (120 × .65 = 78; 120 × .75 = 90.)
4. Add resting heart rate to results obtained in step 3 to give lower and upper heart rates of target zone. (Lower limit: 78 + 80 = 158; upper limit: 90 + 80 = 170.)

The pattern of the preferred exercise session is shown in the following figure:

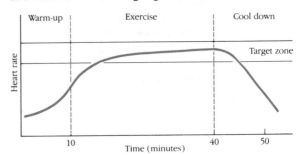

Tips for Joggers

1. Always warm up before jogging. Be sure to stretch the muscles in the back of your legs.
2. Wear good running shoes and comfortable clothes.
3. Avoid running on concrete and asphalt, if possible; running tracks and grass (watch for holes!) do less damage to feet and legs.
4. Avoid running in temperatures above 85°F.
5. Avoid blisters by wearing shoes and socks that fit properly; coat blister "hot spots" with petroleum jelly and cover with gauze or moleskin.
6. A good running pace is one that allows you to be able to carry on a conversation while running.

For proper running posture:

1. Keep your back straight.
2. Keep your head up, looking straight ahead about 20 feet.
3. Bend your arms at the elbows and keep your forearms parallel to the ground; keep your elbows close to your body (no "wings").
4. Your hands should be loose. Let the tips of your thumb and first or second fingers touch; do not make a fist.
5. Run heel-to-toe, not on the balls of your feet.

Massage

Everyone experiences tense muscles and soreness in parts of the body occasionally. Some parts of the body, such as the neck, shoulders, and back, are prime locations for accumulated tension. Mental and emotional distress can cause muscle tension and physical discomfort.

Massage is an excellent way to reduce physical tension and relax body muscles. In turn, a relaxed body facilitates a relaxed state of mind. All human beings need physical contact with other people. Babies and children are constantly seeking ways to be held, touched, and massaged by their caregivers. Mothers instinctively stroke and rub their infants. Unfortunately, as we grow older we tend to give and receive less physical contact.

Giving a Back Massage

Anyone can give a massage to another person. All that's required is the desire to make another person feel more comfortable and a willingness to be sensitive to another person's stiff muscles.

Learn by exchanging massages with friends and persons you are comfortable with and trust. The person being massaged can be sitting up or lying down. The area to be massaged should be free of clothing. Begin with the neck, using your thumbs to press the muscles on either side of the spine. Press firmly and smoothly away from the spine. Work down the back, always pressing down and away from the spine. Be sensitive to sore places or knots of tense muscles. Apply steady gentle pressure to these areas until you feel the person relax or the muscles soften. As you become more experienced, you can use the heels of your hands or your knuckles to knead tense muscles. Always be sensitive to what the other person is feeling.

It helps to use a small amount of skin oil on your hands to reduce friction. You may want to play soft music or encourage the person to relax while you are massaging him or her.

Giving a Foot Massage

A foot massage is a relaxing, pleasant experience. The foot is a sensitive part of the body and often has places that are stiff or sore. Most people feel greatly relaxed after receiving a foot massage.

Begin by washing the person's feet with warm water. Rub the whole foot and ankle with a small amount of massage oil. Massage each toe and between each toe. Gently pull each toe to stretch the muscles and joints. You may hear the joint make a small cracking sound; this is normal. Massage the foot with your thumbs, fingers, or knuckles from top to bottom. Do one foot and then the other. It's easier if you cradle the foot in your lap. Be sensitive and gentle. Ask the person to tell you if any part hurts. Spend more time in places that are sore by gently pressing, rubbing, and massaging the area.

Always give a massage with your whole being—not just your hands. Be gentle, caring, and sensitive to what the other person is experiencing. A massage is an ideal way for two persons to become more in touch with their bodies and to release physical tension.

Appendix D

Health Emergencies

The Role of Imagery in Emergency Healing
Bleeding Emergencies
Burns
Choking
First Aid for Sports Injuries

The Role of Imagery in Emergency Healing

Your initial mental reaction to a minor injury such as a gashed finger or a stubbed toe is usually annoyance at being clumsy or anger directed at the injured part of the body. Fear and anger inhibit natural healing processes and usually increase pain, too.

Following the injury, do whatever is necessary to provide immediate relief (see following information). Then, close your eyes. Become calm. Let your mind focus on a familiar scene or memory in which you feel comfortable and relaxed. Notice that your body is healthy and strong in your mind. Allow your mind to travel through all the parts of your body, relaxing any tension you become aware of in any muscles or organs. Let your mind enter a dreamlike state. Know that when you emerge from this pleasant, dreamlike, relaxed state of mind, your body will have begun to heal itself. Your discomfort will be much less. The injured part of your body will already feel more comfortable, thus reassuring you that recovery has begun and that healing will proceed quickly.

Bleeding Emergencies

1. Control bleeding with direct pressure over the wound. Apply firm, steady pressure with a sterile gauze pad, clean handkerchief, or even the bare hand if necessary. You can slow the bleeding from a hand, arm, foot, or leg by elevating the limb above the level of the heart.

2. Visualize the cut or wound in your mind. See the wound or cut closing and the skin sealing off the flow of blood. Feel the injured area becoming cool and comfortable. Notice that there is no redness or sign of infection in the area. Imagine examining the injury a week or so from now and noticing that there is hardly any scar or discomfort in the area. The area has become completely normal again.

3. Bleeding from the ear after a head injury or bleeding from the scalp must be treated by a professional. Apply pressure gently to any scalp wound. Do not bend the neck.

4. Coughing or vomiting blood requires immediate professional attention.

Burns

Minor burns caused by fire, covering only a small areas of the body, can be treated with cold running water or an ice pack applied for 20–30 minutes to relieve swelling and pain. Do not use grease of any kind. Cold running water is the best first aid.

Serious burns require prompt professional care. *Call for help immediately.* Wrap the victim in a clean, wet sheet or towel moistened at room temperature. Burn victims need fluid. Give the victim all the water he or she desires. Do not attempt to clean the burns or remove clothing or other particles attached to the burned area. Keep the victim lying down, calm and reassured.

If you suffer a burn, do *not* become angry at the pain and stinging feeling. Allow your mind to comfort the injured area as if that part of the body belonged to another person. Talk to the injured area in soothing words if that seems to help. Close your eyes and imagine that snow or ice is packed over the burned area. Begin to see healthy new skin covering the area. Imagine showing the burn to a friend in a couple of weeks and describing how fast you were able to heal the part that had been burned.

Choking

Anything stuck in the throat blocking the air passage can stop breathing and cause unconsciousness and death within minutes. Do not interfere with a choking victim who can speak, cough, or breathe. But if a conscious person cannot speak, cough or breathe:

1. Stand just behind and to the side of the victim. Support the victim with one hand on the chest. The victim's head should be lowered. Give four sharp blows between the shoulder blades.

2. If unsuccessful, stand behind the victim and wrap your arms around his or her middle, just above the navel. Clasp your hands together in a double fist and press in and up in quick thrusts. Repeat several times.

3. If still unsuccessful, make your pointer finger into a hook shape. Reach down the victim's throat in a sweeping motion, feeling for the object.

Note: If the object has not been retrieved but the swallower suddenly seems all right, play it safe. Take him or her directly to the hospital. This is especially critical if the swallowed object is a fish bone, chicken bone, or other jagged object that could do internal damage as it passes through the victim's system.

First Aid For Sports Injuries

Nearly all common sports injuries involve the release of fluids and other tissue substances from damaged muscles, tendons, and ligaments. Immediate treatment requires limiting swelling and internal blood loss as much as possible. This is accomplished by applying ice to the injured region, wrapping the injured region in elastic, elevating it, and possibly immobilizing the injured region. These measures will speed healing and decrease pain.

To ice an injury, fill a plastic bag with ice cubes or crushed ice and place the ice directly on the injured region for about 5–10 minutes, three times a day. The cold treatments should be applied for 24–72 hours, depending on the extent of the injury. A foot, hand, or forearm can be placed directly in a bowl or bucket of ice water.

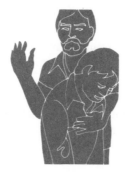
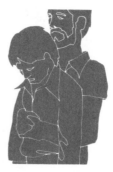
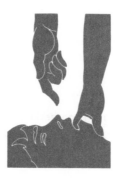

Appendix E

Medical Care

A Schedule for Immunizing Children
The Patient's Guide for a Successful Doctor's Visit
Describing a Personal Medical Problem
Personal Medical History
Drug Information Checklist

A Schedule for Immunizing Children

The following schedule is advised by the Immunization Division of the Centers for Disease Control in Atlanta, a part of the United States Public Health Service.

Your child should receive at the age indicated:

- 2 months — diphtheria, tetanus, pertussis, (DTP, first dose); oral polio (first dose).

- 4 months — DTP (second dose); oral polio (second dose).

- 6 months — DTP (third dose).

- 15 months — measles, mumps, rubella (these three may be combined in a single injection).

- 18 months — DTP (fourth dose); oral polio (third dose).

- 4–6 years — DTP (fifth dose, at school entry); oral polio (fourth dose).

- 14–16 years — tetanus-diphtheria booster and every 10 years thereafter.

The Patient's Guide for a Successful Doctor's Visit

Take Pertinent Information with You

1. Write a description of your present problem (see following section).
2. Have a written personal health history.

Discuss Nonmedical Concerns Beforehand

1. If you wish, inquire about the doctor's credentials and training.
2. You have the right to inquire about the fee and to expect to see an itemization of any additional charges (such as for tests and medications).

Ask About Examinations and Tests

1. Ask if an examination is a complete physical exam. If not, ask which body systems are being examined.
2. Inquire as to significant findings.
3. Satisfy yourself that any tests that are ordered are relevant to your problem and that benefits outweigh any risks.
4. Keep a record of how many x-rays you've had in the past year (including dental x-rays) and ask whether your exposure is in the safe range.
5. Ask the technical names of any tests; have the doctor, nurse, or technician write the names down.
6. Write down the results of any tests, including a pathologist's report. Ask your doctor to compare your results to what is considered normal.

Ask About the Diagnosis

1. Write down the diagnosis in medical terms.
2. Ask the doctor or nurse to explain the diagnosis in terms you can understand.
3. Ask what caused the illness and what is happening to you.
4. Ask whether you are contagious.
5. Ask how the problem can be prevented.

Ask About the Treatment

1. Ask about the pros and cons of all possible treatments.
2. Ask what will happen if you choose not to treat the problem.
3. Obtain pertinent information (from a doctor or pharmacist) about any drug or medicine that is recommended.

Know What to Do After You Leave

1. Ask about return visits.
2. Ask about special instructions to follow at home.
3. Ask whether you are to telephone for lab reports.
4. Ask about possible signs of the problem worsening and what to do.

Describing a Personal Medical Problem

When visiting a doctor, be prepared to describe in your own words why you have come for care. Don't let fear, shame, pride, or embarrassment prevent you from telling the facts. Don't discount any worry or pain. Be sure to mention even the little things that bother you, even if you think they are unrelated to your present problem.

Describe your problem by indicating:

1. All your symptoms (complaints, changes, pains) in the order in which they appeared.
2. In what region of the body a symptom is located.
3. What a symptom is like (a stabbing pain, a knot).
4. A symptom's intensity (unbearable, manageable).
5. When a symptom began to occur.
6. How often a symptom occurs.
7. Whether a symptom is constant or intermittent.
8. What brings a symptom on.
9. How long a symptom lasts.
10. What makes a symptom better.
11. What makes a symptom worse.
12. What symptoms occur together.
13. Any changes in your lifestyle or habits that coincide with the beginning of the present problem.

Personal Medical History

Height: _____   Blood type: ABO _____   Rh _____

Weight now: _____ a year ago _____ highest _____ when _____

Blood pressure: now _____ a year ago _____ highest _____ when _____

Alcohol consumption: never _____ seldom _____ moderate _____ daily _____

Cigarette smoking: cigarettes per day _____ for how long _____

Illness History

Illness	No	Yes	When	Treatment	Special problems
German measles					
Mumps					
Chicken pox					
Scarlet fever					
Diphtheria					
Pneumonia, bronchitis, asthma					
Arthritis					
Rheumatic fever					
Heart disease or heart murmur					
Anemia					
Bleeding problem					
Ulcer, colitis					
Epilepsy					
Severe headaches					
Mononucleosis					
Jaundice or hepatitis					
Eye injury					
Ear disease or injury					
Skin disease					
Varicose veins					
Kidney or bladder problem					

Surgical History

What	When	Where	Physician

Accidents

Date	Cause	Type	Treatment	Physician

Travel Outside U.S.A.

Where	When	How long

Drug Allergies

Drug	Reaction	Date

Other Allergies

☐ Asthma   ☐ Food   Which? _____

☐ Eczema   ☐ Insect   Which? _____

☐ Hay fever   ☐ Pollens   Which? _____

☐ Hives   ☐ Other   State _____

Laboratory Tests and Procedures

	Date	Date	Date	Date	Date	Date	Date	Date
Blood chemistry								
EKG								
Glaucoma test								
Pap smear								
Urinalysis								
X-ray								

Medications Presently Taking

Drug	Dose	How long?

Family History

Disease

	Cancer	Diabetes	Heart disease	Hypertension	Stroke	Other	If deceased, age at death	Cause of death
Father								
Mother								
Brother								
Brother								
Brother								
Sister								
Sister								
Sister								

Drug Information Checklist

Name of physician _____ Telephone number _____

Name of pharmacist _____ Telephone number _____

Name of drug _____ Prescription number _____

Purpose for taking the drug _____

Prescription can be renewed _____ times

Physical description of the drug (color, pill, powder, liquid, tube, capsule) _____

Instructions for use:

Take _____ every _____
       (amount)   (how often)

Foods and other substances this drug should *NOT* be taken with: _____

_____

Foods and other substances this drug should be taken with: _____

_____

Possible side effects: _____

_____

Contact physician or pharmacist if these side effects occur: _____

_____

_____

_____

_____

_____

Glossary

A

acetylcholine a neurotransmitter.

acupuncture a Chinese healing art that uses tiny, thin needles inserted at specific spots on the body to block pain and cure disease.

addiction physical and psychological dependence on a drug. *See also* positive addiction.

adenoidectomy surgical removal of adenoids.

adipocytes cells that store body fat.

aerobic capacity the maximum amount of oxygen the body can process in a given time.

affective disorders certain kinds of severe mental illnesses that are characterized by unusually deep moods, especially depression.

agammaglobulinemia a genetic disease that results in the body's inability to manufacture antibodies.

ageism age-related prejudice.

alcoholism loss of control over drinking alcohol.

allopathic medicine conventional medicine.

alveoli the air sacs in the lungs that exchange oxygen and carbon dioxide.

amenorrhea the absence of menstrual periods.

amino acids biological molecules used in the synthesis of proteins, neurotransmitters, and some hormones.

amniocentesis removal of a small amount of amniotic fluid from a pregnant woman's uterus and examination of fetal cells in the fluid for possible genetic defects.

amygdalin a substance containing cyanide found in laetrile.

anaphylaxis a severe, sometimes fatal, reaction to a drug or allergen.

anemia a deficiency of red blood cells; often caused by an iron deficiency.

anesthetics drugs that inhibit pain.

aneurysm a ballooning out of an artery or vein whose walls have been weakened or damaged.

angina pectoris intermittent chest pains caused by decreased blood flow and oxygen to the heart.

ankylosing spondylitis a degenerative, arthritis-like disease of the spine.

antibody a protein molecule, synthesized by the body's immune system, that recognizes and inactivates foreign substances in the body.

antigen any substance that stimulates antibody production by the body's immune system.

antimetabolite a drug that interferes with a chemical reaction in cells and prevents growth.

aorta the main artery from the heart that carries blood to body tissues.

arterial thrombosis a blood clot within an artery. Because it blocks circulation of blood, the clot can cause a heart attack or stroke.

arteriosclerosis any disease of the arteries; hardening of the arteries.

arthritis a disease, thought to be at least partly of autoimmune origin, in which the joints become stiff and movement painful.

atherosclerosis a disease characterized by formation of fatty, fibrous lesions in the lining of arteries; the major cause of cardiovascular disease. The term is often used interchangeably with arteriosclerosis.

atria the heart chambers that receive oxygen-depleted blood; also called auricles.

autogenic training a system of physical and mental relaxation that employees "autogenic suggestions" (autosuggestive phrases) to effect a physiological change through changes in the autonomic nervous system.

autonomic nervous system (ANS) the portion of the nervous system that plays a key role in maintaining homeostasis by regulating involuntary physiological processes, such as breathing, digestion, and so on.

autoimmune disease a disease caused by the body's immune system attacking the body's own cells.

B

balance study   a way to determine the amount of a particular nutrient required by a given individual.

basal metabolic rate (BMR)   the minimal amount of energy needed to keep the body functioning.

bender   a several days' binge of drinking alcohol.

benign tumor   a tumor in which growing cells remain localized at the site of origin.

beri-beri   a disease caused by deficiency of vitamin B_1.

bile acids   substances produced in the gallbladder that aid in the digestion of fats.

blood alcohol content (BAC)   the percentage of alcohol in the blood.

body work   a regularly practiced physical activity designed to increase physical, psychological, and spiritual dimensions of health.

bran   the outer husk of the wheat kernel.

bronchitis   imflammation of the bronchi of the lungs as a result of irritation; often accompanied by a chronic cough.

Burkitt's lymphoma   a form of cancer, found mainly among Africans, that is associated with the presence of a particular viral infection.

C

calorie   the amount of energy required to raise the temperature of 1 gram of water from 14.5°C to 15.5°C. One thousand calories (a kilocalorie) is a nutritional calorie.

cancer   a group of diseases characterized by unregulated cell multiplication.

capillaries   tiny blood vessels that carry blood to tissues and cells.

carbohydrates   biological molecules consisting of one or more sugar molecules.

carcinogen   a chemical that can cause cancer.

carcinomas   cancers arising from skin and from cells that cover or line body organs.

cardiologist   a physician who specializes in heart and blood vessel diseases.

cardiovascular disease   disease of the heart or blood vessels.

cerebral cortex   the outer part of the human brain, which is responsible for perception and the higher functions of reason, logic, language, creativity, and so on.

cervical cap   a contraceptive device that covers the cervix.

cervix   the lower part of the uterus.

chancre   a painless ulcer or sore that signals the onset of syphilis.

chi   a Chinese term for the vital energy in the human body.

chiropractic   medical treatment by spinal manipulation as well as other healing techniques.

chlamydia   a sexually transmitted disease caused by the bacterium *Chlamydia trachomatis*.

chronic degenerative diseases   diseases that tend to persist for life and that progressively worsen with time.

chronic obstructive pulmonary diseases (COPD)   diseases that restrict the ability of the body to obtain oxygen through the respiratory structures (bronchi and lungs). These diseases include asthma, bronchitis, and emphysema.

cilia   tiny, hairlike projections in the breathing passageways that filter out microscopic organisms and particles before air reaches the lungs.

circumcision   a surgical procedure to remove the foreskin from the penis.

cirrhosis   a severe liver disease often caused by alcohol abuse.

clitoris   a sexually sensitive organ in the female analogous to the penis in the male.

communicable disease   a disease that is passed from person to person, usually by close contact.

condom   a sheath that covers the end of the penis to prevent the movement of sperm into the vagina; it also helps prevent the transmission of organisms that cause some diseases.

congenital defect   any physical abnormality present at birth.

congeners   flavorings, colorings, and other chemicals present in alcoholic beverages.

contraceptive sponge   a device that is impregnated with spermicide and placed in the vagina before intercourse.

contraindication   any medical reason for not taking a particular drug.

coping strategies   ways people devise to help prevent, avoid, or control emotional distress.

coronary arteries   blood vessels that supply oxygenated blood to the heart itself.

culpotomy   a type of tubal ligation procedure.

cystitis   infection of the urinary bladder.

D

delirium tremens (DT's)   hallucinations and uncontrollable shaking caused by withdrawal of alcohol in alcohol-dependent individuals.

diabetes   a disease characterized by imbalance in blood sugar; usually associated with insulin deficiency.

diaphragm   a dome-shaped contraceptive device that is placed in the vagina.

diastole   relaxation of the heart in each heartbeat.

diethylstilbestrol (DES)   a synthetic hormone prescribed for women. If taken during pregnancy, it may cause abnormalities in the reproductive organs of the fetus.

digestive system   the group of organs that digest and absorb food and eliminate waste products.

dilatation and curettage (D and C)   a procedure for removing material from the uterus; a method of abortion.

disease   signs of sickness diagnosed by a physician.

diuretics   drugs that increase urine production.

Down's syndrome   a chromosomal abnormality that produces a disease characterized by severe mental retardation; formerly called "mongolism."

drug   a single chemical substance in a medicine that alerts the structure or function of some of the body's tissues.

drug abuse   persistent or excessive use of a drug for no medical or health reasons.

drug tolerance   adaptation of the body and brain to repeated exposure of a drug.

dysmenorrhea   painful menstruation.

E

ectopic pregnancy   a pregnancy occurring outside the uterus.

electroconvulsive therapy   electric shocks applied to the brain to treat certain forms of mental illness, especially severe depression. A controversial procedure.

emergency response   the coordinated discharge of hormones and activity of the autonomic nervous system to prepare the body to fight or flee in a threatening situation. Also known as the "fight or flight" response.

emotional distress   feelings of frustration, anger, fear, anxiety, or depression that occur when emotional needs are not being met.

emphysema   a progressive degeneration of the lung alveoli, causing breathing and oxygen assimilation to become more and more difficult.

endocrine system   the group of glands in the brain and body that manufacture and secrete hormones.

endometrium   the inner lining of the uterus.

endorphins and enkephalins   small molecules synthesized in the brain that influence the sensation of pain.

energy balance   the state that exists when caloric intake equals caloric expenditure.

environment   all external factors that can affect people.

episiotomy   a small, reversible surgical incision to enlarge the vagina to permit easier passage of a baby out of the mother's body during childbirth.

essential amnio acids   the eight amnio acids that the body cannot synthesize and that must, therefore, be supplied in the diet.

essential hypertension   high blood pressure for which there is no medically known cause.

etiology   the causes or origins of a disease.

F

fallopian tubes   a pair of tubelike structures that transport ova from the ovaries to the uterus and that are the usual site of fertilizaton.

familial pattern   the higher-than-average occurrence of a disease among members of a family.

fermentation   conversion of sugar to ethyl alcohol by yeast.

fertilization   the fusion of a sperm cell and an ovum.

fetal alcohol syndrome   birth defects caused by ingestion of alcohol during pregnancy.

fiber   nondigestible vegetable material; also called dietary fiber or roughage.

fibrillation   highly irregular heartbeat.

fibrinopeptide A   a protein; high levels in the blood may indicate cancer.

foreskin   a fold of skin over the end of the penis.

fructose   a simple sugar found in fruits and honey.

G

G spot   a hypothetical region in the vagina that may be an area of sexual sensitivity in some women.

galactose   a simple sugar.

galvanic skin response (GSR)   changes in the skin's electrical resistance in response to changes in a person's emotional state or arousal level.

gastrointestinal (GI) tract   *see* digestive system.

gender identity   the awareness of being either male or female.

general adaptation syndrome (GAS)   a three-stage physiological reaction to stress.

genetic disease   a hereditary disease; one that is passed from parents to children.

gerontology   the branch of science that studies aging.

glucose   the principal source of energy in all cells, also called dextrose.

glucose tolerance test   a clinical test designed to measure a person's ability to regulate blood sugar levels.

glycogen long chains of glucose molecules stored in animal tissue to provide reserve energy.

goiter an enlargement of the thyroid gland; often caused by an iodine deficiency.

gonadotropins pituitary hormones that regulate many aspects of sexual reproduction.

gonorrhea A sexually transmitted disease caused by gonococcal bacteria.

H

habituation psychological dependence on a drug without physical addiction.

hal old English root of the word "health"; meaning sound or whole.

hangover nausea, headache, fatigue, weakness, irritability, and other symptoms experienced the morning after drinking alcohol.

heart attack obstruction of the coronary arteries, depriving the heart of blood and oxygen.

hemophilia a genetic disease, almost exclusively of males, that slows blood coagulation; as a result the person bleeds excessively when injured.

herbal medicine use of plants and natural substances to treat disease.

herpes genitalis a sexually transmitted disease caused by the *Herpes simplex* virus.

Hippocratic oath the ethical principles governing the practice of medicine, as stated by the Greek physician Hippocrates.

histamine a chemical that is released by cells in response to foreign substances and that causes inflammation.

histocompatibility the degree of similarity between tissues from different individuals, as determined by the classes of antigens on cell surfaces; it is greatest between tissues of identical twins. Matching histocompatibility is essential in organ and tissue transplants and in the transfusion of blood.

HLA antigens substances on the surface of white blood cells that are used to measure how similar tissues are between individuals.

holistic health an approach to health that recognizes the interrelatedness of physical, mental, emotional, spiritual, social, and environmental factors in the attainment of health. The holistic philosophy also emphasizes self-reliance for health as much as possible.

holistic medicine an approach to medical therapy that considers the life situation of the unwell person and not merely the elimination of a specific symptom.

homeopathy a type of therapy that emphasizes stimulation of the body's defenses by administration of a substance that can simulate the disease.

homeostasis the automatic regulation of physiological processes to maintain them in a steady state; the maintenance of a normal, dynamic balance among the various body systems.

hormones "messenger" molecules, produced in endocrine glands, that regulate cellular functions in other parts of the body.

hospice a place for the terminally ill that attends to the physical, psychological, and spiritual needs of the dying.

human chorionic gonadotropin (HCG) a hormone produced during the first stages of pregnancy; it is used as the basis of pregnancy tests.

Huntington's chorea a genetic disease resulting in degeneration of nerve tissue, usually in midlife.

hyperglycemia a condition characterized by blood sugar levels that are persistently too high.

hypertension high blood pressure.

hypnoanesthesia insensitivity to pain and discomfort as a result of hypnosis.

hypnosis a state of forced mental attention in which the mind is particularly open to suggestion.

hypnotherapy the medical use of hypnosis for treating physical and emotional disturbances.

hypoglycemia a condition characterized by blood sugar levels that are persistently too low. *See also* reactive hypoglycemia.

hypothalamus the area of the brain responsible for regulating many of the body's essential functions.

hysterectomy surgical removal of the uterus.

I

iatrogenic illness illness caused by improper medication or medical care.

illness symptoms or ill-feelings experienced by an unwell person.

immune responses the production of antibodies by B-lymphocytes in response to an antigen; also, direct attack on antigens by T-lymphocytes.

immune surveillance hypothesis the proposal that specific cells of the immune system are able to detect and destroy cancer cells as they arise in the body.

immunosuppressive drugs drugs that prevent the immune system from responding to foreign tissues and organisms.

infertile unable to become pregnant or to impregnate.

inflammation a general reaction of tissue to infecting microorganisms or foreign substances.

insulin a hormone secreted by the pancreas that regulates blood sugar (glucose) levels.

insulin rebound   *see* reactive hypoglycemia.

interferon   a substance produced in response to viral infections; it inhibits viral growth.

intrauterine device (IUD)   a small plastic contraceptive device placed in the cavity of the uterus; its precise mode of action is not known.

ionizing radiation   electromagnetic radiation (x-rays, gamma rays) and atomic particles (neutrons, protons) that are energetic enough to knock electrons from elements and produce ions. These electrically charged ions can cause biological damage.

K

karyotype   visualizing and arranging all the chromosomes in a cell.

L

labia majora   a pair of fleshy folds that cover the labia minora.

labia minora   a pair of fleshy folds that cover the vagina.

lactose   a molecule of glucose and galactose chemically bonded together; found primarily in milk.

lactose intolerance   the inability to digest the sugar lactose.

laetrile   an extract of almond or apricot pits used by some to treat cancer.

laparotomy   a type of tubal ligation procedure.

learned behavioral tolerance   apparently "normal" behavior in someone with a high blood alcohol content.

leukemia   abnormal production of white blood cells; a cancer of the blood.

leukocytes   white blood cells that combat infectious organisms and foreign substances in the body.

lifestyle   activities that are a regular part of an individual's daily pattern of living.

lipids   fats, such as cholesterol and triglycerides.

lupus erythematosus   an autoimmune disease in which the body destroys its own tissues.

lymphatic system   a glandular system involved in the immune response.

lymphocytes   white blood cells that can produce antibodies and interferon.

lymphoma   an unregulated (cancerous) proliferation of lymphocytes.

M

macrophages   specialized phagocytic cells that ingest and destroy foreign substances and organisms.

malignant tumor   a tumor in which cells grow rapidly and may spread throughout the body.

mandala   an artistic, religious design used as an object of meditation.

mantra   a sound or phrase that is repeated in the mind to help produce a meditative state.

masturbation   self-induced sexual stimulation.

maximum life span   the age at which there are no survivors of population.

mean life span   the age by which half of the individuals in a population have died.

meditation   a quiet, passive state in which the mind is alert and awake and yet calm and relaxed.

menopause   the cessation of menstruation in midlife.

menstrual cycle   the nearly monthly cycle of ovum production and menstruation.

menstruation   the monthly sloughing of the uterine lining via the vagina.

metabolism   the process of obtaining energy from the breakdown of molecules.

metastasis   the process by which tumor cells are carried by the blood and lymph to diverse parts of the body to form new tumors.

migraine headache   a headache caused by altered blood flow to the brain.

minerals   inorganic substances necessary for cellular functions.

Minamata disease   a disease caused by mercury poisoning.

mutation   a change in genetic material that is then passed on to progeny.

myocardial infarction   the death of a portion of heart muscle; often used synonymously with heart attack or coronary thrombosis.

myocardium   the muscular wall of the heart.

N

neoplasm   a cancer or tumor; unregulated cell multiplication.

nervous system   the brain, spinal cord, and all the nerves of the body.

neuroses   conditions characterized by behaviors and feelings that are considered abnormal but that are not severe enough to prevent most kinds of normal functioning.

neurotransmitters   small molecules in nerve cells that, when released, bind to adjoining nerve cells, causing an electrical signal to be transmitted along the nerve fiber.

nicotine   a chemical constituent in tobacco that produces rapid pulse, increased alertness, and a variety of other physiological effects.

nitrosamines cancer-causing substances that are found in some food and that can also be synthesized in the body.

nutritional deficiency disease a disease caused by the lack of an essential nutrient.

O

oncogene hypothesis the idea that mammalian cell chromosomes harbor unexpressed viral DNA and that virus growth can be initiated by ionizing radiation or by carcinogens, causing the cells in which the viruses grow to become cancerous.

oncogenic pertaining to the cancer-causing potential of a virus.

opiates a group of physically addicting drugs, such as heroin, morphine, and codeine, that are extracted from opium.

organic brain syndrome abnormal mental functioning brought about by degeneration or injury of brain tissue.

orgasm the climax of sexual responses and release of physiological and sexual tensions.

orthomolecular medicine treating a disease by determining whether it is caused by chemical imbalances and correcting them by nutrition.

orthomolecular nutrition supplying a person with a chemically perfect diet for his or her individual needs.

orthomolecular psychiatry correcting mental disorders with nutrition.

osteopathy medical treatment by manipulating the spine and body.

ovaries a pair of almond-shaped organs in the female abdomen that produce egg cells (ova) and female sex hormones.

P

Pap smear a test for cervical cancer.

pathogen an organism causing disease.

pedigree analysis the pattern of inheritance of a trait among all family members over several generations.

pelvic inflammatory disease (PID) a bacterial infection of the internal structures of the pelvis.

penis the male's organ of copulation and urination.

pesticide any substance that kills or limits the growth of insects, rodents, and other pests.

phagocytosis the ingestion and destruction of foreign particles and organisms by specialized kinds of white blood cells.

phencyclidine (PCP) an animal tranquilizer used by people for its psychoactive effects.

phenylketonuria (PKU) a genetically caused metabolic disorder that can usually be controlled nutritionally.

phobia a powerful and irrational fear of something.

phocomelia congenital deformation of limbs, arms, and legs.

pica an appetite for unusual substances, such as paint flakes.

pineal gland a gland in the brain that possibly regulates some body biorhythms.

pituitary gland a hormone-producing gland of the endocrine system.

placebo effect healing that results from a person's belief in the efficacy of a pill, treatment, or other measures when there is no known medicinal value in the substances taken or treatments given.

plague an infectious epidemic disease caused by a bacterium that is carried by rat fleas. Plague killed millions of people during the Middle Ages.

plaque a deposit consisting of fibrous tissue, cholesterol, and other substances that can build up in arteries.

plumbism lead poisoning.

porphyria a disease involving abnormally high blood levels of porphyrin, a component of the hemoglobin molecule.

positive addiction the compelling desire to engage in a health-promoting behavior instead of a health-harming one.

progeria a rare genetic disease in which individuals age prematurely and die young.

progressive relaxation a system of physical and mental relaxation in which portions of the body are relaxed one by one, causing the mind to relax at the same time.

prostaglandins small hormones produced by many tissues in the body.

protein complementarity mixing foods so that all eight essential amino acids are ingested in the diet in proper amounts and proportions.

proteins biological molecules composed of chains of amino acids.

psychoactive drug a substance that primarily alters mood, perception, and other brain functions.

psychophysiological disorders physical illnesses that are the result of emotional states. Also known as psychosomatic disorders.

psychoses conditions characterized by severely abnormal thoughts, moods, or behaviors and a loss of contact with reality.

psychosomatic illness illness caused mainly by mental states and attitudes that change physiology and produce disease.

pubic lice small insects that live in the genital-rectal region.

pus a mixture of white blood cells and cellular debris.

R

rapid eye movement (REM) sleep the stage of sleep characterized by fluttering of the eyes under the closed eyelids and the experience of dreaming.

reactive hypoglycemia lowering of blood glucose levels below normal after eating a lot of sugar.

Recommended Dietary Allowance (RDA) standards for the daily intake of certain nutrients and calories.

refractory period the period in the human sexual response following orgasm and during which a person cannot be sexually stimulated.

relaxation response the physiological opposite of the emergency response; characterized by reduction in metabolic activity and increased feelings of relaxation and calm.

releasing factors hormones produced in the hypothalamus that control the release of hormones from the pituitary gland.

risk factors elements of a person's life that may predispose him or her to illness and disease.

roughage *see* fiber.

S

sarcomas cancers arising from bone and fibrous tissues.

schizophrenia a particular type of psychosis characterized by highly unusual thoughts and behaviors.

scrotum a sac of skin that contains the testes.

self-actualization the need for emotional and spiritual growth.

senescence the process of aging or becoming old.

serotonin neurotransmitter.

sex role a set of expected gender-specific behaviors.

sexually transmitted diseases infections or infestations passed from person to person by sexual contact.

sickle-cell anemia an inherited disease of the blood in which hemoglobin is altered so that red blood cells become sickle-shaped.

side effects unintended and often harmful actions of a drug.

sinoatrial node a region in the right atrium of the heart that regulates heartbeat.

skin the body's first line of defense against disease; it prevents organisms and disease-producing substances from entering the body.

smallpox a severe viral disease that has killed millions of people. It has been eradicated by worldwide vaccination.

smegma a white, cheesy substance that accumulates under the foreskin of the penis.

smog air polluted by chemicals, smoke, particles, dust, and so on.

starch long chains of glucose molecules.

stress an extreme or prolonged disruption in mind-body harmony that can lead to the onset of a variety of physical illnesses.

stressor any condition that elicits the specific phychological and physiological responses characteristic of stress.

stroke an obstruction or rupture of arteries in the brain, resulting in brain damage or death.

sucrose common refined "table" sugar; a molecule of glucose and a molecule of fructose chemically bonded together.

synergism the interaction of drugs to produce an effect that is greater than that of either drug taken alone.

syphilis a sexually transmitted disease caused by spirochete bacteria.

systole the contraction of the heart in each heartbeat.

T

t'ai chi ch'uan Chinese exercises that produce physical and mental harmony.

tar the yellowish-brown residue of tobacco smoke.

tension headache a headache caused by persistent contraction of the muscles in the neck and scalp.

teratogen a drug that affects the development of embryos and causes birth defects.

testes the pair of male reproductive organs that produce sperm cells and male sex hormones.

thalamus the region of the brain that integrates sensory and motor responses.

thalidomide a prescribed sedative that caused congenital defects when taken by pregnant women.

thymosin a hormone secreted by the thymus that may be important in the aging process.

tonsillectomy surgical removal of the tonsils.

toxemia a high blood pressure disease that occasionally occurs in pregnancy.

training effect beneficial physiological changes as a result of exercise.

triglycerides types of lipid (fat) molecules that are specialized for storing energy.

tubal ligation cutting and tying of the fallopian tubes to prevent conception.

tuberculosis an infectious bacterial disease that often affects the lungs.

tumor a mass of abnormal cells growing without regulation. *See also* benign tumor; malignant tumor.

tumor promoters substances that enhance the development of cancer cells without actually causing genetic changes.

tumor virus any virus that can produce a cancer in an organism.

type A behavior a harried, impatient, aggressive, stressful way of living.

typhus a disease caused by a microorganism carried by body lice.

U

urethra the tube that carries urine from the bladder to the outside.

urethritis irritation or infection of the urethra caused by bacteria or women in which a fetus develops.

V

vacuum curettage a procedure used in early abortion.

vagina a woman's organ of copulation and the exit pathway for the fetus at birth.

varicose veins a condition caused by defective valves in veins, usually in the legs.

vasectomy cutting the vas deferens or sperm duct to prevent the passage of sperm (but not seminal fluid) from the body.

vector an animal, often an insect, that carries a disease-causing organism and serves to transmit it.

vegetarians people who eat no animal flesh. Some vegetarians do not eat dairy foods or eggs.

veins blood vessels that return oxygen-depleted blood from the body to the heart.

venereal disease (VD) *see* sexually transmitted disease.

ventricles chambers that pump blood out of the heart.

vital statistics data reporting the number of illnesses or deaths due to particular causes.

vitamin dependency illness a disease characterized by the need for higher-than-normal amounts of a particular vitamin.

vitamins biological substances that assist in chemical reactions in cells.

W

withdrawal uncomfortable and sometimes life-threatening reactions that occur when a person stops taking a physically addicting drug.

Y

yellow fever a viral disease transmitted to humans by mosquito bites.

Yin and Yang in certain Asian philosophies, the opposing forces that, when in balance, produce healthful harmony in people and in nature.

Z

zygote the first cell of a new person, formed at fertilization.

Bibliography

Achterberg, J. *Imagery in Healing.* Boston: New Science Library, 1986.

Agras, W. S. "Relaxation Therapy in Hypertension." *Hospital Practice,* May 1983, 129-137.

Altman, I., and Taylor D. *Social Penetration: The Development of Intimate Relationships.* New York: Holt, Rinehart and Winston, 1973.

Altschule, M. D. "Foreword to Symposium on Atherosclerosis." *Medical Clinics of North America,* 58 (1974), 243-44.

Alter, J. *Stretch and Strengthen.* Boston: Houghton Mifflin, 1986.

American Cancer Society. *Cancer Facts and Figures,* 1987.

Ames, B. N. "Environmental Chemicals Causing Cancer and Genetic Birth Defects: Developing a Strategy in Minimizing Human Exposure." *Journal of Supramolecular Structure,* Supp. 2, 1978.

Ames, B. N. "Identifying Environmental Chemicals Causing Mutations and Cancer." *Science,* 204 (1979), 587-593.

Ames, B. N. "Dietary Carcinogens and Anticarcinogens." *Science,* 221 (1983), 1256-1263.

Amsterdam, E. A., and Holmes, A. M. *Take Care of Your Heart,* New York: Facts on File Publications, 1984.

Anderson, R. M., and May R. M. "Population Dynamics of Human Helminth Infections: Control by Chemotherapy." *Nature,* 297 (1982), 587-563.

Anderson, T. W. "Large Scale Trials of Vitamin C." *Annals of the New York Academy of Sciences, 2nd Conference on Vitamin C,* 258 (1975), 498-504.

Arcos, J. C. "Cancer: Chemical Factors in the Environment." *American Laboratory,* 10 (1978); No. 6: 65-73, No. 7: 29-41.

Babineau, R. "Sexual Counseling for College Students." *Medical Aspects of Human Sexuality,* 12 (1978), 129.

Barbach, L. G. *For Yourself.* New York: Doubleday, 1975.

Barbacid, M. "Mutagens, Oncogenes and Cancer." *Trends in Genetics,* July 1986.

Barber, T. X. "Self-Control: Temperature, Biofeedback, Hypnosis, Yoga, and Relaxation." In *Biofeedback and Self-Control.* Chicago: Aldine, 1976/1977.

Barber, T. X. "Hypnosis, Suggestions, and Psychosomatic Phenomena: A New Look from the Standpoint of Recent Experimental Studies." In J. L. Fosshage and P. Olsen (Eds.), *Healing.* New York: Human Sciences Press, 1977.

Bartrop, R. W., et al. "Depressed Lymphocyte Function After Bereavement." *The Lancet,* 1 (1977), 834-836.

Basmajian, J. V. "Control and Training of Individual Motor Units." In E. Peper, S. Ancoli, and M. Quinn (Eds.), *Mind/Body Integration,* New York: Plenum Press, 1979.

Baum, A.; Fleming, R.; and Reddy, R. M. "Unemployment Stress: Loss of Control, Reactive and Learned Helplessness." *Social Science and Medicine,* 22 (1986), 509-516.

Bedworth, A., and D'Elia, J. A. *Basics of Drug Education.* Farmingdale, N.Y.: Baywood Publishing, 1973.

Belloc, N.; Breslow, L.; and Hochstim, J. "Measurement of Physical Health in a General Population Survey." *American Journal of Epidemiology,* 93 (1971), 328-336.

Bender, G. A. "Great Moments in Medicine." Detroit: Northwood Institute Press/Parke Davis Co., 1966.

Benditt, E. P. "The Origin of Atherosclerosis." *Scientific American,* 236 (February 1977), 74-84.

Benfante, R.; Reed, D.; and Brody, J. "Biological and Social Predictors of Health in an Aging Cohort." *Journal of Chronic Disease,* 38 (1985), 385-395.

Benowitz, N. L. "Smokers of Low-Yield Cigarettes Do Not Consume Less Nicotine." *New England Journal of Medicine,* 309 (1983), 139-142.

Benson, H. *The Relaxation Response.* New York: Wm. Morrow, 1975.

Benson, J.; Koth, J. B.; and Crans, K. D. "The Relaxation Response: A Bridge Between Psychiatry and Medicine." *The Medical Clinics of North America,* 61 (1977), 929-937.

Berkman, P. L. "Measurement of Mental Health in a General Population Survey." *American Journal of Epidemiology,* 94 (1971), 105–111.

Bernstein, R. K. "Psychological Stress and Metabolic Control in Type I Diabetes Mellitus." *New England Journal of Medicine,* 315 (1986), 1293.

Berwick, D. M., and Komaroff, A. L. "Cost Effectiveness of Lead Screening." *New England Journal of Medicine,* 306 (1982), 1392–1398.

Bishop, J. M. "Oncogenes." *Scientific American,* March 1982, 81–92.

Blackman, D. *Operant Conditioning.* London: Methuen, 1974.

Bliss, S. (Ed.). *Berkeley Holistic Health Handbook.* Brattleboro, Vt.: Stephen Greene Press, 1984.

Blumenthal, J. A.; Williams, R. S.; Needles, T. L.; and Wallace, A. G. "Psychological Changes Accompany Aerobic Exercise in Middle-Aged Adults." *Psychosomatic Medicine,* 44 (1982), 529–536.

Bobroff, A. *Eczema: Its Nature, Cure and Prevention.* Springfield, Ill.: Charles C. Thomas, 1962.

Boston Women's Health Book Collective. *New Our Bodies, Ourselves.* Rev. ed. New York: Simon and Schuster, 1985.

Boston Women's Health Book Collective. *Ourselves and Our Children.* New York: Random House, 1978.

Bourne, P. "Foreword." In F. J. Whittington and B. P. Payne, *Drugs and the Elderly.* Springfield, Ill.: Charles C. Thomas, 1979.

Bowes, A., and Church, C. F. *Food Values of Portions Commonly Used.* 12th ed. Philadelphia: J. P. Lippincott, 1975.

Bowes, A., and Charles, C. F. *Food Values of Portions Commonly Used.* 13th ed. Rev. by J. A. T. Pennington and H. N. Church. New York: Harper & Row, 1980.

Bradley, M. O., and Sharkey, N. A. "Mutagenicity and Toxicity of Visible Fluorescent Light to Cultured Mammalian Cells." *Nature,* 266 (1977), 724–726.

Brecher, E. M. *Love, Sex, and Aging.* Boston: Little, Brown, 1984.

Bresler, D. E., and Trubo, R. *Free Yourself from Pain.* New York: Simon and Schuster, 1979.

Breslow, L. "A Quantitative Approach to the World Health Organization Definition of Health: Physical, Mental and Social Well-Being." *International Journal of Epidemiology,* 1 (1972), 347–355.

Breslow, L., and Enstrom, J. E. "Persistence of Health Habits and Their Relationship to Mortality." *Preventive Medicine,* 9 (1980), 469–483.

Brodeur, P. "Annals of Chemistry." *New Yorker,* April 7, 1975.

Bross, I. D. J., and Natarajan, J. "Leukemia from Low-Level Radiation." *New England Journal of Medicine,* 287 (1972), 107.

Bross, I. D. J.; Ball, M.; and Falen, S. "A Dose Response Curve for the One Rad Range: Adult Risks from Diagnostic Radiation." *American Journal of Public Health,* 69 (1979), 130–136.

Brown, B. B. *New Mind, New Body.* New York: Harper & Row, 1974.

Brown, B. B. *Stress and the Art of Biofeedback.* New York: Harper & Row, 1977.

Brown, M. S., and Goldstein, J. L. "How LDL Receptors Influence Cholesterol and Atherosclerosis." *Scientific American,* November 1984.

Bunker, J. P.; Barnes, B. A.; and Mosteller, F. *Costs, Risks, and Benefits of Surgery.* New York: Oxford University Press, 1977.

Burnet, F. M. *Immunology, Aging, and Cancer.* San Francisco: W. H. Freeman, 1976.

Butler, R. N., and Lewis, M. I. *Aging and Mental Health.* St. Louis: C. V. Mosby, 1977.

Cairns, J. *Cancer, Science and Society.* San Francisco: W. H. Freeman, 1979.

Calabrese, E. J. *Pollutants and High-Risk Groups.* New York: Wiley Interscience, 1978.

Califano, J. A., Jr. *America's Health Care Revolution.* New York: Random House, 1986.

Callen, K. E. "Mental and Emotional Aspects of Long-Distance Running." *Psychosomatics,* 24 (1983), 133–151.

Cameron, E., and Pauling, L. "Supplemental Ascorbate in the Supportive Treatment of Cancer: Prolongation of Survival Times in Terminal Human Cancer." *Proceedings of the National Academy of Sciences,* 73 (1976), 3685–3689.

Cannon, W. B. *The Wisdom of the Body.* New York: W. W. Norton, 1932.

Capra, F. "The New Physics as a Model for a New Medicine." *Journal of Social Biology,* 1 (1978), 71–77.

Carlton, W. *In Our Professional Opinion.* South Bend, Ind.: University of Notre Dame Press, 1978.

Carter, H., and Glick, P. C. *Marriage and Divorce: A Social and Economic Study.* Cambridge, Mass.: Harvard University Press, 1970.

Cassell, E. J. *The Healer's Art: A New Approach to the Doctor-Patient Relationship.* Philadelphia: J. B. Lippincott, 1976.

Castelli, W. P. "Hypertension: A Perspective from the Framingham Experience." In P. Sleight and E. Freis (Eds.), *Hypertension.* London: Butterworths, 1982.

Centers for Disease Control. *1975 Abortion Surveillance Report.* Washington, D.C.: U.S. Government Printing Office, April 1977.

Centers for Disease Control and National Institute of Child Health and Human Development. "Oral Contraceptive Use and the Risk of Breast Cancer." *New England Journal of Medicine,* 315 (1986), 405–411.

Chambers, C. D.; Inciardi, J. A.; and Siegel, H. A. *Chemical Coping.* New York: Spectrum Publications, 1975.

"Chernobyl—An Early Report." *Environment,* June 1986.

Chisholm, R. "On the Trail of the Magic Bullet." *High Technology,* January 1983, 57–63.

Christian, J. J. "Love Canal's Unhealthy Voles." *Natural History,* October 1983, 8–16.

Cimino, J. A., and Demopoulos, H. B. "Determinants of Cancer Relevant to Prevention, in the War on Cancer." In H. B. Demopoulos and M. A. Mehlman (Eds.), *Cancer and the Environment.* Park Forest South, Ill.: Pathotox, 1980.

Cobb, S., and Rose, R. M. "Hypertension, Peptic Ulcer, and Diabetes in Air Traffic Controllers." *Journal of the American Medical Association,* 224 (1973), 489–492.

Cohen, N. W., and Estner, L. J. *Silent Knife—Cesarean Prevention and Vaginal Birth After Cesarean.* South Hadley, Mass.: Bergin and Garvey Publishers, 1983.

Cohen, S., and Stillman, R. C. (Eds.). *The Therapeutic Potential of Marihuana.* New York: Plenum Press, 1976.

Coles, R. "Medical Ethics and Living a Life." *The New England Journal of Medicine,* 301 (1979), 444–446.

Comfort, A. *A Good Age.* New York: Crown, 1976.

Comfort, A. *The Biology of Senescence.* 3rd ed. New York: Elsevier, 1979.

Commission of Inquiry. "Chiropractic in New Zealand." Report of the Commission of Inquiry, 1979. (Available from Palmer College of Chiropractic, Davenport, IA 52803.)

Committee on Diet, Nutrition and Cancer, National Research Council. *Diet, Nutrition and Cancer,* Washington, D.C.: National Academy Press, 1982.

Connell, E. B. "The Crisis in Contraception." *Technology Review,* May/June 1986.

Conniff, R. "Living Longer." *Next,* May/June 1981, 38–48.

Connolly, G. N., et al. "The Reemergence of Smokeless Tobacco." *New England Journal of Medicine,* 314 (1986), 1020–1027.

Connor, W. E. "Too Little vs. Too Much: The Case for Preventive Nutrition." *The American Journal of Clinical Nutrition,* 32 (1979), 1975–1978.

Conry, T.; Fry, D.; Fry, N.; and Okagaki, A. *Consumer Guide to Cosmetics.* New York: Anchor-Doubleday, 1980.

Consumers Union. "Salt and High Blood Pressure." *Consumer Reports,* March 1979, 147–149.

Consumers Union. "Ready-To-Eat Cereals." *Consumer Reports,* October 1986, 628–637.

Cooper, C. L. (Ed.). *Stress Research,* New York: John Wiley & Sons, 1983.

Cooper, K. *The New Aerobics.* New York: M. Evans, 1970.

Cooper, K. *The Aerobics Way.* New York: M. Evans, 1977.

Cooper, K., and Cooper, M. *Aerobics for Women.* New York: Bantam Books, 1973.

Cooper, M. J., and Aygen, M. M. "A Relaxation Technique in the Management of Hypercholesterolemia." *Journal of Human Stress,* 5 (1979), 124–127.

Cousins, N. "The Mysterious Placebo: How Mind Helps Medicine Work." *Saturday Review,* October 1, 1977, 9–16.

Cousins, N. "What I Have Learned from 3000 Doctors." *Saturday Review,* February 1978, 12–15.

Cunningham, A. J. "Information and Health in the Many Levels of Man." *Advances,* 3 (1986), 32–45.

Danowski, T. S.; Nolan, S.; and Stephan, T. "Obesity." *World Review of Nutrition and Dietetics,* 22 (1975), 270–279.

Davidson, W. "Stress in the Elderly." *Physiotherapy,* 64 (1978), 113–115.

Davis, R. M. "Current Trends in Cigarette Advertising and Marketing." *New England Journal of Medicine,* 316 (1987), 725–32.

DeBakey, M., and Gotto, A. *The Living Heart.* New York: David McKay, 1977.

Deliman, T., and Smolowe, J. S. (Eds.). *Holistic Medicine: Harmony of Body Mind Spirit.* Reston, Va.: Reston Publishing Company, 1982.

Delza, S. *T'ai Chi Ch'uan.* New York: Cornerstone Library, 1961.

Dershowitz, A. "Bad Ideas Have Rights Too." *San Francisco Chronicle,* September 7, 1986, This World Section, p. 19.

Deyo, R. A., et al. "How Many Days of Bed Rest for Acute Low Back Pain?" *New England Journal of Medicine,* 315 (1986), 1064–1070.

DeYoung, H. G. "Acid Rain Regulators Shift into Low Gear." *High Technology,* September/October 1983, 82–86.

DeYoung, H. G. "State of the Heart." *High Technology,* May 1984, 33–42.

Dishman, R. K. "Medical Psychology in Exercise and Sport." *Medical Clinics of North America,* 69 (1985), 123–144.

Dobihal, E. "Talk or Terminal Care?" *Connecticut Medicine,* 38 (1974), 365.

Doll, R., and Peto, R. "The Causes of Cancer: Quantitative Estimates of Avoidable Risks of Cancer in the United States Today." *Journal of the National Cancer Institute,* 66 (1981), 1191–1308.

Donnison, C. P. *Civilization and Disease.* New York: Wood, 1938.

Dryfoos, J. G. "Contraceptive Use, Pregnancy Intention, and Pregnancy Outcomes Among U.S. Women." *Family Planning Perspectives,* 14 (March/April 1982), 81–94.

Dubos, R. *Man Adapting.* New Haven: Yale University Press, 1965.

Dubos, R. *Man, Medicine, and Environment.* New York: Praeger, 1968.

Dunn, W. L. (Ed.). *Smoking Behavior: Motives and Incentives.* Washington, D.C.: V. H. Winston and Sons, 1972.

Eagan, A. "The Selling of Premenstrual Syndrome." *Ms,* 11 (1983), 24–31.

Eckholm, E. P. *The Picture of Health.* New York: W. W. Norton, 1977.

Eddy, M. B. *Science and Health: A Key to the Scriptures.* Boston: Christian Science Society, 1890.

Edwards, D. D. "Nicotine: A Drug of Choice." *Science News,* January 18, 1986, 44.

Eisdorfer, C. "The Conceptualization of Stress and a Model for Further Study." In Michael R. Zales (Ed.), *Stress in Health and Disease.* New York: Brunner/Mazel, 1985.

Eisenberg, L. "The Social Imperatives of Medical Research." *Science,* 198 (1977), 1105–1112.

Engel, G. L. "The Need for a New Medical Model: A Challenge for Biomedicine." *Science,* 196 (1977), 129–137.

Engelhardt, H. T., Jr. "Allocating Scarce Medical Resources and the Availability of Organ Transplantation." *New England Journal of Medicine,* 311 (1984), 66–67.

Esdaile, J. *Mesmerism in India and Its Practical Application in Surgery and Medicine.* Hartford, England: Silus Andrus and Son, 1850.

Evans, F. J. "Unravelling Placebo Effects." *Advances,* 1 (1984), 11.

Evans, H. J., et al. "Radiation-Induced Chromosome Aberrations in Nuclear-Dockyard Workers." *Nature,* 277 (1979), 531.

Eyer, J. "Hypertension as a Disease of Modern Society." In *Stress and Survival.* St. Louis: C. V. Mosby, 1979.

Faraday, A. *Dream Power,* New York: Berkeley Medallion, 1972.

Farley, D. "Test-Tube Skin and Other High-Tech Treatments for Burns." *FDA Consumer Magazine,* June 1987.

Feldman, S. *Choices in Childbirth.* New York: Grosset & Dunlap, 1978.

Felig, P. "Very-Low-Calorie Protein Diets." *New England Journal of Medicine,* 310 (1984), 589–591.

Ferguson, M. *The Brain Revolution.* New York: Taplinger, 1973.

Ferguson, T. "The Best Bet Yet for Worried Smokers." *Prevention,* June 1987.

Fettner, A. G., and Weintraub, P. "Elixirs of Youth." *Omni,* October 1986.

Ficher, I. "Causes of Low Sex Drive." *Medical Aspects of Human Sexuality,* 12 (1978), 31.

Fielding, J. E. "Smoking: Health Consequences and Control." *New England Journal of Medicine,* 313 (1985), 491–498 and 555–561.

Fielding, J. E., and Yankauer, A. "The Pregnant Smoker and the Pregnant Drinker." *American Journal of Public Health,* 68 (1978), 835–838.

Fiennes, R. N. *The Environment of Man.* New York: St. Martin's, 1978.

Finn, S. B., and Glass, R. B. "Sugar and Dental Decay." *World Review of Nutrition and Dietetics,* 22 (1975), 304–326.

Fischman, J. "Type A on Trial." *Psychology Today,* February 1987.

Fish, J. M. *Placebo Therapy.* San Francisco: Jossey-Bass, 1973.

Fitzgerald, F. T. "Science and Scam: Alternative Thought Patterns in Alternative Health Care." *New England Journal of Medicine,* 309 (1983), 1066–1067.

Flint, M. B. "All About Holistic Medicine." *Business Week,* January 15, 1986, 9.

Folan, L. *Lilias, Yoga and You.* Cincinnati: WCET, 1972.

Folkman, S. "Personal Control and Stress and Coping Processes: A Theoretical Analysis." *Journal of Personality and Social Psychology,* 46 (1984), 839–852.

Fontana, V. J.; Holt, L. E., Jr.; and Mainland, D. "Effectiveness of Hyposensitization Therapy in Ragweed Hayfever in Children." *Journal of the American Medical Association,* 195 (1966), 109.

Ford, C. S., and Beach, A. *Patterns of Sexual Behavior.* New York: Harper & Row, 1951.

Forrest, J. D., and Henshaw, S. K. "What U.S. Women Think and Do About Contraception." *Family Planning Perspectives,* 151 (1983), 157–163.

Forrest, J. D.; Tietze, C.; and Sullivan, E. "Abortion in the United States." *Family Planning Perspectives,* 10 (1978), 271–279.

Fossel, E. T., et al. "Detection of Malignant Tumors." *New England Journal of Medicine,* 315 (1986), 1369–1376.

Fosshage, J. L., and Olsen, P. *Healing — Implications for Psychotherapy.* New York: Human Sciences Press, 1978.

Foster, K. R., and Guy, A. W. "The Microwave Problem." *Scientific American,* September 1986.

Frank, J. D. *Persuasion and Healing.* Baltimore: Johns Hopkins University Press, 1973.

Frank, J. D. "Mind-Body Relationships in Illness and Healing." *Journal of the International Academy of Preventive Medicine,* 2 (1975), 46–59.

Fraser, L. "Food Irradiation — Zapping What You Eat." *Science for the People Magazine,* March/April 1986.

Friederick, M. A. "Concerns About the Vagina." *Medical Aspects of Human Sexuality,* 12 (1978), 53–54.

Friedman, M. "Premature Ejaculation." *Medical Aspects of Human Sexuality,* 12 (1978), 131.

Friedman, M., and Rosenman, R. H. *Type A Behavior and Your Heart.* New York: Alfred A. Knopf, 1974.

Friedman, S. B., and Glasgow, L. A. "Psychological Factors—And Resistance to Infectious Disease." *Pediatric Clinic of North America,* 13 (1966), 315–335.

Frumkin, K., et al. "Nonpharmacological Control of Essential Hypertension in Man." *Psychosomatic Medicine,* 40 (1978) 294–317.

Gallo, R. C. "The First Human Retrovirus." *Scientific American,* December 1986.

Gallwey, W. T. *The Inner Game of Tennis.* New York: Random House, 1976.

Gambrell, R. D. "The Menopause: Benefits and Risk of Estrogen and Progestogen Replacement Therapy." *Fertility and Sterility,* 37 (1982), 457–474.

Garfield, C. A. *Stress and Survival: The Emotional Realities of Life-Threatening Illness.* St. Louis: C. V. Mosby, 1979.

Garfield, S. R. "The Delivery of Medical Care." *Scientific American,* (April 1970), 15.

Garmon, L. "Puzzled over PCBs." *Science News,* May 29, 1982, 361–363.

Garmon, L. "Dioxin in Missouri: Troubled Times." *Science News,* January 22, 1983, 59–62.

Gatchell, R. J., and Price, K. P. *Clinical Applications of Biofeedback Appraisal and Status.* New York: Pergamon Press, 1979.

Gaylin, W. "The Patient's Bill of Rights." *The Saturday Review of the Sciences,* March 1973, 22–25.

Gibbons, E., and Gibbons, J. *Feast on a Diabetic Diet.* New York: Fawcett Crest, 1973.

Gilbert, R. "The Nicotine Habit." *Addictions,* 24 (1977), 63–77.

Gittelsohn, A. M., and Weinberg, J. E. "On the Incidence of Tonsillectomy and Other Common Surgical Procedures." In J. P. Bunker, B. A. Barnes, and F. Mosteller (Eds.), *Costs, Risks, and Benefits of Surgery.* New York: Oxford University Press, 1977.

Glass, D. C. *Behavior Patterns, Stress, and Coronary Disease.* New York: John Wiley & Sons, 1977.

Glasser, W. *Positive Addiction.* New York: Harper & Row, 1976.

Glymour, D. and Stalker, D. "Engineers, Cranks, Physicians, Magicians." *New England Journal of Medicine,* 308 (1983), 960–961.

Golas, Thaddeus. *The Lazy Man's Guide to Enlightenment.* Palo Alto, Calif.: Seed Center, 1971.

Gold, M. "The Radiowave Syndrome." *Science 80,* January 1980, 79–84.

Goldbaum, E. "Irradiation Prompts Food for Thought." *Industrial Chemical News,* August 1986.

Goldstein, J. H. "A Laugh a Day." *The Sciences,* August/September 1982, 12–15.

Goldstein, S., and Podolsky, S. "The Genetics of Diabetes Mellitus." *Medical Clinics of North America,* 62 (1978), 639–654.

Good, R. A., and Day, N. K. "Influence of Nutrition on Diseases of Aging." In R. J. Marin and R. J. Bing (Eds.), *Frontiers in Medicine.* New York: Human Sciences Press, 1985.

Goodfriend, M., and Wolpert, E. A. "Death from Fright: Report of a Case and Literature Review." *Psychosomatic Medicine,* 38 (1976), 348–353.

Goodwin, D. W. *Is Alcoholism Hereditary?* New York: Oxford University Press, 1976.

Goodwin, D. W. *Alcoholism: The Facts.* New York: Oxford University Press, 1981.

Gordon, S. *Lonely in America.* New York: Simon & Schuster, 1976.

Gori, G. B., and Peters, J. A. "Etiology and Prevention of Cancer." *Preventive Medicine,* 4 (1975), 239–260.

Gorlin, R., and Zucker, H. D. "Physicians' Reaction to Patients." *New England Journal of Medicine,* 308 (1983) 1059–1060.

Grace, W. I., and Graham D. T. "Relationship of Specific Attitudes and Emotions to Certain Bodily Diseases." *Psychosomatic Medicine,* 14 (1952), 243–251.

Graff, G. "Food Irradiation Comes Down to Earth." *High Technology,* March 1984.

Graves, F. 'How Safe Is Your Diet Soft Drink?" *Common Cause Magazine,* July/August 1984.

Green, E. "Biofeedback for Mind-Body Self-Regulation: Healing and Creativity." In D. Shapiro (Ed.), *Biofeedback and Self-Control.* Chicago: Aldine, 1972.

Green, E. E.; Green, A. M.; and Norris, P. A. "Self-Regulation Training for Control of Hypertension." *Primary Cardiology,* 6 (1980), 126–137.

Greenberg, R. A., et al. "Measuring the Exposure of Infants to Tobacco Smoke." *New England Journal of Medicine,"* 310 (1984), 1075–1078.

Greydanus, D. E., and Hofmann, A. D. "Psychological Factors in Diabetes Mellitus." *American Journal of Diseases in Children,* 133 (1979), 1061–1066.

Grinspoon L. *Marihuana Reconsidered.* Cambridge, Mass.: Harvard University Press, 1977.

Grinspoon, L., and Bakalar, J. B. *Psychedelic Drugs Reconsidered.* New York: Basic Books, 1979.

Grundy, S. M. "Cholesterol and Coronary Heart Disease." *Journal of the American Medical Association,* 256 (1986), 2849–2858.

Hadler, N. M. "Regional Back Pain." *New England Journal of Medicine,* 315 (1986), 1090–1092.

Hales, D. "Mind over Body: Old Theories, New Proof." *Medical World News,* October, 10, 1983, 58–72

Hall, C. *The Meaning of Dreams.* New York: McGraw-Hill, 1966.

Hammond, C. B., et al. "Effects of Long Term Estrogen Replacement Therapy." *American Journal of Obstetrics and Gynecology,* 133 (1979), 537–547.

Hampson, J. L., and Hampson, I. G. "The Ontogenesis of Sexual Behavior in Man." In W. C. Young (Ed.), *Sex and Internal Secretions.* 3rd ed. Baltimore: Williams, & Wilkins, 1961.

Harris, J. E. "The AIDS Epidemic: Looking into the 1990s." *Technology Review,* July 1987.

Harrison, R. M., and Laxen D. P. H., "Natural Source of Tetraalkyllead in Air." *Nature,* 275 (1978), 738–741.

Hatcher, R. A., et al. *Contraceptive Technology, 1984–1985.* New York: Irvington Publishers, 1984.

Hawking, Stephen. Quoted in *Quest,* April 1979.

Hawkins, R. C., and Clement, P. F. "Development and Construct Validation of a Self-report Measure of Binge Eating Tendencies." *Addictive Behaviors,* 5(1980), 219–226.

Haynes, S. G., et al. "The Relationship of Psychosocial Factors to Coronary Heart Disease in the Framingham Study." *American Journal of Epidemiology,* 107 (1978), 362–385.

Hecht, F.; Hecht, B. K.; and Bixenman, H. A. "Caution About Chorionic Villi Sampling in the First Trimester." *New England Journal of Medicine,* 310 (1984), 1388–1395.

Hegsted, D. M. "Remarks on Nutrition and Health." In Select Senate Committee on Nutrition and Human Needs, *Dietary Goals for the United States.* Washington, D.C.: U.S. Government Printing Office, 1977.

Hendee, W. R. (Ed.). *Health Effects of Low Level Radiation.* Norwalk, N.J.: Appleton-Century-Crofts, 1984.

Heneson, N. "The Selling of P.M.S." *Science 84,* May 1984, 67–71.

Hennes, J. D. "The Measurement of Health."*Medical Care Review,* 29 (1972), 1268–1288.

Henry, J. P., and Stephens, P. M. *Stress, Health, and the Social Environment.* New York: Springer-Verlag, 1977.

Hickey, J. L. S., and Kearney, J. J. *The Development of an Engineering Control Research and Development Plan for Carcinogenic Materials.* Washington, D.C.: U.S. Government Printing Office, 1977.

Higgenson, J. "The Face of Cancer Worldwide." *Hospital Practice,* November 1983, 145–157.

Hilfiker, D. "Allowing the Debilitated to Die." *New England Journal of Medicine,* 308 (1983), 716–719.

Hilgard, E. R.; Atkinson, R. C.; and Atkinson, R. *Introduction to Psychology.* New York: Harcourt Brace Jovanovich, 1975.

Hilgard, E. R., and Hilgard, J. R. *Hypnosis in the Relief of Pain.* Los Altos, Calif.: William Kaufmann, 1975.

Hillman, A. L., et al. "Managing the Medical-Industrial Complex." *New England Journal of Medicine,* 315 (1986), 511–513.

Hirayama, T. "Nonsmoking Wives of Heavy Smokers Have a Higher Risk of Lung Cancer: A Study from Japan." *British Journal of Medicine,* 282 (1981), 183–185.

Hodgkinson, N. *Will to Be Well.* London: Hutchinson, 1984.

Hodgson, M. J., and Parkinson, D. K. "Diagnosis of Organophosphate Intoxication." *New England Journal of Medicine,* 313 (1985), 329.

Holden, C. "Holistic Health Concepts Gaining Momentum." *Science,* 200 (1978), 1029.

Holmes, T. H., and Rahe, R. H. "The Social Readadjustment Rating Scale." *Journal of Psychosomatic Research,* 11 (1967), 213–218.

Holmgren, J. "Actions of Cholera Toxin and the Prevention and Treatment of Cholera." *Nature,* 292 (1981), 413–418.

Hook, E. B. "Differences Between Rates of Trisomy 21 (Down's Syndrome) and Other Chromosomal Abnormalities Diagnosed in Live Births and in Cells Cultured After Second Trimester Amniocentesis — Suggested Explanations and Implication for Genetic Counseling and Program Planning." In D. Bergsma and R. L. Summitt (Eds.), *Proceedings of the 1977 Birth Defects Conference,* New York: Alan R. Liss, Inc., 1977.

Hopson, J. L. "Battle at the Isle of Self." *Science 80,* March/April 1980, 77–82.

Horne, H. H. *A Philosophy of Safety and Safety Education.* New York: Safety Education Digest, 1940.

House, J. D.'s; Strecher, V.; Metzner, H. L.; and Robbins, C. A. "Occupational Stress and Health Among Men and Women in the Tecumseh Community Study." *Journal of Health and Social Behavior,* 27 (1986) 62–77.

Howe, G. M. *A World Geography of Human Disease.* New York: Academic Press, 1977.

Hughes, R.; Javanovich, B.; and Brewin, R. *The Tranquilizing of America.* New York: Harcourt Brace Jovanovich, 1979.

Hume, W. I. *Biofeedback,* vol. III. New York: Human Sciences Press, 1981.

Ikard, F. F.; Green, D.; and Horn, D. "A Scale to Differentiate Between Types of Smoking as Related to the Management of Affect." *International Journal of Addictions,* 4 (1969), 649–659.

Illich, I. *Medical Nemesis.* New York: Pocket Books, 1976.

Ingelfinger, F. J. "Cancer! Alarm! Cancer!" *New England Journal of Medicine,* 293 (1975), 1319–1320.

Inglis, B., and West, R. *The Alternative Health Guide.* New York: Alfred A. Knopf, 1983.

Insel, P. M., and Moos, R. *Health and the Social Environment.* Lexington, Mass.: Lexington Books, 1974.

Israel, L., and Chahinian, A. R. *Lung Cancer.* New York: Academic Press, 1976.

Issels, J. *Cancer: A Second Opinion.* London: Hadder and Stoughton, 1975.

Jaco, D. "Colon Cancer." *Preventive Medicine,* 6 (1977), 535–544.

Jacobs, B. L. "How Hallucinogenic Drugs Work." *American Scientist,* July/August 1987.

Jacobs, B. L., and Trulson, M. E. "Mechanisms of Action of LSD." *American Scientist,* 67 (1979), 396–404.

Jacobson, C. K., and Ettlinger, C. *How to Be Wrinkle-Free: Look Younger Longer Without Plastic Surgery.* New York: Putnam, 1986.

Jacobson, E. *Progressive Relaxation.* Chicago: University of Chicago Press, 1938.

Jarrett, R. J. *Nutrition and Disease.* London: Croom Helm Ltd., 1979.

Jarrett, R. J. "Diabetes Mellitus and Nutrition." In J. Rose (Ed.), *Nutrition and Killer Diseases.* Park Ridge: Noyes Publishing, 1982.

Jaspe, M. *The Placebo Effect in Healing.* Lexington, Mass.: Lexington Books, 1978.

Jeffers, J. M. The Effects of Physical Conditions on Locus of Control, Body Image, and Interpersonal Relationship Orientations/University Males and Females." *Dissertation Abstracts,* 37 (1977), 3289.

Jellinek, E. M. *The Disease Concept of Alcoholism.* New Haven: College and University Press, 1960.

Jemmott, J. B. "Academic Stress, Power Motivation, and Decrease in Secretion Rate of Salivary Secretory Immunoglobin A." *The Lancet,* June 25, 1983, 46–55.

Jenkins, C. D. "Behaviorial Risk Factors in Coronary Artery Disease." *The Annual Review of Medicine,* 29 (1978), 543–562.

Jensen, G. D., and Robbins, M. B. "Multiple Orgasms in Men." *Medical Aspects of Human Sexuality,* 11 (1977), 8.

Jonas, S. *Medical History—The Training of Doctors in the U.S.* New York: W. W. Norton, 1978.

Jones, B. M., and Jones, M. K. "Women and Alcohol: Intoxication, Metabolism, and the Menstrual Cycle." In M. Greenblatt and M. A. Schuckit (Eds.), *Alcoholism Problems in Women and Children.* New York: Grune & Stratton, 1976.

Jourard, S. M. *The Transparent Self.* New York: Van Nostrand Reinhold, 1971.

Kahn, D. "Religious Roots of a Medical Crisis." *Harvard Magazine,* March–April 1978, 42–46.

Kales, A., and Kales, J. D. *Evaluation and Treatment of Insomnia.* New York: Oxford University Press, 1984.

Kanin, G. "To Rest Is to Rust." *Quest,* June 1979, 65–68.

Kannel, W. B. and Sorlie, P. "Some Health Benefits of Physical Activity." *Archives of Internal Medicine,* 139 (1979), 857–861.

Kanner, A. D.; Coyne, J. C.; Schaefer, C.; and Lazarus, R. S. "Comparison of Two Modes of Stress Measurement: Daily Hassles and Uplifts Versus Major Life Events." Journal of Behavioral Medicine, 4 (1981), 1–27.

Kaplan, H. S. *The New Sex Therapy.* New York: Brunner/Mazel, 1974.

Kaslof, L. J. *Wholistic Dimensions in Healing.* New York: Doubleday, 1978.

Katch, F. I., and McArdle, W. D. *Nutrition, Weight Control, and Exercise.* Philadelphia: Lea and Febiger, 1983.

Kaufman, D. W. "Constituents of Cigarette Smoke and Cardiovascular Disease." *New York State Journal of Medicine,* December 1983, 1267–1268.

Kazemi, J. *Disorders of the Respiratory System.* New York: Grune & Stratton, 1976.

Kelsey, J. L., et al. "Oral Contraceptives and Breast Disease." *American Journal of Epidemiology,* 107 (1978), 236–245.

Kemmer, F. W., et al. "Psychological Stress and Metabolic Control in Patients with Type I Diabetes Mellitus." *New England Journal of Medicine,* 314 (1986), 1078–1084.

Kermode, G. O. "Food Additives." *Scientific American,* 226 (March 1972), 15–21.

Kiecolt-Glaser, J. K., and Glaser, R. "Psychological Influences on Immunity." *Psychosomatics,* 27 (1986), 621–624.

King, B. J. *Billie Jean.* New York: Harper & Row, 1974.

King, J. C., and Fabio, S. "Alcohol Consumption and Cigarette Smoking: Effect on Pregnancy." *Clinical Obstetrics and Gynecology,* 26 (1983), 437–448.

Kinsey, A. C.; Pomeroy, W.; and Martin C. *Sexual Behavior in the Human Male.* Philadelphia: Saunders, 1948.

Kinsey, A. C.; Pomeroy, W.; Martin, C.; and Gebhardt, P. *Sexual Behavior in the Human Female.* Philadelphia: Saunders, 1953.

Kitzinger, S. *Your Baby Your Way.* New York: Pantheon, 1987.

Kleinmetz, B. *Essentials of Abnormal Psychology.* New York: Harper & Row, 1974.

Kleitman, N. "Patterns of Dreaming." *Scientific American,* 203 (1960), 82–103.

Klopfer, B. "Psychological Variables in Human Cancer." *Journal of Projective Techniques,* 21 (1957), 331–340.

Kobasa, S. C; Maddi, S. R.; and Kahn, S. "Hardiness and Health: A Prospective Study." *Journal of Personality and Social Psychology,* 42 (1982), 168–177.

Kohn, H. I., and Fry, R. J. M. "Radiation Carcinogenesis." *New England Journal of Medicine,* 310 (1984), 504–511.

Kolata, G. "Value of Low-Sodium Diets Questioned." *Science,* 216 (1982), 38.

Kolata, G. "Some Bypass Surgery Unnecessary." *Science,* 222 (1983), 605.

Korchin, S. J. *Modern Clinical Psychology.* New York: Basic Books, 1976.

Krebs, J. "Clocks, Pineals and Compasses." *Nature,* 274 (1978), 115–119.

Kristein, M. M.; Arnold, C. B.; and Wynder, E. L. "Health Economics and Preventive Care." *Science,* February 4, 1977.

Kroger, W. S. *Clinical and Experimental Hypnosis.* Philadelphia: J. B. Lippincott, 1977.

Kromhout, D.; Bosschieter, E. B.; and de Lezenne Coulander, C. "The Inverse Relation Between Fish Consumption and 20-Year Mortality from Coronary Heart Disease." *New England Journal of Medicine,* 312 (1985), 1205-1209.

Kübler-Ross, E. *On Death and Dying.* New York: Macmillan, 1969.

Kübler-Ross, E. *Death: The Final Stage of Growth.* New York: Prentice-Hall, 1975.

Kuhn, M. "To Rest Is to Rust." *Quest,* June 1979, 66.

Ladas, A. K.; Whipple, B.; and Perry, J. D. *The G Spot and Recent Discoveries About Human Sexuality.* New York: Holt, Rinehart and Winston, 1982.

Lamb, D. R. *Physiology of Exercise.* New York: Macmillan, 1978.

Lander, L. *Defective Medicine: Risk, Anger and the Malpractice Crisis.* New York: Farrar, Straus & Giroux, 1978.

Landy, D. *Culture, Disease and Healing.* New York: Macmillan, 1977.

Laurence, D. R., and Black, J. W. *The Medicine You Take.* London: Croom Helm, 1978.

Lazarus, R. S. "A Strategy for Research on Psychological and Social Factors in Hypertension." *Journal of Human Stress,* 2 (1978), 35-40.

Leaf, A. "New Perspectives on the Medical Consequences of Nuclear War." *New England Journal of Medicine,* 315 (1986), 905-912.

Leboyer, F. *Birth Without Violence.* New York: Alfred A. Knopf, 1975.

Lederer, W. J., and Jackson, D. *The Mirages of Marriage.* New York: W. W. Norton, 1968.

Leigh, H., and Reiser, M. F. "Major Trends in Psychosomatic Medicine: The Psychiatrist's Evolving Role in Medicine." *Annals of Internal Medicine,* 87 (1977), 233-239.

Leonard, G. *The Ultimate Athlete.* New York: Viking, 1974.

Leonard, G. "The Holistic Health Revolution." *New West,* May 1976, 39-43.

LeCron, L. M. *Experimental Hypnosis.* New York: Macmillan, 1952.

Levine, J. D.; Gordon, N. C.; and Fields, H. L. "The Mechanism of Placebo Analgesia." *The Lancet,* 2 (1978), 654-657.

Levy, R. I., and Moskowitz, J. "Cardiovascular Research: Decades of Progress, a Decade of Promise." *Science,* 217 (1982), 121-129.

Levy, S. M. *Behavior and Cancer: Life-style and Psychosocial Factors in the Initiation and Progression of Cancer.* San Francisco: Jossey-Bass, 1985.

Lewin, R. *Hormones.* New York: Doubleday, 1973.

Lewis, J. P. "Laetrile." *Western Journal of Medicine,* 127 (1977), 55-61.

Lilly, J. C. *Programming and Metaprogramming in the Human Biocomputer.* New York: Bantam, 1974.

Linder, R. L. *PCP: The Devil's Dust.* Belmont: Wadsworth Publishing, 1981.

Linn, S. "Lack of Association Between Contraceptive Usage and Congenital Malformations in Offspring." *American Journal of Obstetrics and Gynecology,* 147 (1983), 923-927.

Lipnick, R. J., et al. "Oral Contraceptives and Breast Cancer." *Journal of the American Medical Society,* 255 (1986), 58-61.

Loftus, E. F., and Fries, J. F. "Informed Consent May Be Hazardous to Your Health." *Science,* 204 (1979), 11.

Lowrence, W. M. *Of Acceptable Risk.* Los Altos, Calif.: William Kaufmann, 1976.

Lykken, D. T. "Polygraph Interrogation." *Nature,* 307 (1984), 681-684.

Lynch, J. J. *The Broken Heart: The Medical Consequences of Loneliness.* New York: Basic Books, 1977.

Lyon, J. L., et al. Childhood Leukemias Associated with Fallout from Nuclear Testing." *New England Journal of Medicine,* 300 (1979), 397-402.

Makinodan, T., and Yunis, E. *Immunology and Aging.* New York: Plenum Medical Books, 1977.

Mann, F. *Acupuncture: The Ancient Chinese Art of Healing.* New York: William Heineman, 1978.

Mann, F. *Scientific Aspects of Acupuncture.* London: William Heinemann, 1983.

Mann, G. V. "Diet-Heart: End of an Era." *New England Journal of Medicine,* 297 (1977), 644-649.

Margarey, C. "Holistic Cancer Therapy." *Journal of Psychosomatic Research,* 27 (1983), 181-184.

Margren, S., and Caan, B. "Applied Nutrition in Clinical Medicine." *Medical Clinics of North America,* 63 (1979).

Margo, C. E. "Selling Surgery." *New England Journal of Medicine,* 314 (1986), 1575-1576.

Marmot, M. G., et al. "Epidemiological Studies of Coronary Heart Disease and Stroke in Japanese Men Living in Japan, Hawaii, and California." *American Journal of Epidemiology,* 102 (1975), 514-525.

Martell, E. A. "Alpha-Radiation Dose at Bronchial Bifurcations of Smokers from Indoor Exposure to Radon Progeny." *Proceedings of the National Academy of Science,* 80 (1983), 1285-1289.

Marx, J. "Neurobiology: Researchers High on Endogenous Opiates." *Science,* 193 (1976), 1227.

Marx, J. "Coronary Spasms and Heart Disease." *Science,* 208 (1980), 1127-1130.

Marx, J. L., and Kolata, G. B. *Combatting the #1 Killer: The Science Report on Heart Research.* Washington,

D.C.: American Association for the Advancement of Science, 1978.

Maslow, A. W. *Motivation and Personality.* New York: Harper & Row, 1970.

Masters, W. H. "Sex and Aging—Expectations and Reality." *Hospital Practice,* August 15, 1986.

Masters, W. H., and Johnson, V. E. *Human Sexual Response.* Boston: Little, Brown, 1966.

Masters, W. H., and Johnson, V. E. *Human Sexual Inadequacy.* Boston: Little, Brown, 1970.

Masters, W. H., and Johnson, V. E. *Homosexuality in Perspective.* Boston: Little, Brown, 1979.

Maugh, T. H. "Chemical Carcinogens: The Scientific Basis for Regulation." *Science,* 201 (1978), 1200.

Maugh, T. H., and Marx, J. L. *Seeds of Destruction.* New York: Plenum Press, 1975.

Mayer, J., and Bullen, B. "Nutrition and Athletic Performance." *Physiological Reviews,* 40 (1960), 374.

McCabe, O. L. *Changing Human Behavior.* New York: Grune & Stratton, 1977.

McCann, J. "In Vitro Testing for Cancer-Causing Chemicals." *Hospital Practice,* September 1983, 73–85.

McCarty, D., and Kaye, M. "Reasons for Drinking: Motivational Patterns and Alcohol Use Among College Students." *Addictive Behaviors,* 9 (1984), 185–188.

McLean, P. D. "Depression as a Specific Response to Stress." *Stress and Anxiety,* 3 (1976), 297–320.

McPherson, K., and Fox, M. S. "Treatment of Breast Cancer." In J. P. Bunker, B. A. Barnes, and F. Mostelle (Eds.), *Costs, Risks, and Benefits of Surgery.* New York: Oxford University Press, 1977.

Medical Letter. "Nutrition in Pregnancy." *Medical Letter,* 20 (1978), 65–66.

Medical World News. "Breast Feeding." *Medical World News,* February 5, 1979, 62–72.

Mendelsohn, R. S. *Mal(e) Practice.* Chicago: Contemporary Books, 1981.

Metzner, H. L.; Carman, W. J.; and House, J. "Health Practices, Risk Factors, and Chronic Disease in Tecumseh." *Preventive Medicine,* 12 (1982), 491–507.

Miller, N. "Biofeedback and Visceral Learning." *Annual Review of Psychology,* 29 (1978), 373–404.

Miller, W. B. "Why Some Women Fail to Use Their Contraceptive Method: A Psychological Investigation." *Family Planning Perspectives,* 18 (1986), 27–32.

Mills, I. H. "Coping with the Stress of Modern Society." *Physiotherapy,* 64 (1978), 109–112.

Moertel, C. G., et al. "A Clinical Trial of Amygadalin (Laetrile) in the Treatment of Human Cancer." *New England Journal of Medicine,* 306 (1982), 201–206.

Moertel, C. G., et al. "High-Dose Vitamin C Versus Placebo in the Treatment of Patients with Advanced Cancer Who Have Had No Prior Chemotherapy." *New England Journal of Medicine,* 312 (1985), 137–141.

Money, J., and Ehrhardt, A. *Man and Woman: Boy and Girl.* Baltimore: Johns Hopkins University Press, 1972.

Moore, M. C., and Moore, L. J. *The Complete Handbook of Holistic Health.* New York: Prentice-Hall, 1983.

Moorefield, C. W. "The Use of Hypnosis and Behavior Therapy in Asthma." *American Journal of Clinical Hypnosis,* 13 (1971), 162.

Morris, I. N., et al. "Coronary Heart Disease and Physical Activity at Work." *The Lancet,* 2 (1953), 1053–1057.

Mortimer, C. H., and Bresser, G. M. "Endocrinology of the Hypothalamus." *Recent Advances in Medicine,* 17 (1977).

"Multiple Risk Factor Intervention Trial." *Journal of the American Medical Association,* 248 (1982), 1465–1477.

Murozumi, M.; Chow, T. J.; and Patterson, C. "Chemical Concentrations of Pollutant Lead Aerosols, Terrestrial Dusts, and Sea Salts in Greenland and Antarctica Snow Strata." *Geochimica Cosmochimica Acta,* 33 (1969), 1247–1254.

National Research Council. *Lead: Airborne Lead in Perspective.* Washington, D.C.: National Academy of Sciences, 1972.

Needleman, H. L., and Piomelli, S. *The Effects of Low Level Lead Exposure.* New York: National Resources Defense Council, 1978.

Neel, J. V., et al. *Diabetes Mellitus.* PHS Publication No. 1163, February 1965.

Nerem, R. M.; Levesque, M. J.; and Cornhill, J. F. "Social Environment as a Factor in Diet-Induced Atherosclerosis." *Science,* 208 (1980), 1475–1476.

Nero, A. V., Jr. "The Indoor Radon Story." *Technology Review,* January 1986.

New York Times. "Study Shows Sharp Increase in Breast Feeding in a Decade." March 25, 1984, 71.

Newborne, P. M. *Trace Substances and Health.* New York: Marcel Dekker, 1976.

Nicholi, A. M., Jr. "PCP Use Among College Students." *Journal of American College Health,* April 1983, 197–200. (a)

Nicholi, A. M. Jr. "Recent Patterns of Psychoactive Drug Use Among College Students: The Inhalants." *Journal of American College Health,* August 1983, 41–43. (b)

Nicholi, A. M., Jr. "The College Student and Marijuana: Research Findings Concerning Adverse Biological and Psychological Effects." *Journal of American College Health,* October 1983, 73–77. (c)

Noone, R. *In Search of the Dream People.* New York: Wm. Morrow, 1972.

Nossal, G. J. V. *Antibodies and Immunity.* New York: Basic Books, 1978.

Notkins, A. L. "The Causes of Diabetes." *Scientific American,* November 1979.

Nowell, P. C. "The Clonal Evolution of Tumor Cell Populations." *Science,* 194 (1976), 23–28.

Nriagu, J. O. "Did Lead Poisoning Contribute to the Fall of the Empire?" *New England Journal of Medicine,* 308 (1983), 660–663.

Nuclear War Letters. *New England Journal of Medicine,* 316 (1987), 688–690.

O'Connor, J., and O'Connor, D. "Premature Orgasm in Women." *Medical Aspects of Human Sexuality,* 12 (1978), 131.

Olds, J. "Hypothalamic Substrates of Reward." *Physiological Reviews,* 42 (1962), 554–604.

Oliver, M. F. "Diet and Coronary Heart Disease." In J. Yudkin (Ed.), *Diets of Man: Needs and Wants.* London: Applied Science Publishers, 1978.

Ory, H. W. "The Noncontraceptive Health Benefits from Oral Contraceptive Use." *Family Planning Perspectives,* 14 (July–August 1982), 182–184.

"Osteoporosis Protection Plan." National Institutes of Health recommendations. *Prevention,* August 1987.

Ottens, A. J. "The Effects of Transcendental Meditation upon Modifying the Cigarette Smoking Habit." *Journal of School Health,* 44 (1975), 577–583.

Paffenbarger, R. S.; Hyde, R. T.; Wing, A. L.; and Hseih, C.-C. "Physical Activity, All-Cause Mortality, and Longevity of College Alumni." *New England Journal of Medicine,* 314 (1986), 605–613.

Paffenbarger, R. S.; Hyde, R. T.; Wing, A. L.; and Steinmetz, C. H. "A Natural History of Athleticism and Cardiovascular Health." *Journal of the American Medical Association,* 252 (1984), 491–495.

Pardridge, W. M. "Potential Effects of the Dipeptide Sweetener Aspartame on the Brain." *Nutrition and the Brain,* 7 (1986), 199–241.

Pariser, H. "Frequently Overlooked Signs of the Early Stages of Venereal Disease in Men." *Medical Aspects of Human Sexuality,* 12 (1978), 121–122.

Parkes, C. *Bereavement: Studies of Grief in Adult Life.* New York: International Universities Press, 1972.

Parlee, M. B. "New Findings: Menstrual Cycles and Behavior." *Ms,* 10 (1982), 126–127.

Parons, L., and Sommers, S. C. *Gynecology.* 2nd ed. Philadelphia: Saunders, 1978.

Pauling, L. *Vitamin C and the Common Cold.* San Francisco: W. H. Freeman, 1970.

Pauling, L. "Are Recommended Daily Allowances for Vitamin C Adequate?" *Proceedings of the National Academy of Sciences,* 71 (1974), 4442–4446.

Paulson, D. "Psychogenic Infertility in Men." *Medical Aspects of Human Sexuality,* 12 (1978), 136–137.

Pearlin, L. I., and Schooler, C. "The Structure of Coping." *Journal of Health and Social Behavior,* 19 (1978), 2–21.

Pelletier, K. *Mind as Healer, Mind as Slayer.* New York: Delta, 1977. (a)

Pelletier, K. "Mind as Healer, Mind as Slayer." *Psychology Today,* 10 (February 1977), 35. (b)

Pelletier, K. *Holistic Medicine.* New York: Delta, 1980.

Perlow, D. L. and Perlow, J. S. *Herpes: Coping with the New Epidemic.* Englewood Cliffs, N.J.: Prentice-Hall, 1983.

Perry, P. "Are We Having Fun Yet?" *American Health,* March 1987, 58–63.

Peterkin, B. B.; Kerr, R. L.; and Shore, C. J. "Diets That Meet Dietary Goals." *Journal of Nutrition Education,* 10 (1978), 15–18.

Petersen, D. M.; Whittington, F. J.; and Payne, B. P. *Drugs and the Elderly.* Springfield, Ill.: Charles C. Thomas, 1979.

Peterson, L., and Renstrom, P. *Sports Injuries: Their Prevention and Treatment.* Chicago: Year Book Medical Publishers, 1986.

Petrich, J.; and Holmes, T. H. "Life Changes and the Onset of Illness." *The Medical Clinics of North America,* 61 (1977), 825–838.

Pihl, R. O., and Parkes, M. "Hair Element Content on Learning Disabled Children." *Science,* 198 (1977), 204–206.

Pincus, J. H., and Tucker, G. J. *Behavioral Neurology.* New York: Oxford University Press, 1978.

Pinhas, V. "Sex Guilt and Sexual Control in Alcoholic Women in Early Sobriety." *Sexual and Disability Journal,* 3 (Winter 1980).

Platt, R.; Polk, B. F.; Murdock, B.; and Rosner, B. "Mortality Associated with Nosocomial Urinary-Tract Infection." *New England Journal of Medicine,* 307 (1982), 637.

Pollock, M. L.; Wilmore, J. H.: and Fox, S. M. *Health and Fitness Through Physical Activity.* New York: John Wiley & Sons, 1978.

Population Reports, Series H, Number 7, January/February 1984.

Pozen, M. W., et al. "A Predictive Instrument to Improve Coronary-Care Unit Admission Practice in Acute Ischemic Heart Disease." *New England Journal of Medicine,* 310 (1984), 1275–1278.

Prasad, A. S. *Trace Elements and Iron in Human Metabolism.* New York: Plenum Medical Books, 1978.

Prescott, D. M., and Flexer, A. S. *Cancer: The Misguided Cell.* 3rd ed. New York: Charles Scribner's Sons, 1986.

Pugliese, M. T.; Lifshitz, F.; Grad, G.; Fort, P.; and Marks-Katz, M. "Fear of Obesity." *New England Journal of Medicine,* 309 (1983), 513–518.

Raloff, J. "Noise Can Be Hazardous to Our Health." *Science News,* June 5, 1982. 377–381.

Raloff, J. "Agent Orange: What Isn't Settled." *Science News,* May 19, 1984, 314–317.

Ramsey, P. *The Patient as Person—Explorations of Medical Ethnics.* New Haven: Yale University Press, 1970.

Reading, A. "Illness and Disease." *Medical Clinics of North America,* 61 (1977), 703.

Reid, R. L., and Yen, S. S. C. "The Premenstrual Syndrome." *Clinical Obstetrics and Gynecology,* 26 (1983), 710–717.

Relman, A. S. "Marijuana and Health." *New England Journal of Medicine,* 306 (1982), 603–605.

Relman, A. S. "Dealing with Conflicts of Interest." *New England Journal of Medicine,* 313 (1983), 749–751.

Renshaw, D. C. "I'm Just Not Interested in Sex, Doctor." *Medical Aspects of Human Sexuality,* 12 (1978), 32.

Restak, R. "The Brain Makes Its Own Narcotics." *Saturday Review,* March 5, 1977, 7–11.

Ricaurte, G., et al. "Hallucinogenic Amphetamine Selectively Destroys Brain Serotonin Nerve Terminals." *Science,* 229 (1985), 986.

Richards, V. *The Wayward Cell: Cancer.* Berkeley: University of California Press, 1978.

Rickert, W. S. "Less Hazardous Cigarettes: Fact or Fiction?" *New York State Journal of Medicine,* December 1983, 1269–1272.

Riggs, B. L., and Melton, L. J. "Involutional Osteoporosis." *New England Journal of Medicine,* 314 (1986), 1676–1684.

Riley, V. "Psychoneuroendocrine Influences on Immunocompetence and Neoplasia." *Science,* 212 (1981), 1100–1110.

Robinson, A. B. "Orthomolecular Medicine: Diagnosis and Therapy." Address Given at the 6th Annual Meeting of the National Society for Autistic Children, June 1974.

Rockstein, M., and Sussman, M. L. *Nutrition, Longevity, and Aging.* New York: Academic Press, 1976.

Rodger, J. C., and Drake, B. L. "The Enigma of the Fetal Graft." *American Scientist,* January/February 1987.

Rogers, C. R. *Becoming Partners.* New York: Delacorte, 1972.

Rogers, D. E. *American Medicine: Challenges for the 1980s.* Cambridge: Ballinger, 1978.

Rogers, E. S. *Human Ecology and Health.* New York: Macmillan, 1960.

Rosenbaum, E. H., et al. *Health Through Nutrition.* San Francisco: Alchemy Books, 1978.

Rosenberg, I. H.; Solomons, N. W.; and Levin, D. M. "Interaction of Infection and Nutrition: Some Practical Concerns." *Ecology of Food and Nutrition,* 4 (1976), 203.

Rosenfield, A. "Oral and Intrauterine Contraception: A 1978 Risk Assessment." *American Journal of Obstetrics and Gynecology,* 132 (1978), 92–106.

Roth, D. L., and Holmes, D. S. "Influence of Physical Fitness in Determining the Impact of Stressful Life Events on Physical and Psychological Health." *Psychosomatic Medicine,* 47 (1985), 164–173.

Rotter, J. I., and Rimoin, D. L. "The Genetics of Diabetes." *Hospital Practice,* May 15, 1987.

Rowe, J. W., and Kahn, R. L. "Human Aging: Usual and Successful." *Science,* July 10, 1987.

Rudman, D., and Williams, P. J. "Megadose Vitamins." *New England Journal of Medicine,* 309 (1983), 488–496.

Salk, J. *Man Unfolding.* New York: Harper & Row, 1972.

Samuels, M., and Bennett, H. Z. *Well Body, Well Earth.* San Francisco: Sierra Club Books, 1983.

Samuels, M., and Samuels, N. *Seeing with the Mind's Eye.* New York: Random House, 1975.

Sarason, I. G.; Sarason, B. R.; and Johnson, J. H. "Stressful Life Events: Measurement, Moderators, and Adaptation." In Susan R. Burchfield (Ed.), *Stress.* Washington, D.C.: Hemisphere, 1985.

Sarker, I. M., and Zimmer, M. A. *Dying to Be Thin.* New York: Warren, 1987.

Sarrel, P., and Sarrel, L. "How Couples Can Learn to Share Their Inner Feelings." *Redbook,* 180, 46–49.

Scarf, M. *Intimate Partners.* New York: Random House, 1987.

Schacter, S., and Rodin, J. *Obese Humans and Rats.* Washington, D.C.: Erlbaum/Halstead, 1974.

Schafer, W. *Stress, Distress and Growth.* Davis, Calif.: International Dialogue Press, 1978.

Schell, O. *Modern Meat.* New York: Random House, 1984.

Schildkraut, J. "The Biochemistry of Affective Disorders: A Brief Summary." In A. M. Nicholi, Jr. (Ed.), *The Harvard Guide to Modern Psychiatry.* Cambridge, Mass.: Harvard University Press, 1978.

Schmidt, F. "Health Risks of Passive Smoking." *World Smoking and Health,* 3 (1978), 19–24.

Scholl, T. O.; Sobel, E.; Tanfer, K.; Soefer, E. F.; and Saidman, B. "Effects of Vaginal Spermicides on Pregnancy Outcome." *Family Planning Perspectives,* 15 (1983), 244–250.

Schwartz, J. L. "Successes and Failures in Smoking Cessation: Insights from Personal Interviews." *World Smoking and Health,* 3 (1978), 11–18.

Schrock, P. "Exercise and Physical Activity During Pregnancy." In J. J. Sciarra (Ed.), *Gynecology and Obstetrics.* New York: Harper & Row, 1978.

Schultz, J., and Luthe, W. *Autogenic Training: A Psychophysiologic Approach in Psychotherapy.* New York: Grune & Stratton, 1959.

Scrimshaw, N., and Young, V. R. "The Requirements of Human Nutrition." *Scientific American,* 235 (1976), 51–64.

Selye, H. *The Stress of Life.* Rev. ed. New York: McGraw-Hill, 1976.

Selye, H. "The Stress Concept: Past, Present and Future." In C. O. Cooper (Ed.), *Stress Research.* New York: John Wiley & Sons, 1983.

Selzer, R. *Mortal Lessons: Notes on the Art of Surgery.* New York: Simon and Schuster, 1976.

Serban, G. (Ed.). *The Social and Medical Aspects of Drug Abuse.* New York: Spectrum Publications, 1984.

Shangold, M. M. "Causes, Evaluation, and Management of Athletic Oligo-/Amenorrhea." *Medical Clinics of North America,* 69 (1985), 83-96.

Shapiro, A. K. "Factors Contributing to the Placebo Effect." *American Journal of Psychotherapy,* Supp. 1, 18 (1964), 73-88.

Shapiro, J. L. *When Men Are Pregnant.* San Luis Obispo, Calif.: Impact Publishers, 1987.

Shealy, C. N. *90 Days to Self-Health.* New York: Bantam, 1977.

Shealy, C. N. "Freedom from Pain." *Quest,* June 1979, 33-38.

Shell, E. R. "The Guinea Pig Town." *Science 82,* December 1982, 58-63.

Shock, N. W. "The Physiology of Aging." *Scientific American,* 206 (1962), 110.

Shor, R. E., and Orne, M. T. *The Nature of Hypnosis.* New York: Holt, Rinehart and Winston, 1965.

Short, R. V. "Breast Feeding." *Scientific American,* 250 (1984), 35-41.

Siegel, F. P., and Siegal, M. *AIDS: The Medical Mystery.* New York: Grave Press, 1983.

Silverman, M., and Lee, P. R. *Pills, Profits, and Politics.* Berkeley: University of California Press, 1974.

Simonelli, C., and Eaton, R. P. "Cardiovascular and Metabolic Effects of Exercise." *Postgraduate Medicine,* 63 (1978), 71-77.

Simonton, O. C., and Simonton, S. M. "Belief Systems and Management of Emotional Aspects of Malignancy." *Journal of Transpersonal Psychology,* 7 (1975), 29-40.

Simonton, O. C.; Simonton, S. M.; and Creighton, J. *Getting Well Again.* Los Angeles: J. P. Tarcher, 1978.

Simonton, S. M., and Shook, R. L. *The Healing Family: The Simonton Approach for Families Facing Illness.* New York: Bantam Books, 1986.

Slater, P. "Sexual Adequacy in America." *Intellectual Digest,* November 1973.

Smith, D. E., and Gay, G. R. *It's So Good, Don't Even Try Once.* New York: Prentice-Hall, 1972.

Smith, D. W.; Bierman, E. L.; and Robinson, N. M. *The Biologic Ages of Man.* Philadelphia: Saunders, 1978.

Smith, N. J. "Excessive Weight Loss and Food Aversion in Athletes Simulating Anorexia Nervosa." *Pediatrics,* 66 (1980), 139-142.

Smith, R. E., and Ascough, J. C. "Induced Affect in Stress-Management Training." In Susan R. Burchfield (Ed.), *Stress.* Washington, D.C.: Hemisphere, 1985.

Smith, R. J. "Jere Goyan Brings Innovative Record to FDA." *Science,* 206 (1979), 200-201.

Snyder, S. "Matter over Mind: The Big Issues Raised by Newly Discovered Brain Chemicals." *Psychology Today, June 1980.*

Solnick, R. I. *Sexuality and Aging.* Los Angeles: University of Southern California Press, 1978.

Sprague, K. *The Gold's Gym Book of Strength Training.* Los Angeles: J. P. Tarcher, 1979.

Stallones, R. A. "Ischemic Heart Disease and Lipids in Blood and Diet." *Annual Review of Nutrition,* 3 (1983), 155-185.

Stapf, S. E. "A Propaganda War Against Cigarettes." *New York Times,* January 4, 1987, Section 3, p. 2.

Steel, K.; Gertman, P. M.; Crescenzi, B. S.; and Anderson, J. "Iatrogenic Illness on a General Medical Service at a University Hospital." *New England Journal of Medicine,* 304 (1981), 638-642.

Stein, M.; Schiavi, R. C.; and Camerino, M. "Influence of Brain and Behavior on the Immune System." *Science,* 191 (1976), 435.

Sterman, M. B. "Biofeedback and Epilepsy." *Human Nature,* May 1978, 50-55.

Stoll, B. H. (Ed.). *Mind and Cancer Prognosis.* New York: John Wiley & Sons, 1979.

Stout, C., et al. "Unusually Low Incidence of Death from Myocardial Infarction Study of an Italian American Community in Pennsylvania." *Journal of the American Medical Association,* 188 (1964), 845-849.

Strauss, M. J. "The Political History of the Artificial Heart." *New England Journal of Medicine,* 310 (1984), 332-334.

Stuart, R. B., and Davis, B. *Slim Chance in a Fat World.* Champaign, Ill.: Research Press, 1972.

Sun, M. "Missouri's Costly Dioxin Lesson." *Science,* 219 (1983), 367-369. (a)

Sun, M. "Dioxin's Uncertain Legacy." *Science,* 219 (1983), 468-469. (b)

Sun, M. "EDB Contamination Kindles Federal Action." *Science,* 223 (1984), 464-466. (a)

Sun, M. "Renewed Interest in Food Irradiation." *Science,* 223 (1984), 667-668. (b)

Surgeon General of the United States. *Healthy People.* Washington, D.C.: U.S. Government Printing Office, 1979. (a)

Surgeon General of the United States. *Report on Smoking and Health.* Washington, D.C.: U.S. Government Printing Office, 1979. (b)

Surgeon General of the United States. *The Health Consequences of Smoking: Cancer.* Washington, D.C.: U.S. Government Printing Office, 1982.

Surgeon General of the United States. *The Health Consequences of Smoking: Cardiovascular Disease.* Washington, D.C.: U.S. Government Printing Office, 1984.

Szasz, T. *Ceremonial Chemistry.* New York: Anchor Books, 1974.

Tager, I. B., et al. "Longitudinal Study of the Effects of Maternal Smoking on Pulmonary Function in Children." *New England Journal of Medicine,* 309 (1983), 699–703.

Tapp, J. T. "Multisystems Holistic Model of Health, Stress, and Coping." In Tiffany M. Field, Philip M. McCabe, and Neil Schneiderman (Eds.), *Stress and Coping.* Hillsdale, N. J.: Lawrence Erlbaum, 1985.

Tessler, R., and Mechanic, D. "Psychological Distress and Perceived Health Status." *Journal of Health and Social Behavior,* 19 (1978), 254–262.

Thomas, L. "On the Science and Technology of Medicine." In J. Knowles (Ed.) *Doing Better and Feeling Worse.* New York: W. W. Norton, 1977.

Thomas, L. "On Magic in Medicine." *New England Journal of Medicine,* August 1978.

Thomas, L. *The Medusa and the Snail.* New York: Viking-Penguin, 1979.

Thompson, T. L.; Moran, M. G.; and Nies, A. S. "Psychotropic Drug Use in the Elderly." *New England Journal of Medicine,* 308 (1983), 134–138.

Thomson, R. *Natural Medicine.* New York: McGraw-Hill, 1978.

Thurow, L. C. "Medicine Versus Economics." *New England Journal of Medicine,* 313 (1985), 1569.

Train, R. E. "The Environment Today." *Science,* 201 (1978), 320–324.

Trungpa, C. "Acknowledging Death." In P. Olson and J. L. Fosshage (Eds.), *Healing: Implications for Psychotherapy.* New York: Human Sciences Press, 1977.

Trussell, J., and Westoff, C. F. "Contraceptive Practice and Trends in Coital Frequency." *Family Planning Perspectives,* 12 (September/October 1980), 246–249.

Truswell, A. S. "Letter to the Editor." *New England Journal of Medicine,* 315 (1986), 709.

Tschirley, F. H. "Dioxin." *Scientific American,* February 1986.

Tubesing, D. A. *Wholistic Health: A Whole Person Approach to Primary Health Care.* New York: Human Sciences Press, 1979.

Turco, R. P., et al. "Nuclear Winter: Global Consequences of Multiple Nuclear Explosions." *Science,* 222 (1983), 1283–1292.

Underwood, E. J. *Trace Elements in Human and Animal Nutrition.* 4th ed. New York: Academic Press, 1977.

Urbain, W. M. *Food Irradiation.* New York: Academic Press, 1986.

U.S. Congress, Office of Technology Assessment. "Passive Smoking in the Workplace." Washington, D.C.: U.S. Government Printing Office, 1986.

U.S. Department of Health and Human Services. *Drug-Utilization in Office-Based Practice, A Summary of Findings.* Hyattsville, Md: National Center for Health Statistics, Public Health Service, 1983.

U.S. Department of Health, Education, and Welfare. "Chart Book on Smoking, Tobacco, and Health." Washington, D.C.: U.S. Government Printing Office, 1972.

U.S. Environmental Protection Agency. "Air Quality Criteria for Lead, Vol. II." EPA 600/8-77-017, December 1977, 13–25.

U.S. Senate Select Committee on Nutrition and Human Needs. *Dietary Goals for the United States.* Washington, D.C.: U.S. Government Printing Office, 1977.

Usdin, G., and Hofling, C. K. *Aging: The Process and the People.* New York: Brunner/Mazel, 1978.

Van den Bosch, R. *The Pesticide Conspiracy.* New York: Doubleday, 1978.

Vaux, K. L. *This Mortal Coil: The Meaning of Health and Disease.* San Francisco: Harper & Row, 1978.

Verbrugge, L. M. "Marital Status and Health." *Journal of Marriage and the Family,* 41 (1979), 267–285.

Verbrugge, L. M. "Multiple Roles and Physical Health of Women and Men." *Journal of Health and Social Behavior,* 24 (1983), 16–30.

"Viruses." *Time,* November 3, 1986.

Wagoner, J. K. "Occupational Carcinogenesis: The Two Hundred Years Since Percivall Pott." *Annals of the New York Academy of Sciences,* 271 (1976), 1–4.

Walker, S. *Help for the Hyperactive Child.* Boston: Houghton Mifflin, 1977.

Walker, W. J. "Changing U.S. Life Style and Declining Vascular Mortality." *New England Journal of Medicine,* 308 (1983), 649–651.

Wallerstein, E. *Circumcision: An American Health Fallacy.* New York: Springer, 1980.

Wanzer, S. H., et al. "The Physician's Responsibility Toward Hopelessly Ill Patients." *New England Journal of Medicine,* 310 (1984), 955–960.

Ward, B. and Dubos, R. *Only One Earth.* New York: W. W. Norton, 1972.

Warner, K. E. "Cigarette Advertising and Media Coverage of Smoking and Health." *New England Journal of Medicine,* 312 (1985), 384–388.

Warner, K. E. "A Ban on the Promotion of Tobacco Products." *New England Journal of Medicine,* 316 (1987), 745–748.

Weill, A. *Health and Healing.* New York: Houghton Mifflin, 1983.

Weiner, H. *Psychology and Human Disease.* New York: Elsevier, 1977.

Weiner, H. "The Illusion of Simplicity: The Medical Model Revisited." *American Journal of Psychiatry,* 135 (July 1978), supp.

Weis, W. L. "Can You Afford to Hire Smokers?" *Personnel Administrator,* May 1981, 71–78.

Weis, W. L. "Clearing the Air on Office Smoke." *Business Week,* February 7, 1983, 4.

Weisburd, S. "Food for Mind and Mood." *Science News,* April 7, 1984, 216–219.

Weisman, A. D. *Coping with Cancer.* New York: McGraw-Hill, 1979.

Weiss, J. M. "Psychological Factors in Stress and Disease." *Scientific American,* June 1972, 104–113.

Weiss, R. S. *Loneliness: The Experience of Emotional and Social Isolation.* Cambridge, Mass.: MIT Press, 1973.

Wekstein, L. *Handbook of Suicidology.* New York: Brunner/Mazel, 1979.

Welch, B. L., and Welch, A. S. *Physiological Effects of Noise.* New York: Plenum Press, 1970.

Wennberg, J., and Gittlesohn, A. "Variations in Medical Care Among Small Areas." *Scientific American,* April 1981, 120–134.

Wertheimer, A. I. "An Empirical Overview of the Prescription Drug Market." In J. P. Morgan and D. V. Kagan (Eds.), *Society and Medication: Conflicting Signals for Prescribers and Patients.* Lexington, Mass.: D. C. Heath, 1983.

White, J. R., and Froeb, H. F. "Small Airways Dysfunction in Nonsmokers Chronically Exposed to Tobacco Smoke." *New England Journal of Medicine,* 302 (1980), 720–723.

White, L.; Tursky, B.; and Schwartz, G. E. *Placebo.* New York: Guilford Press, 1985.

Whitehouse, F. W. "The Diagnosis of Diabetes." *Medical Clinics of North America,* 62 (1978), 627–637.

Wildavsky, A. "Doing Better and Feeling Worse: The Political Pathology of Health Policy." *Daedalus,* Winter 1976, 105–123.

Willaims, A. R. *Ultrasound: Biological Effects and Potential Hazards.* New York: Academic Press, 1983.

Willaims, J. F. *Personal Hygiene Applied.* Philadelphia: Saunders, 1934.

Williams, M. E., and Hadler, N. M. "The Illness as the Focus of Geriatric Medicine." *New England Journal of Medicine,* 308 (1983), 1357–1359.

Williams, R. J. *The Wonderful World Within You.* New York: Bantam, 1977.

Wing, J. K. *Reasoning About Madness.* Oxford, England: Oxford University Press, 1978.

Woods, J. S. "Drug Effects on Human Sexual Behavior." In N. F. Woods and J. S. Woods (Eds.), *Human Sexuality in Health and Illness.* St. Louis: C. V. Mosby, 1975.

Woolley, F. R. "Ethical Issues in the Implantation of the Total Artificial Heart." *New England Journal of Medicine,* 310 (1984), 292–296.

Worick, W. W., and Schaller, W. E. *Alcohol, Tobacco and Drugs.* Englewood Cliffs, N.J.: Prentice-Hall, 1977.

World Health Organization. "Smoking and Its Effect on Health." Technical Report No. 568, 1975.

Wurtman, R. J. "The Effect of Light on the Human Body." *Scientific American,* 233 (1975), 69–78.

Wurtman, R. J. "Brain Muffins." *Psychology Today,* October 1978, 140–145.

Wurtman, R. J. "Nutrients That Modify Brain Function." *Scientific American,* April 1982, 50–60.

Wynder, E., and Hoffman, D. *Tobacco and Tobacco Smoke.* New York: Academic Press, 1967.

Yano, K.; Reed, D. M.; and McGee, D. L. "Ten-Year Incidence of Coronary Heart Disease in the Honolulu Heart Program." *American Journal of Epidemiology,* 119 (1984), 653–666.

Yudkin, J. *Sweet and Dangerous.* New York: Bantam, 1972.

Zilbergeld, B. *Male Sexuality.* Boston: Little, Brown, 1978.

Index

579